The Biology
of Idiotypes

The Biology
of Idiotypes

Edited by
Mark I. Greene
Harvard Medical School
Boston, Massachusetts

and

Alfred Nisonoff
Rosenstiel Research Center
Brandeis University
Waltham, Massachusetts

Plenum Press • New York and London

Library of Congress Cataloging in Publication Data

Main entry under title:

The Biology of idiotypes.

Includes bibliographies and index.
1. Immunoglobulin idiotypes. I. Greene, Mark I. II. Nisonoff, Alfred. [DNLM: 1. Immunoglobulin Idiotypes. QW 601 B615]
QR186.7.B57   1984   591.2′9   84-13474
ISBN 0-306-41646-8

© 1984 Plenum Press, New York
A Division of Plenum Publishing Corporation
233 Spring Street, New York, N.Y. 10013

Printed in the United States of America

Contributors

ABUL K. ABBAS, Departments of Pathology, Harvard Medical School and Brigham and Women's Hospital, Boston, Massachusetts 02115

ANDREW ARNOLD, Metabolism Branch, National Cancer Institute, Bethesda, Maryland 20205

AJAY BAKHSHI, Metabolism Branch, National Cancer Institute, Bethesda, Maryland 20205

JEFFREY A. BLUESTONE, Transplantation Biology Section, Immunology Branch, National Cancer Institute, Bethesda, Maryland 20205

CONSTANTIN A. BONA, Department of Microbiology, Mount Sinai School of Medicine, New York, New York 10029

ALFRED L. M. BOTHWELL, Department of Pathology, Division of Immunology, and The Howard Hughes Medical Institute, Yale University School of Medicine, New Haven, Connecticut 06510

KIM BOTTOMLY, Department of Pathology, Yale University Medical School, New Haven, Connecticut 06510

J. DONALD CAPRA, Department of Microbiology, The University of Texas Health Science Center, Dallas, Texas 75235

PIERRE-ANDRÉ CAZENAVE, Unité d'Immunochimie Analytique, Institut Pasteur, 75015 Paris, France

JAN CERNY, Department of Microbiology, University of Texas Medical Branch, Galveston, Texas 77550

J. LATHAM CLAFLIN, Department of Microbiology and Immunology, The University of Michigan Medical School, Ann Arbor, Michigan 48109

JOSEPH M. DAVIE, Departments of Microbiology and Immunology and of Pathology, Washington University School of Medicine, St. Louis, Missouri 63110

MARTIN E. DORF, Department of Pathology, Harvard Medical School, Boston, Massachusetts 02115

EILEEN DUNN, Department of Pathology, Yale University Medical School, New Haven, Connecticut 06510

K. EICHMANN, Max Planck Institute for Immunobiology, Freiburg, Federal Republic of Germany

SUZANNE L. EPSTEIN, Transplantation Biology Section, Immunology Branch, National Cancer Institute, Bethesda, Maryland 20205

ANN J. FEENEY, Institute for Cancer Research, Philadelphia, Pennsylvania 19111

K. FEY, Max Planck Institute for Immunobiology, Freiburg, Federal Republic of Germany

MICHEL FOUGEREAU, Centre d'Immunologie INSERM-CNRS de Marseille-Luminy, 13288 Marseille Cedex 9, France

BARBARA G. FROSCHER, Department of Immunology, Scripps Clinic and Research Foundation, La Jolla, California 92037

R. JERROLD FULTON, Departments of Microbiology and Immunology and of Pathology, Washington University School of Medicine, St. Louis, Missouri 63110. *Present address:* Department of Microbiology, University of Texas Health Science Center, Dallas, Texas 75235

MARK I. GREENE, Department of Pathology, Harvard Medical School, Boston, Massachusetts 02115

NEIL S. GREENSPAN, Departments of Microbiology and Immunology and of Pathology, Washington University School of Medicine, St. Louis, Missouri 63110

EDGAR HABER, Cardiac Unit, Department of Medicine , Massachusetts General Hospital and Harvard Medical School, Boston, Massachusetts 02114

SUSAN HUDAK, Department of Microbiology and Immunology, The University of Michigan Medical School, Ann Arbor, Michigan 48109

TOSHIHIRO ITO, Department of Immunology, School of Medicine, Chiba University, Chiba, 280 Japan

CHARLES A. JANEWAY, JR., Department of Pathology, Immunology Division, and The Howard Hughes Medical Institute, Yale University School of Medicine, New Haven, Connecticut 06510

SHYR-TE JU, Department of Pathology, Harvard Medical School, Boston, Massachusetts 02115

DOMINIQUE JUY, Unité d'Immunochimie Analytique, Institut Pasteur, 75015 Paris, France

ELVIN A. KABAT, Departments of Microbiology, Human Genetics and Development, and Neurology, and Cancer Center/Institute for Cancer Research, Columbia University College of Physicians and Surgeons, New York, New York 10032, and National Institute of Allergy and Infectious Diseases, National Institutes of Health, Bethesda, Maryland 20205

MASAMOTO KANNO, Department of Immunology, School of Medicine, Chiba University, Chiba, 280 Japan

NORMAN R. KLINMAN, Department of Immunology, Scripps Clinic and Research Foundation, La Jolla, California 92037

NORMAN R. KLINMAN, Department of Immunology, Scripps Clinic and Research Foundation, La Jolla, California 92037

HEINZ KOHLER, Department of Molecular Immunology, Roswell Park Memorial Institute, Buffalo, New York 14263

STANLEY J. KORSMEYER, Metabolism Branch, National Cancer Institute, Bethesda, Maryland 20205

HENRY G. KUNKEL, (Deceased) The Rockefeller University, New York, New York

ADAM LOWY, Department of Pathology, Harvard Medical School, Boston, Massachusetts 02115

RICHARD G. LYNCH, Department of Pathology, University of Iowa College of Medicine, Iowa City, Iowa 52242

MARY MCNAMARA, Department of Molecular Immunology, Roswell Park Memorial Institute, Buffalo, New York, 14263

ANNE MADDALENA, Department of Microbiology and Immunology, The University of Michigan Medical School, Ann Arbor, Michigan 48109

MICHAEL N. MARGOLIES, Department of Surgery, Massachusetts General Hospital and Harvard Medical School, Boston, Massachusetts 02114

I. MELCHERS, Max Planck Institute for Immunobiology, Freiburg, Federal Republic of Germany

GARY L. MILBURN, Department of Pathology, University of Iowa College of Medicine, Iowa City, Iowa 52242

JOHN MONROE, Department of Pathology, Harvard Medical School, Boston, Massachusetts 02115

GINA MOSER, Departments of Pathology, Harvard Medical School and Brigham and Women's Hospital, Boston, Massachusetts 02115

D. E. MOSIER, Institute for Cancer Research, Philadelphia, Pennsylvania 19111

MOON H. NAHM, Departments of Microbiology and Immunology and of Pathology, Washington University School of Medicine, St. Louis, Missouri 63110

MICHAEL J. ONYON, Department of Pathology, Harvard Medical School, Boston, Massachusetts 02115

FRANCES L. OWEN, Department of Pathology and Cancer Research Center, Tufts University School of Medicine, Boston, Massachusetts 02111

ROGER M. PERLMUTTER, Division of Biology, California Institute of Technology, Pasadena, California 91125. *Present address:* Department of Medical Genetics, University of Washington School of Medicine, Seattle, Washington 98195

ROBERTO J. POLJAK, Département d'Immunologie, Institut Pasteur, 75724 Paris Cedex 15, France

DANIÉLÉ PRIMI, Unité d'Immunochimie Analytique, Institut Pasteur, 75015 Paris, France

KLAUS RAJEWSKY, Institute for Genetics, University of Cologne, D-5000 Cologne 41, Federal Republic of Germany

RICHARD L. RILEY, Department of Immunology, Scripps Clinic and Research Foundation, La Jolla, California 92037

JOSÉ ROCCA-SERRA, Centre d'Immunologie INSERM-CNRS de Marseille-Luminy, 13288 Marseille Cedex 9, France

HANS-DIETER ROYER, Department of Biological Chemistry, Harvard Medical School, Boston, Massachusetts 02115

STUART RUDIKOFF, Laboratory of Genetics, National Cancer Institute, Bethesda, Maryland 20205

DAVID H. SACHS, Transplantation Biology Section, Immunology Branch, National Cancer Institute, Bethesda, Maryland 20205

CLAUDINE SCHIFF, Centre d'Immunologie INSERM-CNRS de Marseille-Luminy, 13288 Marseille Cedex 9, France

DAVID H. SHERR, Department of Pathology, Harvard Medical School, Boston, Massachusetts 02115

KATHERINE A. SIMINOVITCH, Metabolism Branch, National Cancer Institute, Bethesda, Maryland 20205

M. M. SIMON, Max Planck Institute for Immunobiology, Freiburg, Federal Republic of Germany

GREGORY W. SISKIND, Divison of Allergy and Immunology, Department of Medicine, Cornell University Medical College, New York, New York 10021

CLIVE A. SLAUGHTER, Department of Microbiology, The University of Texas Health Science Center, Dallas, Texas 75235

SUSAN SMYK, Department of Molecular Immunology, Roswell Park Memorial Institute, Buffalo, New York 14263

TAKAYUKI SUMIDA, Department of Immunology, School of Medicine, Chiba University, Chiba, 280 Japan

MASATOSHI TAGAWA, Department of Immunology, School of Medicine, Chiba University, Chiba, 280 Japan

IZUMI TAKEI, Department of Immunology, School of Medicine, Chiba University, Chiba, 280 Japan

MASARU TANIGUCHI, Department of Immunology, School of Medicine, Chiba University, Chiba, 280 Japan

G. JEANETTE THORBECKE, Department of Pathology, New York University School of Medicine, New York, New York 10016

CÉCILE TONNELLE, Centre d'Immunologie INSERM-CNRS de Marseille-Luminy, 13288 Marseille Cedex 9, France

THOMAS A. WALDMANN, Metabolism Branch, National Cancer Institute, Bethesda, Maryland 20205

JACQUELINE WOLFE, Department of Microbiology and Immunology, The University of Michigan Medical School, Ann Arbor, Michigan 48109

DORITH ZHARHARY, Department of Immunology, Scripps Clinic and Research Foundation, La Jolla, California 92037

Preface

The phenomenon of idiotypy was discovered almost thirty years ago, but it was only during the past decade that it attracted widespread interest and became the subject of numerous research investigations. From the outset, much of the interest in idiotypy was based on its implications with respect to the repertoire of antibodies. Kunkel showed, for example, that idiotypes associated with certain human myeloma or Bence–Jones proteins were present in normal human globulins at levels of less than one part per million. Also, Oudin's original definition of idiotypy implied that idiotypes could be uniquely associated with individual rabbits as well as with particular antigen-binding specificities. Such observations provided some of the earliest evidence for an extensive repertoire of immunoglobulin molecules. The implications of these findings have been amply confirmed by recent studies of protein structure and molecular genetics; many of these studies are reviewed in the present volume. It is known now that the diversity of antibodies is based on the presence of numerous V_L and V_H genes, on recombinatorial events involving D and J segments, on somatic mutations, and on processes involving deletion of DNA followed by repair with errors, including insertions. Each of these parameters is capable of influencing the idiotype expressed by the final immunoglobulin product.

Regulation of the immune response is another area in which idiotypy has significantly influenced modern immunology. That regulation can be mediated through idiotypic determinants is readily demonstrated by the ability of anti-idiotypic antibodies to selectively suppress, or under certain conditions enhance the idiotypic component of the immune response. Similarly, idiotype-bearing or anti-idiotypic T cells and T-cell factors have been shown to have suppressive effects on the subsequent expression of an idiotype, and at least one class of T cells appears to enhance such expression. This area of research has been greatly stimulated by Jerne's provocative network theory, which is discussed in several contributions to this volume.

The purpose of this book is to provide, through the contributions of leading investigators, a description of the current status of the field of idiotypy. The text is organized into two broad areas. One includes the relationship of idiotypy to molecular structure, as analyzed at the level of protein or DNA. The second focuses on regulation of the immune response mediated through idiotypic or anti-idiotypic determinants on immunoglobulins, T-cell receptors, or T-cell-derived factors.

Mark I. Greene
Alfred Nisonoff

Contents

PART IV. STRUCTURES ON T CELLS

The Biology
of Idiotypes

PART I
MOLECULAR GENETIC ASPECTS OF IDIOTYPES

1

Idiotypic Determinants, Minigenes, and the Antibody Combining Site

ELVIN A. KABAT

1. Definition, General Principles, and Significance

Idiotypic determinants, idiotopes, are best defined as antigenic determinants located on the Fv fragment of an antibody molecule. Since the demonstration that myeloma antibodies from different individuals showed characteristic distinct antigenic specificities[1,2] and the subsequent findings that such antigenic determinants were present on induced antibodies[3-5] they have posed a structural and genetic problem, the solution of which is crucial to our understanding not only of the three-dimensional aspects of antibody structure but also of the regulation of antibody synthesis, the maintenance of antibody levels, and the rise and fall of antibody populations with combining sites of slightly different specificities. Most intriguing is the possibility that nature has made use of similar principles in other ligand–receptor interactions. Although there is little evidence for this at the moment, recent studies[6-11] indicate that anti-idiotypic antibodies formed against antibodies to hormones, agonists, and antagonists, which interact with specific receptors on the cell surface, show a specificity which may structurally resemble a portion of the hormone. Alternatively, the antibodies and the receptors may have sites which might be similar in sequence and in three-dimensional structure.

Another area which may well revolutionize our knowledge of the immune system rests on the observation that immunization with anti-idiotypic antibody (antibody 2) induces the formation of immunoglobulins bearing the idiotype (antibody 3) some of which may have combining sites specific for the antigen which produced the original idiotypic antibody (antibody 1) used to induce the anti-idiotype (antibody 2).[12-17] Thus, one becomes able to

ELVIN A. KABAT • Departments of Microbiology, Human Genetics and Development, and Neurology, and Cancer Center/Institute for Cancer Research, Columbia University College of Physicians and Surgeons, New York, New York 10032, and National Institute of Allergy and Infectious Diseases, National Institutes of Health, Bethesda, Maryland 20205.

induce antibody in an animal which has never been injected with the antigen; the nature, repertoire, quantity, and fine specificities of such antibodies remain to be established. It should be borne in mind that in all instances one is dealing with active immunization with Freund's adjuvant to induce the formation of antibody 1, 2, and 3 and the effects are all in these actively immunized animals. Indeed insufficient attention has been given to characterizing the specificities and biologic properties and effects of the serum antibodies thus induced except for the use of anti-idiotype in suppressing idiotype and thus changing the spectrum of the antibodies induced by immunization.[18−22] Anti-idiotypic antibody to individual myeloma proteins also specifically suppresses growth of the myeloma tumors *in vivo*[23,24] and induces the formation of T-helper cells.[25,26]

It is obvious that the ability to identify and distinguish between the amino acid residues responsible for idiotypic determinants and those determining antibody specificity and complementarity is a crucial first step. The seminal observation in this direction was made by Oudin and Cazenave[27,28] and has subsequently been extensively verified with many antigens.[29−36] They showed that, in single animals immunized with crystalline ovalbumin, similar idiotypic determinants were present on antibodies to different antigenic determinants on the ovalbumin molecule and even on immunoglobulin molecules with no detectable antiovalbumin specificity. These idiotypic specificities were not found in any measurable amount in a preimmunization sample of serum from the same animal. The implications of this finding were profound for they established that there were two distinct but somehow interrelated universes associated with Fv fragments, a universe of antibody combining sites and a universe of idiotypic specificities. They also provided insight into the oft-confirmed findings that immunization resulted in a substantial rise in immunoglobulin not reacting with the antigen.[37]

A second crucial finding was that of Rodkey[38−41] (see Refs. 42–45) who showed that animals immunized with a given antigen which developed antibodies of a given idiotype subsequently produced anti-idiotypic antibodies either spontaneously or on further immunization. These antibodies reacted with the earlier serum samples which contained antibody bearing the idiotype. This raised the question of idiotype–anti-idiotype interaction in regulating the levels of antibody of a given idiotype. The Jerne network theory[46] was in part based on these two findings.

A third important contribution came when it was recognized[47] that antibodies to a given antigenic determinant could show many individual (private) idiotypic determinants (IdI).* This was most strikingly demonstrated with human antibodies to blood group A substance. Anti-idiotypic antibodies produced in rabbits to purified anti-A from four different individuals showed entirely different and individual idiotypic specificities reacting only with the immunizing anti-A and not with isolated human anti-A antibodies from 28 persons. Among mouse monoclonal proteins binding $\beta 2 \rightarrow 6$ and $\beta 2 \rightarrow 1$ fructosans, 10 distinct IdI and 11 patterns of IdX reactivities were found.[48] Thus, the universe of idiotypic

---

*Abbreviations: IdI, individual idiotypic determinants or idiotopes unique to a given monoclonal immunoglobulin; IdX, cross-reactive idiotypic determinant shared by monoclonal immunoglobulins; class II dextrans, dextran with alternating $\alpha 1 \rightarrow 3$ $\alpha 1 \rightarrow 6$ glucoses as the basic structural unit[73] with a small number of short side chains of $\alpha 1 \rightarrow 6$ linked glucose[74]; class I dextrans, dextran composed largely of $\alpha 1 \rightarrow 6$ linked glucose with short branches of $\alpha 1 \rightarrow 2$, $\alpha 1 \rightarrow 3$, and $\alpha 1 \rightarrow 4$ linked glucoses substituted on the $\alpha 1 \rightarrow 6$ linked chains in a comb-like arrangement.[75−77]

determinants even in antibodies to one or a few structurally related antigenic determinants in an outbred or even in an inbred population is extremely large.

In addition to this large number of unique idiotypes, cross-reactive idiotypic specificities, IdX, have been found among human IgM antibodies to IgG,[49] rheumatoid factors with specificity for histone,[50] monoclonal antibodies to streptolysin O,[51] human IgG cryoglobulins,[52] and human cold agglutinins with blood group I, i specificity; other cold agglutinins with anti-Pr specificity showed cross-reactive idiotypic specificity unrelated to the I and i cold agglutinins.[53]

A monoclonal anti-idiotypic antibody to the V_κ chain of TEPC15, a phosphocholine-binding antibody, cross-reacted with a Thy-1 determinant on mouse T cells.[54] Weak idiotypic cross-reactions between myeloma antibodies binding phosphorylcholine of human and mouse,[55] between goat and sheep antibodies which distinguish sickle cell from normal hemoglobin,[56] and with horse, goat, pig, and chicken antibodies to human serum albumin[57] with rabbit auto-anti-idiotypic antibody to serum albumin have been reported. Human C-reactive protein in the presence of Ca^{2+} and mouse myeloma protein HOPC8 both bind phosphocholine[58,59] and C-reactive protein cross-reacted with an anti-idiotypic serum to HOPC8[59] if Ca^{2+} was present. These findings too suggest similarities in parts of their combining sites. Thus, what are being recognized as idiotypic determinants may be revealing a much broader spectrum of structure and/or sequence similarities among receptors which may have profound implications for the way in which complementarity is generated. It may be that certain small peptide segments, such as the Phe-Tyr-Met-Glu and Phe-Tyr-Met-Asp so strikingly associated with phosphorylcholine binding[60-62] might prove to be the functional units determining antibody site specificity; others may confer idiotypic specificity, etcetera, regardless of whether they occur in immunoglobulins or in other receptor proteins of related specificities.

An important issue to be resolved which is crucial to the precise location of idiotypic determinants to the Fv region is the finding that expression of the idiotype is almost always much greater when V_H and V_L are assembled than when either is tested separately, although idiotypic determinants of monoclonal antibodies associated with heavy chains[63-65] or with the light chains[65,66] have been reported in outbred as well as in inbred animals; in some instances immunization has been carried out with the isolated chains or with the isolated H chain recombined with light chains from normal mouse serum.[67-69]

It should always be borne in mind that even in those instances in which an isolated H or L chain shows substantial idiotypic specificity, a small contamination with the other chain will substantially augment the amount of idiotype found. Thus, isolated H and L chains of MOPC173(IgG2a) showed no idiotypic determinants, as assayed with syn-, allo-, and xenogeneic antisera,[70] on extensive purification although after initial separation on G-100 Sephadex, substantial cross-contamination remained. Idiotype was not regenerated by combination of H_{173} or L_{173} with L or H chains from other myelomas.

The role of H and L chains was also illustrated in the Ars system by matings of A/J mice with strains that do not produce light chains essential for the expression of the Ars-associated idiotype (CRI_A).[71] Mice were bred that were homozygous for $Igh-C^e$ (characteristic of A/J) and $Lyt-2^a,3^a$. (The κ V gene required for expression of CRI_A is closely linked to the genes controlling T-cell differentiation antigens $Lyt-2^a,3^b$ and $Lyt-2^b,3^b$ but is not found in strains expressing $Lyt-2^a,3^a$.) When such CRI_A-negative mice were mated with BALB/c or C57BL/6 mice (which produce the requisite L but not the H chains) the offspring responded to immunization with Ars-KLH by producing anti-Ars with the CRI_A idiotype; when mated with strains that lacked the appropriate genes controlling L chains no CRI_A was produced by the offspring. Thus, expression required both the proper H chain (Igh-C^e) with the proper L chain. Similar findings were seen with other idiotypic systems.[72]

A substantial body of data has been accumulated that shows linkage of idiotype expression to the heavy-chain C-region allotypes and that attempts to establish an order for the various idiotypic markers (see reference 17). In these studies the IdI is presumed to be a marker for the whole V_H-D_H-J_H region. However, no IdI studied has been localized in the V_H region, the only one for which sequence data are definitive being the anti-$\alpha1\rightarrow3$ $\alpha1\rightarrow6$ dextran[73-77] associated with the D_H minigene.[78-81] Since there is overwhelming evidence of assortment of V_H with the D_H and J_H minigenes and of V_κ and J_κ in V-region assembly[82-89] it becomes very difficult to determine what these idiotype–allotype linkages involve. Indeed, the high frequency of about 10% true recombinants in backcrosses in some systems (see ref. 17) is consistent with their being a consequence of somatic heavy-chain assembly. Until linkage can be shown with idiotypes located in V_H, the ordering of V-region genes is fictitious. The linkage being seen may be only a reflection of D_H and/or J_H assortment.

Indeed, Juszczak and Margolies[90] found that all CRI^- hybridomas of the 36-60 type assort with J_H3 and those with the CRI^+ hybridomas of the 36-65 type use J_H2. Recent data in the mouse[91] have located 12 D_H minigenes from 80 to 1 kilobase 5′ to the four J_H minigenes; the distance between V_H and D_H is unknown. Moreover, there is no information as to how the D_H minigenes may assort with V_H and with J_H. There is therefore no way in the absence of an IdI marker which is in V_H and not in J_H to establish linkage. Since there is now substantial evidence from the human and rabbit heavy-chain sequences, that runs of 14,[92] 13,[93] and 8[94] nucleotides homologous to the human D minigenes[95] are found in CDR2, since a human V_H-D_H-J_H clone with a deletion corresponding closely to CDR2 has been described,[96] since extra nucleotides may be inserted during the process of D_H-J_H joining[97] which may also occur between rabbit V_κ and J_κ,[98] and an extra amino acid numbered as [95A] has been found in a human Bence–Jones protein MEV[99] at the site of V_κ-J_κ joining, the problem becomes even more complicated. Moreover, the role of heavy–light-chain association appears to be substantial and is difficult to explain. It may well be that the use of inbred lines has introduced some reduction in the scope of the assortment process and provided on one-sided body of linkage data. It seems quite reasonable that further studies using IdI determinants localized to CDR1 and CDR2 will make linkage studies more informative unless additional evidence of insertion or deletion in the CDRs is obtained.

The study of idiotypes of antibodies made in inbred lines of mice and with monoclonal mouse myeloma[100] and hybridoma[101] proteins of a given specificity has provided additional insights into the nature of idiotypic determinants and has also made experimental investigations much simpler. For the study of cross-reacting idiotypic specificities (IdX) among these monoclonal proteins and to differentiate them from the homologous individual idiotype–anti-idiotype reaction (IdI), it is necessary in inhibition assays to use a monoclonal antibody other than the one used to produce the anti-idiotype; otherwise the tight binding of the IdI–anti-IdI reaction prevents inhibition and obscures or reduces the ability to detect fine differences in IdX, the cross-reacting idiotype.[47-53] Such systems have substantially simplified the study of cross-reacting idiotypes and have revealed them to have a more restricted repertoire.

Thus, for example, in assays of the QUPC52 individual idiotypic specificity of 11 BALB/c hybridoma antibodies to $\alpha1{\rightarrow}6$ dextran,[101] all with groove-type sites,[102,103] two gave no reaction and the others cross-reacted with binding affinities varying over about one log; a C57BL/6JA hybridoma protein did not react nor did a BALB/c myeloma protein W3129 with a cavity-type site.[103] Using a cross-reacting system, one of the same two non-reactors in the IdI system did not react, the other gave a very weak reaction, whereas the others cross-reacted and the range of variation was somewhat more restricted, 0.40 to 1.0 of the inhibition obtained with the cross-reacting inhibitor used in the system and a different pattern of inhibition emerged. Indeed, one hybridoma reacted better than did QUPC52. Similar results have been obtained in other cross-reacting idiotypic systems with myeloma and hybridoma proteins.

2. Correlation of Idiotypic Determinants with Amino Acid Sequence

Despite extensive sequencing of myeloma antibodies and more recently of hybridoma antibodies (see Ref. 62) the identification of amino acid residues associated with or responsible for idiotypic specificity is extremely limited. The most definitive data come from the myeloma and hybridoma antibodies[81] to the highly branched class II dextran B1355S with alternating $\alpha1{\rightarrow}3$ and $\alpha1{\rightarrow}6$ glucoses[73] for which a considerable number of V_H domains have been sequenced.[78,79] These monoclonal antibodies fall into five groups by quantitative precipitin studies[81] based on the extent to which a large number of class I dextrans cross-react. Group 1 reacts only with three class II dextrans; groups 2, 3, 4, and 5 also react best with the three class II dextrans but each successive group not only cross-reacts with more class I dextrans but shows progressively increasing capacities of the dextrans which cross-react to precipitate antibody. Among these mouse myeloma and hybridoma antibodies, two individual idiotypic specificities (IdI) have been recognized with rabbit anti-idiotypic sera,[79] one for myeloma protein J558 and the other for myeloma protein MOPC104E. A cross-reacting idiotypic specificity (IdX) has also been found.

Table I shows the correlation between precipitin group, IdX, IdI(J558), IdI(MOPC104E), and V_H sequences.[81] For simplicity the V_H region (excluding the D_H and J_H minigenes) has been classified into four groups 1, 1', 3, and 4; all V_H 1 sequences are identical; V_H 1' (Hdex 12) differs from group 1 with Asn (N) replacing Lys (K) at position 63 [62]; V_H 3 (Hdex 9) has Arg, His, Asn, and Phe (R, H, N, and F) at positions 63 [62], 73 [72], 77 [76], and 80 [79], and V_H 4 has Lys-Lys (KK) at positions 54, 55 [53, 54]. (Values in brackets are homologized aligned numbering[62]; other values are sequential numbering.) The various myeloma and hybridoma antibodies differ substantially in D_H and J_H. It is evident that IdX is V_H region associated since it is present in all V_H regions except Hdex 14, V_H 4, in which Lys (K) replaces Asn (N) at positions 54, 55 [53, 54] in CDR2. Both IdI(J558 and MOPC104E) correlated with D_H positions 100, 101 [96, 97]. Anti-IdI(J558) gives strong reactions with Hdex 31, Hdex 36, Hdex 9, and J558, three proteins with Arg-Tyr (RY) (Hdex 36 not sequenced), and a weaker reaction with Hdex 1 and Hdex 2 with Asn-Tyr (NY) at these positions. These myeloma and hybridoma proteins fall into all five precipitin groups. The IdI(MOPC104E) is thus far assoicated only

TABLE I

Association of Specificity, Sequence, and Idiotype[a]

Specificity	Sequence				Idiotype		
	V_H 1–99 [1–95][b]	D_H 100, 101 [96, 97]	J_H 102–117 [98–113]		IdX	IdI(J558)	IdI(MOPC104E)
Group 1							
Hdex 12	1'	GN	Y R - A Y - - Q - - - V - - - -	J_3	++	–	–
Hdex 25	1	SY	- - - - - - Q - - - - - - - -	J_1	++	–	–
Hdex 31	1	RY	Y A M - Y - - Q - - - S - - -	J_4	++	++	–
Group 2							
Hydex 36	?	?	?		++	++	–
Group 3							
Hdex 6	1	SH	- - - - - - - - - - - - -	J_1	++	–	–
Hdex 9	3	RY	- - - - - - - - - - - - -	J_1	++	++	–
J558	1	RY	- - - - - - - - - - - - -	J_1	++	++	–
Group 4							
Hdex 1	1	NY	H - - - - V - - - - - - -	J_1'	++	+	–
Hdex 24	1	SS	Y - - - Y - - Q - - - L - - -	J_2	++	–	–
Hdex 3	1	RD	- - - - - - - - - - - - -	J_1	++	–	–
Group 5							
MOPC104E	1	YD	W Y F D V W G A G T T V T V S S	J_1	++	–	++
Hdex 14	4	YD	- - - - - - - - - - - - -	J_1	– –	–	++
Hdex 11	1	YD	F - - - Y - - Q - - - L - - -	J_2	++	–	++
Hdex 2	1	NY	- - - - - - - - - - - - -	J_1	++	+	–

[a] From Reference 81.

[b] The V_H1 sequence of MOPC104E is reported[80] (see reference 62. V_H1' of Hdex 12 differs with N at position 63 [62] instead of K; V_H3 of Hdex 9 has R, H, N, and F at positions 63 [62], 73 [72], 77 [76], and 80 [79], respectively, instead of K, D, S, and Y; V_H4 of Hdex 14 has K, K at positions 54, 55 [53, 54] instead of N, N.

with precipitin group 5, Hdex 14, Hdex 11, and MOPC104E all with Tyr-Asp (YD) at these positions. Proteins lacking both IdI specificities fall into groups 1, 3, and 4 with Gly-Asn (GN), Ser-Tyr (SY), Ser-His (SH) and Ser-Ser (SS), and Arg-Asp (RD) at these positions. These might represent other IdI specificities.

Since some IdI(J558) cross-reactivity occurs in five precipitin groups, the residues determining IdI(J558) specificity would seem largely independent of those involved in determining the site differences determining the precipitin groups, findings consistent with those in the Ars system showing that monoclonal antibodies possessing the cross-reacting idiotype but which bind or did not bind Ars showed very few sequence differences in the first 52 amino acids of their V_L and V_H chains and were apparently using the same V-region genes.[104]

With a monoclonal mouse anti-IdI(J558),[105] Hdex 24 which lacked IdI(J558) with the rabbit antiserum, and J558 showed an interesting relationship. Diazotization and coupling of p-aminobenzoic acid to these antibodies blocked binding of J558 and of Hdex 24 to the anti-IdI. However, if the coupling was carried out in the presence of the hapten, 1 M α-methyl-D-glucoside, the loss of binding of IdI of J558 was prevented, i.e., the IdI was retained, whereas Hdex 24 lost its IdI determinant; the IdX of both was unaffected. The D_H of Hdex 24 has Ser-Ser rather than the Arg-Tyr related to the rabbit anti-IdI(J558) but it has two Tyr in J_H at 102 [98] and 106 [102], and both Hdex 24 and J558 have Tyr at 103 [99], all in CDR3. Since the diazonium compound couples to Tyr residues, it would appear that J558 and Hdex 24 share an idiotypic determinant other than that recognized by the rabbit anti-IdI, that it is site related and located in CDR3 since α-methyl-D-glucoside inhibited the diazotization reaction with J558. Neither the immunodominant idiotypic residue recognized by the hybridoma monoclonal anti-idiotype nor the Tyr to which the diazonium group has been coupled has been defined. Examination of positions [98], [99], and [102] on the two Fab fragments which have been studied crystallographically[106,107] (see Ref. 62) shows positions [98] and [99] to be at or close to the mouth of the combining site. One might speculate that Tyr [99] is immunodominant in both but that in Hdex 24, the diazonium group preferentially attaches to Tyr [98] which might account for its continuing to block the site even in the presence of hapten. In J558, however, the coupling would take place on Tyr [99] which would not react because it was contacting the hapten.

One of two splenic clones of anti-DNP antibody reacted with rabbit anti-T15 idiotype but not with mouse anti-T15 while another showed the reverse behavior.[108] Thus, fine-structure mapping of residues determining idiotypic specificity and antibody specificity will require use of several species of anti-idiotype. This and the previous finding raise the question of how many idiotypic determinants are present on a monoclonal immunoglobulin.

Attempts to define residues involved in determining idiotype in other systems involve additional assumptions and are limited in that only a few sequences have been compared. Based on the early findings in the $\alpha1\rightarrow3$ $\alpha1\rightarrow6$ dextran system,[78,79] an analysis of the V_L and V_H sequences involved in the idiotypic specificity of MOPC173 of unknown antibody specificity[109] inferred that residue 100 in V_L was involved in specificity since V_L MOPC21 and V_H of MOPC173 associated to form an idiotypic determinant whereas V_L of XRPC24 did not. V_L of MOPC21 shows many amino acid differences from V_L of MOPC173 but has an identical J_L whereas V_L of XRPC24 has a different J_L in which Gly 100 is replaced by Ser. Since there are reported to be V_H-J_L contacts in this region the role of J_L is hypothesized to be conformational by analogy with IdX of the $\alpha1\rightarrow6$ $\alpha1\rightarrow3$ dextan system residues 54 and 55 [53, 54] of CDR2 of V_H.

Although seven V_H and five V_L anti-inulin ($\beta2{\rightarrow}1$ fructosan)-binding myelomas have been completely sequenced, one V_L has been partially sequenced, and although, using mouse anti-idiotypic sera, distinct anti-IdX specificities have been recognized eight of which are inhibitable by hapten, inferences as to the amino acid residues involved in IdX specificity are difficult to make. One V_L IdX, IdXB, present on UPC61 and on W3082 and not on the other six anti-inulin myelomas was correlated with Ile 53-Asp 56 on these two chains[110]; the sequence beyond residue 35 was not determined for AMPC1 which shares IdXF with UPC61 and W3082. Since IdXB and IdXF differ in that AMPC1 does not possess IgXB, its sequence could aid materially in defining both these determinants. IdXC is present on all V_L chains except ABPC47N and J606, and IdXD is on all chains except ABPC47N, J606, and ABPC4. In view of this difference, IgXC and IgXD appeared to correlate with Ile 53 of V_L but were thought to involve other residues.[110] If Ile 53 occurred on one or on both AMPC1 and ABPC4, this might shed light on its role and on the specificity difference between IgXC and IgXD. If the above inferences prove to be correct this would implicate one amino acid Ile 53 in three distinct cross-reacting specificities, resembling in part the findings with the IdI of anti-$\alpha{\rightarrow}3$ $\alpha1{\rightarrow}6$ dextrans discussed above. Indeed, J606 and UPC61 differ by only one amino acid in the CDRs of V_L, residue 53, and by two amino acids, one in CDR2, residue 53, and one in FR3, residue 110, of V_H,[110] again indicating that a single amino acid may be involved in several idiotypic determinants. If idiotypic determinants are no different than other antigenic determinants in size and shape they could well exhibit specificity differences due to involvement of adjacent amino acids either altering conformation or contributing to the binding energy of interaction. These findings suggest that CDR1 and CDR2 of V_L and V_H are important in IdX specificity. Since each of the anti-inulin myeloma proteins had a unique IdI[48] which could be assayed using the mouse antisera from which the anti-IdX had been absorbed, it remains a problem to define these IdI and their relation to the various IdX considering the limited numbers of substitutions. It would seem that the IdI and IdX determinants might involve some of the same regions of an Fv fragment, with the IdX and IdI antibodies showing different degress of fitting to the idiotypic determinant. A study of IdI and IdX using monoclonal anti-idiotypic sera could be very informative.

A most extensive study of idiotypic specificities has recently been carried out for four myeloma and seven hybridoma antibodies specific for the $\beta1{\rightarrow}6$ galactans using mouse anti-idiotypic sera to each[111] and is discussed in detail in Chapter 7 of this volume. In general agreement with the $\alpha1{\rightarrow}3$ $\alpha1{\rightarrow}6$ antidextran system[78,79,81] all but one[112] of the IdI and IdX are associated with CDR3 (D). A hypothetical model of the anti-$\beta1{\rightarrow}6$ galactan[113] shows the D segment to be at the surface of the molecule.

The analysis of idiotypes in the NP system[114,115] has become more interesting and complicated by the findings that changes in idiotype expression involved recombination in which CDR1 and CDR2 of one gene and CDR3 of another were used indicating that V_H (CDR1 and CDR2) and D_H (CDR3) are of importance.[115] A change of one amino acid in D could alter one idiotypic determinant and abolish another without affecting binding specificity. The sequence data in the oxazolone system have not yet permitted identification of residues involved in idiotypic specificity.[69]

A rabbit antiserum to a 68,000-dalton V_H-related product of a marmoset T-cell line was found to react with the Fab fragments but not with L chains or C regions of certain human and mouse myeloma proteins and not to react with others by passive hemagglutination, radioimmune precipitation, or ELISA. Since the V_H of four of these, two which reacted and two which did not, had been completely sequenced, it was possible[116] to correlate the amino acid residues associated with the immunological specificity of this T-cell-derived product. The reactivity of the antiserum was associated with Asp[31] in CDR1; Asn[53], Thr[57], Tyr[65], Gly[65] in CDR2; and with Tyr[96] and Val[102] in CDR3. It was also associated with Ile[48] in FR1, Ser[76], Tyr[79], Gln[81], and Arg[94] in FR3, and Ala[105] in FR4. The location of these residues on a hypothetical three-dimensional model showed residues 94, 102, and 105 to be internal and all others were at the surface of the molecule and might be involved in the determinant; as other sequences become available further definition of the antigenic determinant may become possible. Although additional examination of this line is needed to ascertain the nature of the reacting substance and to be sure that immunoglobulin, possibly bound to Fc receptors, etcetera, is absent, the principle of establishing specificity by comparisons of reactivity and nonreactivity with known sequenced light and heavy chains is a useful approach.

3. Where Are Idiotypic Determinants Located?

The three existing X-ray structures of Fab fragments McPC603,[117] Newm,[118] and KOL[119,120] show the antibody combining site of McPC603 to be essentially a fairly deep cavity (see Ref. 121) whereas Newm[118] and KOL[119] are grooves (see Ref. 122). Attempts to model other types of sites by retaining the crystallographic structure of the FR and replacing the CDR of McPC603[117] or of Newm[118] by those of known antibodies have led to additional insights. Thus, the combining site of a type III antipneumococcal antibody so constructed[121] was found to be a groove complementary to six sugars in agreement with immunochemical findings.[123] In studies of myeloma[102] and hybridoma antibodies[103] to α $1{\rightarrow}6$ dextrans, immunochemical mapping established two types of sites—groove-type in which $\alpha 1{\rightarrow}6$ chains of six and seven $\alpha 1{\rightarrow}6$ glucoses fitted into the site and a cavity-type site in myeloma protein W3129[102] most complementary to five glucoses which was specific for the terminal nonreducing ends of chains. The terminal one or two sugars contributed over 50% of the total binding energy of the five $\alpha 1{\rightarrow}6$ glucoses making up the determinant[102,124] indicating that they were firmly held in three dimensions, e.g., at the base of a cavity. In studies of the effects of the isomaltose oligosaccharides in inhibiting the W3129 idiotype—rabbit anti-idiotype reaction[125] there was a remarkable parallelism between the two sets of data; in both instances the inhibition was maximal with the pentasaccharide and the disaccharide showed substantial inhibition unlike that seen with groove-type sites in which the first two glucoses contribute less than 5% of the total binding energy.[102] These data almost of necessity establish that the idiotype determinants at least in a cavity-type site are located on the outside of the antibody combining cavity and that filling the site with oligosaccharide causes a conformational change by which the configuration of the idiotype determinant is altered. The reasoning is as follows. If the site is saturated with disaccharide which positions itself at the base of the antibody combining cavity where it is bound most strongly (50% of the total binding energy of the pentasaccharide) one might expect no interference with the anti-idiotype reacting at the tip of the combining site. Thus, the disaccharide should not be a very good inhibitor of idiotype–anti-idiotype interaction. That the relative inhibiting power of the oligosaccharides in inhibiting dextran–antibody and idiotype–anti-idiotype runs parallel suggests that the extent of the conformational change as the combining site adjusts to fit around the oligosaccharides of increasing size distorts the idiotypic patch to comparable extents. Whether in a groove-type site the anti-idiotype could sterically block the entrance to the site and prevent hapten from entering and whether the effects are also conformational remain to be established (see reference 126).

A recent report[127] demonstrating that a series of myeloma and hybridoma antibodies to phosphocholine of the IgA isotype reacted with an anti-idiotypic antiserum to TEPC15 whereas those of the IgM and IgG isotypes did not, was interpreted as indicating that "not only V regions but also the constant region of the immunoglobulin molecule contribute to the formation of an idiotypic determinant."

It is evident that much additional work will be needed for a comprehensive understanding of idiotype structure.

ACKNOWLEDGMENTS. Work in the laboratories is supported by Grant PCM 81-02321 from the National Science Foundation and by Cancer Center Support Grant CA-13696 to Columbia University. Work with the PROPHET computer system is supported by the National Cancer Institute, National Institute of Allergy and Infectious Diseases, National Institute of Arthritis, Diabetes and Digestive and Kidney Diseases, the National Institute of General Medical Sciences, and the Division of Research Resources (Contract NO1-RR-8-2118) of the National Institutes of Health.

References

1. Lohss, F., Weiler, E., and Hillmann, G., 1953, Myelom-Plasma-Proteine. III. Mitteilung zur Immunochemie der γ-myelom-Proteine, *Z. Naturforsch. Teil B* **8**:625–631.
2. Slater, R. J., Ward, S. M., and Kunkel, H. G., 1955, Immunological relationships among the myeloma proteins, *J. Exp. Med.* **101**:85–108.
3. Oudin, J., and Michel, M., 1963, Une nouvelle forme d'allotypie des globulines γ du serum de lapin apparemment liee a le fonction et a la specificite anticorps, *C.R. Seances Soc. Biol. Paris* **257**:805–808.
4. Kunkel, H. G., Mannik, M., and Williams, R. C., 1963, Individual antigenic specificity of isolated antibodies, *Science* **140**:1218–1219.
5. Gell, P. G. H., and Kelus, A. S., 1964, Anti-antibody or clone-product?, *Nature* **201**:687–689.
6. Sege, K., and Peterson, P. A., 1978, Use of anti-idiotypic antibodies as cell-surface receptor probes, *Proc. Natl. Acad. Sci. USA* **75**:2443–2447.
7. Schreiber, A. B., Couraud, P. O., André, C., Vray, B., and Strosberg, A. D., 1980, Anti-alprenolol anti-idiotypic antibodies bind to β-adrenergic receptors and modulate catecholamine-sensitive adenylate cyclase, *Proc. Natl. Acad. Sci. USA* **77**:7385–7389.
8. Marasco, W. A., and Becker, E. L., 1982, Anti-idiotype as antibody against the formyl peptide chemotaxis receptor of the neutrophil, *J. Immunol.* **128**:963–968.
9. Wassermann, N. H., Penn, A. S., Freimuth, P. I., Treptow, N., Wentzel, S., Cleveland, W. L., and Erlanger, B. F., 1982, Anti-idiotypic route to anti-acetylcholine receptor antibodies and experimental myasthenia gravis, *Proc. Natl. Acad. Sci. USA* **79**:4810–4814.
10. Cleveland, W. L., Wassermann, N. H., Sarangaran, R., Penn, A. S., and Erlanger, B. F., 1983, Monoclonal antibodies to the acetylcholine receptor (AChR) by a normally functioning auto-anti-idiotypic mechanism, *Nature* **305**:56–57.
11. Schechter, Y., Maron, R., Elias, D., and Cohen, I. R., 1982, Autoantibodies to insulin receptor spontaneously develop as anti-idiotypes in mice immunized with insulin, *Science* **216**:542–545.
12. Ubain, J., 1976, Idiotypes, expression of antibody diversity and network concepts, *Ann. Immunol. (Inst. Pasteur)* **127C**: 357–374.

13. Cazenave, P.-A., 1977, Idiotypic anti-idiotypic regulation of antibody synthesis in rabbits, *Proc. Natl. Acad. Sci. USA* **74**:5122–5125.

14. Sachs, D. H., Berzofsky, J. A., Pisetsky, D. S., and Schwartz, R. H., 1978, Genetic control of the immune response to staphylococcal nuclease, *Springer Semin. Immunopathol.* **1**:51–83.

15. Wysocki, L. J., and Sato, V. L., 1981, The strain A anti-*p*-azophenylarsonate major cross-reactive idiotypic family includes members with no reactivity toward *p*-azophenylarsonate, *Eur. J. Immunol.* **11**:832–839.

16. Armo, M., Mariamé, B., Voegtlé, D., and Cazenave, P.-A., 1982, The idiotypic network: The murine MOPC315 anti-DNP system, *Ann. Immunol. (Inst. Pasteur)* **133D**:255–262.

17. Sachs, D. H., 1980, Genetic control of idiotype expression, in: *Immunology 80* (M. Fougereau and J. Dausset, eds.), Academic Press, New York, pp. 478–495.

18. Cosenza, H., and Köhler, H., 1972, Specific suppression of the antibody response by antibodies to receptors, *Proc. Natl. Acad. Sci. USA* **69**:2701–2705.

19. Hart, D. A., Wang, A. L., Pawlak, L. L., and Nisonoff, A., 1972, Suppression of idiotypic specificities in adult mice by administration of anti-idiotypic antibody, *J. Exp. Med.* **135**:1293–1300.

20. Ju, S. T., Gray, A., and Nisonoff, A., 1977, Frequence of occurrence of idiotypes associated with anti-*p*-azophenylarsonate antibodies arising in mice immunologically suppressed with respect to a cross-reactive idiotype, *J. Exp. Med.* **145**:549–556.

21. Bach, B. A., Greene, M. I., Benacerraf, B., and Nisonoff, A., 1979, Mechanisms of regulation of cell-mediated immunity. IV. Azobenzenearsonate-specific suppressor factor(s) bear cross-reactive idiotypic determinants the expression of which is linked to the heavy-chain allotype linkage group of genes, *J. Exp. Med.* **149**:1084–1098.

22. Bona, C., Lieberman, R., House, S., Green, I., and Paul, W. E., 1979, Immune response to levan. II. T-independence of suppression of cross-reactive idiotypes by anti-idiotype antibodies, *J. Immunol.* **122**:1614–1619.

23. Lynch, R. G., Graff, R. J., Sirisinha, S., Simms, E. S., and Eisen, H. N., 1972, Myeloma proteins as tumor-specific transplantation antigens, *Proc. Natl. Acad. Sci. USA* **69**:1540–1544.

24. Jorgensen, T. O., 1982, Lymphocyte specificity for an isologous mouse myeloma protein, Thesis, Department of Immunology, Institute of Medical Biology, University of Tromso, Norway, pp. 1–41.

25. Eichmann, K., and Rajewsky, K., 1975, Induction of T and B cell immunity by anti-idiotypic antibody, *Eur. J. Immunol.* **5**:661–666.

26. Miller, G. G. P., Nadler, P. I., Hodes, R. J., and Sachs, D. H., 1982, Modification of T cell antinuclease idiotype expression by *in vivo* administration of anti-idiotype, *J. Exp. Med.* **155**:190–200.

27. Oudin, J., and Cazenave, P.-A., 1971, Similar idiotypic specificities in immunoglobulin fractions with different antibody functions or even without detectable antibody function, *Proc. Natl. Acad. Sci. USA* **68**:2616–2620.

28. Cazenave, P.-A., Ternynck, T., and Avrameas, S., 1974, Similar idiotypes in antibody-forming cells and in cells synthesizing immunoglobulins without detectable antibody function, *Proc. Natl. Acad. Sci. USA* **71**:4500–4502.

29. Metzger, D. W., Miller, A., and Sercarz, E. E., 1980, Sharing of an idiotypic marker by monoclonal antibodies specific for distinct regions of hen lysozyme, *Nature* **287**:540–542.

30. Kohno, Y., Berkower, I., Minna, J., and Berzofsky, J. A., 1982, Idiotypes of anti-myoglobin antibodies: Shared idiotypes among monoclonal antibodies to distinct determinants of sperm whale myoglobin, *J. Immunol.* **128**:1742–1748.

31. Enghofer, E., Glaudemans, C. P. J., and Bosma, M. J., 1979, Immunoglobulins with different specificities have similar idiotypes, *Mol. Immunol.* **16**:1103–1110.

32. Eichmann, K., Coutinho, A., and Melchers, F., 1977, Absolute frequencies of lipopolysaccharide-reactive B cells producing A5A idiotype in unprimed, streptococcal A carbohydrate-primed, anti-A5A idiotype-sensitized and anti-A5A idiotype-suppressed A/J mice, *J. Exp. Med.* **146**:1436–1449.

33. Hiernaux, J., and Bona, C. A., 1982, Shared idiotypes among monoclonal antibodies specific for different immunodominant sugars of lipopolysaccharide of different gram-negative bacteria, *Proc. Natl. Acad. Sci. USA* **79**:1616–1620.

34. Sakato, N., Fujio, H., and Amano, T., 1980, Idiotypic analysis of antibodies to hen egg-white lysozyme (HEL). I. Occurrence of species-specific cross-reactive idiotypes of antibodies directed to distinct regions of HEL in guinea pigs, *J. Immunol.* **124**:1866–1873.

35. Liu, Y., Bona, C. A., and Schulman, J. L., 1981, Idiotype of clonal responses to influenza virus hemagglutinin, *J. Exp. Med.* **154**:1525–1538.
36. Ju, S.-T., Benacerraf, B., and Dorf, M. E., 1980, Genetic control of a shared idiotype among antibodies directed to distinct specificities, *J. Exp. Med.* **152**:170–182.
37. Boyd, W. C., and Bernard, H., 1937, Quantitative changes in antibodies and globulin fraction in sera of rabbits injected with several antigens, *J. Immunol.* **33**:111–122.
38. Rodkey, L. S., 1974, Studies on idiotypic antibodies: Production and characterization of autoantiidiotypic antisera, *J. Exp. Med.* **139**:712–720.
39. Binion, S. B., and Rodkey, L. S., 1982, Naturally induced auto-anti-idiotypic antibodies: Induction by identical idiotopes in some members of an outbred rabbit family, *J. Exp. Med.* **156**:860–872.
40. Rodkey, L. S., 1976, Studies of idiotypic antibodies: Reactions of isologous and autologous anti-idiotypic antibodies with the same antibody preparations, *J. Immunol.* **117**:986–989.
41. Rodkey, L. S., 1980, Autoregulation of immune responses via idiotype network interactions, *Microbiol. Rev.* **44**:631–659.
42. Kluskens, L. and Köhler, H., 1974, Regulation of immune response by autogeneous antibody against receptor, *Proc. Natl. Acad. Sci. USA* **71**:5083–5087.
43. Bona, C. A., Heber-Katz, E., and Paul, W. E., 1981, Idiotype–anti-idiotype regulation. I. Immunization with a levan-binding myeloma protein leads to the appearance of auto-anti-(anti-idiotype) antibodies and to the activation of silent clones, *J. Exp. Med.* **153**:951–967.
44. Kelsoe, G., and Cerny, J., 1979, Reciprocal expansions of idiotypic anti-idiotypic clones following antigen stimulation, *Nature* **279**:333–334.
45. Schrater, A. F., Goidl, E. A., Thorbecke, J., and Siskind, G. W., 1979, Production of auto-anti-idiotypic antibody during the normal immune response to TNP-Ficoll. III. Absence in *nu/nu* mice: Evidence for T-cell dependence of the anti-idiotypic antibody response, *J. Exp. Med.* **150**:808–817.
46. Jerne, N. K., 1974, Towards a network theory of the immune system, *Ann. Immunol. (Inst. Pasteur)* **125C**:373–389.
47. Kunkel, H. G., Killander, J., and Mannik, M., 1966, Current trends in immune globulin research, *Acta Med. Scand. Suppl.* **445**:63–73.
48. Lieberman, R., Potter, M., Humphrey, W., Jr., Mushinski, E. B., and Vrana, M., 1975, Multiple individual and cross-specific idiotypes on 13 levan-binding myeloma proteins of BALB/c mice, *J. Exp. Med.* **142**:106–119.
49. Kunkel, H. G., Agnello, V., Joslin, F. G., Winchester, R. J., and Capra, J. D., 1973, Cross idiotypic specificity among monoclonal IgM proteins with anti-γ-globulin activity, *J. Exp. Med.* **137**:331–342.
50. Agnello, V., Arbetter, A., Ibanez de Kasep, G., Powell, R., Tan, E. M., and Joslin, F., 1980. Evidence for a subset of rheumatoid factors that cross-react with DNA-histone and have a distinct cross-idiotype, *J. Exp. Med.* **151**:1514–1527.
51. Riesen, W. F., Braun, D. G., Škvăril, F., and Mansa, B., 1982, Idiotypic and structural analysis of monoclonal human immunoglobulins with anti-streptolysin O activity, *Int. Arch. Allergy Appl. Immunol.* **67**:86–92.
52. Abraham, G. N., Podell, D. N., Welch, E. H., and Johnston, S. L., 1983, Idiotypic relatedness of human monoclonal IgG cryoglobulins, *Immunology* **48**:315–320.
53. Feizi, T., Kunkel, H. G., and Roelcke, D., 1974, Cross idiotypic specificity among cold agglutinins in relation to combining activity for blood group-related antigens, *Clin. Exp. Immunol.* **18**:283–293.
54. Pillemer, E., and Weissman, I. L., 1981, A monoclonal antibody that detected a V_κ-TEPC15 idiotypic determinant cross-reactive with a Thy-1 determinant, *J. Exp. Med.* **153**:1068–1079.
55. Riesen, W. F., 1979, Idiotypic cross-reactivity of human and murine phosphorylcholine-binding immunoglobulins, *Eur. J. Immunol.* **9**:421–425.
56. Karol, R. A., Reichlin, M., and Nobel, R. W., 1977, Evolution of an idiotypic determinant: Anti-Val, *J. Exp. Med.* **146**:435–444.
57. Jackson, S., Kulhavy, R., and Mestecky, J., 1981, Shared idiotypes among anti-albumin antibodies of different species, *Scand. J. Immunol.* **14**:31–37.
58. Young, N. M., and Williams, R. E., 1978, Comparison of the secondary structures and binding sites of C-reactive protein and the phosphorylcholine-binding murine myeloma proteins, *J. Immunol.* **121**:1893–1898.
59. Volanakis, J. E., and Kearney, J. F., 1981, Cross-reactivity between C-reactive protein and idiotypic determinants on a phosphocholine-binding murine myeloma protein, *J. Exp. Med.* **153**:1604–1614.

60. Kabat, E. A., Wu, T. T., and Bilofsky, H., 1976, Attempts to locate residues in complementarity-determining regions of antibody combining sites that make contact with antigen, *Proc. Natl. Acad. Sci. USA* **73:**617–619.

61. Kabat, E. A., 1978, The structural basis of antibody complementarity, *Adv. Protein Chem.* **32:**1–75.

62. Kabat, E. A., Wu, T. T., Bilofsky, H., Reid-Miller, M., and Perry, H., 1983, *Sequences of Proteins of Immunological Interest,* Tabulation and analysis of amino acid and nucleic acid sequences of precursors, V-regions, C-regions, J-chain, β_2-microglobulins, major histocompatibility antigens, Thy-1, complement, C-reactive protein, thymopoietin, post-gamma globulin, and α_2-macroglobulin, National Institutes of Health, Bethesda.

63. Childs, R., and Feizi, T., 1975, Cross idiotypic specificity among heavy chains of macroglobulins with blood group I and i specificities, *Nature* **255:**562–564.

64. Milner, E. C. B., and Capra, J. D., 1983, Structural analysis of monoclonal anti-arsonate antibodies: Idiotypic specificities are determined by the heavy chain, *Mol. Immunol.* **20:**39–46.

65. Lieberman, R., Vrana, M., Humphrey, W., Chien, C. C., and Potter, M., 1977, Idiotypes of inulin-binding myeloma proteins localized to variable region light and heavy chains: Genetic significance, *J. Exp. Med.* **146:**1294–1304.

66. Nahm, M. H., Clevinger, B. L., and Davie, J. M., 1982, Monoclonal antibodies to streptococcal group A carbohydrates. I. A dominant idiotypic determinant is located in V_κ, *J. Immunol.* **129:**1513–1518.

67. Sogn, J. A., Yarmush, M. L., and Kindt, T. J., 1976, An idiotypic marker for the V_L region of an homogeneous antibody, *Ann. Immunol. (Inst. Pasteur)* **127C:**397–408.

68. Yarmush, M., Sogn, J. A., Mudgett, M., and Kindt, T. J., 1977, The inheritance of antibody V regions in the rabbit: Linkage of an H-chain-specific idiotype to immunoglobulin allotypes, *J. Exp. Med.* **145:**916–930.

69. Kaartinen, M., Griffiths, G. M., Hamlyn, P. H., Markham, A. F., Karjalainen, K., Pelkonen, J. L. T., Makela, O., and Milstein, C., 1983, Anti-oxazolone hybridomas and the structure of the oxazolone idiotype, *J. Immunol.* **130:**937–945.

70. Schiff, C., Boyer, C., Milili, M., and Fougereau, M., 1979, The idiotypy of the MOPC 173 (IgG_{2a}) mouse myeloma protein: Characterization of syngeneic, allogeneic and xenogeneic anti-idiotypic antibodies. Contribution of the H and L chains to the idiotypic determinants, *Eur. J. Immunol.* **9:**831–841.

71. Brown, A. R., Gottlieb, P. D., and Nisonoff, A., 1981, Role and strain distribution of genes controlling light chains needed for the expression of an intrastrain cross-reactive idiotype, *Immunogenetics* **14:**85–99.

72. Sommé, G., Sera, J. R., Leclercq, L., Moreau, J.-L., Mazie, J.-C., Moinier, D., Fugereau, M., and Thèze, J., 1982, Contribution of the H- and L-chains and of the binding site to the idiotypic specificities of mouse anti-GAT antibodies, *Mol. Immunol* **19:**1011–1019.

73. Misaki, A., Torii, M., Sawai, T., and Goldstein, I. J., 1980, Structure of the dextran of *Leuconostoc mesenteroides* B-1355, *Carbohydr. Res.* **84:**273–285.

74. Seymour, F., Knapp, R. D., Chen, E. C. M., Bishop, S. H., and Jeanes, A., 1979, Structural analysis of Leuconostoc dextrans containing 3-O-α-D-glucosylated α-D-glucosyl residues in both linear-chain and branch-point positions or only in branch-point positions by methylation and by ^{13}C-NMR spectroscopy, *Carbohydr. Res.* **74:**41–62.

75. Sidebotham, R. L., 1974, Dextrans, *Adv. Carbohydr. Chem. Biochem.* **30:**371–444.

76. Jeanes, A., Haynes, W. C., Wilham, C. A., Rankin, J. C., Melvin, E. H., Austin, M. J., Cluskey, J. E., Fisher, B. E., Tsuchiya, H. M., and Rist, C. E., 1954, Characterization and classification of dextrans from ninety-six strains of bacteria, *J. Am. Chem. Soc.* **76:**5041–5052.

77. Jeanes, A., and Seymour, F., 1979, The α-D-glucopyranosidic linkages of dextrans: Comparison of percentages from structural analysis by peridoate oxidation and by methylation, *Carbohydr. Res.* **74:**31–40.

78. Schilling, J., Clevinger, B., Davie, J. M., and Hood, L., 1980, Amino acid sequence of homogeneous antibodies to dextran and DNA rearrangements in heavy chain V-region gene segments, *Nature* **283:**35–40.

79. Clevinger, B., Schilling, J., Hood, L., and Davie, J. M., 1980, Structural correlates of cross-reactive and individual idiotypic determinants on murine antibodies to α-(1→3) dextran, *J. Exp. Med.* **151:**1059–1070.

80. Kehry, M., Sibley, L., Fuhrman, J., Schilling, J., and Hood, L., 1979, Amino acid sequence of a mouse immunoglobulin μ chain, *Proc. Natl. Acad. Sci. USA* **76:**2932–2936.

81. Newman, B., Sugii, S., Kabat, E. A., Torii, M., Clevinger, B. L., Schilling, J., Bond, M., Davie, J. M.,

and Hood, L., 1983, Combining site specificities of mouse hybridoma antibodies to dextran B1355S, *J. Exp. Med.* **157**:130–140.

82. Kabat, E. A., Wu, T. T., and Bilofsky, H., 1978, Variable region genes for the immunoglobulin framework are assembled from small segments of DNA—A hypothesis, *Proc. Natl. Acad. Sci. USA* **75**:2429–2433.

83. Weigert, M., Gatmaitan, L., Loh, E., Schilling, J., and Hood, L., 1978, Rearrangement of genetic information may produce immunoglobulin diversity, *Nature* **276**:785–790.

84. Valbuena, O., Marcu, K. B., Weigert, M., and Perry, R. P., 1978, Multiplicity of germline genes specifying a group of related mouse κ chains with implications for the generation of immunoglobulin diversity, *Nature* **276**:780–784.

85. Kabat, E. A., Wu, T. T., and Bilofsky, H., 1979, Evidence supporting somatic assembly of the DNA segments (minigenes), coding for the framework, and complementarity determining segments of immunoglobulin variable regions, *J. Exp. Med.* **149**:1299–1313.

86. Wu, T. T., Kabat, E. A., and Bilofsky, H., 1979, Some sequence similarities among mouse DNA segments that code for λ and κ light chains of immunoglobulins, *Proc. Natl. Acad. Sci. USA* **76**:4617–4621.

87. Kabat, E. A., Wu, T. T., and Bilofsky, H., 1980, Evidence indicating independent assortment of framework and complementarity-determining segments of the variable regions of rabbit light chains: Delineation of a possible J minigene, *J. Exp. Med.* **152**:72–84.

88. Kabat, E. A., 1980, Antibodies, hypervariable regions and minigenes, *J. Immunol.* **125**:961–969.

89. Kabat, E. A., 1982, Antibody diversity versus antibody complementarity, *Pharmacol. Rev.* **34**:23–38.

90. Juszczak, E. C., and Margolies, M., 1983, Amino acid sequence of the heavy chain variable regions of the A/J mouse anti-arsonate monoclonal antibody 36/60 bearing a minor idiotype, *Biochemistry* **22**:4291–4296.

91. Wood, C., and Tonegawa, S., 1983, Diversity and joining segments of mouse immunoglobulin heavy chain genes are closely linked and in the same orientation: Implications for the joining mechanism, *Proc. Natl. Acad. Sci. USA* **80**:3030–3034.

92. Wu, T. T., and Kabat, E. A., 1982, Fourteen nucleotides in the second complementarity-determining region of a human heavy-chain variable region gene are identical with a sequence in a human D minigene, *Proc. Natl. Acad. Sci. USA* **79**:5031–5032.

93. Rechavi, G., Ram, D., Glazer, L., Zakut, R., and Givol, D., 1983, Evolutionary aspects of immunoglobulin heavy chain variable regions (V_H) gene subgroups, *Proc. Natl. Acad. Sci. USA* **80**:855–859.

94. Bernstein, K. E., Reddy, E. P., Alexander, C. B., and Mage, R. G., 1982. A cDNA sequence encoding a rabbit heavy chain variable region of the V_Ha2 allotype showing homologies with human heavy chain sequences, *Nature* **300**:74–76.

95. Siebenlist, U., Ravetch, J. V., Korsmeyer, S., Waldmann, T., and Leder, P, 1981, Human immunoglobulin D segments encoded in tandem multigenic families, *Nature* **294**:631–635.

96. Takahashi, N., Noma, T., and Honjo, T., 1984, Rearranged immunoglobulin V_H pseudogene that deletes the second complementarity determining region *Proc. Natl. Acad. Sci. USA* **81**: (in press).

97. Alt, F. W., and Baltimore, D., 1982, Joining of immunoglobulin heavy chain gene segments: Implications from a chromosome with evidence of three D–J_H fusions, *Proc. Natl. Acad. Sci. USA* **79**:4118–4122.

98. Dreher, K. L., Emorine, L., Kindt, T. J., and Max, E. E., 1983, A cDNA clone encoding a complete rabbit immunoglobulin κ light chain of b4 allotype, *Proc. Natl. Acad. Sci. USA* **80**:4489–4493.

99. Eulitz, M., and Linke, R. P., 1982, Primary structure of the variable part of an amyloidogenic Bence–Jones protein (Mev.): An unusual insertion in the third hypervariable region of a human κ-immunoglobulin light chain, *Hoppe-Seyler's Z. Physiol. Chem.* **363S**:1347–1358.

100. Potter, M., 1977, Antigen binding myeloma proteins of mice, in: *Advances of Immunology,* Vol 25 (H. G. Kunkel and F. J. Dixon, eds.), Academic Press, New York, pp. 141–211.

101. Sharon, J., D'Hoostelaere, L., Potter, M., Kabat, E. A., and Morrison, S. L., 1982, A cross-reactive idiotype, QUPC52 IdX, present on most but not all anti-α(1→6) dextran-specific IgM and IgA hybridoma antibodies with combining sites of different sizes, *J. Immunol.* **128**:498–500.

102. Cisar, J., Kabat, E. A., Dorner, M., and Liao, J., 1975, Binding properties of immunoglobulin combining sites specific for terminal or non-terminal antigenic determinants in dextran, *J. Exp. Med.* **142**:435–459.

103. Sharon, J., Kabat, E. A., and Morrison, S. L., 1982, Immunochemical characterization of binding sites of hybridoma antibodies specific for α(1→6) linked dextran, *Mol. Immunol.* **19**:375–388.

104. Margolies, M. N., Wysocki, L. J., and Sato, V. L., 1983, Immunoglobulin idiotype and anti-anti-idiotype utilize the same variable region genes irrespective of antigen specificity, *J. Immunol.* **130**:515–517.

105. Dickerman, J., Clevinger, B., and Friedenson, B., 1981, Loss of an individual idiotype on chemical modification: A strategy for assigning idiotypic determinants, *J. Exp. Med.* **153**:1275–1285.
106. Segal, D. M., Padlan, E. A., Cohen, G. H., Rudikoff, S., Potter, M., and Davies, D. R., 1974, The three-dimensional structure of a phosphorylcholine-binding mouse immunoglobulin Fab and the nature of the antigen binding site, *Proc. Natl. Acad. Sci. USA* **71**:4298–4302.
107. Saul, F. A., Amzel, L. M., and Poljak, R. J., 1978, Preliminary refinement and structural analysis of the Fab fragment from human immunoglobulin New at 2 Å resolution, *J. Biol. Chem.* **253**:585–595.
108. Sigal, N. H., 1977, Novel idiotypic and antigen-binding characteristics in two anti-dinitrophenyl monoclonal antibodies, *J. Exp. Med.* **146**:282–286.
109. Schiff, C., Boyer, C., Milili, M., and Fougereau, M., 1981, Structural basis for M-173 idiotypic determinants distinctively recognized in syngeneic and allogeneic immunization: Contribution of DH, JH and Jκ regions to an idiotope recognized by allogeneic antisera, *Ann. Immunol. (Inst. Pasteur)* **132C**:113–129.
110. Johnson, N., Slankard, J., Paul, L., and Hood, L., 1982, The complete V domain amino acid sequences of two myeloma inulin-binding proteins, *J. Immunol.* **128**:302–307.
111. Rudikoff, S., Pawlita, M., Pumphrey, J., Mushinski, E., and Potter, M., 1983, Galactan binding antibodies: Diversity and structure of idiotypes, *J. Exp. Med.* **158**:1385–1400.
112. Rudikoff, S., 1983, Immunoglobulin structure–function correlates: Antigen binding and idiotypes, in: *Contemporary Topics in Molecular Immunology,* Vol. 9 (F.P. Inman and T. J. Kindt, eds.), Plenum Press, New York, pp. 169–209.
113. Pawlita, M., Mushinski, E., Feldmann, R. J., and Potter, M., 1981, A monoclonal antibody that defines an idiotope with two subsites in galactan-binding myeloma proteins, *J. Exp. Med.* **154**:1946–1956.
114. Rajewski, K., and Takemori, T., 1983, Genetic expression and function of idiotypes, in: *Annual Review of Immunology,* Vol. 1 (W. E. Paul, C. G. Fathman, and H. Metzger, eds.), Annual Reviews, Inc., Palo Alto, pp. 569–607.
115. Dildrop, R., Bruggemann, M., Radbruch, A., Rajewsky, K., and Beyreuther, K., 1982, Immunoglobulin V region variants in hybridoma cells. II. Recombination between V genes, *EMBO J.* **1**:635–640.
116. Marchalonis, J. J., Wang, A.-C., and Wu, T. T., 1983, Identification of amino acid residues implicated in the cross-reaction between immunoglobulin V_H and a T cell receptor molecule, *Exp. and Clinical Immunogenetics* **1**: (in press).
117. Segal, D. M., Padlan, E. A., Cohen, G. H., Rudikoff, S., Potter, M., and Davies, D. R., 1974, The three-dimensional structure of a phosphorylcholine-binding mouse immunoglobulin Fab and the nature of the antigen binding site, *Proc. Natl. Acad. Sci. USA* **71**:4298–4302.
118. Saul, F. A., Amzel, L. M., and Poljak, R. J., 1978, Preliminary refinement and structural analysis of the Fab fragment from human immunoglobulin New at 2 Å resolution, *J. Biol. Chem.* **253**:585–595.
119. Marquart, M., Deisenhofer, J., Huber, R., and Palm, W., 1980, Crystallographic refinement and atomic models of the intact immunoglobulin molecule Kol and its antigen-binding fragment at 3.0 Å and 1.9 Å resolution, *J. Mol. Biol.* **141**:369–391.
120. Marquart, M., and Deisenhofer, J., 1983, The three-dimensional structure of antibodies, *Immunol. Today* **3**:160–166.
121. Davies, D. R., and Padlan, E. A., 1977, Correlations between antigen-binding specificity and the three-dimensional structure of the antibody combining sites, in: *Antibodies in Human Diagnosis and Therapy* (E. Haber and R. M. Krause, eds.), Raven Press, New York, pp. 119–143.
122. Davies, D. R., and Metzger, H., 1983, Structural basis of antibody function, in: *Annual Review of Immunology,* Vol. 1 (W. E. Paul, C. G. Fathman, and H. Metzger, eds.), Annual Reviews, Inc., Palo Alto, pp. 87–117.
123. Mage, R. G., and Kabat, E. A,, 1963, The combining regions of the type III pneumococcus polysaccharide and homologous antibody, *Biochemistry* **2**:1278–1288.
124. Bennett, L. G., and Glaudemans, C. P. J., 1979, The affinity of a linear, α-D-(1→6)-linked D-glucopyranan (dextran) for homogeneous immunoglobulin A W3129, *Carbohydr. Res.* **72**:315–319.
125. Weigert, M., Raschke, W. C., Carson, D., and Cohn, M., 1974, Immunochemical analysis of the idiotypes of mouse myeloma proteins with specificity for levan or dextran, *J. Exp. Med.* **139**:137–147.
126. Ekborg, G., Ittah, Y., and Glaudemans, C. P. J., 1983, Monoclonal IgA J539 binds galactopyranosyl antigens on its surface, *Mol. Immunol.* **20**:235–238.
127. Morahan, G., Berek, C., and Miller, J. F. A. P., 1983, An idiotypic determinant formed by both immunoglobulin constant and variable regions, *Nature* **301**:720–722.

2

The Genes Encoding Anti-NP Antibodies in Inbred Strains of Mice

ALFRED L. M. BOTHWELL

1. Introduction

The phenomenon of recurrent idiotypes has provided access to immunological interactions of various kinds. By definition, the antigenic structures which specify the variable regions of heavy and light chains of antibodies form the idiotypic determinants. They must be generated by B cells yet are apparently recognized and perhaps mimicked by T cells. The expression of idiotypes on B cells poses many questions. Most important to our investigation is determining the nature of the mechanisms causing the selection for the generation of an idiotype. Do the idiotypic structures form a focal point for lymphocyte interactions or are they primarily the consequence of other types of biological regulation?

The generation of an idiotype is increasingly an operational definition. Initially, it seemed that the dominant expression of families of antigenically related antibodies reflected something unique. Now, as we study idiotypic responses, there are major and minor families. Any frequently occurring antigenic structures found in serum antibodies can be identified and studied using serological reagents. The combination of serological analysis of serum antibodies and chromosomal DNA characterization is now permitting a rapid definition of basic components and structural characteristics of idiotype-bearing antibody families.

It is hoped that the description of the gene usage will suggest more definitive rules which can describe the expression of genes. These rules are not necessarily rigid and must accommodate the development of an antibody response over time. The factors which could influence the quality and quantity of antibodies during an immune response are many. However, a major goal is understanding the relative contribution of regulatory influences

ALFRED L. M. BOTHWELL • Department of Pathology, Division of Immunology, and The Howard Hughes Medical Institute, Yale University School of Medicine, New Haven, Connecticut 06510.

of T or B cells on B cells versus the role of antigen selection in inducing antibody-producing cells.

The commonly studied idiotypic systems include the responses to (4-hydroxy-3-nitro-phenyl)acetyl (NP), $(Glu^{60}Ala^{30}Tyr^{10})_n$ (GAT), phosphocholine (PC), p-azophenylarson-ate (Ars), group A streptococcal carbohydrate (A5A), dextran, and, most recently, oxazo-lone. The germ-line V_H genes for the major NP^b idiotypic family in C57BL/6 mice and PC in BALB/c mice were the first characterized.[1,2] Since the NP^b idiotype bearing anti-bodies all bear λ light chains, their description was complete with the identification of all the genes encoding λ chains.[3,4] The three κ light chains that associate with the single V_H gene product that form anti-PC antibodies have been well characterized.[5] Subsequently, the genes for the Ars response in A/J[6,7] and BALB/c mice (Near and Gefter, unpub-lished), and the NP^a response in BALB/c[8] have been identified. Recently, the gene sequences encoding the anti-GAT antibodies in C57BL/6[9] and BALB/c[10–12] and antioxazolone[13] and the MOPC460 idiotype in BALB/c (E. Dzierzak, C. Janeway, Jr., and A. Bothwell, unpublished data) have been identified.

The primary focus of these studies is to offer a molecular account of the genes used and detailed description of the expressed genes by DNA sequencing methods. Some of these studies are facilitated by the recent observations that some of the same V_H or V_L genes are used in the different idiotypic systems. Most notable is the use of the same V_H gene in C57BL/6 to make either anti-NP antibodies or anti-GAT antibodies. A very similar if not identical V_H is used in BALB/c to make anti-NP or anti-GAT antibodies. The anti-GAT antibodies use a κ light chain and not the λ chains characteristic of anti-NP antibodies. The equivalent BALB/c allele for a minor or CRI$^-$ class of anti-Ars antibodies in A/J mice corresponds to the gene for the major anti-Ars response in BALB/c. The significance of this common usage of a small number of V genes found in the various idiotypic systems is unclear but may provide some clues which will be discussed later.

At the present time, the mechanisms that contribute to the selection of resting B lym-phocytes for expression or clonal expansion have certainly been outlined, but precise answers are not available. The molecular description of an idiotype should be ideally suited for this purpose. There is a reproducible expression of a limited number of gene products. The task of defining the germ-line-encoded sequences for the majority of the relevant anti-bodies is feasible. Furthermore, the potential regulatory roles of T cells or B cells should be more apparent and definable.

2. Experimental Approach and Initial Findings Concerning Anti-NP Antibodies

The study of the genes encoding anti-NP antibodies was initiated using the C57BL/6 mouse strain. The primary goal was a study of the generation of antibody diversity and a molecular characterization of genes used to generate idiotype-bearing antibodies. These antibodies have four general properties, which suggested a very close relationship between V genes would be apparent and give useful comparisons. The antibodies all bear λ chains, have similar affinities for related haptens, common isoelectric focusing patterns, and reac-tivity to a polyspecific anti-idiotypic antiserum.

Studies on serum idiotype-bearing antibodies have been refined by the derivation of monoclonal antibodies. The majority of these antibodies show an antigenic relatedness, but some classification or subdivision has been attempted. Six groups of antibodies have been designated.[14] These groups presumably reflect heavy-chain variable-region differences (perhaps mainly D_H) since all of the antibodies bear λ light chains and most were from a primary response. Few somatic mutations would be expected in these antibodies. The first four groups are more closely related to each other serologically than the remaining two groups and represent the majority of the serum idiotype. The fifth and sixth groups are more closely related to each other than to any of the first four and are a minor component of the idiotype found in serum. Group six is the only one that shows a significant serological relationship to BALB/c and anti-NP antibodies. Thus far, the analysis of functional DNA sequences encoding six antibodies has been performed. Three of these belong to groups I or II. Of the remaining three, one could not be classified (S43) and two have not been analyzed serologically.

The molecular studies were initiated prior to the availability of probes for the J_H regions so molecular cDNA clones were constructed from poly(A)-containing RNA. We chose two proteins which were very different from each other idiotypically.[15] The hybridoma B1-8 produced an IgM antibody and was generated by fusion 7 days after a primary immunization. The S43 hybridoma produced an IgG2a antibody and was obtained from the spleen of a hyperimmunized animal. Another hybridoma producing an IgG1 antibody obtained from the same fusion as B1-8 designated B1-48 has been characterized by cloning the rearranged V_H gene.

The amino acid sequences translated from the DNA sequences encoding the C57BL/6 V_H genes[1] and the BALB/c 17.2.25 gene[8] are shown in Fig. 1. Several features of the C57BL/6 sequences were noticed immediately and substantiated by the comparison with the other V_H germ-line sequences and the BALB/c sequence. The most variable portions of the expressed antibody genes in C57BL/6 were the D_H and J_H regions. The only obvious common feature was the occurrence of the tyrosine residue at the first position in the D_H region. The total length of D_H varied, being 4, 5, or 7 amino acid residues in these sequences and varied extensively beyond the first position in primary sequence. The total length of D_H plus J_H also varied, being 20 or 22 residues in these examples. The S43 antibody, a somatic variant, contained seven replacement changes which were located at many different sites in the molecule. This antibody has a 4.5-fold affinity for the hapten than the B1-8 antibody, so these alterations probably do not affect residues that make contact with hapten. This suggested that residues in the CDRs at positions 33 and 59–65 were not contact residues. Further comparisons were made with the MOPC104E and MOPC315 sequences and we suggested that the Met-His sequence at positions 34 and 35, and perhaps the Arg and Asp residues at the beginning of CDR2 might also be involved as contact residues.[16] The His-35 residue is more likely to be the actual contact residue in CDR1 since the Met-34 is probably directed inward.[17,18] In the λ light chain, the tryptophan residue at position 93 or 98 is a good candidate for a contact residue since there is evidence for a charge transfer complex with the aromatic hapten.[16]

From these studies, we also realized that very closely related sequences existed in the germ line and yet were not used. This suggests that the framework portion of the antibody must have some very subtle structural features which, when combined with the more variable structures (D_H and J_H), produce an expressed antibody. Thus, in a functional and also structural sense, the V domains are constructed using segments whose individual ident-

```
                                       -19                             1                  10                  20                        30
                                        * *
B1-8      M G W S C I M L F L A A T A T G V H S Q V Q L Q Q P G A E L V K P G A S V K L S C K A S G Y T F T
B1-48     - - - - - - - - - - - - - - - - - - - - - - - - - - - - - - - - - - - - - - - - - T - - - - - -
S43       - - - - - - - - - - - - - - - - - - - - - - - - - - - - - - - - - - - - - - - - - T - - - - - -
17.2.25   - K C - W V I F F - M - V V - - - N - E - - - - - S - - - - - R - - - - - - - - - - - - F N I K

          CDR1  * *                40                    * *         CDR2            60                       70
B1-8      S Y W M H W V K Q R P G R G L E W I G R I D P N S G G T K Y N E K F K S K A T L T V D K P S S T A
B1-48     - - - - - - - - - - - - - - - - - - - - - - - - - - - - - - - - - - - - - - - - - - - - - - - -
S43       - - L - - - - - - - N - - - - - - - - - - - - - - - T - - - - - H - R - - - I - - - - - - - - - -
17.2.25   D T Y - - - - - - - E Q - - - - - - - A N - N - - - D P - - I - A - T S T N - -

          80                              *           90        D                              J
B1-8      Y M Q L S S L T S E D S A V Y Y C A R Y D Y Y G S S . . Y F D Y W G Q G T T L T V S S
B1-48     - - - - - - - - - - - - - - - - - - - L L G . . . W - - V - - T - - V - - -
S43       - - - - - - - - - - - - - - - - - - - R L G R - - . . Y R - - V - - T - - V - - -
17.2.25   - L - - - - - - - - - - - - - - - - - T - - Y R - P . . Y Y A M - - - S V - - -
```

FIGURE 1. Amino acid sequences of anti-NP V_H regions. All sequences were predicted from the DNA sequence. The DNA sequences except for B1-48 have been published.[1,8] An asterisk indicates residues currently believed to be contact residues. The B1-8 and S43 antibodies use J_H2, B1-48 uses J_H1, and 17.2.25 uses J_H4.

ities become obscured. There may be isolated residues, such as Tyr-99 and His-35 in the V_H or Trp 98 in V_L which are critical contact residues, but regions which form individual idiotopes may be rather complex. This is very nicely illustrated in this set of antibodies. The B1-8 antibody was used to generate monoclonal anti-idiotopes. One such antibody, Ac38, has been used to characterize variants of the B1-8 antibody. One can lose Ac38 binding of B1-8 by a single mutation in the middle of the D_H region (B1-8.V3).[19] Yet it is also possible to maintain the B1-8 D_H region and substitute about 10 amino acids in the first 65 residues (B1-8.V1) and retain the Ac38 idiotope.[19] Thus, sequences which are very distant in the primary sequence must participate in forming idiotopes.

Our recently completed studies on the BALB/c V_H gene[8] used in an anti-NP response appear to confirm our observations of the C57BL/6 sequences (see Fig. 1). That is, the Met-His in the CDR1 sequence was maintained in spite of a completely different sequence in the preceding seven codons. In addition, the CDR2 region beyond codon 53 was very different from the C57BL/6 sequences characterized while codon 99 was still a tyrosine residue.

These data suggested, even from the beginning, the subtle features that may occur in this family of antibodies between the antigen and the antibody. Thus, a critical chemical interaction may result in a dominant selection for antibodies of this type. This, although admittedly intuitive, is shaping the next phase of our work. Certainly, we can learn more by studying the structure of a few more of the prototypic antibodies. However, this type of analysis does tend to give only structural information and its biases. We need now to probe the response again to determine the relationship of memory cells and κ-bearing antibodies to the response. Since there is a predominance of κ-bearing antibodies after extensive hyper-immunization,[15] why are they not seen earlier? Is there something special about the inter-action of the λ-bearing immunoglobulin on a resting B lymphocyte with NP that results in a more efficient or complete activation of B cells into plasma cells? Perhaps the cells bearing κ antibodies are only partially activated and are preferentially diverted to the memory state.

The initial findings dramatically revealed at the DNA level that an IgM antibody could possess a germ-line V_H DNA sequence while an IgG2a antibody was encoded by a V_H gene that had undergone extensive somatic mutation.[1] The generalization was made that this might reflect a general property of antibodies, namely, that non-IgM antibodies might frequently possess somatic mutations while IgM antibodies might only rarely contain them. The process of gene rearrangement would occur during B-cell development in the bone marrow and somatic variants would be generated primarily after antigenic stimulation in the periphery of the lymphoid system. A more extensive survey of anti-PC myeloma and hybridoma protein sequences resulted in similar conclusions.[5]

The actual mechanism of somatic mutation is still a mystery and the subject of much speculation. The process may be a progressive one which is initiated after the primary response to antigen. The encounter with antigen may result in the clonal expansion of resting B lymphocytes. Some of the progeny of such clones may differentiate directly to produce antibody-secreting cells and others give rise to longer-lived memory B cells. The process of mutation may occur in such cells and be associated with any proliferation that occurs. Any stimulus to this set of cells such as proliferation by T-helper cells might result in a broader spectrum of specificities represented in the memory cells. Occasionally, these cells may differentiate into antibody-producing cells without reexposure to antigen. After a repeated immunization the products of these memory cells become apparent.

A hint of the progressive nature of the response may be seen in our studies of anti-NP antibodies. The S43 hybridoma was obtained after extensive hyperimmunization. The V_H region encoding the S43 antibody contained 10 bp which were mutated from the germ-line *186-2* gene.[1] Since the sequence was determined from a cDNA clone, we do not know the extent of somatic mutation in the flanking sequences but assume it is extensive. Studies of two anti-PC V_H regions revealed extensive somatic mutation, especially in the 3′ region which flanked a heavily mutated V_H gene.[20] We have cloned the rearranged V_H gene from another hybridoma derived early in the anti-NP response, designated B1-48. The DNA sequence of the entire 4.6-kb EcoRI fragment containing the rearranged V_H gene has been determined. The $V(186-2)$ gene is rearranged into J_H1 so that there are about 1500 bp 5′ and about 3000 bp 3′ to the rearranged *VDJ* segment. The exons and the entire 5′ flanking region have been compared with the $V(186-2)$ DNA sequence. The 3′ flanking region has been compared with the published BALB/c sequences[21,22] and our unpublished sequence of the C57BL/6 J_H region. A clone of the C57BL/6 J_H region was obtained from C. Nottenberg and I. Weissman, Stanford University. The entire B1-48 V_H rearranged EcoRI fragment possesses a germline sequence except at a single location. There is a deletion of 10 bp (TCATTTATTG) which contains the canonical nonameric recognition sequence for *VDJ* rearrangement just 5′ to J_H3. The germ-line C57BL/6 clone was shown to possess this sequence. There are no sequences similar to this in the immediate vicinity, so we doubt that this deletion arose subsequent to molecular cloning of this gene. This hybridoma was isolated early during an immune response (day 7) but synthesizes an IgG1 antibody. This may be a spleen cell that was trapped very early in the process of somatic diversification.

3. Germline V_H Genes Related to the NP^b Idiotype

These initial studies revealed general features about genes encoding idiotypically related antibodies. Initially, seven V_H genes which showed a high degree of homology by hybridization were chosen for DNA sequence determination. Thus far, only one, designated $V(186-2)$, has been found functional in an idiotype-bearing anti-NP hybridoma and six hybridomas have been examined. The germline DNA sequences were very similar[1] and this is evident in the translated amino acids shown in Fig. 2. The $V(186-2)$ sequence is used as a reference. There are several points to be noted. First, the $V(145)$ sequence was identical to the $V(186-2)$ sequence except at codon 22 where serine was encoded instead of a cysteine. We suggested that this gene was probably not functional since it could not make an intra-V-region disulfide bond.[1] Another sequence that was extremely close to $V(186-2)$ is $V(186-1)$. There were only three codons which were different and yet there is no indication that it is ever used to make anti-NP antibodies. The remaining sequences show extensive variation in CDR2 but few differences elsewhere. Gene $V(6)$ has a deletion in codon 22 and cannot give rise to an intact translational reading frame. The DNA sequences showed some striking segmental homologies which raised the possibility that a process related to gene conversion might have occurred in the evolution of this multigene family.[1] Because somatic mechanisms can alter rearranged genes we might encounter some unexpected genes expressed. Recently, a double recombination event between $V(102-1)$ and $V(186-2)$ was shown to occur *in vitro*.[23,24] The net result is that approximately 65 N-terminal residues are fused to the rest of the B1-8 protein. It may be that some events

```
                        1          10        20        30        40        50
                                                     CDR1
186-2    Q V Q L Q Q P G A E L V K P G A S V K L S C K A S G Y T F T S Y W M H W V K Q R P G R G L E W I G R
145      - - - - - - - - - - - - - - - - - - - - - - - - - - - - - - - - - - - - - - - - - - - - - - - - -
186-1    - - - - - - - - - - - - - - - - - - - - S - - - - - - - - - - - - - - - - - - - - - - - - - - - N
23       - - - - - - - - - - T - - - - - - - - - - - - - - - - - - - - - - - - - - - - - - - - - - - - - N
6        - - - - - - - - - - - - - - - - - - - V - - * - - - - - - - - - - - - - - - - Q - - - - - - - - -
102-1    - - - - - - - - - - R - - - - - - S - - - - - - - - - - - - - - - - - - - - - - E - - - - - - - - N
3-1      - - - - - - - - - - - - - - - - - - - - - - - - - - - - - - - - D - - - - - - - Q - - - - - - - - N

                       60         70        80        90
            CDR2
186-2    I D P N S G G T K Y N E K F K S K A T L T V D K P S S T A Y M Q L S S L T S E D S A V Y Y C A R
145      - - - - - - - - - - - - - - - - - - - - - - - - - - - - - - - - - - - - - - - - - - - - - -
186-1    - - - - - - - - - - - - - - - - - - - - - - - - - - T S - - - - - - - - - - - - - - - - H - -
23       - N - G N - - - - - - - - - - - - - - - V - - - - - S S - - - - - - - - - - - - - - - - - - -
6        - Y - G - S S - - - - - - - - - - - - - - - - - - - - T - - - - - - - - - - - - - - - - - - -
102-1    - H - S D S D - - - - Q - - - - - - - - - - - G - - - S - - - - - - - - - - - - - I - - - - -
3-1      - Y - S D S E - - - - Q - - - - - - - - - D - - - - - S - - - - - - - - - - - - - - - - - - -
```

FIGURE 2. Predicted amino acid sequence of V_H genes of the 186-2 family. The translated sequences are derived from previously published DNA sequences.[1] The asterisk in the V(6) sequence indicates the inability to predict a codon since a deletion of one base occurs at this position.

that occur in these V_H genes occur less frequently in other V_H genes. This might be related to the large number of very homologous sequences both in exons and in introns.

When a V_H probe was used to detect cross-hybridizing genes using the Southern blot procedure, 10 major bands were seen.[1] Some of these bands have three to six genes in them and minor bands are evident. The total number of related sequences is probably 35–50. Since the total number of V_H genes in the mouse is approximately 100, this cross-hybridizing family of genes is the largest such family comprising 40–50% of the V_H repertoire.

Initially, 15 V_H genes were found on 10 recombinant phages. More recently, nine new phages have been isolated containing one V_H gene per clone. Thus, we have potentially 24 unique V_H genes cloned. A summary of the EcoRI DNA fragments present in the recombinant phages is shown in Table I. They are grouped according to the largest EcoRI fragment that contains a V_H gene. It is clear that there are five different phages that contain a 6.5-kb fragment bearing a V_H gene and potentially six. The uncertainty exists because phage 1 has one EcoRI site deleted (see footnote a of Table I). There are four 5-kb DNA fragments that contain V_H genes. In addition, there are some common EcoRI DNA fragments which do not contain V_H genes. In many of the phages a 6.5- and/or a 1.85-kb fragment is found. In most and perhaps all cases this is indicative of extensive DNA sequence homology in the regions flanking the actual exon regions. It is possible that in

TABLE I
EcoRI DNA Fragments Contained in Cross-Hybridizing λ VNPB Phages[a]

λVNPB-3	21.0, 1.0
λVNPB-147	16.0, 2.0
λVNPB-104	12.0, 1.0, 0.5, 0.1
λVNPB-6	8.0, 5.5, 1.0
λVNPB-130	8.0, 5.0, 0.46
λVNPB-23	6.5, 6.5, 1.85, 1.6
λVNPB-145	6.5,, 6.5, 0.38
λVNPB-17	6.5, 6.5, 3.5*, 1.85, 1.6
λVNPB-12	6.5, 2.3*, 1.85
λVNPB-2	6.5, 2.4*, 1.85
λVNPB-1	>5.0, 6.5, 1.85, 0.35
λVNPB-168	5.5, 6.5, 2.2, 0.35
λVNPB-102	5.0, 5.5, 2.3, 2.2, 0.25
λVNPB-186	5.0, 5.0, 5.5, 1.85, 1.7, 1.0, 0.38
λVNPB-20	5.0, 2.4*, 1.85, 1.0
λVNPB-22	4.4, 4.0, 1.5, 0.5, 0.4
λVNPB-4	3.5, 4.5, 2.9, 2.1, 1.6, 1.5, 0.6
λVNPB-16	1.6, 5.0, 3.5, 1.9, 1.8, 1.7, 1.65*
λVNPB-5	1.6, 5.0, 3.5, 1.9, 1.8, 1.7

[a]The phages 1, 2, 4, 5, 12, 16, 17, 20, and 22 were constructed using the Charon 30 vector. A partial MboI-digested C57BL/6 DNA fraction was used. The other phages were generated using Charon 4A and a sized DNA fraction of partial EcoRI-digested C57BL/6 DNA. The EcoRI fragment that is fused to the left arm of the Charon 30 phage is indicated with an asterisk. The numbers refer to the size of a DNA fragment in kb and the underlined fragment sizes indicate the presence of a V gene. Phages 3 and 104 contain two V genes on each EcoRI fragment underlined.

several cases this homology could be due to actual chromosomal overlap in the cloned sequences. In the original collection of 10 recombinant phages there are only two possible locations for overlap between cloned segments. The restriction endonuclease maps of these phages are shown in Fig. 3. The maps are oriented such that the orientation of the exons is identical. Transcription of the exons (5' to 3') would proceed from left to right in all of these sequences. The two sites of possible overlap in cloned segments are between phages 23 and 186 and between phages 6 and 3. In the first case the common $EcoRI$ fragment is the 1.85-kb fragment that is also found in phages 17, 12, 2, and 1. More phage clones or cosmid clones will be needed to complete the linkage of this repetitive segment of chromosomal DNA. In some cases actual DNA sequence analysis may be needed to complete the gene linkage. The overlap between the 1-kb fragment found in phages 6 and 3 is very likely. The mobility of this DNA fragment in agarose gels is identical and detectably different from similarly sized DNA fragments found in phages 104, 186, and 20 (A. Bothwell, unpublished data). Assuming this linkage to be accurate, the three closely related V_H genes are physically linked in the chromosomal DNA. From the restriction maps presented in Fig. 3, 10 out of 15 of the V_H gene isolates (two-thirds) were found linked to another related V_H gene. Thus, we expect most if not all of the V_H genes to be physically linked. A common distance between four of the five V_H gene pairs is about 12 kb. The distance in phage 3 is about 18 kb. Thus, some variability is already apparent. Increasingly there is evidence that the V_H genes may have the same relative orientation (5' to 3') along the chromosome. There is not even a hint of a gene or a flanking region with opposite polarity. Our bank of V_H gene isolates probably represents 15–25% of the total V_H repertoire.

The extent of flanking sequence homology is readily apparent when comparing restriction endonuclease maps of these regions (see Fig. 4). The maps were drawn after alignment of the V_H exon regions. The first 12 V_H genes show a homology which extends several kilobases into the flanking regions. The *186-2* family can be considered at present to consist of the top 12 V_H genes. Notable features of this family are the occurrence of $AccI$ sites within and immediately flanking the exons, a $PstI$ site at codon 4, and the $SstI$, $KpnI$, $BglI$, and $BglII$ sites in the flanking regions. Several of the remaining V_H genes are closely related to each other, expecially $V(104-1)$, $V(104-2)$, $V(102-2)$, $V(147-1)$, $V(147-2)$, and $V(168)$. There is a common $HinfI$ site just 5' to the leader sequence and also at codon 90 and several $PstI$ sites both in and adjacent to exons. Another characteristic feature of these two families is the identity of codon 7. In the *186-2* family it is exclusively proline while in all other genes studied codon 7 is a serine residue. It is probably that the *186-2* family is very closely linked together. However, some interspersion must occur. This is evident from the restriction maps presented in Fig. 3. In phages 102 and 3 the genes $V(102-1)$ and $V(3-1)$ are members of the *186-2* family while the other genes on these phages $V(102-2)$ and $V(3-2)$ are not. If all of these V_H genes have the same polarity, then as one proceeds 5' (referring to transcriptional orientation) to one of these phages one must eventually encounter the other phage. The $V(102-2)$ gene or the $V(3-2)$ gene would then interrupt the *186-2* family.

In some of these phages extensive DNA sequence analysis of flanking regions has been performed. For example, DNA sequence of the 3 kb 3' to both $V(102-1)$ and $V(186-2)$ is about 95% complete. The actual DNA sequences have only 5% sequence differences which are scattered over the entire flanking region. Approximately 80% of the differences were single base changes with the remainder being single, double, or triple base insertions

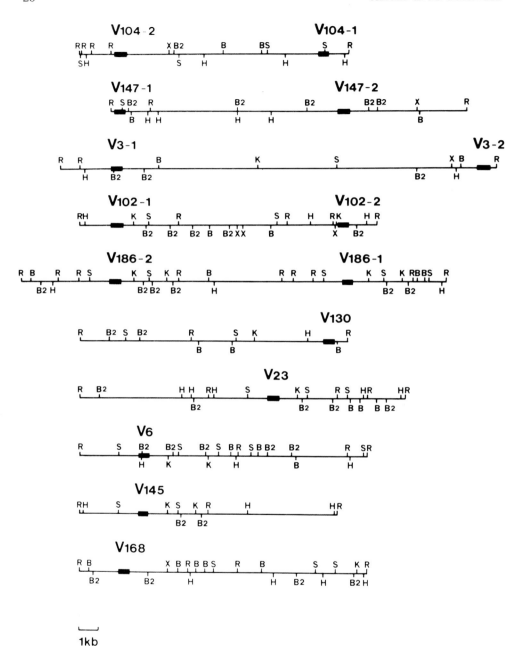

Figure 3. Restriction maps of NP^b V_H genes. The V_H clone designation is given above each solid block of approximately 600 bp which represents the exon regions. From DNA sequence studies (Bothwell, to be published) the orientation of all V_H genes is such that the RNA transcription would occur left to right in the 5' to 3' direction. The following abbreviations are used to designate restriction endonuclease sites: R, EcoRI; B, BamH1; B1, BglI; B2, BglII; H, HindIII; K, KpnI; S, SstI; X, Xba; A, AccI; P, PstI.

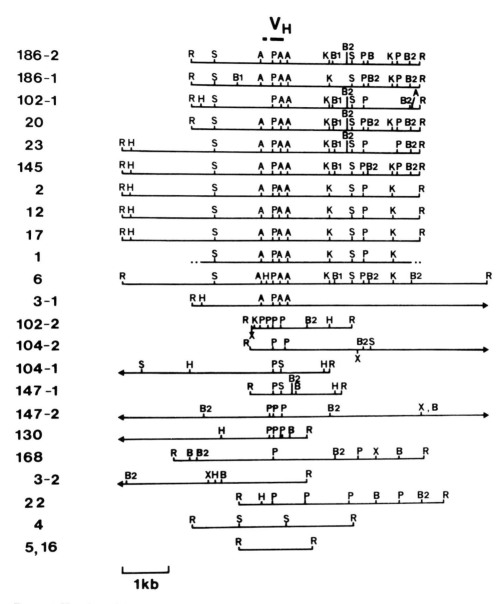

FIGURE 4. Homology of DNA flanking V_H regions. The restriction maps of the EcoRI fragments or a portion of the EcoRI fragment are aligned relative to the V_H gene. If an EcoRI fragment extends greater than 3–4 kb in either direction it is indicated with an arrow. For many of the phages the complete restriction map is given in Fig. 3. Abbreviations to denote sites are used as in Fig. 3. In phage 1 the precise location of the EcoRI site is unknown at present. For all phages except 22, 4, 5, and 16 the orientation of transcription of the exons would be in the 5' to 3' direction from left to right. In these four phages the location of the V gene is known but the orientation is uncertain.

or deletions or in one case a 10-bp deletion. These characteristics observed in regions flanking V_H germ-line genes are qualitatively very similar to the differences seen in somatic
variants. Since these germ-line V_H genes are so homologous they must have arisen by some
gene duplication mechanism. We can therefore compare these related sequences and
assume there was at least a common progenitor. The differences are then a measure of the
normal process of molecular evolution over this region of the chromosome. It is possible
that the processes of normal molecular evolution are similar to those giving rise to somatic
mutations in B lymphocytes. This suggests that the normal processes of generation of DNA
replication errors can be dramatically amplified in lymphocytes to produce somatic variants.
The mechanism of somatic mutation may involve a localized amplification of DNA replication which would increase the replication errors in a localized region. An onion skin
model of replication localized in a V region seems an attractive analogy. Considerable
homology is also seen at the DNA sequence level between regions in which the homology
is not so apparent from the restriction endonuclease maps. This information is not immediately relevant for our understanding of the function of a subset of these genes and our
data are limited. As we continue toward our goal of complete linkage of this multigene
family some of that information may be sought.

The DNA sequences of these 24 V_H genes are nearing completion and the close relationships that exist are remarkable. The first seven V_H gene sequences[1] raised the possibility that a process related to gene conversion might have occurred in this multigene family.
The occurrence of such a process in immunoglobulin genes was further substantiated by
our work on the IgG2a genes.[25] It is more obvious now with many more V_H gene
sequences and a more detailed description of V_H gene evolution will be forthcoming when
the DNA sequencing is completed and more physical linkage is available. It is possible that
the predicted double recombination or gene conversion event might occur in vivo during an
immune response. We are screening newly generated anti-NP hybridomas with this in
mind. It is possible that interactions between such homologous chromosomal segments may
be more common in this V gene family. About 20% of these V_H genes are pseudo-V_H
regions. Perhaps some could be corrected by somatic mechanisms or be functional as
sequence donors.

There is, at present, one gene that seems relatively unique. The first hybridization
studies on $V(130)$ indicated it was significantly different,[1] but the DNA sequencing studies were more informative (A. Bothwell, unpublished data). The surprise was that it has a
DNA sequence nearly identical to the gene which was used in BALB/c to produce anti-
NP antibodies[8] (NP^a idiotype). As mentioned in the introduction, the BALB/c gene, or
one nearly identical to it, is also used to make another family of idiotypically related antibodies to the synthetic polypeptide antigen GAT. The translated amino acid sequences of
V(130), the NP^a gene, and the GAT gene are shown in Fig. 5. The similarity between
these sequences is remarkable. Only six codons differ between the expressed NP^a (17.2.25)
sequence and $V(130)$. If the NP^a sequence is derived from the same gene as the anti-GAT
sequences, then codons 13 and 76 in the NP^a sequence have probably been altered by
somatic mutation. Considering the similarity in these predicted protein sequences, one won-
ders why the $V(130)$ sequence has not been found in the anti-NP antibodies from C57BL/
6. Perhaps the sample size has been too small and, indeed, we will find that it is used with
a certain frequency. Alternatively, there may be some hidden defect that inactivates its

```
                1                    10                   20                   30
130    E  I  Q  L  Q  Q  S  V  A  E  L  V  R  P  G  A  S  V  K  L  S  C  T  A  S  G  F  N  I  K
NPa    -  -  -  -  -  -  -  G  -  -  -  -  -  -  -  -  -  -  -  -  -  -  -  -  -  -  -  -  -  -
GAT    -  -  -  -  -  -  -  G  -  -  -  K  -  -  -  -  -  -  -  -  -  -  -  -  -  -  -  -  -  -
                                                                        CDR1

                                     40                   50                   60
130    N  T  Y  M  H  W  V  K  Q  R  P  E  Q  G  L  E  W  I  G  R  I  D  P  A  N  G  N  T  K  Y
NPa    D  -  -  -  -  -  -  -  -  -  -  -  -  -  -  -  -  -  -  -  -  -  -  -  -  -  -  -  -  -
GAT    D  -  -  -  -  -  -  -  -  -  -  -  -  -  -  -  -  -  -  -  -  -  -  -  -  -  -  -  -  -
                                                           CDR2

                                     70                   80                   90
130    A  P  K  F  Q  G  K  A  T  I  T  A  D  T  S  S  N  T  A  Y  L  Q  L  S  S  L  T  S  E  D
NPa    D  -  -  -  -  -  -  -  -  -  -  -  -  -  -  -  T  -  -  -  -  -  -  -  -  -  -  -  -  -
GAT    D  -  -  -  -  -  -  -  -  -  -  -  -  -  -  -  -  -  -  -  -  -  -  -  -  -  -  -  -  -
                CDR2

       91
130    T  A  I  Y  Y  C  A  R
NPa    -  -  V  -  -  -  -  -
GAT    -  -  V  -  -  -  -  -
```

FIGURE 5. Comparison of a C57BL/6 V_H gene with closely related and expressed BALB/c sequences. The NP^a sequence was derived from the DNA sequence of the BALB/c 17.2.25 anti-NP hybridoma.[8] The GAT sequence represents the most likely germ-line-encoded sequence of BALB/c anti-GAT hybridomas.[10]

function. Recently, missense changes in exon regions have been shown to be responsible for loss of secretion.[26] This situation is reminiscent of the $V(186-2)$ family where a gene very closely related to the expressed gene, $V(186-1)$, may not be used to make anti-NP antibodies.

This emphasizes the subtle nature of the *in vivo* selection process unless for very obscure reasons many of the germ-line V_H genes are not functional. The majority of C57BL/6 anti-NP antibodies must come from the $V(186-2)$ gene. Since the germ-line genes are so similar it is possible that a small number of genes may be used in generating a small fraction of anti-NP antibodies. Understanding the structures of these antibodies and comparing them with other expressed and unexpressed genes may suggest a structural basis for expression if it exists.

The apparent selectivity seen in the genes used to generate the NP^b idiotype is contrasted by the observation that the $V(182-2)$ gene is also used to generate anti-GAT antibodies in C57BL/6 mice.[9] The same is true in the BALB/c response to NP[8] or GAT.[9-12] It is possible that the two antigens may have a similar structure, perhaps the tyrosine in GAT resembles the aromatic ring in NP. Another possibility is that there is a preferential expression of these V_H genes. The most attractive possibility is that there is a preferential rearrangement of certain V_H genes. Until we can say with certainty that there are no more surprises related to the molecular processes of V gene expression we must reserve judgment on the significance of idiotypes in regulating the immune response.

4. Summary

The analysis of the NP idiotypic response has already played a central role in our understanding of antibody expression. One original goal was to determine the breadth of the functional NP^b V gene repertoire by analysis of antibodies that were very different idiotypically. We learned really for the first time that major idiotypically related families of antibodies can be expected to originate fron one V_H and one V_L gene. In several cases minor families have been detected and usually come from different but related V genes. The notion that the IgM antibodies are primarily germ line encoded and non-IgM somatic variants arise as derivatives of the same genes was realized in both the NP[1] and the PC[2] system. The heavy- and light-chain DNA sequences have contributed to the description of the occurrence of somatic mutations.[1,27] This knowledge now permits a more refined analysis of idiotypes expressed in serum and suggests ways of probing for the functional significance of somatic variants. So far studies have only involved λ-bearing antibodies. These studies have contributed to our knowledge of the λ genes[3,27-29] and also the heavy-chain genes.[25,30] Both V_H- and C_H-region sequences suggested that a process perhaps related in some form to a gene conversion event was occurring in these gene families. The structural analysis has suggested alterations in the genome can occur both over evolutionary time and over a much shorter time (somatic point mutation and gene conversion). We would like to determine if there is a functional overlap in these processes. The focus of our studies will be to determine precisely the relationship of somatic mutation to the development of the response and to the generation and expression of immunological memory.

References

1. Bothwell, A. L. M., Paskind, M., Reth, M., Imanishi-Kari, T., Rajewsky, K., and Baltimore, D., 1981, Heavy chain variable region contribution to the NP^b family of antibodies: Somatic mutation evident in a γ2a variable region, *Cell* **24:**625–637.
2. Crews, S., Griffin, J., Huang, H., Calame, K., and Hood, L., 1981, A single V_H gene segment encodes the immune response to phosphoryl choline: Somatic mutation is correlated with the class of the antibody, *Cell* **25:**59–66.
3. Miller, J., Bothwell, A., and Storb, U. 1981, Physical linkage of the constant region genes for immunoglobulins λI and λIII, *Proc. Natl. Acad. Sci. USA* **78:**3829–3833.
4. Blomberg, B., Traunecker, A., Eisen, H., and Tonegawa, S. 1981, Organization of four mouse λ light chain immunoglobulin genes, *Proc. Natl. Acad. Sci. USA* **78:**3765–3769.
5. Gearhart, P. J., Johnson, N. D., Douglas, R., and Hood, L., 1981, IgG antibodies to phosphoryl choline exhibit more diversity that their IgM counterparts, *Nature* **291:**29–34.
6. Sims, J., Rabbitts, T. H., Estess, P., Slaughter, C., Tucker, P. W., and Capra, J. D., 1982, Somatic mutation in genes for the variable portion of the immunoglobulin heavy chain, *Science* **216:**309–311.
7. Siekevitz, M., Huang, S. Y., and Gefter, M. L., 1983, The genetic basis of antibody production: A single heavy chain variable region gene encodes all molecules bearing the dominant anti-arsonate idiotype in the strain A mouse, *Eur. J. Immunol.* **13:**123–132.
8. Loh, D. Y., Bothwell, A. L. M., White-Scharf, M. E., Imanishi-Kari, T., and Baltimore, D., 1983, Molecular basis of a mouse strain-specific anti-hapten response, *Cell* **33:**85–93.
9. Rocca-Serra, J., and Fougereau, M., 1983, Two monoclonal antibodies against different antigens using the same V_H germ-line gene, *Nature* **304:**353–355.
10. Rocca-Serra, J., Matthes, H. W., Kaartinen, M., Milstein, C., Theze, J., and Fougereau, M., 1983, Analysis of antibody diversity: V-D-J mRNA nucleotide sequence of four anti-GAT monoclonal antibodies: A paucigene system using alternate D-J recombinations to generate functionally similar hypervariable regions, *EMBO J.* **2:**867–872.
11. Schiff, C., Milili, M., and Fougereau, M., 1983, Immunoglobulin diversity: Analysis of the germ-line V_H gene repertoire of the murine anti-GAT response, *Nucleic Acids Res.* **11:**4007–4017.
12. Kraig, E., Kronenberg, M., Kapp, J. A., Pierce, C. W., Abruzzini, A. F., Sorensen, C. M., Samelson, L. E., Schwartz, R. H., and Hood, L. E., 1983, T and B cells that recognize the same antigen do not transcribe similar heavy chain variable region gene segments, *J. Exp. Med.* **158:**192–209.
13. Kaartinen, M., Griffiths, G. M., Hamlyn, P. H., Markham, A. F., Karjalainen, K., Pelkonen, J. L. T., Makela, O., and Milstein, C., 1983, Anti-oxazolone hybridomas and the structure of the oxazolone idiotype, *J. Immunol.* **130:**937–945.
14. White-Scharf, M. E., and Imanishi-Kari, T., 1982, Cross-reactivity of the NP^a and NP^b idiotypic responses of BALB/c and C57BL/6 mice to (4-hydroxy-3-nitrophenyl) acetyl (NP), *Eur. J. Immunol.* **12:**935–942.
15. Reth, M., Hammerling, G. J., and Rajewsky, K., 1978, Analysis of the repertoire of anti-NP antibodies in C57BL/6 mice by cell fusion. I. Characterization of antibody families in the primary and hyperimmune response, *Eur. J. Immunol.* **8:**393–400.
16. Reth, M., Bothwell, A. L. M., and Rajewsky, K., 1981, Structural properties of the hapten binding site and of idiotypes in the NP^b antibody family, in: *Immunoglobulin Idiotypes and Their Expression* (C. Janeway, H. Wigzell, and C. F. Fox, eds.), Academic Press, New York, pp. 169–178.
17. Segal, D. M., Padlan, E. A., Cohen, G. H., Rudikoff, S., Potter, M., and Davies, D. R., 1974, The three-dimensional structure of a phosphorylcholine-binding mouse immunoglobulin Fab and the nature of the antigen binding site, *Proc. Natl. Acad. Sci. USA* **71:**4298–4302.
18. Davies, D. R., Padlan, E. A., and Segal, D. M., 1975, Immunoglobulin structures at high resolution, in: *Contemporary Topics in Molecular Immunology,* Volume 4 (F. P. Inman and W. J. Mandy, eds.), Plenum Press, New York, pp. 127–155.
19. Rajewsky, K., and Takemori, T., 1983, Genetics, expression, and function of idiotypes, in: *Annual Review of Immunology,* Vol. 1 (W. E. Paul, C. G. Fathman, and H. Metzger, eds.), Annual Reviews Inc., Palo Alto, Calif., pp. 569–607.

20. Kim, S., Davis, M., Sinn, E., Patten, P., and Hood, L., 1981, Antibody diversity: Somatic mutation may be extensive and is localized in and around the rearranged V_H gene, *Cell* **27:**573–581.
21. Sakano, H., Maki, R., Kurosawa, Y., Roeder, W., and Tonegawa, S., 1980, Two types of somatic recombination are necessary for the generation of complete immunoglobulin heavy-chain genes, *Nature* **286:**676–683.
22. Gough, N. M., and Bernard, O., 1981, Sequences of the joining region genes for immunoglobulin heavy chains and their role in generation of antibody diversity, *Proc. Natl. Acad. Sci. USA* **78:**509–513.
23. Dildrop, R., Bruggemann, M., Radbruch, A., Rajewsky, K., and Beyreuther, K., 1982, Immunoglobulin V region variants in hybridoma cells. II. Recombination between V genes, *EMBO J.* **5:**635–640.
24. Krawinkel, U., Zoebelein, G., Bruggemann, M., Radbruch, A., and Rajewsky, K., 1983, Recombination between antibody heavy chain V-region genes: Evidence for gene conversion, *Proc. Natl. Acad. Sci. USA* **80:**4997–5001.
25. Schreier, P. H., Bothwell, A. L. M., Mueller-Hill, B., and Baltimore, D., 1981, Multiple differences between the nucleic acid sequences of the IgG2a^a and IgG2a^b alleles of the mouse, *Proc. Natl. Acad. Sci. USA* **78:**4495–4499.
26. Wu, G. E., Hozumi, N., and Murialdo, H., 1983, Secretion of a λ2 immunoglobulin chain is prevented by a single amino acid substitution in its variable region, *Cell* **33:**77–83.
27. Bothwell, A. L. M., Paskind, M., Reth, M., Imanishi-Kari, T., Rajewsky, K., and Baltimore, D., 1982, Somatic variants of murine lambda light chains, *Nature* **298:**380–382.
28. Bothwell, A. L. M., Paskind, M., Schwartz, K. C., Sonenshein, G. E., Gefter, M. L., and Baltimore, D., 1981, Dual expression of λ genes in the MOPC-315 plasmacytoma, *Nature* **290:**65–67.
29. D'Eustachio, P., Bothwell, A. L. M., Takaro, T. K., Baltimore, D., and Ruddle, F. H., 1981, Chromosomal location of the structural genes encoding murine immunoglobulin lambda light chains, *J. Exp. Med.* **153:**793–800.
30. Schreier, P. H., Quester, S., and Bothwell, A. L. M., 1984, Allotypic differences in murine IgM genes, (in preparation).

3

Structural and Genetic Basis of the Major Cross-Reactive Idiotype of the A Strain Mouse

CLIVE A. SLAUGHTER AND J. DONALD CAPRA

1. Introduction

Structural features peculiar to the variable regions of antibodies are widely believed to interact with regulatory forces which help to control and fine-tune the specific immune responses in which these antibodies participate.[1] The serologically recognized features of antibody variable regions known as idiotypes[2,3] constitute structurally definable analogs of the sites which interact with regulatory forces in this way, and they may in some cases be identical to such sites. Over the last decade, a number of laboratories have devoted considerable effort to the detailed chemical characterization of idiotypic determinants on antibody molecules. Most of this research has centered on structural comparisons of antibodies or myeloma proteins which belong to families of related molecules sharing a common specificity for antigen but differing in their expression of a cross-reactive idiotype. Antibodies elicited in the mouse in response to the hapten *p*-azophenylarsonate (Ars) have been particularly well studied in this regard and illustrate many of the problems involved in the structural characterization of idiotypes in general.

2. Murine Antiarsonate Antibodies May Be Classified into at Least Three Families

When coupled to the protein carrier keyhole limpet hemocyanin (KLH), Ars stimulates a vigorous antihapten response in all mouse strains. Monoclonal antibodies specific

CLIVE A. SLAUGHTER AND J. DONALD CAPRA • Department of Microbiology, The University of Texas Health Science Center, Dallas, Texas 75235.

for Ars, isolated by the hybridoma technique,[4,5] may be classified into three families[6] (Fig. 1). These families, designated Ars-A, Ars-B, and Ars-C, are defined by the N-terminal amino acid sequences of their heavy-chain variable regions (V_H regions*), which belong to different subgroups. The families delineated in this way are further distinguished both by various serological characteristics[6] and by their use of light-chain variable regions (V_L regions) belonging to different subgroups.[6] The three families are believed to be encoded by different sets of germ-line genes, and the ability of a mouse strain to recruit a particular family into its response to Ars is an inherited characteristic. This situation exemplifies the frequently observed expression of multiple sets of germ-line genes in response to a single antigenic determinant.

While only three families of antiarsonate antibodies have been delineated so far, it is likely that more will be described in the future. Some may arise by the subdivision of the existing families. For example, preliminary evidence obtained in our laboratory suggests that the Ars-B family contains antibodies which can be ascribed to at least two sets of germ-line genes (K. Meek, personal communication). Other families may eventually be recognized through the discovery of sets of antibodies having novel structures or properties which do not allow them to be placed in one of the existing families. For example, after hyperimmunization of A strain mice with KLH-Ars, the predominant component of the hapten-specific antibody mixture which appears in the serum has markedly different amino acid sequence[7,8] from the antibodies so far identified among hybridomas.[9,10] The sequence of this predominant component appears to contain residues which cannot be accounted for simply as deriving from an inhomogeneous mixture of antibodies belonging to the currently recognized antibody families, and further investigation may require the creation of one or more new families to accommodate the anti-Ars antibodies found in hyperimmune serum. Although other families may be identified, however, the three so far described probably account for the bulk of the response at the hybridoma level in A/J mice immunized according to currently standard protocols.

3. The Major Antiarsonate Cross-Reactive Idiotype of the A Strain Mouse Is Associated with the Ars-A Family

Inbred strains of mice may vary genetically in the spectrum of antibodies which are elicited by hapten. A strain mice, for example, respond to Ars at the serum level with antibodies of which a major portion bears a cross-reactive idiotype (CRI).[11] The CRI is conventionally identified using a polyclonal rabbit antiserum which is raised against A/J mouse anti-Ars serum antibodies and rendered idiotypically specific by absorption on preimmune A/J immunoglobulin.[11] The CRI is measured in a radioimmunoassay which determines the degree of inhibition of the reaction between the rabbit anti-CRI and radiolabeled A/J anti-Ars serum antibodies.[11] The immunodominant component of the A/J

---

*"V_H region" here refers to amino acid residues 1–121 of the heavy chain, which are encoded by three separate genes, V_H, D_H, and J_H. "V_H segment," in contrast, is used to denote amino acid residues 1–98 of the heavy chain, which are encoded by the V_H gene alone. Similarly, "V_L region" refers to amino acid residues 1–108 of the light chain, which are encoded by two separate genes, V_κ and J_κ (or V and J). "V_κ segment" is used for amino acid residues 1–95, which are encoded by the V_κ gene alone.

```
                                10            20            30      CRI

Ars A    93G7    E V Q L Q Q S G A E L V R A G S S V K M S C K A S G Y T F T   +
         R16.7   _____  +
         123E6   _____ T _____ T _____ T _____  +
         124E1   _____ T _____  +
         3D5-2   _____  +
         36-65   _____  +
         31-62   _____ P _____  +
         91A3    _____ T _____  -
         45-49   _____ M _ P _____ T _____ A I _    -

Ars-B    96B8*   E V Q L Q Q S G P E L V K P G A S V K I S C K T S G Y T F T   -
         4AC7*   _____ M _____ A( )___( )_( )   -
         1AD10*  _____ M _____ A _____( )_( )   -
         44-1-3  < _____ R _____ A _____   -
         31-41   < ____ V _____ D A _____ A _____    -
         45-112  < _____ D A _____ A _____   -
         45-165  < I ____ V _____ K _____ E T _____ A( )_____( )  -

Ars-C    94B10   D V Q L Q E S G P G L V N P S Q S L S L T C S V T G Y S I T   -
         92D5    _____ K _____(                 )  -
         36-60   E _____ S ___ K _____ T _____ D _____  -
         31-64   E _____ S ___ K _____  -

                 * BALB/c
```

FIGURE 1. Families of murine antiarsonate antibodies. Comparison of the N-terminal V_H amino acid sequences of antiarsonate hybridoma products within families. ———, identical residues; ( ), region in which no assignments are available. A, Ala; C, Cys; D, Asp; E, Glu; F, Phe; G, Gly; H, His; I, Ile; K, Lys; L, Leu; M, Met; N, Asn; P, Pro; Q, Gln; R, Arg; S, Ser; T, Thr; V, Val; W, Trp; Y, Tyr. The expression of the CRI is noted for each molecule. All antibodies are derived from the A/J mouse strain unless otherwise indicated. The sequences of 93G7, 123E6, 124E1, 91A3, 94B10, and 92D5 are revised from those in Ref. 21; 3D5-2 is from Ref. 23; 36-65, 31-62, 45-49, 44-1-3, 31-41, 45-112, 45-165, 36-60, and 31-64 are from Ref. 22; R16.7 is from Ref. 9. The sequences of 96B8, 4AC7, and 1AD10 are the unpublished data of C. A. Slaughter.

serum response to Ars which is measured by this assay is normally lacking in the immune sera of most other mouse strains.[11] Such strains are said to be CRI-negative. Breeding studies between the CRI-positive A/J mouse strain and CRI-negative strains such as BALB/c show that expression of the CRI in the serum response to Ars is inherited as if it were determined by a single autosomal dominant gene at a locus linked to the *Igh* gene complex.[12] Linkage to *Igh* is a feature common to many such idiotypic systems.[13] Crosses involving the relatively few mouse strains with a heritable variant κ light-chain phenotype[14,15] also demonstrate a requirement for an appropriate gene linked to the *Igk* complex.[16,17] These results exemplify the commonly observed "allelic" diversity in expression of shared idiotypic specificities.

The expression among hybridomas of one of the three structurally defined anti-Ars families, Ars-A, shows the same restriction to the A strain as does expression of the CRI in the serum response, and so far all A/J monoclonal antibodies bearing the CRI have been found to belong to the Ars-A family.[6] However, the amino acid sequence of the A/J anti-Ars hyperimmune serum pool referred to above, despite having been enriched for the CRI-positive component by isoelectric focusing,[18] is very different from the sequences of Ars-A antibodies.[9,10] This suggests that expression of the CRI may be associated with more than one antibody family in the A/J strain. Furthermore, it has been shown that mice from strains such as BALB/c, nominally classified as CRI-negative on the basis of their serum response to Ars, can produce CRI-positive antibodies at the monoclonal level both in response to antigenic challenge[19] and in response to administration of anti-CRI antibodies.[20] Preliminary amino acid sequence analysis in our laboratory of two CRI-positive antibodies from BALB/c supplied by J. Urbain indicates that these antibodies utilize a subset of heavy-chain variable regions normally associated with the Ars-B rather than the Ars-A family and that this is a subset closely similar to one which has already been identified in the A/J (K. Meek, personal communication). This result provides strong evidence that different sets of germ-line genes may provide vehicles for the expression of the CRI. Nevertheless, most of the currently available information pertaining to the structural and genetic basis of CRI expression has been obtained by study of the Ars-A family of the A strain mouse and it is this information which forms the principal subject of the present chapter.

4. Members of the Ars-A Family Show Variation as Well as Commonality in Their Serological Properties

Although members of the Ars-A antibody family are similar in many respects, several lines of evidence suggest that structural differences exist among them. There is, for example, variation in the N-terminal amino acid sequences of their heavy and light chains,[21-23] in their affinities for Ars,[24,25] and in their fine-specificity patterns for antigen.[24] However, one of the most intensively studied aspects of the diversity between Ars-A antibodies is the variation they show in the degree of expression of the CRI in the conventional radioimmunoassay.[21,26,27] Individual hybridoma products may be classified as CRI-positive or CRI-negative depending on their capacity to inhibit the interaction between radiolabeled A/J serum anti-Ars (CRI) and rabbit anti-CRI antibodies by an arbitrary 50% under a standard set of conditions. According to this definition, most Ars-A antibodies can be designated CRI-positive but some are found to be CRI-negative. Furthermore, among those classified as CRI-positive, there is a broad quantitative range of capacity to inhibit in the assay. Table I (column A) shows examples of Ars-A hybridoma products (HP) ranging from the very strongly CRI-positive HP93G7 and HPR16.7, through the progressively more weakly CRI-positive HP123E6 and HP124E1, to the CRI-negative HP91A3. The structural differences which give rise to this variability are generally assumed to produce their serological effects through alterations of determinants in the hypervariable regions, since the interaction between CRI and anti-CRI in the conventional assay is sensitive to inhibition by hapten[27] (Table I, column A).

The serological relationships of these antibodies have been further studied with anti-

TABLE I
Inhibition of Binding in Various Assay Systems by Purified Hybridoma Products[a]

	ng required for 50% inhibition		
Unlabeled inhibitor	A Rabbit anti-CRI/CRI*	B Rabbit anti-Id 123E6/93G7*	C Rabbit anti-Id 91A3/93G7*
A/J antiarsonate	15	200	25
HP93G7	12	32	12
HPR16.7	9	not done	10
HP123E6	50	87	86
HP124E1	2,900	48	16
HP91A3	>20,000	>20,000	25
Arsonate (mM)	10	2	>100

[a]Assay A: Canonical assay for CRI, showing diversity of degree of CRI expression (Ref. 21) and high sensitivity to hapten.[26,27] Antibodies capable of inhibiting by 50% (all except HP91A3) are designated CRI-positive. Assay B: Heterologous assay for idiotypic specificities shared by HP93G7 and HP123E6, showing commonality among CRI-positive antibodies and high sensitivity to hapten inhibition[66] Assay C: Heterologous assay for idiotypic specificities shared by HP93G7 and HP91A3, showing commonality among all Ars-A antibodies[6] and relative insensitivity to hapten inhibition (E. Milner, personal communication).
*Radiolabeled. Assays utilized 10 ng ^{125}I-labeled tracer antibody and slightly less than an equivalent amount of anti-idiotype.

idiotypic reagents made against homogeneous hybridoma products rather than against the modestly heterogeneous mixture of antibodies from the different families present in A/J anti-Ars serum. When such reagents are used in competition radioimmunoassays with the homologous hybridoma product (the one used to generate the anti-idiotypic reagent) as radiolabeled ligand, cross-reactivities with other hybridoma products are typically very limited.[26] Such assays are, therefore, said to measure "private" or "individual" idiotypes. Specificities of this kind, which are restricted to one or a few hybridoma products, attest further to the existence of structural variation within the Ars-A family. However, if these same anti-idiotypic reagents are used in competition radioimmunoassays with a heterologous hybridoma product (one different from the monoclonal antibody used to generate the reagent) as radiolabeled ligand, a broad measure of commonality between Ars-A antibodies is revealed[27] (Table I, columns B and C). Nonetheless, the precise pattern of cross-reactivities which is observed depends on the particular combination of anti-idiotype and labeled ligand employed. For example, in an assay using anti-Id 123E6 in conjunction with HP93G7 as radiolabeled ligand, all CRI-positive antibodies compete approximately equally strongly, but the CRI-negative HP91A3 fails to compete significantly (P. Estess, personal communication) (Table I, column B). On the other hand, in an assay using anti-Id 91A3 in conjunction with HP93G7 as radiolabeled ligand, all Ars-A antibodies compete approximately equally strongly whether they are CRI-positive or CRI-negative.[6] Although these heterologous assay systems measure cross-reactive idiotypes in the broadest sense, the relationship between the determinants they detect and the determinants comprising the CRI as conventionally defined has in no case been precisely established. In some cases, such as the anti-Id 123E6/93G7* assay (Table I, column B), the determinants may overlap substantially those comprising the CRI, since the assay offers clearcut discrimination between CRI-positive and CRI-negative antibodies and is sensitive to hapten inhibition. In other cases, such as the anti-Id 91A3/93G7* assay (Table I, column C), the determinants probably overlap minimally with those comprising the CRI, since the reactivity patterns which the assay generates and the low level of sensitivity to hapten inhibition which it shows are both quite different from the characteristics of the conventional assay for the CRI. Nonetheless, such heterologous assay systems have proved extremely useful for identifying selected structurally distinct subsets of anti-Ars antibodies[6] and are used in preference to the conventional CRI assay for many purposes.

More recently, the antigenic structure of the Ars-A antibody family has begun to be dissected with monoclonal anti-idiotypic reagents.[28] These are generated by immunizing a mouse either with serum anti-Ars antibodies which bear the CRI or with an Ars-A hybridoma product. Monoclonal antibodies which recognize some or all members of the Ars-A family are then isolated by the hybridoma technique. Anti-idiotypic reagents with a variety of reactivity patterns, some entirely novel, have already been generated in this way,[28] suggesting that a large number of different determinants, including ones which are distinct from the immunodominant determinants comprising the CRI, will become accessible to study by this procedure. Although it is not clear whether these reagents can assist substantially in establishing the structural basis of the CRI as classically defined, they do provide further evidence for structural variation within the Ars-A family and will doubtless become increasingly important as tools for fine discrimination between closely similar Ars-A antibodies.

Variation within antibody families of the kind displayed by the Ars-A family is a general phenomenon and is sometimes very extensive. It has been demonstrated in structural studies of antibodies against $\alpha1 \rightarrow 3$ dextran,[29] (4-hydroxy-3-nitrophenyl)acetyl (NP),[30] phosphocholine (PC),[31] 2-phenyloxazolone,[32] and the synthetic polymers GAT and GA,[33] and has also been characterized in families of closely related myeloma proteins sharing specificity for antigen, including galactan-binding myeloma proteins[34] and inulin-binding myeloma proteins.[35,36] The structural and genetic basis for such variation is the subject of intense interest both for the study of idiotypy and for the study of antibody diversity as a whole.

5. Differences in Expression of the CRI among Members of the Ars-A Family Are Due to Structural Variation in the Heavy Chain

The question of whether structural differences in the light-chain variable region or the heavy-chain variable region are responsible for the differences between members of the Ars-A family in expression of the CRI has been addressed in chain recombination experiments.[37] In these experiments, hybrid immunoglobulin molecules are constructed from the isolated heavy and light chains of hybridoma products which differ in their expression of the CRI. Table II shows, as an example, recombinations between HP93G7, a strongly

---

*Radiolabeled.

TABLE II

Expression of CRI by Reconstituted Hybridoma Products in Which Heavy and Light Chains Were Derived from a CRI-Positive and a Structurally Related CRI-Negative Antibody [37]

Heavy chain	Light chain	Anti-CRI/CRI*, % inhibition by 50 ng
	93G7 untreated	84
	91A3 untreated	10
93G7	93G7	79
91A3	91A3	0
91A3	93G7	9
93G7	91A3	77
93G7	—	13
—	93G7	11
91A3	—	0
—	91A3	1

*Radiolabeled.

CRI-positive molecule, and HP91A3, a CRI-negative molecule also belonging to the Ars-A family. The light chain of HP91A3 can completely restore the CRI to the heavy chain of HP93G7, showing that in this combination of molecules the heavy chain determines the presence or absence of the CRI.[37] Similarly, hybrid molecules constructed from two CRI-positive hybridoma products of the Ars-A family which differ quantitatively in the degree of expression of the idiotypic character express the CRI at a level which correlates with that of the heavy-chain donor.[37] Although light chains of both CRI-positive and CRI-negative members of the Ars-A family are capable of restoring the CRI to an appropriate Ars-A heavy chain, light chains from the Ars-B or Ars-C families cannot produce this effect.[37] That light chains of certain CRI-negative HP can restore CRI is in agreement with the findings of Gill-Pazaris et al.[37a]

6. Amino Acid Sequence Comparison of Ars-A Light Chains Reveals a High Degree of Uniformity in Structure, and a Commonality in Genetic Repertoire between Strains

In light of the serological differences and other differences between members of the Ars-A family, total amino acid sequence analysis of the heavy- and light-chain variable regions of five Ars-A hybridoma products was undertaken in our laboratory. This was done in order to assess the extent and distribution of amino acid replacements and hence to establish the structural basis of the variation in expression of the CRI. The antibodies chosen for analysis were selected to represent the full range of quantitative expression of the CRI, extending from the most strongly CRI-positive HP93G7 and HPR16.7, through the progressively more weakly CRI-positive HP123E6 and HP124E1, to a CRI-negative member of the family, HP91A3 (Table I). These antibodies also differ in their expression of "private" idiotypes,[26] in their reactivity with monoclonal anti-idiotypic antibodies,[28] and in their fine specificity for antigen,[24] but show similar affinities for the immunizing hapten, *p*-azophenylarsonate.[24] These and all other Ars-A antibodies so far subjected to detailed structural analysis are IgG1, κ. Hybridomas 93G7 and 91A3 were derived in a single fusion, but since the spleens of two different mice were employed, it is not known whether they arose from the same animal or different animals. Hybridomas 123E6 and 124E1 rose in a second fusion, and again, the spleens of two different mice were pooled. Hybridoma R16.7 was derived in a third fusion and was the gift of A. Nisonoff.

The amino acid sequences of the five light-chain variable regions[9] are shown in Fig. 2. Also included in Fig. 2 are two A/J light chains derived independently from CRI-positive hybridomas 10K26 and 10K44 and sequenced by Ball *et al.*[38] Figure 2 also shows the light chain from a CRI-positive hybridoma derived from the C.AL-20 strain, a congenic mouse strain in which the genes encoding immunoglobulin heavy chains are derived from the A strain and the genes encoding immunoglobulin light chains are derived from BALB/c.[10] All the chains are strikingly similar in sequence and show less than 3% overall variation. This high degree of similarity is consistent with the observation that any one of these light chains will substitute for any other in serological analyses for the CRI (Section 4). It is possible that all the chains are the products of a single A/J germ-line V_κ gene or, in the case of the C.AL-20, the BALB/c homolog of this gene. Certain repeated replacements which occur at positions 30, 92, and 93 (Fig. 2) may be attributed to parallel but independent somatic mutational events under this hypothesis. The alternative possibility,

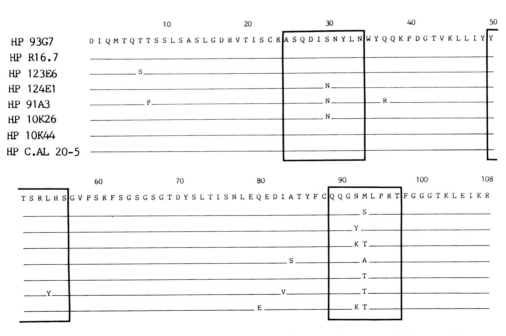

FIGURE 2. Antiarsonate hybridoma light chains. Comparison of amino acid sequences of light-chain V regions with that of HP93G7. ⸺, identical residues. Numbering is sequential. Complementarity-determining regions are outlined. For single-letter code for amino acid residues, see legend to Fig. 1. Hybridoma products 93G7, R16.7, 123E6, 124E1, and 91A3 are from Ref. 9; 10K26 and 10K44 are from Ref. 38; C.AL-20-5 is from Ref. 10.

that they indicate the existence of separate germ-line genes which encode the sequences of antibodies bearing the appropriate alternative residues at the positions which show repeated replacements, is rendered unattractive by examples of discordancy in the occurrence of the repeated replacements in different chains.

The overall similarity between these light-chain sequences is interrupted by a prominent focus of variability at positions 92 and 93, located centrally within the third hypervariable region (Fig. 2). The origin of this diversity is probably somatic, but the precise mechanism which gives rise to such a localized area of sequence variation is unknown.

Although differences are apparent throughout the V_κ segments, which extend from positon 1 to 95 of the mature polypeptide, the J_κ segments, which extend from position 96 to 108, are identical in all the chains. The Ars-A antibodies appear to utilize a single germline J_κ gene, identified as the homolog of either $J_\kappa 1$ or $J_\kappa 2$ in BALB/c.[39,40] $J_\kappa 1$ and $J_\kappa 2$ encode the same amino acid sequence, except for the first positon, at which $J_\kappa 1$ encodes a tryptophan and $J_\kappa 2$ encodes a tyrosine. In all the Ars-A antibodies there is an arginine at position 96. The codon for this arginine may be derived from the 3' end of the V_κ gene or it may be produced as result of a consistent intracodonic recombination event during $V_\kappa - J_\kappa$ joining.[9]

The similarity between the C.AL-20 light chain and the light chains from the A/J shows that the BALB/c can contribute V_κ chains essentially identical to those of the A/J to make a CRI-positive antibody in response to Ars. This equivalence of the light-chain repertoire in A/J and BALB/c accounts for the lack of dependency of CRI expression on the segregation of κ-chain genes in crosses involving the BALB/c and A/J strain (Section 2). It is interesting that a light chain virtually identical to those of the Ars-A family has recently been reported in another BALB/c antibody elicited in response to the hapten 2-phenyloxazolone.[41] A similar chain has also been found in a BALB/c myeloma protein (MOPC173) of unknown antigen specificity.[42] Both proteins have heavy chains which differ from each other and from those of the Ars-A family. These appear to be examples of the long-predicted production of novel antigen specificities by combinatorial association of V_H and V_L segment genes to form novel variable-region pairs. Recently, it has been shown in our laboratory that light chains with N-terminal amino acid sequences almost identical to those of the Ars-A family are used by two CRI-positive hybridoma products from BALB/c mice (K. Meek, personal communication). In these antibodies, the light chains are associated with heavy chains which use variable regions presently classified within the Ars-B family (Section 2). Isolated light chains from one of these CRI-positive molecules from BALB/c have been successfully used to restore expression of the CRI to the isolated heavy chains of HP93G7, a CRI-positive member of the Ars-A family, thus further illustrating the similarity of the light chains in these two families of antibodies (D. Jeske, personal communication).

7. The Different V_H Segments Probably Arise from a Single Germline V_H Gene by Somatic Mutation

The V_H-region amino acid sequences of the set of five Ars-A antibodies[10,43-46] are shown in Fig. 3, together with that of a sixth member of the family, HP101F11, which is strongly CRI-positive but shows a markedly reduced level of binding to antigen.[47] All the

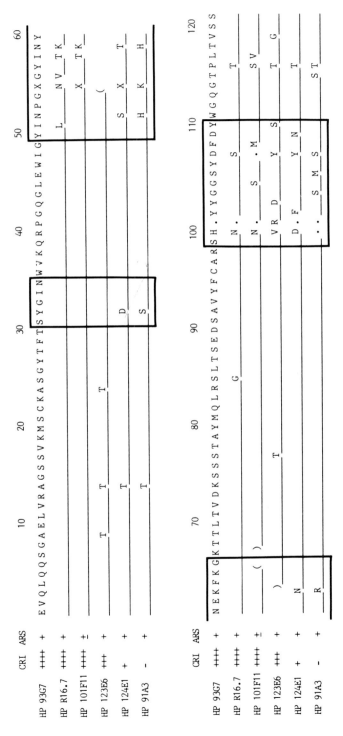

Figure 3. Antiarsonate hybridoma heavy chains. Comparison of amino acid sequences of heavy-chain V regions with that of HP93G7. (———), identical residues; (·), gap introduced to maximize homology; [( )], region in which no assignments are available. Numbering is sequential. Complementarity-determining regions are outlined. For single-letter code for amino acid residues, see legend to Fig. 1. X, secondarily modified Asn residue.[46] The expression of the CRI and the level of arsonate binding are noted for each molecule. The sequences of hybridoma products 93G7, R16.7, 123E6, 124E1, and 91A3 are from Ref. 46; 101F11 is from Ref. 47.

chains fall within the $V_H V$ subgroup[48] and, although they are more variable than the corresponding light chains (Fig. 2), they constitute a closely related set in which no one heavy chain differs from the prototypic sequence of HP93G7[44] at more than 12 positions. The V_H-region amino acid sequence of the CRI-positive A/J anti-Ars antibody HP36-65, which has been deduced from a DNA sequence,[49] also belongs to this family.

In antibodies of the Ars-A family, the segment encoded by the V_H gene apparently extends from position 1 to 98 of the mature heavy chain[50] (see below). The demonstration of multiple sequence differences within this region raises the question of how many A/J germ-line V_H genes are involved in coding for members of the Ars-A family. Southern filter hybridization studies of germ-line DNA from A/J mice, carried out using V_H-segment DNA probes from Ars-A hybridomas, have revealed several V_H genes closely related to members of the Ars-A family.[44,49] However, use of a J_H probe to detect the rearranged gene in hybridoma DNA has shown that productive rearrangements give rise to restriction fragments of the same size in most hybridomas making Ars-A antibodies.[50,51] This suggests that V_H DNA from only one of the restriction fragments distinguished in digests of genomic DNA is used to make antibodies of this family. The identity of the related genes on the other restriction fragments has not yet been established. However, there is a close, general evolutionary relationship between the V_H segments of antibodies in the Ars-A family and V_H segments of heavy chains belonging to the $V_H II$ subgroup.[48] For example, the DEX-positive myeloma protein MOPC104E[52] differs from HP93G7 by 21 V_H-segment amino acid residues, the NP^b-positive antibody HPB1-8[30] differs from it by 22 amino acid residues, and the BALB/c myeloma protein MPC11[53] differs from it by 20 amino acid residues. Genes encoding proteins such as these may be sufficiently closely related to cross-hybridize with Ars-A V_H segment probes under the conditions employed for Southern filter hybridization.

Siekevitz et al. have cloned EcoRI restriction fragments of embryonic A/J DNA,[50] and among inserts which hybridized most strongly to a V_H-segment DNA probe made from the CRI-positive cell line 36-65, they distinguished three different genes by restricton mapping and DNA sequencing, all of which are present on restriction fragments of the same size. One had a sequence corresponding exactly to the amino acid sequence of the V_H segment expressed by the 36-65 cell line. The amino acid sequences described in the present chapter are best interpreted as having been derived from this germ-line gene. The other two genes, although extremely similar to the first, encode at least eight amino acids which are different from it. Only one of these amino acids has been found in any sequence of a member of the Ars-A family. This result represents the strongest evidence currently available that a single germ-line V_H gene is utilized by members of the Ars-A family, and that differences in their V_H-segment sequences must be ascribed predominantly to somatic mutation. However, it does not exclude the possibility that sequence information from portions of more remotely related genes is occasionally used by the Ars-A family after unequal crossing over or gene conversion events.

A thorough investigation of the number of germ-line V_H genes which contribute to intrafamily variation has also been conducted for BALB/c anti-PC antibodies of the T15 family[54] and for C57BL/6 anti-NP antibodies of the NP^b family.[30] In these cases, too, the amino acid or DNA sequences of the family of expressed V_H segments were compared to the nucleotide sequences of the set of most closely related germ-line V_H genes. Although several closely similar V_H genes were identified and sequenced in each family, it was apparent in both cases that the expressed proteins nearly always derived from only one germ-line gene of the set. These observations form the basis of an emerging consensus of opinion that somatic mutation plays a dominant role in diversification of the V-segment sequences within many such antibody families.

8. Loss of the CRI Is Due to Mutational Divergence from the Germline Sequence

Figure 4 shows the V_H-segment amino acid sequences of the six hybridoma products illustrated in Fig. 3 compared to the sequence endoded by $\lambda Id^{CR}11$, a genomic clone representative of clones bearing the V_H gene utilized by members of the Ars-A family.[50] The series of six expressed antibodies shows differences from the germ-line sequence at a total of 13 positions of the 98 in the V_H segment (13%). All of the replacements can be accounted for by single nucleotide substitutions. The number of differences shown by each antibody ranges from zero for HP101F11 to seven for HP91A3. It is noteworthy that the antibodies which are most strongly CRI-positive show fewer differences from the germ-line sequence than antibodies which are weakly CRI-positive or CRI-negative. This observation is consistent with the hypothesis that the germ line encodes the amino acid sequence of a strongly CRI-positive antibody, and that reduction in the level of CRI expression in members of the Ars-A family is due to divergence from this sequence by somatic mutation.

This result has a parallel among the corresponding V_L segments.[9] Direct information about DNA sequences of V_L genes utilized by members of the Ars-A family is not yet available. However, if it is assumed that a single germ-line gene encodes all known V_L segments in this family, and if it is further assumed that the most common amino acid at each position is encoded by this germ-line gene, then the most strongly CRI-positive antibodies are again found to have the fewest differences from the putative germ-line sequence.[9,38,45]

9. The Distributon of Substitutions in the V_H Segments Is Nonrandom

The linear distribution of V_H-segment positions bearing substitutions from the germ-line sequence is clearly different from that expected on the basis of a random distribution of mutations. Counting only those residues for which firm identifications are available, the incidence of amino acid replacements within the first and second complementarity-determining regions (CDR) (12.3%) is 8.0 times higher than the corresponding incidence in the framework regions (1.5%). The second CDR provides a special focus of variability, with an incidence of replacements (14.1%) which is 7.6 times higher than the incidence in the remainder of the V_H segment (1.9%). Historically, the hypervariable regions in the V_H and V_L chains were delineated by comparison of molecules which belonged to the same variable-region subgroup but which had been selected without regard to the antigen specificity of the parent myeloma proteins.[55–57] The localization of differences could thus be interpreted as due, at least in part, to differences in antigen specificity, since most of the hypervariable regions were subsequently shown to contain complementarity-determining amino acids. More recent comparisons have focused on antibodies which belong to the same family.

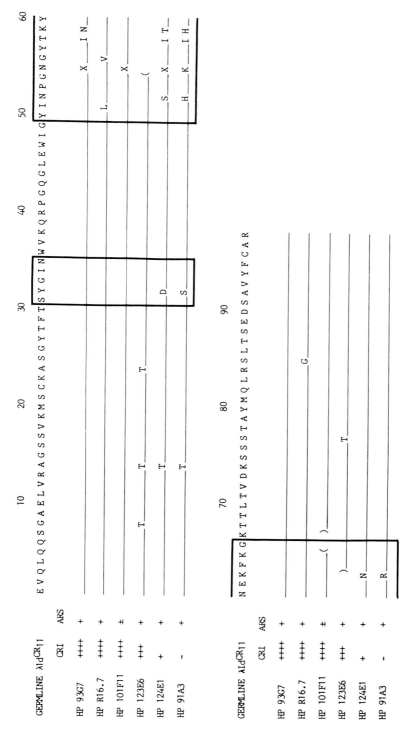

FIGURE 4. Relationship of antiarsonate hybridoma V_H segments to a germ-line V_H-segment gene. Comparison of amino acid sequences of V_H segments of molecules shown in Fig. 3 with the sequence encoded by the genomic clone $\lambda Id^{CR}11.^{(50)}$ (———), identical residues. Numbering is sequential. Complementarity-determining regions are outlined. For single-letter code for amino acid residues, see legend to Fig. 1. X, secondarily modified Asn residue. [46] The expression of the CRI and the level of arsonate binding are noted for each expressed antibody.

These antibodies share not only V_H and V_L subgroups in common, but also specificity for the same antigen. In some of these studies, hypervariability in CDR3 of the heavy chain has been observed,[29,31] but variability in CDR1 and CDR2 has in no case been prominent. There is thus a general trend toward diminution of hypervariability in the CDRs and this has usually been attributed to selection against mutations in these regions based on the requirement for binding to the same antigen.[58] The present set of anti-Ars V_H chains provides a significant departure from this trend, since CDR2, as well as CDR3 (Sections 9 and 10), provides a conspicuous focus for variability. It may be important that these chains, unlike the ones sequenced in other studies, have been drawn from antibodies showing a very broad range of idiotypic expression. This unusual result may thus be associated with variation in CRI expression. Such an interpretation receives support from the observation that the binding of CRI to anti-CRI antibodies is largely inhibitable by hapten, suggesting that residues in the CDRs play a role in expression of the CRI.[27]

A second aspect of the nonrandom distribution of replacements in these chains is the clustering of differences in "hot spots" of variation. The 22 amino acid residues which differ from the germ-line V_H sequence are located at just 13 positions. Seven of these positions bear replacements in one V_H segment only. However, three bear replacements in two V_H segments and three bear replacements in three V_H segments. Examples of such "hot spots" are found in both framework and hypervariable regions. Once again, since this set of antibodies was selected to maximize variation in the degree of expression of the CRI, some positions may owe their high incidence of replacements directly or indirectly to selection for loss of the CRI. At least two of the multiply substituted positions, 14 and 58, show identical repeated replacements. At position 14, three V_H segments (HP123E6, HP124E1, and HP91A3) have a variant Thr in place of the germ-line-encoded Ala, and at position 58, three V_H segments (HP93G7, HP124E1, and HP91A3) have a variant Ile in place of the germ-line-encoded Thr. In both cases, the substitutions are found in V_H segments drawn from at least two different animals in independent fusion experiments (Section 5). Such repeated substitutions are likely to be a common feature of antibodies belonging to the Ars-A family, since examples of substitutions identical to the ones described here have also been discovered at five positions in chains sequenced independently by Margolies *et al.*[22,50] (M. Margolies, personal communication). It is noteworthy, however, that no correlation between the presence of these repeated substitutions at different positions is yet discernible. Other examples of repeated substitutions have previously been observed among V_L segments of the Ars-A family[9,45] (Section 5) and among chains from other systems such as the V_L segments of inulin-binding myeloma proteins.[36] The V_H segments from anti-Ars antibodies of the Ars-A family, however, provide the best evidence so far that the phenomenon may arise from repeated yet independent somatic mutation events.

10. D_H-Segment Diversity Adds Greatly to Structural Variability within the Ars-A Family and Is Probably Generated Somatically

The D_H segment, which encompasses a portion of CDR3, provides another focus for differences between members of the Ars-A family. Comparison of the nucleotide sequence of the V_H gene believed to be involved in coding for the Ars-A antibodies[50] with the amino acid sequences described here for the expressed proteins indicates that the N-terminal boundary of the D_H segment lies between position 98 and 99, such that the codon for position 98 is supplied by the V_H gene and the codon for position 99 is supplied by the D_H gene. This, in turn, suggests that there is no junctional diversity at the V_H–D_H boundary, since all six chains have the same amino acid, Ser, at position 99. The C-terminus of the D_H segment is located at position 107, which marks the site of joining between the D_H and the J_H gene. At this position there are four different residues in the six molecules. This example of junctional diversity will be discussed in Section 10.

Between the boundaries of the D_H segment the six chains differ in both sequence and length. After the introduction of gaps in the shorter sequences to maximize homology (Fig. 3), it becomes clear that a "core" segment of relatively conservative sequence can be distinguished from a highly variable "N" segment.[59] The core segment extends from position 101 to 106, and the N segment includes positions 99, 100, and 100a. The latter is the region in which all the variation in length and 5 of the 10 D_H-segment residues differing from the HP93G7 prototype are confined.

Although there exists no direct information on germ-line D_H genes in the A/J mouse, nucleotide sequences are available for 12 BALB/c D_H genes, probably the complete set in the BALB/c.[60,61] These fall into three families, D_{FL16}, and D_{SP2}, and D_{52}. The prototype gene for the D_{FL16} family, $D_{FL16.1}$, is the most closely homologous to the D_H core segments of the Ars-A antibodies. A comparison is shown in Fig. 5. The core sequence of HP101F11 is identical to the corresponding sequence encoded by $D_{FL16.1}$, but the core sequences of the remaining Ars-A antibodies differ at between one and three positions. One of these differences, the substitution of a Met for a Ser at position 105 in HP91A3, requires a double base change. All the antibodies except HP101F11 bear a common replacement in the sequence encoded by $D_{FL16.1}$, a Gly for a Ser at position 104. Since this Gly is present in the majority of the antibodies, it is likely to be encoded in the germ-line gene or genes which give rise to the expressed set of D_H segments. This suggests that a hitherto undescribed

GERMLINE $D_{FL16.1}$			Y Y Y G S S Y
	CRI	ARS	
HP 93G7	++++	+	S H＿＿＿ G ＿＿
HP R16.7	++++	+	S N＿＿＿ G ＿＿
HP 101F11	++++	±	S N ＿＿＿＿＿
HP 123E6	+++	+	S V R ＿ D ＿ G ＿＿
HP 124E1	+	+	S D F ＿＿ G ＿＿
HP 91A3	–	+	S＿＿ S G M ＿

FIGURE 5. Relationship of antiarsonate hybridoma D_H segments to a germ-line D_H-segment gene. Comparison of amino acid sequences of D_H segments of molecules shown in Fig. 3 with the sequence encoded by the $D_{FL16.1}$ gene of BALB/c.[60] (———), identical residues. For single-letter code for amino acid residues, see legend to Fig. 1. The expression of the CRI and the level of arsonate binding are noted for each expressed antibody.

germ-line member of the D_{FL16} gene family is recruited in these antibodies. The number of germ-line D_{FL16} genes encoding the different D_H segments in the Ars-A family is unknown, but an attractive possibility is that a single gene, which encodes the prototype core sequence found in HP93G7 and HPR16.7, is employed by all the molecules. Under this hypothesis the amino acid differences from the prototype seen in HP101F11, HP123E6, HP124E1, and HP91A3 result from somatic mutation, and the smallest numbers of mutations are once again found in the most strongly CRI-positive antibodies, as is the case in the V_H segments (section 6). The relationship between this hypothetical single gene and $D_{FL16.1}$ is, of course, unknown. It may represent the A/J allelic counterpart to the BALB/c $D_{FL16.1}$ gene or it may define a new locus within the D_{FL16} complex.

Although $D_{FL16.1}$ encodes a Tyr in the position immediately preceding the N-terminal boundary of the D-segment core sequence (position 100a), Tyr has been identified in none of the Ars-A antibodies at this position, but is always replaced by another amino acid. It is not known to what extent nucleotides from the germ-line codon at this position are utilized to create this diversity but it is interesting to note that while the second and third nucleotides of a hypothetical Tyr condon are appropriate for creating a codon for the His in HP93G7, the Asn in HPR16.7 and HP101F11, and the Asp in HP124E1, they are inappropriate for creating codons for the Arg in HP123E6 and the Ser in HP91A3. Amino acids at the N-terminus or the C-terminus of a D_H core segment, which are determined by codons unknown as parts of any germ-line D_H gene related to the one encoding the core sequence, have been described in several systems.[59,60] These amino acids are now generally thought to result from the template-independent addition of nucleotides at the DNA level during V_H–D_H joining or D_H–J_H joining, catalyzed by a terminal deoxynucleotidyl transferase, thus creating a so-called N segment.[59,62] It is not yet clear whether this mechanism alone is capable of giving rise to the same amino acid, Ser, at the N-terminus of every N segment at the V_H–D_H junction in the Ars-A antibodies, or whether other factors are selecting for Ser in this position, such as the requirement that the antibodies must be capable of combining with antigen.

The most common length for the N segment in the present set of antibodies is two residues, but HP123E6 and HP91A3 have N segments with the atypical lengths of three residues and one residue, respectively. It is possible that such differences in chain length may produce profound differences in the stereochemical properties of this region of the antibody molecule. However, it is not yet known whether any signficance attaches to the fact that both the antibodies with an N segment of atypical length show reduced levels of expression of the CRI.

11. Most J_H-Segment Diversity Is Somatically Generated, but There Are Also Examples of the Use of an Alternative J_H Gene That Compromises Antigen Binding

The J_H segment extends from the site of D_H–J_H joining at position 107 to the C-terminus of the V_H region at postion 121. All six J_H sequences illustrated in Fig. 3 are different. However, all but the J_H segment of HP101F11 show closest homology to the germ-line J_H2 gene of BALB/c.[63,64] Although data on the germ-line J_H genes in the A/J are incomplete at the DNA level, this result suggests that five of the six J_H segments are the products of a single germ-line gene representing the A/J homolog of BALB/c J_H2. A comparison of the five Ars-A J_H segments with the sequence encoded by J_H2 is included in Fig. 6. The chains differ from the germ-line sequence at one or two positions each. The total of eight amino acid differences is distributed over six positions and the only position which shows more than one replacement is the junctional position, 107. This distribution of substitutions is consistent with the hypothesis that the germ-line J_H gene used by these five antibodies encodes the same amino acid sequence as BALB/c J_H2 and that all differences from this sequence are generated somatically. In the J_H segment there is no correlation between the number of differences from germ line and the degree of expression of the CRI.

The junctional diversity at position 107 in the five antibodies cannot be accounted for solely by variation in the position of D_H–J_H joining. The J_H2 gene has a Tyr codon, TAC, at the first position[63,64] and Tyr is present in two of the five antibodies, HP123E6 and HP124E1. However, HP93G7 has an Asp at this position, encoded by a GAC codon.[44] This could have been generated by a joining event which brought a hypothetical G from the 3' end of the D_H gene into apposition with AC from the Tyr codon at the 5' end of the J_H gene, thus creating a hybrid codon for Asp. Alternatively, it could have been generated from the J_H Tyr codon by a mutational change of the first base from T to G. Both HPR16.7 and HP91A3 have a Ser at position 107, the former encoded by a TCC codon (A. Maxam, personal communication). A Ser codon could have been generated twice by independent mutations of the second base in the Tyr codon from A to C, or it could have arisen by the formation of a hybrid codon between a D_H gene and a J_H gene. However, if the latter mechanism was used, there is no way both the Asp codon in HP93G7 and the Ser codons in HPR16.7 and HP91A3 could have arisen if the same D_H and J_H genes were involved in all three cases, whatever the position of joining might have been.

The J_H segment of HP101F11 is unlike the other five antibodies in that it has an amino acid sequence identical to that determined by a portion of the coding region of the J_H4 gene of BALB/c[63,64] (Fig. 6). Southern filter hybridization studies of 101F11 hybridoma DNA using a J_H3–J_H4 probe reveal that the productively rearranged gene is associated with an EcoRI restriction fragment which is shorter than the corresponding fragments in the other five hybridomas.[47] The latter all share a common size (Section 6). The size difference, 0.8 kb, is that which would be expected under the hypothesis that HP101F11 uses the A/J homolog of the BALB/c J_H4 gene in place of the J_H2 gene utilized by the other hybridoma products.[47] The use of J_H4 correlates with the markedly reduced level of antigen binding shown by HP101F11, a property which probably results from a decreased affinity for hapten.[47] Margolies et al. have also inferred the use of the J_H4 gene in certain Ars-A antibodies with diminished antigen-binding ability (M. Margolies, personal communication). Chain recombination experiments between HP101F11 and the strongly antigen-binding HP93G7 show that the weak binding of antigen by HP101F11 is ascribable exclusively to a defect or defects in the structure of the heavy chain.[47] It is interesting to note that the position of joining between the D_H and the J_H segment in HP101F11 yields a J_H segment which is one residue shorter than the J_H segments of the other five molecules, and that a Met encoded by the J_H4 gene in HP101F11 replaces an otherwise invariant Phe at position 109. These differences may account for the change in antigen-binding behavior. Since HP101F11 is strongly CRI-positive, however, these structural alterations apparently have no effect on the degree of expression of the CRI.

			CRI	ARS	
GERMLINE	J_H2				Y F D Y W G Q G T T L T V S S
HP 93G7			+++	+	D ——————————— P
HP R16.7			+++	+	S
HP 123E6			+++	+	———————— S ——————— G
HP 124E1			+	+	————————— N
HP 91A3			-	+	———— S ——————————— S

GERMLINE	J_H4	Y Y A M D Y W G Q G T S V T V S S
HP 101F11		+++ ±

GERMLINE	J_H1	Y W Y F D V W G A G T T V T V S S
GERMLINE	J_H2	——————— Y —————— Q —————— L —————
GERMLINE	J_H3	W — A Y —— Q ———— L ——————— A
GERMLINE	J_H4	— Y A M — Y —— Q ——— S ————

FIGURE 6. Relationship of aniarsonate hybridoma J_H segments to germ-line J_H-segment genes. Comparison of amino acid sequences of J_H segments of molecules shown in Fig. 3 with the sequences encoded by germ-line J_H-segment genes of BALB/c.[63,64] (———), identical residues. For single-letter code for amino acid residues, see legend to Fig. 1. The expression of the CRI and the level of arsonate binding are noted for each expressed antibody.

12. Many Factors May Interact in a Complex Way to Produce the Diversity Seen among Antibodies of the Ars-A Family

Various aspects of the distribution of substitutions are associated with the loss of CRI in this set of molecules. These include the greater incidence of replacements in antibodies showing diminished expression of the CRI, the unusual degree of clustering of replacements in the CDRs, and the localization of much of the variation in "hot spots" at which antibodies with weakened CRI expression can be distinguished from strongly CRI-positive antibodies. In the three antibodies showing diminished expression of the CRI there are, in total, 20 positions in the heavy chains and 7 positions in the light chains which bear residues not present in one or other of the strongly CRI-positive antibodies. These residues signal positions which possibly have an effect on the structure of the determinants comprising the CRI. However, chain recombination experiments suggest that it is the structural variation in the heavy chain which is responsible for the variation in expression of the CRI in Ars-A antibodies[37] (Section 4).

Some, but almost certainly not all the positions which distinguish antibodies with weakened CRI expression from antibodies with strong CRI expression affect the structure of the determinants comprising the CRI. The CRI itself is defined by a rabbit anti-CRI serum which is polyclonal, and the anti-CRI is conventionally prepared against A/J anti-Ars serum antibodies which are also polyclonal.[11] It is thus impossible on the basis of serology alone to eliminate any of these positions from possible involvement in modifying CRI expression, since the polyclonal anti-idiotypic antibodies may bind to a number of different epitopes. Some of the difficulties inherent in the conventional definition of the CRI can be avoided if idiotypic specificities defined only in terms of monoclonal anti-idiotypic antibodies are considered. It is, however, not clear how to identify the antigenically dominant determinants comprising the CRI by using a panel of monoclonal reagents which recognize a diverse series of determinants, any one of which may contribute only a minor part to the total antigenicity of the V region. Since the proportion of variant residues which have a direct effect on CRI expression is thus unknown, and may be small, it is possible that the pattern of replacements associated with the loss of the CRI in this set of molecules is determined partially by factors only indirectly related to variation in the degree of CRI expression.

One such factor is mutation rate. In the absence of selection, mutations in the V regions accumulate to an extent which is believed to depend on the duration of developmental time in which the expressed V-region genes are subject to a high rate of somatic mutation.[31,41] The distribution of substitutions is controlled to an unknown extent by differences in the rates at which mutational changes and other somatic alterations arise at different sites. It is possible that mutations at positions affecting expression of the CRI occur more rarely than mutations at other positions and, therefore, arise mostly in molecules sharing a high probability of bearing replacements at highly mutable sites irrelevant to expression of the CRI. This may account for the otherwise anomalous observation of concordant variation in the numbers of substitutions in both V_H and V_L chains, despite the lack of any detectable dependency of CRI expression or variation in light-chain structure.[37] It may also account for the existence of hypervariable positions at which the replacements do not appear precisely in accord with the level of CRI expression, such as positions 58 and 100 in the heavy chain. Hypervariability at positions which are probably unimportant for expression of the CRI may also be accounted for in this way. For example, position 14 in the heavy chain bears a substitution in all three molecules showing reduced or absent expression of the CRI, but is located in a framework region where it may be remote from the sites of interaction with anti-idiotypic antibodies.

Another factor which modulates the distribution of mutations is stabilizing selection which suppresses amino acid substitutions at functionally crucial sites and permits only "conservative" changes (substitution of acidic residues by acidic, basic by basic, hydrophobic by hydrophobic, etcetera) at other locations. The requirement for a high level of antigen binding imposed on the molecules chosen for sequence analysis (except HP101F11) is capable of mediating such selection. The replacements which are found in the face of such stabilizing selection are ones which do not compromise the general integrity of the three-dimensional structure and cause no significant alterations in the specific sites which interact with antigen. An indication of the action of this and other kinds of selection may be obtained during sequencing studies at the nucleic acid level, where it will be possible to measure ratios of the incidence of silent and nonsilent base changes and to compare these ratios to those expected on the basis of unselected mutation. A significant elevation of base changes which give rise to amino acid substitutions can be taken as an indication of differential selection.[65]

A third factor controlling the distribution of variation is selection for divergence of amino acid sequences. Although overt selection for loss of CRI expression was imposed on the molecules described here during the choice of antibodies for sequence analysis, the patterns of variation which result from this selection may reflect not only the distribution of mutations affecting the CRI itself, but also the incidence of mutations affecting other, as yet unidentified, properties which are closely correlated with expression of the CRI *in vivo*. Possible examples of such properties are particular fine-specificity patterns or the appearance or disappearance of distinct idiotypic specificities.

These various factors are capable of interacting in a complex way to produce the patterns of variation seen in the Ars-A family and they are presumably also at work in other systems of expressed antibodies. The multiplicity of forces interacting to produce the patterns of structural variation within antibody families of this kind makes the identification of residues affecting idiotypic expression very difficult. Nevertheless, a detailed analysis of the way the patterns of variation are affected by changes in immunization and antibody sampling procedures may provide important information about the forces which exercise physiological control over the production of specific antibodies during immune responses *in vivo*.

ACKNOWLEDGMENTS. We are grateful to Dr. Pila Estess for providing the 93G7, 123E6, 124E1, and 91A3 hybridomas, to Drs. Alfred Nisonoff and Edmundo Lamoyi for their gift of the R16.7 hybridoma, and to Drs. Nisonoff and Isabel Barasoain for their gift of the C.AL-20-5 hybridoma. It is a pleasure to acknowledge the skilled technical assistance of Sandy Graham, Priscilla Presley, and Ana Garcia-Spain and the excellent secretarial services of Kathy van Egmond. This work was supported by Robert A. Welch Foundation Grant I-874.

References

1. Jerne, N. K., 1974, Towards a network theory of the immune system, *Ann. Immunol. (Inst. Pasteur)* **125C**:373–389.
2. Oudin, J., and Michel, M., 1963, Une nouvelle forme d'allotypie des globulines γ du sérum de lapin apparemment liée a la jonction et a la specificité anticorps, *C.R. Acad. Sci.* **257**:805–808.
3. Kunkel, H. G., Mannik, M., and Williams, R. C., 1963, Individual antigenic specificity of isolated antibodies, *Science* **140**:1218–1219.
4. Köhler, G., and Milstein, C., 1976, Derivation of specific antibody-producing tissue culture and tumor lines by cell fusion, *Eur. J. Immunol.* **6**:511–519.
5. Estess, P., Nisonoff, A., and Capra, J. D., 1979, Structural studies on induced antibodies with defined idiotypic specificities. VIII. NH$_2$-terminal amino acid sequence analysis of heavy and light chain variable regions of monoclonal anti-*p*-azophenylarsonate antibodies from A/J mice differing with respect to a cross-reactive idiotype, *Mol. Immunol.* **16**:1111–1118.
6. Milner, E. C. B., and Capra, J. D., 1982, V$_H$ families in the antibody response to *p*-azophenylarsonate: Correlation between serology and amino acid sequence, *J. Immunol.* **129**:193–199.
7. Capra, J. D., Tung, A. S., and Nisonoff, A., 1977, Structural studies on induced antibodies with defined idiotypic specificities. V. The complete amino acid sequence of the light chain variable regions of anti-*p*-azophenylarsonate antibodies from A/J mice bearing a cross-reactive idiotype, *J. Immunol.* **119**:993–999.
8. Capra, J. D., and Nisonoff, A., 1979, Structural studies on induced antibodies with defined idiotypic specificities. VII. The complete amino acid sequence of the heavy chain variable region of anti-*p*-azophenylarsonate antibodies from A/J mice bearing a cross-reactive idiotype, *J. Immunol.* **123**:279–284.
9. Siegelman, M., and Capra, J. D., 1981, Complete amino acid sequence of light chain variable regions derived from five monoclonal anti-*p*-azophenylarsonate antibodies differing with respect to a cross-reactive idiotype, *Proc. Natl. Acad. Sci. USA* **78**:7679–7683.
10. Slaughter, C. A., Siegelman, M., Estess, P., Barasoain, I., Nisonoff, A., and Capra, J. D., 1982, Antibody diversity and idiotypes: Primary structural analysis of monoclonal A/J antiarsonate antibodies, in: *Developmental Immunology: Clinical Problems and Aging* (E. L. Cooper and M. A. B. Brazier, eds.), Academic Press, New York, pp. 45–67.
11. Kuettner, M. G., Wang, A.-L., and Nisonoff, A., 1972, Quantitative investigations of idiotypic antibodies. VI. Idiotypic specificity as a potential genetic marker for the variable regions of mouse immunoglobulin polypeptide chains, *J. Exp. Med.* **135**:579–595.
12. Pawlak, L. L., Mushinski, E. B., Nisonoff, A., and Potter, M., 1973, Evidence for the linkage of the IgC$_H$ locus to a gene controlling the idiotypic specificity of anti-*p*-azophenylarsonate antibodies in strain A mice, *J. Exp. Med.* **137**:22–31.
13. Eichmann, K., 1975, Genetic control of antibody specificity in the mouse, *Immunogenetics* **2**:491–506.
14. Edelman, G. M., and Gottlieb, P. D., 1970, A genetic marker in the variable region of light chains of mouse immunoglobulins, *Proc. Natl. Acad. Sci. USA* **67**:1192–1199.
15. Gibson, D., 1976, Genetic polymorphism of mouse immunoglobulin light chains revealed by isoelectric focusing, *J. Exp. Med.* **144**:298–303.
16. Laskin, J. A., Gray, A., Nisonoff, A., Klinman, N. R., and Gottlieb, P. D., 1977, Segregation at a locus determining an immunoglobulin genetic marker for the light chain variable region affects inheritance of expression of an idiotype, *Proc. Natl. Acad. Sci. USA* **74**:4600–4604.
17. Brown, A. R., Estess, P., Lamoyi, E., Gill-Pazaris, L., Gottlieb, P. D., Capra, J. D., and Nisonoff, A., 1980, Studies of genetic control and microheterogeneity of an idiotype associated with anti-*p*-azophenylarsonate antibodies of A/J mice, *Prog. Clin. Biol. Res.* **42**:231–248.
18. Tung, A. S., and Nisonoff, A., 1975, Isolation from individual A/J mice of anti-*p*-azophenylarsonate antibodies bearing a cross-reactive idiotype, *J. Exp. Med.* **141**:112–126.
19. Sigal, N. H., 1982, Regulation of azophenylarsonate-specific repertoire expression. I. Frequency of cross-reactive idiotype-positive B cells in A/J and BALB/c mice, *J. Exp. Med.* **156**:1352–1365.
20. Moser, M., Leo, O., Hiernaux, J., and Urbain, J., 1983, Idiotypic maniipulation in mice: BALB/c mice can express the cross-reactive idiotype of A/J mice, *Proc. Natl. Acad. Sci. USA* **80**:4474–4478.
21. Estess, P., Lamoyi, E., Nisonoff, A., and Capra, J. D., 1980, Structural studies on induced antibodies

with defined idiotypic specificities. IX. Framework differences in heavy- and light-chain variable regions of monoclonal anti-p-azophenylarsonate antibodies from A/J mice differing with respect to a cross-reactive idiotype, *J. Exp. Med.* **154**:863–875.

22. Margolies, M. N., Marshak-Rothstein, A., and Gefter, M. L., 1981, Structural diversity among anti-p-azophenylarsonate monoclonal antibodies from A/J mice: Comparison of Id$^-$ and Id$^+$ sequences, *Mol. Immunol.* **18**:1065–1077.

23. Alkan, S. S., Knecht, R., and Braun, D. G., 1980, The cross-reactive idiotype of anti-4-azobenzene-arsonate hybridoma-derived antibodies in A/J mice constitutes multiple heavy chains, *Hoppe-Seyler's Z. Physiol. Chem.* **361**:191–195.

24. Kresina, T. F., Rosen, S. M., and Nisonoff, A., 1982, Degree of heterogeneity of binding specificities of antibodies to the phenylarsonate group that share a common idiotype, *Mol. Immunol.* **19**:1433–1439.

25. Rothstein, T. L., and Gefter, M. L., 1983, Affinity analysis of idiotype-positive and idiotype-negative Ars-binding hybridoma proteins and Ars-immune sera, *Mol. Immunol.* **20**:161–168.

26. Lamoyi, E., Estess, P., Capra, J. D., and Nisonoff, A., 1980, Heterogeneity of an intrastrain cross-reactive idiotype associated with anti-p-azophenylarsonate antibodies of A/J mice, *J. Immunol.* **124**:2834–2840.

27. Lamoyi, E., Estess, P., Capra, J. D., and Nisonoff, A., 1980, Presence of highly conserved idiotypic determinants in a family of antibodies that constitute an intrastrain cross-reactive idiotype, *J. Exp. Med.* **152**:703–711.

28. Nelles, M. J., Gill-Pazaris, L. A., and Nisonoff, A., 1981, Monoclonal anti-idiotypic antibodies reactive with a highly conserved determinant on A/J serum anti-p-azophenylarsonate antibodies, *J. Exp. Med.* **154**:1752–1763.

29. Schilling, J., Clevinger, B., Davie, J. M., and Hood, L., 1980, Amino acid sequence of homogeneous antibodies to dextran and DNA rearrangements in heavy chain V region gene segments, *Nature* **283**:35–40.

30. Bothwell, A. L. M., Paskind, M., Reth, M., Imanishi-Kari, T., Rajewsky, K., and Baltimore, D., 1981, Heavy chain variable region contribution to the NP^b family of antibodies: Somatic mutation evident in γ2a variable region, *Cell* **24**:625–637.

31. Gearhart, P. J., Johnson, N. D., Douglas, R., and Hood, L., 1981, IgG antibodies to phosphorylcholine exhibit more diversity than their IgM counterparts, *Nature (London)* **291**:29–34.

32. Kaartinen, M., Griffiths, G. M., Hamlyn, P. H., Markham, A. F., Karjalainen, K., Pelkonen, J. L. T., Mäkelä, O., and Milstein, C., 1983, Anti-oxazolone hybridomas and the structure of the oxazolone idiotype, *J. Immunol.* **130**:937–945.

33. Ruf, J., Tonnelle, C., Rocca-Serra, J., Moinier, D., Pierres, M., Ju, S.-T., Dorf, M. E., Thèze, J., and Fougereau, M., 1983, Structural bases for public idiotypic specificities of monoclonal antibodies directed against poly (Glu^{60} Ala^{30} Tyr^{10}) and poly (Glu^{80} Ala^{60}) random copolymers, *Proc. Natl. Acad. Sci, USA* **80**:3040–3044.

34. Pawlita, M., Potter, M., and Rudikoff, S., 1981, κ-chain restriction in anti-galactan antibodies, *J. Immunol.* **129**:615–618.

35. Vrana, M. S., Rudikoff, S., and Potter, M., 1978, Sequence variation among heavy chains from inulin-binding myeloma proteins, *Proc. Natl. Acad. Sci. USA* **75**:1957–1961.

36. Johnson, N., Slankard, J., Paul, L., and Hood, L., 1982, The complete V domain amino acid sequences of two myeloma inulin-binding proteins, *J. Immunol.* **128**:302–307.

37. Milner, E. C. B., and Capra, J. D., 1983, Structural analysis of monoclonal anti-arsonate antibodies: Idiotypic specificities are determined by the heavy chain, *Mol. Immunol.* **20**:39–46.

37a. Gill-Pazaris, L. A., Lamoyi, E., Brown, A. R., and Nisonoff, A., 1981, Properties of a minor cross-reactive idiotype associated with anti-p-azophenylarsonate antibodies of A/J mice, *J. Immunol.* **126**:75–79.

38. Ball, R. K., Chang, J.-Y., Alkan, S. S., and Braun, D. G., 1983, The complete amino acid sequence of the light chain variable region of two monoclonal anti-p-azobenzene-arsonate antibodies bearing the cross-reactive idiotype, *Mol. Immunol.* **20**:197–201.

39. Sakano, H., Huppi, K., Heinrich, G., and Tonegawa, S., 1979, Sequences of the somatic recombination sites of immunoglobulin light-chain genes, *Nature* **280**:288–294.

40. Max, E. E., Seidman, J. G., and Leder, P., 1979, Sequences of five potential recombination sites encoded close to an immunoglobulin κ constant region gene, *Proc. Natl. Acad. Sci. USA* **76**:3450–3454.

41. Kaartinen, M., Griffiths, G. M., Markham, A. F., and Milstein, C., 1983, mRNA sequences define an unusually restricted IgG response to 2-phenyloxazolone and its early diversification, *Nature* **304**:320–324.

42. Schiff, C., and Fougereau, M., 1975, Determination of the primary structure of a mouse IgG2a immunoglobulin: Amino acid sequence of the light chain, *Eur. J. Biochem.* **59**:525–537.
43. Siegelman, M., Slaughter, C. A., McCumber, L. J., Estess, P., and Capra, J. D., 1981, Primary structural studies of monoclonal A/J anti-arsonate antibodies differing with respect to a cross-reactive idiotype, in: *Immunoglobulin Idiotypes* (C. A. Janeway Jr., E. E. Sercarz, and H. Wigzell, eds.), Academic Press, New York, pp. 135–158.
44. Sims, J., Rabbitts, T. H., Estess, P., Slaughter, C. A., Tucker, P. W., and Capra, J. D., 1982, Somatic mutation in genes for the variable portion of the immunoglobulin heavy chain, *Science* **216**:309–311.
45. Capra, J. D., Slaughter, C. A., Milner, E. C. B., Estess, P., and Tucker, P. W., 1982, The cross-reactive idiotype of A-strain mice: Serological and structural studies, *Immunol. Today* **3**:332–339.
46. Slaughter, C. A., and Capra, J. D., 1983, Amino acid sequence diversity within the family of antibodies bearing the major anti-arsonate cross-reactive idiotype of the A-strain mouse, *J. Exp. Med.* **158**:1615–1634.
47. Slaughter, C. A., Jeske, D. J., Kuziel, W. A., Milner, E. C. B., and Capra, J. D., Use of J_H4 joining segment gene by an anti-arsonate antibody, *J. Immunol.* (in press).
48. Kabat, E. A., Wu, T. T., Bilofsky, H., Reid-Miller, M., and Perry, H., 1983, Sequences of proteins of immunological interest, U.S. Department of Health and Human Services.
49. Siekevitz, M., Gefter, M. L., Brodeur, P., Riblet, R., and A. Marshak-Rothstein, 1982, The genetic basis of antibody production: The dominant anti-arsonate idiotypic response of the strain A mouse, *Eur. J. Immunol.* **12**:1023–1032.
50. Siekevitz, M., Huang, S. Y., and Gefter, M. L., 1983, The genetic basis of antibody production: A single heavy chain variable region gene encodes all molecules bearing the dominant anti-arsonate idiotype in the strain A mouse, *Eur. J. Immunol.* **13**:123–132.
51. Estess, P., Otani, F., Milner, E. C. B., Capra, J. D., and Tucker, P. W., 1982, Gene rearrangements in monoclonal A/J anti-arsonate antibodies, *J. Immunol.* **129**:2319–2322.
52. Kehry, M. R., Fuhrman, J. S., Schilling, J. W., Rogers, J., Sibley, C. H., and Hood, L. E., 1982, Complete amino acid sequence of a mouse μ chain: Homology among heavy chain constant region domains, *Biochemistry* **21**:5415–5424.
53. Zakut, R., Cohen, J., and Givol, D., 1980, Cloning and sequence of the cDNA corresponding to the variable region of immunoglobulin heavy chain MPC 11, *Nucleic Acids Res.* **8**:3591–3601.
54. Crews, S., Griffin, J., Huang, H., Calame, K., and Hood, L., 1981, A single V_H gene segment encodes the immune response to phosphorylcholine: Somatic mutation is correlated with the class of the antibody, *Cell* **25**:59–66.
55. Milstein, C., and Pink, J. L. R., 1970, Structure and evolution of immunoglobulins, *Prog. Biophys. Mol. Biol.* **21**:209–263.
56. Wu, T. T., and Kabat, E. A., 1970, An analysis of the sequences of the variable regions of Bence-Jones proteins and myeloma light chains and their implications for antibody complementarity, *J. Exp. Med.* **132**:211–250.
57. Capra, J. D., and Kehoe, J. M., 1974, Variable region sequences of five immunoglobulin heavy chains of the $V_H III$ subgroup: Definitive identification of four heavy chain hypervariable regions, *Proc. Natl. Acad. Sci. USA* **71**:845–848.
58. Capra, J. D., 1981, Antibody diversity: A somatic model, in: *Immunoglobulin Idiotypes* (C. A. Janeway, Jr., E. E. Sercarz, and H. Wigzell, eds.), Academic Press, New York, pp. 825–830.
59. Alt, F. W., and Baltimore, D., 1982, Joining of immunoglobulin heavy chain gene segments: Implications from a chromosome with evidence of three $D-J_H$ fusions, *Proc. Natl. Acad. Sci. USA* **79**:4118–4122.
60. Kurosawa, Y., and Tonegawa, S., 1982, Organization, structure, and assembly of immunoglobulin heavy chain diversity DNA segments, *J. Exp. Med.* **155**:201–218.
61. Wood, C., and Tonegawa, S., 1983, Diversity and joining segments of mouse immunoglobulin heavy chain genes are closely linked and in the same orientation: Implications for the joining mechanism, *Proc. Natl. Acad. Sci. USA* **80**:3030–3034.
62. Tonegawa, S., 1983, Somatic generation of antibody diversity, *Nature (London)* **302**:575–581.
63. Barnard, O., and Gough, N. M., 1980, Nucleotide sequence of immunoglobulin heavy chain joining segments between translocated V_H and constant region genes, *Proc. Natl. Acad. Sci. USA* **77**:3630–3634.
64. Sakano, H., Maki, R., Kurosawa, Y., Roeder, W., and Tonegawa, S., 1980, Two types of somatic recom-

bination are necessary for the generation of complete immunoglobulin heavy-chain genes, *Nature* **286:**676–683.

65. Loh, D. Y., Bothwell, A. L. M., White-Scharf, M. E., Imanishi-Kari, T., and Baltimore, D., 1983, Molecular basis of a mouse strain-specific anti-hapten response, *Cell* **33:**85–93.

66. Estess, P., 1980, Structural and serologic analyses of monoclonal A/J anti-arsonate antibodies with and without a cross-reactive idiotype. Ph.D. thesis, The University of Texas Health Science Center, Dallas.

4

The Molecular Genetics of Phosphocholine-Binding Antibodies

Roger M. Perlmutter

1. Introduction

Early structural analyses of antibody molecules were confounded by the complex hetero-geneity which typifies most humoral immune responses. The search for homogeneous anti-body populations led to the use of simple bacterial vaccines as immunogens, many of which elicited quite restricted serum antibodies.[1] In the early 1960s, a number of mineral oil-induced murine plasmacytomas were identified which secrete antibodies specific for phosphocholine[2] (PC), the immunodominant determinant on certain rough strains of *Streptococcus pneumoniae*.[3] The murine antibody response to PC has been shown to be quite restricted in isotype[4] and idiotype.[5] In particular, the majority of induced BALB/c anti-PC antibodies bear idiotypic determinants related to those present on a prototype PC-binding plasmacytoma protein, T15, and the expression of this idiotype is inherited as a single Mendelian allele closely linked to the immunoglobulin allotype locus.[6] In addition, neonatal administration of anti-T15 antitypic antibodies completely abrogates the anti-R36A pneumococcal response in mice.[7] These data, coupled with the nearly homogeneous affinities of anti-PC sera as measured by hapten inhibition,[8] suggested that the murine response to PC might be essentially monoclonal.

Using more refined analyses, however, it was possible to define several related clon-otypes of anti-PC antibodies in BALB/c mice. Low levels of antibodies related to the sero-logically distinct PC-binding plasmacytoma proteins M511, M167, and M603 were demonstrated[9,10] and studies of monoclonal anti-PC antibodies generated using a splenic focus technique revealed a large number of different antibodies distinguishable by affinity for PC and PC analogs and by idiotype.[11]

Thus, although inheritance studies suggested that the T15-like PC-binding antibodies

Roger M. Perlmutter • Division of Biology, California Institute of Technolgy, Pasadena, California 91125. *Present Address:* Department of Medical Genetics, University of Washington School of Medicine, Seattle, Washington 98195.

were simply encoded in the germ line, a variety of serological evidence made plain a hidden diversity in murine antibodies to PC. In this context, protein and DNA sequencing strategies could be fruitfully applied to the analysis of PC-binding antibodies in hopes of defining the structural basis of antibody diversity. Data to be reviewed in this chapter clearly illustrate that (1) a small number of germ-line genes are responsible for the generation of anti-PC antibodies bearing the T15 idiotype, (2) the majority of idiotype-negative antibody variants result from a process of somatic mutation acting on a small set of germ-line V_H and V_κ genes, and (3) the T15 idiotype is a complex structure likely reflecting contributions from several germ-line gene segments. In addition, I will review data addressing the evolutionary constraints that affect these genetic elements and that have preserved a uniform T15-like binding site-related idiotype in most murine speices.[12]

2. Structural Diversity of Anti-PC Heavy Chains

Three discrete gene segments, V_H, D, and J_H, which are discontinuous in germ-line DNA, are juxtaposed during B-cell differentiation to form the antibody V_H gene.[13] In order to analyze the contribution of each of these gene segments to the diversity of PC-binding antibody heavy chains, complete amino acid sequences for 20 heavy chains derived from BALB/c hybridoma or plasmacytoma proteins which bind PC were obtained (Fig. 1).[14] Seven of these sequences are identical to the prototype sequence of the T15 plasmacytoma protein, the remaining sequences differ by 1 (HPCG12) to 15 (HPCG15) substitutions. A majority of these differences (39/68) fall within the first 101 amino acids encoded by the V_H gene segment. Other substitutions reflect utilization of multiple D segments and the mechanism of V_H–D–J_H joining as discussed below. To understand the substantial N-terminal diversity of these sequences, it was essential to determine whether differences in the V_H-encoded portion of the heavy chain necessarily reflected the existence of multiple germ-line gene segments for these antibodies.

3. Genes Encoding Anti-PC V_H Regions

A cDNA probe complementary to heavy-chain mRNA from the plasmacytoma S107, which is identical in sequence to T15, was used to estimate the size of the T15-related gene family. Fig. 2 shows the results of a genomic Southern blot (where BALB/c DNA is digested with the restriction endonuclease EcoRI and the resulting fragments are separated by agarose gel electrophoresis and transferred to nitrocellulose) using the S107 cDNA labeled with ^{32}P as a probe. Four strongly hybridizing bands greater than 88% homologous can be identified. Exhaustive screening of a BALB/c genomic phage library yielded at least one phage clone for each band seen on the genomic blot as shown in Fig. 2. Complete DNA sequences for each of the members of this V_H family were then determined and the translated protein sequences derived from these DNA sequences were compared with the previously determined protein sequences for PC-binding antibody heavy chains. Fig. 3 shows this comparison for the four gene sequences, labeled *V1*, *V3*, *V11*, and *V13*, and for variant heavy-chain sequences. The *V1* gene encodes a protein identical to T15; thus, this sequence has its expected germ-line equivalent. None of the variant protein sequences is represented

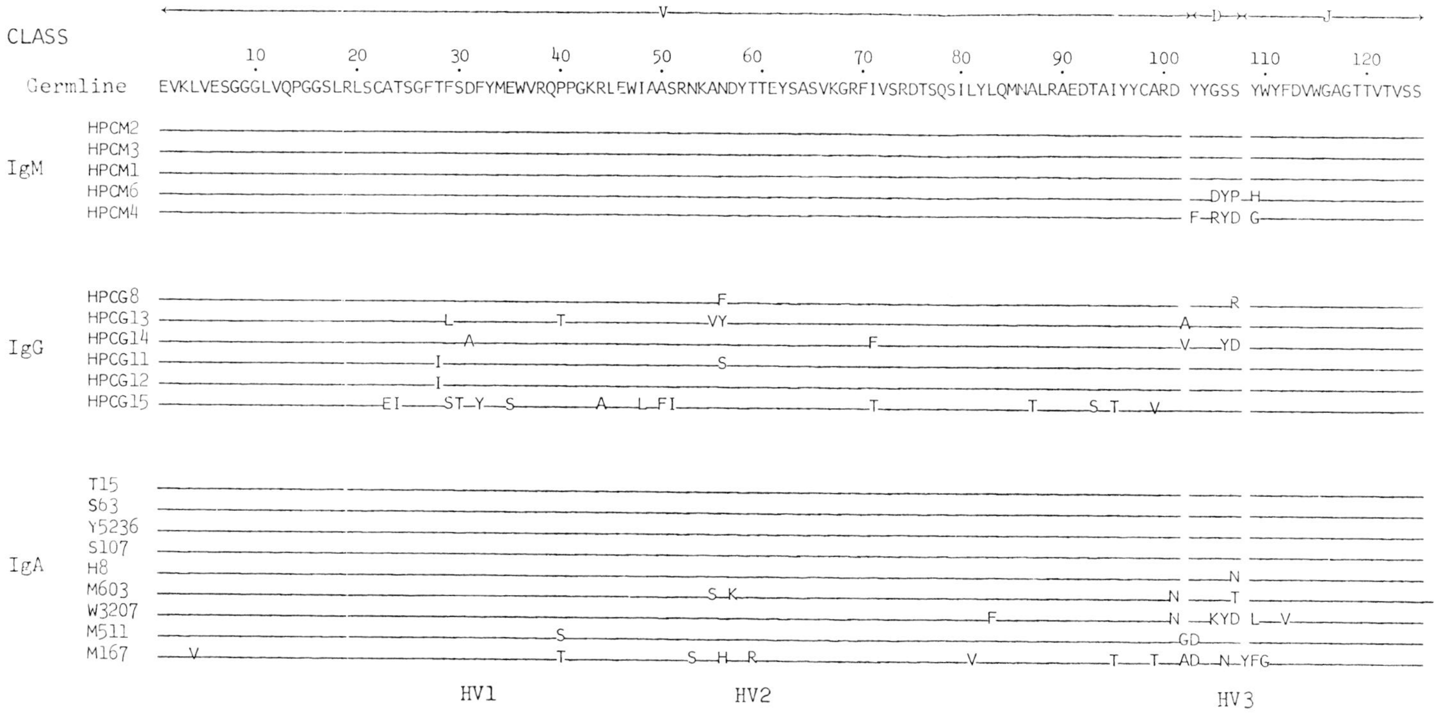

CLASS

Germline

```
                10        20        30        40        50        60        70        80        90       100       110       120
       EVKLVESGGGLVQPGGSLRLSCATSGFTFSDFYMEWVRQPPGKRLEWIAASRNKANDYTTEYSASVKGRFIVSRDTSQSILYLQMNALRAEDTATYYCARD YYGSS YWYFDVWGAGTTVTSS
```

IgM
```
HPCM2  ————————————————————————————————————————————————————————————————————————————————————————————————————
HPCM3  ————————————————————————————————————————————————————————————————————————————————————————————————————
HPCM1  ————————————————————————————————————————————————————————————————————————————————————————————————————
HPCM6  ——————————————————————————————————————————————————————————————————————————————————————————DYP-H————
HPCM4  ——————————————————————————————————————————————————————————————————————————————————————F-RYD G———————
```

IgG
```
HPCG8  ————————————————————————————————————————————————————————————————————————————————————————R——————————
HPCG13 ——————————————————————————————T———————————F—————————————————————————————————————————A——————————————
HPCG14 ———————————————————A———————————————————VY————————————————————————————————————————V—YD—————————————
HPCG11 ———————————————————I————————————————————F———————————————————————————————————————————————————————————
HPCG12 ———————————————————I—————————————————S—————————————————————————————————————————————————————————————
HPCG15 ——————————————EI——ST—Y—S——A——L-FI———————————————T——————————T—S-T—V——————————————————————————————
```

IgA
```
T15    ————————————————————————————————————————————————————————————————————————————————————————————————————
S63    ————————————————————————————————————————————————————————————————————————————————————————————————————
Y5236  ————————————————————————————————————————————————————————————————————————————————————————————————————
S107   ————————————————————————————————————————————————————————————————————————————————————————————————————
H8     ——————————————————————————————————————————————S-K.————————————————————————————————N————————————————
M603   —————————————————————————————————————————————————————————————————————————————————————-T————————————
W3207  ————————————————————————————————————————————————————————————————————F—————————————N——KYD L—V———————
M511   ——————————————————————————S—————————————————————————————————————————————————————————————GD——————————
M167 V ——————————————T——————————————S—H-R————————————————————V————————————————T—T—AD—N-YFG—————————
```

HV1   HV2   HV3

FIGURE 1. Complete heavy-chain variable-region sequences from antibodies binding phosphocholine. Shown are protein sequences for 13 hybridoma and seven myeloma proteins with specificity for phosphocholine. The residues are numbered consecutively and the positions encoded by V_H, D, and J_H gene segments are indicated with arrows. Adapted from Ref. 14 with permission of the authors.

Clone DNA   Sperm DNA
   EcoRI   EcoRI

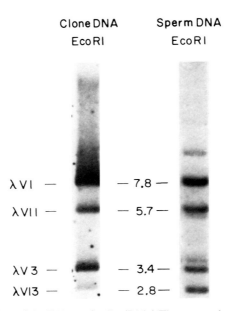

λ V I —   — 7.8 —

λ VII —   — 5.7 —

λ V 3 —   — 3.4 —

λ VI3 —   — 2.8 —

FIGURE 2. Southern blot analysis of the T15 gene family. (Right) The pattern obtained when 10 μg of BALB/ c sperm DNA is completely digested with *EcoRI* and the resulting fragments are separated by agarose gel electrophoresis, blotted onto nitrocellulose, and T15-related sequences identified by hybridization with a ^{32}P-labeled probe complementary to T15. (Left) EcoRI restriction digests of four recombinant phage clones corresponding to the four major V_H segments identified in the right-hand lane. The numbering of clones is derived from Ref. 15 (adapted with permission of the authors).

in the germ line and in fact with a single exception all are most closely related to the V1 sequence. Three independent clones containing this V_H segment were sequenced and were found to be identical; thus, no additional closely related V_H gene segments exist in the germ line of BALB/c mice. The inescapable conclusion is that the 12 observed variant V_H protein sequences must have arisen somatically within individual B-cell clones.[15]

4. Structural Features of Somatic Mutation

Germ-line V_H gene segments exhibit characteristic structural features essential to rearrangement and expression. Each includes two exons separated by an intervening sequence of variable length. The 5′ exon encodes a signal peptide which is cleaved from the mature secreted product. RNA polymerase II promoter signals, termed *CAAT* and *TATA* boxes,[16] are located about 110 and 90 bases upstream from the signal exon.[17] Rearrangement of V_H gene segments is mediated in part by paired recognition sequences located 3′ to the structural exon and 5′ to the D-region gene segments.[18] Similar sequences are found 3′ to D segments and 5′ to J_H segments. Juxtaposition of V_H, D, and J_H gene segments is an early event in pre-B cells[19] which results in the deletion or transposition of intervening DNA separating the V_H, D, and J_H gene segments such that a continuous

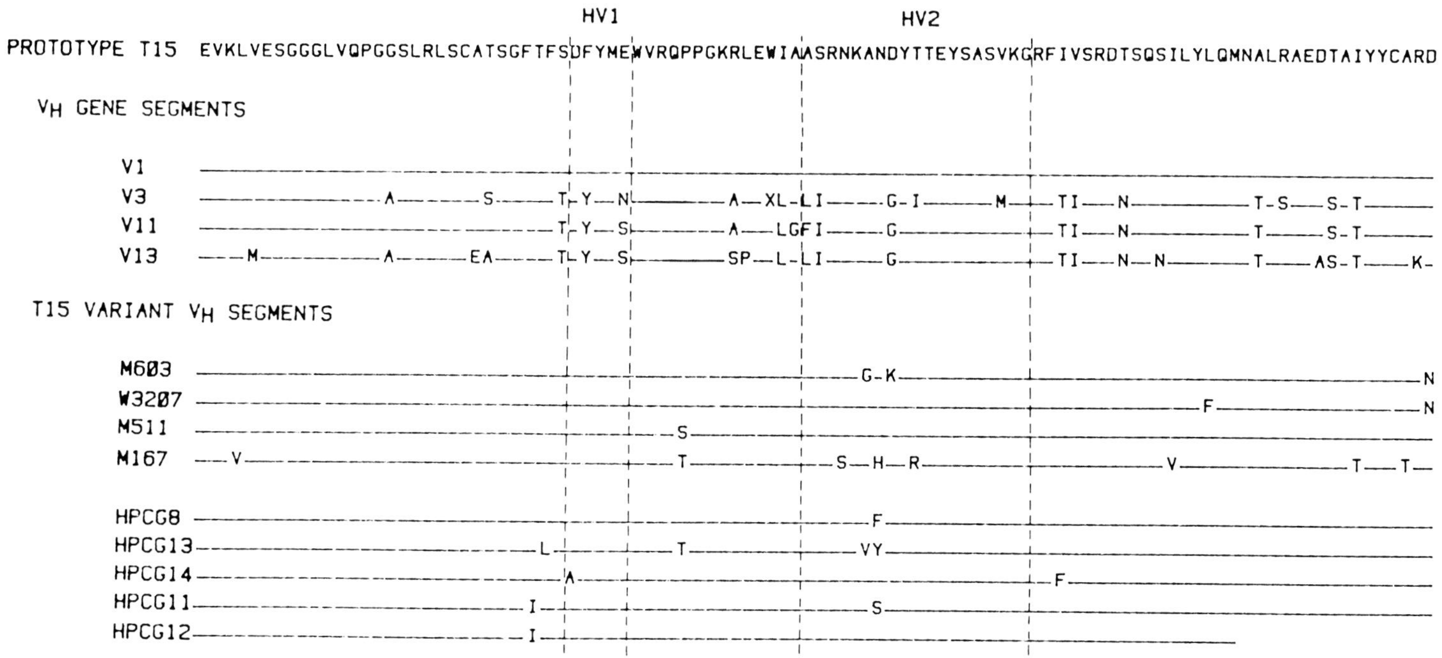

PROTOTYPE T15   EVKLVESGGGLVQPGGSLRLSCATSGFTFSDFYMEWVRQPPGKRLEWIAASRNKANDYTTEYSASVKGRFIVSRDTSQSILYLQMNALRAEDTAIYYCARD

HV1

HV2

V_H GENE SEGMENTS

V1
V3
V11
V13

T15 VARIANT V_H SEGMENTS

M603
W3207
M511
M167
HPCG8
HPCG13
HPCG14
HPCG11
HPCG12

FIGURE 3. Genes encoding PC-binding heavy chains. Shown is a comparison of the sequences of the four germ-line V_H segments identified in Fig. 2, translated into amino acids, with the sequences of variant heavy chains from Fig. 1. The sequence of the NH_2-terminal 101 residues of the T15 myeloma heavy chain is listed at the top. Dashed lines demarcate the positions of first (HV1) and second (HV2) hypervariable regions (see Ref. 39).

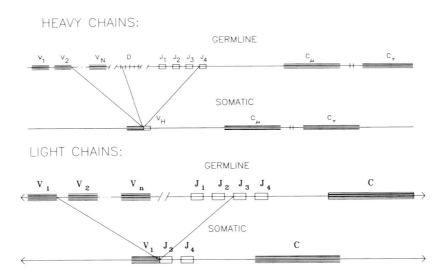

FIGURE 4. The organization and rearrangements of antibody gene segments. The germ-line configurations of antibody heavy- and light-chain gene segments are shown and the rearrangements which result in assembly of a functional variable-region gene are diagrammed.

reading frame is formed. The germ-line structural organization and somatic rearrangements of antibody gene segments are diagrammed in Fig. 4.

In an attempt to characterize the observed variation in V_H sequences of BALB/c anti-PC heavy chains, the rearranged *V1* gene was cloned and sequenced from two PC-binding myelomas, M167 and M603.[20] Careful comparison of these sequences with the germ-line *V1* gene sequence reveals three important features of the somatic mutation process (Fig. 5):

1. Somatic mutation is extensive, e.g., the M167 V_H gene includes 44 substitutions, insertions, or deletions from the germ-line sequence.
2. The observed mutations are entirely localized to the region including and immediately surrounding the V_H gene—sequences 5 kb 5′ and 3′ to the gene are unmutated.[20]
3. The pattern of variation cannot be explained by recombination between the germ-line *V1* gene segment and any other member of the T15 family, and the observed alterations in the J_H region exclude recombinational models of somatic diversification since these sequences are present in the germ line as single copies.

Thus, we find that the variability in heavy-chain sequences from PC-binding antibodies largely reflects the action of a mutational mechanism which is finely focused on the rearranged V_H gene. There are, however, a number of sequence variants which result from other mechanisms.

5. *D* Regions and V_H–*D*–J_H Joining

Although much of the observed sequence heterogeneity in PC-binding heavy chains results from somatic mutation, examination of the complete sequences shown in Fig. 1

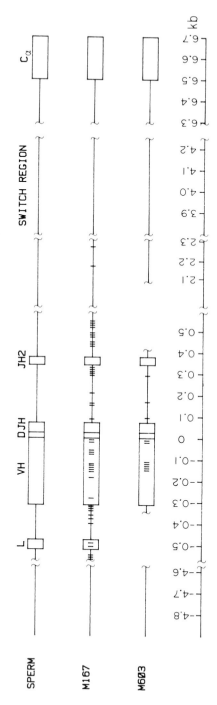

FIGURE 5. The distribution of somatic mutations in rearranged V_H genes. Hatch marks indicate the position of mutations from the germ-line (sperm) sequence in heavy-chain genes of two PC-binding myelomas, M167 and M603. Adapted with permission from Ref. 20.

		V1			DFL 16.1					J$_H$1		
T15:	protein	A	R	D	Y	Y	G	S	S	Y	W	Y
	DNA	GCA	AGA	GAT	TAC	TAC	GGT	AGT	AGC	TAC	TGG	TAC
				*					*			
M167:	DNA	GCA	AGA	AAT	TAC	TAC	GGT	AGT	ACC	[ ]	TGG	TAC
	protein	A	R	N	Y	Y	G	S	T		W	Y

FIGURE 6. Junctional diversity in D–J_H joining. The site of D–J_H joining for the M603 heavy chain is compared with that seen in the T15 heavy chain. Positions marked by an asterisk represent somatic mutations.

reveals that 29 of 68 amino acid substitutions occur within the D-region-encoded sequence or near the sites of V_H–D–J_H joining. All of the BALB/c anti-PC heavy chains utilize the J_H1 gene segment; however, the precise site of D–J_H joining can vary by as many as four nucleotides within the J_H1 region. Fig. 6 illustrates that junctional diversity at the site of D–J_H joining shortens the variable region of one heavy chain, M603, by one residue when compared with the prototype T15 sequence even though both heavy chains utilize identical germ-line V_H, D, and J_H segments.

A minimum of three different germ-line D segments (as defined by Kurosawa and Tonegawa[21]) are used in the formation of PC-binding heavy chains. The majority (16/20) employ the $DFL16.1$ gene segment, while the remaining four proteins utilize either $DSP2.2$ or a member of the $DSP2.3$ D-segment family. As in the case of the J_H1 segment, junctional diversity occurs at the sites of D joining and may occur at both the 5' and the 3' end of the D segment. In addition, as shown in Figs. 6 and 7, somatic mutation may also occur within the D segment. Thus, sequence heterogeneity in or near the D-region-encoded portion of PC-binding heavy chains results from utilization of multiple germ-line D gene segments, somatic mutation of these germ-line sequences (assuming no additional D-region gene segments exist in the germ line), and junctional diversity at the sites of V_H–D and D–J_H joining. Occasionally, the observed nucleotide sequence at the sites of D-region recombination does not reflect any known germ-line sequence and seems to have arisen *de novo*. In M167, for example, two guanine nucleotides are appended at the site of V_H–D joining and four nucleotides (three thymidine and one guanine) appear to have been added at the site of D–J_H1 joining (Fig. 7). Similar short repetitive sequences, termed *N regions*, have

		V1				DFL 16.1					J$_H$1		
T15:	protein	A	R	D		Y	Y	G	S	S	Y	W	Y
	DNA	GCA	AGA	GAT		TAC	TAC	GGT	AGT	AGC	TAC	TGG	TAC
		*							*				
M167:	DNA	ACA	AGA	GAT	GCG	GAC	TAC	GGT	AAT	AGC	TAC	TTT	GGG	TAC
	protein	T	R	D	A	D	Y	G	N	S	Y	F	G	Y

FIGURE 7. N-region diversity in V_H genes. The germ-line sequences of $V1$,[15] $D_{FL16.1}$,[21] and J_H1[18] are compared with the sequence of the rearranged V_H gene from the M167 myeloma.[20] Nucleotides not encoded in the germ line and apparently added somatically are underlined. (*) Changes likely secondary to somatic mutation.

been found at V_H-D-J_H joining sites in other heavy chains[22] and may be an important feature of the joining mechanism.

6. Structural Diversity of PC-Binding Light Chains

Three major groups of κ variable-region sequences, resembling T15, M603, and M167, respectively, participate in the formation of PC-binding antibodies. The M167-like light chains have been examined in some detail and have been shown to employ a single germ-line V_κ gene segment joined in each case to $J_\kappa 5$[23,24] (Fig. 8). Sequence substitutions in these light-chain variable regions, as in the heavy chains previously described, result from a process of localized, clustered somatic mutation.[25] It is likely that the T15 and M603-like light-chain groups are also encoded by single germ-line V_κ genes. For the M167-like light-chain group, there is no evidence of junctional diversity at the site of $V_\kappa-J_\kappa 5$ joining which may reflect the importance of a J_κ-encoded leucine at postion 101, which is a contact residue for PC.[26]

7. Selection of Variant Antibodies

One striking feature of somatic mutation in PC-binding antibodies is its close association with antibody isotype: variant sequences are restricted to IgG and IgA antibody classes while IgM anti-PC antibodies employ the germ-line variable-region sequence (Fig. 1). Since the progenitor lymphocyte for all B cells secreting anti-PC antibodies is an IgM-bearing cell[27] likely synthesizing heavy and light chains which are identical in sequence to the germ-line-encoded molecules, it is reasonable to suggest that subsequent somatic mutation of these germ-line sequences would generate multiple variant clones and that some of these may be selectively expanded on the basis of increased affinity for antigen. Using diazophenylphosphocholine (DPPC), a PC analog thought to more closely resemble the haptenic determinant on PC-derivatized protein conjugates, the variant antibodies shown in Fig. 1 which were isolated from PC-KLH-primed fusion products show a significantly higher affinity for antigen than does the germ-line-encoded molecule, T15.[28] Close association of somatic mutation with antibody class may thus be an artifact reflecting cycles of antigen selection; those clones most likely to undergo a class switching event are also those most exposed to the selective pressure of antigen. Indeed, NH_2-terminal sequences apparently demonstrating somatic mutation of the V1 germ-line sequence in IgM anti-PC heavy chains have been reported by others.[29] Alternatively, or perhaps in addition, the somatic mutation process may be initiated or accelerated by isotype switching.

In accord with theories which propose antigen-driven selection of spontaneously occurring somatic mutations, comparison of the DNA sequences of V_H[20] and V_κ[25] rearranged genes reveals a rough concordance between the extent of somatic mutation in V_H and the extent of somatic mutation in V_κ. Thus, the mechanism responsible for the production of somatic variants appears to act simultaneously on both heavy and light chains.

Another population of variant antibodies, defined in PC-KLH hyperimmune animals, binds DPPC much more avidly than PC and invariably lacks the T15 idiotype.[30] These

$J_\kappa 5$

```
                      ←——HV1——→              ←——HV2——→
      10        20        30        40        50        60        70        80        90        100       110
GERMLINE
GENE  DIVITQDELSNPVTSGESVSISCRSSKSLLYKDGKTYLNWFLQRPGQSPQLLIYLMSTRASGVSDRFSGSGSGTDFTLEISRVKAEDVGVYYCQQLVEYP LTFGAGTKLELKR

M167  ————————————————————————————————————————————————————————————————————————————————————————————————— —————————————

M511  —————————————K———————————————————————————————————————————R—————————————————————————————————————————— —————————————

HPCG9 ————————————————————————————————————————————————————————S——————————————————————————————————————————— —————————————

HPCG22 ———————————————————————————————————————————————————————————————————————————————————————————————————— —————————————

HPCG10 ———————————————————————————————————————————————————————————————————————————————————————————————————— —————————————

HPCG13 ————————————N——————————————————————————————————————————————————————————————————————————————————————— —————————————
```

FIGURE 8. Variations in the protein sequences of BALB/c light chains from PC-binding antibodies. The germ-line sequences of the V_κ gene segment encoding M167-like light chains[23,24] and of the $J_\kappa 5$ gene segment translated into amino acids[18] are compared with the sequences of six κ light chains from PC-binding antibodies. The protein sequences have been corrected according to the recently obtained nucleotide sequences.[25] The sequence is numbered consecutively with HV1 and HV2 indicating first and second hypervariable regions.[39]

"group II" antibodies have been shown to contain a heavy chain which is not encoded by any member of the T15 gene family[31] and a light chain which is unlike any observed in typical PC-binding antibodies.[32] Interestingly, these different groups of variable-region sequences are expressed in an isotype-restricted fashion. Serum anti-PC antibodies utilizing the T15 V_H are restricted to IgM and IgG3 classes in BALB/c mice[33] whereas group II antibodies utilizing a different V_H gene segment are restricted to IgG1[31] and occasionally IgE classes. The mechanism of selective association of specific variable regions with particular isotypes is obscure. It is of interest that IgG3 antibodies bearing T15-like variable regions are most protective against *in vivo* challenge with viable pneumococcoal organisms.[34]

8. Molecular Basis of the T15 Idiotype

Although the T15 idiotype has been identified as a potential site for regulation of the immune response to PC,[7] attempts to correlate protein sequence data with serological reactivity of anti-T15 reagents reveal that the T15 idiotype is a complex structure. This analysis is further complicated by heterogeneity in existing anti-T15 sera which may not recognize identical determinants.[35,36] Close genetic linkage of T15 idiotypic markers to *Ig-1* locus allotypes[6] appears to localize the T15 idiotype to the heavy chain. T15 and an Ig-1^b PC-binding antibody, C3, are idiotypically distinct although differing by only four residues in V_H and a single substitution in J_H regions.[36] This result would imply that the D region plays no role in the formation of the T15 idiotype. Conversely, T15 and HPCM6 heavy chains differ only in their D regions and yet HPCM6 lacks the T15 idiotype[14] (Fig. 1). Further evidence for the involvement of multiple gene segments in directing synthesis of the T15 idiotype results from comparison of T15 and HPCM3 antibodies which share identical heavy-chain variable regions although HPCM3 lacks the T15 idiotype. It is thus likely that the T15 idiotype reflects contributions from V_H, V_κ, J_H, and D gene segments. Nevertheless, the predominant binding site-related idiotype of PC-binding antibodies is clearly a germ-like structure and the importance of idiotype-specific helper T cells,[37] viewed in this context, is not obvious. The ill-defined nature of T15 idiotypes is apparent in the demonstration of a monoclonal T15-specific reagent which recognizes the T-cell surface marker Thy-1.[38]

9. Evolution of the T15 Gene Family

Four V_H gene segments that are more than 88% homologous comprise the T15 gene family in BALB/c mice. As we have seen, all of the BALB/c anti-PC heavy chains employ the *V1* gene segment with two exceptions: HPCG13 (Fig. 1) is probably encoded by the *V11* gene segment after substantial somatic mutation,[15] and group II antibodies with high affinity for DPPC are encoded by an unrelated V_H gene segment.[31] The *V11* gene segment also contributes to the formation of antibodies specific for influenza virus hemagglutinin (W. Gerhard, personal communication) and the translated *V11* sequence is identical to the V_H-region sequence of the M47A myeloma heavy chain.[39] The *V13* gene segment encodes a protein identical to the 38C myeloma heavy chain (R. Riblet, personal communication) and is thus a functional sequence. In contrast, the *V3* gene segment is a pseudogene in that it contains two in-phase termination codons and an aberrant 3′ recognition sequence.[40] *V3* is located 16 kb 5′ to the *V1* gene segment on chromosome 12[15] and there is evidence from classical recombination studies that *V11* and *V13* are located 5′ to *V3* (R. Riblet, personal communication), although these have not been physically linked.

The T15 gene family provides an ideal proving ground for the evaluation of evolutionary theories since one of these gene segments *(V1)* encodes a heavy chain that is likely to be important for the protection of mice against bacterial infection[34] and thus presumably subject to strong selection pressures, while a closely related and physically linked gene segment *(V3)* is a pseudogene. Sequence comparisons of PC-binding heavy chains from other mouse strains indicate that the *V1* gene segment is indeed closely conserved[41] and a structural equivalent may well exist in human DNA.[42]

Southern blot analysis of genomic DNA from a number of mouse strains and from inbred Lewis rats shows that all strains have apparently retained both *V1* and *V13* elements and that most strains also contain *V11* and *V3* (Fig. 9). Germ-line rat DNA includes a large number of sequences homologous to the S107 probe, probably reflecting expansion of the T15 gene family during the approximately 10 million years since divergence of rats and mice. Nucleotide sequence analysis of the *V1* gene from B10.P mice confirms that this

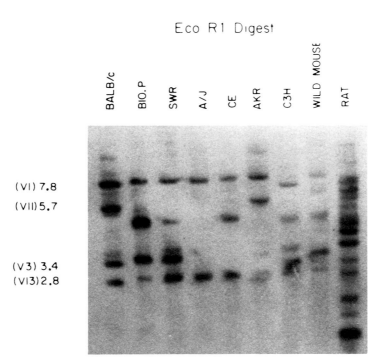

FIGURE 9. Southern blot results obtained using a ^{32}P-labeled probe complementary to the T15 V_H gene segment to detect homologous sequences in *Eco*RI-digested DNA from the indicated mouse strains and from Lewis rats. Ten μg of DNA was used in each case. The numbering of the positive fragments reflects Fig. 2.

sequence has been strongly conserved since divergence of the Ig-1^a and Ig-1^b chromosomes and a similar analysis of the *V3* gene in B10.P mice has allowed us to construct a detailed history of the evolution of this pseudogene (R. M. Perlmutter, J. A. Griffin, B. Berson, and L. Hood, manuscript in preparation). Thus, the preeminence of somatic mutation in the generation of variant PC-binding antibodies does not appear to reduce the importance of individual germ line V_H genes. In fact, the *V1* gene may have been selected for binding to PC as represented in bacterial carbohydrates, and the somatic mutations observed after immunization with PC-KLH may be an example of adaptive immunity to an antigen infrequently encountered during normal life.

10. The Extent of Antibody Diversity

Examination of the anti-PC antibodies and the genes which encode them illuminates the multiple strategies employed by higher vertebrates to amplify a limited amount of germline information encoding immunoglobulins. All of the described mechanisms which contribute to antibody heterogeneity are utilized in PC-binding antibodies, specifically:

1. Combinatorial association of heavy and light chains, as in the productive association of two different light chains with structurally identical heavy chains in T15 and HPCM3
2. Combinatorial joining of germ-line gene segments, manifested by the use of at least three different *D* segments joined to *V1* and J_H1 in PC-binding heavy chains
3. Junctional diversity, which can alter the length (Fig. 6) as well as the sequence (Fig. 1) of anti-PC variable regions
4. N-region diversity, which appears to generate novel sequences through the additon of nucleotides at the sites of V_H–D and D–J_H joining (Fig. 7)
5. Somatic mutation operating coordinately on V_H, D, J_H, V_κ, and J_κ gene segments, which is responsible for the majority of substitutions in anti-PC antibodies

The PC-binding antibodies that have been analyzed are encoded by as few as nine germ line gene segments (*V1*, V_κM167, V_κM603, V_κT15, J_H1, $J_\kappa5$, and three *D* segments) and yet NH_2-terminal analyses of 42 heavy and light chains have identified 21 variants (R. M. Perlmutter, S. Crews, P. Gearhart, and R. Douglas, unpublished observations). Since new IgG anti-PC variants have been accruing steadily without repetition, we infer that the potential diversity in this system is very large indeed. Extrapolating this result to the total V_H and V_κ repertoire of the mouse, it appears that antibody diversity is essentially unlimited.

In some ways, the detailed molecular dissection of the BALB/c anti-PC antibodies has left us with the misleading impression of structural chaos within this highly restricted population. But in fact, with the exception of group II antibodies which share a very different specificity[30] and origin,[31] the variation in anti-PC antibodies represents a kind of microheterogeneity. The vast majority of PC-binding antibodies induced by carbohydrate vaccines are IgM and IgG3 molecules which bear common serological determinants and are structurally homogeneous. The initial demonstration of a dominant C_H-linked idiotype[5] in anti-PC sera quite correctly predicted the existence of a highly restricted set of germ line genes encoding anti-PC antibodies. Thus, we need look no further than the germ-line V_H and V_κ genes to explain the uniform expression of the T15 idiotype despite the complexity of the specific structure of this determinant.

11. Diversity in Other Antibody Populations

It is as yet too early to tell whether the lessons learned from analysis of PC-binding antibodies will be strictly generalizable to other antibody systems; however, evidence presented elsewhere in this volume in general confirms that restricted antibody populations with a predominant serum idiotypic profile are generated through the use of a small number of germ-line gene segments.[43-45] Murine antibodies induced by group A streptococcal carbohydrate (GAC), for example, constitute a highly restricted population in which hyperimmune animals produce large quantities of extremely homogeneous GAC-binding antibody and no two individuals produce identical molecules.[46] Thus, although the GAC-specific repertoire of each individual mouse is quite small, the repertoire of every mouse strain is quite large. Molecular analysis of the genes encoding GAC-binding antibodies indicates that here, as in the PC system, the observed restriction in antibody heterogeneity reflects the use of a small number of germ-line V_H and V_κ gene segments (R. M. Perlmutter, J. Klotz, M. Bond, M. Nahm, J. M. Davie, and L. Hood, 1984). These results further emphasize the importance of somatic mutation in the generation of antibody diversity.

12. Summary

Murine anti-PC antibodies elicited by immunization with pneumococcal vaccine represent a homogeneous population which shares V_H serological determinants and a limited light-chain repertoire. Application of protein and DNA sequencing strategies to the study of these antibodies provides an extraordinarily detailed view of the generation of antibody diversity. In particular we have learned that:

1. Virtually all of the PC-binding heavy chains utilize a single germ-line V_H gene segment, nevertheless fully half of the completely sequenced anti-PC heavy chains contain sequence substitutions within the region encoded by the V_H gene segment.
2. A majority of substitutions in anti-PC antibodies result from a process of somatic mutation which operates concordantly on both rearranged V_H and V_κ genes.
3. Although the specific structure which defines the T15 idiotype is complex, its predominance in PC-specific antibodies probably reflects the small number of germ-line gene segments which interact to produce efficient PC-binding molecules.
4. The importance of the T15 V_H gene segment can be inferred from the close conservation of this genetic element in rodents.

ACKNOWLEDGMENTS. I thank Connie Katz for secretarial assistance, Dr. Stephen Crews and Jerry Siu for valuable discussions, and Dr. Lee Hood for critical reading of the manuscript. I am the recipient of a New Investigator Award (AI-18088) from the NIH.

References

1. Krause, R. M., 1970, The search for antibodies with molecular uniformity, *Adv. Immunol.* **12**:1-56.
2. Potter, M., 1972, Immunoglobulin-producing tumors and myeloma proteins of mice, *Physiol. Rev.* **52**:631-719.
3. Leon, M. A., and Young, N. M., 1971, Specificity for phosphorylcholine of six murine myeloma proteins reactive with pneumococcus C polysaccharide and B-lipoprotein, *Biochemistry* **10**:1424-1429.
4. Lee, W., Cosenza, H., and Kohler, H., 1974, Clonal restriction of the immune response to phosphorylcholine, *Nature* **247**:55-57.
5. Lieberman, R., Potter, M., Mushinsky, F., Humphrey, W., and Rudikoff, S., 1974, Genetics of a new IgV$_H$ (T15 idiotype) marker in the mouse regulating natural antibody to phosphorylcholine, *J. Exp. Med.* **139**:983-988.
6. Lieberman, R., Rudikoff, S., Humphrey, W., Jr., and Potter, M., 1981, Allelic forms of anti-phosphorylcholine antibodies, *J. Immunol.* **126**:172-176.
7. Cosenza, H., and Kohler, H., 1972, Specific suppression of the antibody response by antibodies to receptors, *Proc. Natl. Acad. Sci. USA* **69**:2701-2705.
8. Claflin, J. L., and Davie, J. M., 1974, Clonal nature of the immune response to phosphorylcholine. III. Species-specific binding characterisitcs of rodent anti-phosphorylcholine antibodies, *J. Immunol.* **113**:1678-1684.
9. Claflin, J. L, and Rudikoff, S., 1976, Uniformity in the clonal repertoire for the immune response to phosphorylcholine in mice: A case for a germline basis of antibody diversity, *Cold Spring Harbor Symp. Quant. Biol.* **41**:725-734.
10. Ruppert, V. J., Williams, K., and Claflin, J. L., 1980, Specific clonal regulation in the immune response to phosphocholine. I. Genetic analysis of the response of a distinct idiotype (M511Id), *J. Immunol.* **124**:1068-1074.
11. Gearhart, P., Sigal, N., and Klinman, N., 1975, Heterogeneity of the BALB/c anti-phosphorylcholine antibody response at the precursor cell level, *J. Exp. Med.* **141**:56-74.
12. Claflin, J. L., and Davie, J. M., 1974, Specific isolation and characterization of antibody directed to binding site antigenic determinants, *J. Immunol.* **114**:70-75.
13. Early, P. W., Huang, H., Davis, M. M., Calame, K., and Hood, L., 1980, An immunoglobulin heavy chain variable region is generated from three segments of DNA: V$_H$, D, and J$_H$, *Cell* **19**:981-992.
14. Gearhart, P., Johnson, N., Douglas, R., and Hood, L., 1981, IgG antibodies to phosphorylcholine exhibit more diversity than their IgM counterparts, *Nature* **291**:29-34.
15. Crews, S., Griffin, J., Huang, H., Calame, K., and Hood, L., 1981, A single V$_H$ gene segment encodes the immune response to phosphorylcholine: Somatic mutation is correlated with the class of the antibody, *Cell* **25**:59-66.
16. Clarke, C., Berenson, J., Goverman, J., Boyer, P. D., Crews, S., Siu, G., and Calame, K., 1982, An immunoglobulin promoter region is unaltered by DNA rearrangement and somatic mutation during B cell development, *Nucleic Acids Res.* **10**:7731-7749.
17. Breathnach, R., and Chambon, P., 1981, Organization and expression of eukaryotic split genes coding for proteins, *Annu. Rev. Biochem.* **50**:349-383.
18. Honjo, T., 1983, Immunoglobulin genes, *Annu. Rev. Immunol.* **1**:499-528.
19. Maki, R., Kearney, J., Paige, C., and Tonegawa, S., 1980, Immunoglobulin gene rearrangement in immature B cells, *Science* **209**:1366-1369.
20. Kim, S., Davis, M. M., Sinn, E., Patten, P., and Hood, L., 1981, Antibody diversity: Somatic hypermutation of rearranged V$_H$ genes, *Cell* **27**:573-581.
21. Kurosawa, Y., and Tonegawa, S., 1982, Organization, structure and assembly of immunoglobulin heavy chain diversity DNA segments, *J. Exp. Med.* **155**:201-218.
22. Alt, F., and Baltimore, D., 1982, Joining of immunoglobulin heavy chain gene segments: Implications from a chromosome with evidence of three D–J$_H$ fusions, *Proc. Natl. Acad. Sci. USA* **79**:4118-4122.
23. Selsing, E., and Storb, U., 1981, Somatic mutation of immunoglobulin light chain variable region genes, *Cell* **25**:47-58.
24. Gershenfeld, H., Tsukamoto, A., Weissman, I. L., and Joho, R., 1981, Somatic diversification is required to generate the V$_\kappa$ genes of MOPC 511 and MOPC 167 myeloma proteins, *Proc. Natl. Acad. Sci. USA* **78**:7674-7678.

25. Gearhart, P. J., and Boganhagen, D., 1983, Clusters of point mutations are found exclusively around rearranged antibody variable genes, *Proc. Natl. Acad. Sci. USA* **80:**3439–3443.

26. Padlan, E. A., Segal, D. M., Spande, T. R., Davies, D. R., Rudikoff, S., and Potter, M., 1973, Structure at 4.5 Å resolution of a phosphorylcholine-binding Fab, *Nature New Biol.* **245:**165–167.

27. Gearhart, P., Sigal, N., and Klinman, N., 1975, Production of antibodies of diverse immunoglobulin classes by cells derived from a single stimulated B cell, *Proc. Natl. Acad. Sci. USA* **72:**1707–1711.

28. Rodwell, J., Gearhart, P., and Karush, F., 1983, Restriction in IgM expression. IV. Affinity analysis of monoclonal anti-phosphorylcholine antibodies, *J. Immunol.* **130:**313–316.

29. Kocher, H. P., Borek, C., and Jaton, J.-C., 1981, The immune response of BABL/c mice to phosphoryl-choline is restricted to a limited number of V_H and V_L isotypes, *Mol. Immunol.* **18:**1027–1033.

30. Chang, S. P., Brown, M., and Rittenberg, M. B., 1982, Immunologic memory to phosphorylcholine. II. PC-KLH induces two antibody populations that dominate different isotypes, *J. Immunol.* **128:**702–710.

31. Chang, S. P., Perlmutter, R. M., Brown, M., Heusser, C. H., Rittenberg, M. B., and Hood, L., 1984, Immunologic memory to phosphorylcholine. IV. Hybridomas representative of group I and group II antibodies utilize distinct V_H genes, *J. Immunol.* **132:**1550–1555.

32. Todd, I., Chang, S. P., Perlmutter, R. M., Aebersold, R., Heusser, C., Hood, L., and Rittenberg, M. B., 1984, Immunologic memory to phosphorylcholine V. Hybridomas representative of group II antibodies utilize V_{κ}1–3 gene(s), *J. Immunol.* **132:**1556–1560.

33. Perlmutter, R. M., Hansburg, D., Briles, D. E., Nicolotti, R. A., and Davie, J. M., 1978, Subclass restriction of murine anti-carbohydrate antibodies, *J. Immunol.* **121:**566–572.

34. Briles, D. E., Forman, C., Hudak, S., and Claflin, J. L., 1982, Antiphosphorylcholine antibodies of the T15 idiotype are optimally protective against *Streptococcus pneumoniae, J. Exp. Med.* **156:**1177–1185.

35. Perlmutter, R. M., and Davie, J. M., 1977, Characterization of molecular heterogeneity and multispecificity in homologous idiotypic antisera, *J. Immunol.* **118:**769–774.

36. Clarke, S. H., Claflin, J. L., and Rudikoff, S., 1982, Polymorphisms in immunoglobulin heavy chains suggesting gene conversion, *Proc. Natl. Acad. Sci. USA* **79:**3280–3284.

37. Bottomly, K., Mathieson, B., and Mosier, D., 1978, Anti-idiotype regulation of helper cell function for the response to phosphorylcholine in adult BALB/c mice, *J. Exp. Med.* **148:**1216–1227.

38. Pillemer, E., and Weissman, I. L., 1981, A monoclonal antibody that detects a V_{κ}-TEPC 15 idiotypic determinant cross-reactive with a Thy-1 determinant, *J. Exp. Med.* **153:**1068–1079.

39. Kabat, E. A., Wu, T. T., Bilofsky, H., Reid-Miller, M., and Perry, H., 1983, *Sequences of Proteins of Immunological Interest,* U.S. Department of Health and Human Services, Public Health Service, National Institutes of Health.

40. Huang, H., Crews, S., and Hood, L., 1918, An immunoglobulin V_H pseudogene, *J. Mol. Appl. Genet.* **1:**93–101.

41. Clarke, S. H., Claflin, J. L., Potter, M., and Rudikoff, S., 1983, Polymorphisms in anti-phosphorylcholine antibodies reflecting evolution of immunoglobulin families, *J. Exp. Med.* **157:**98–113.

42. Riesen, W., Braun, D., and Jaton, J.-C., 1976, Human and murine phosphorylcholine-binding immunoglobulins: Conserved subgroup and first hypervariable region of heavy chains, *Proc. Natl. Acad. Sci. USA* **73:**2096–2100.

43. Bothwell, A. L. M., Paskind, M., Reth, M., Imanishi-Kari, T., Rajewsky, K., and Baltimore, D., 1981, Heavy chain variable region contribution to the NP^b family of antibodies: Somatic mutation evident in a γ2a variable region, *Cell* **24:**625–637.

44. Sims, J., Rabbitts, T. H., Estess, P., Slaughter, C., Tucker, P. W., and Capra, J. D., 1982, Somatic mutation in genes for the variable portion of the immunoglobulin heavy chain, *Science* **216:**309–311.

45. Kaartinen, M., Griffiths, G. M., Hamlyn, P. H., Markham, A. F., Karjalainen, K., Pelkonen, J. L. T., Mäkelä, O., and Milstein, C., 1983, Anti-oxazolone hybridomas and the structure of the oxazolone idiotype, *J. Immunol.* **130:**937–945.

46. Perlmutter, R. M., Briles, D. E., and Davie, J. M., 1977, Complete sharing of light chain spectrotypes by murine IgM and IgG anti-streptococcal antibodies, *J. Immunol.* **118:**2161–2166.

5

Genetic Rearrangements of Human Immunoglobulin Genes

STANLEY J. KORSMEYER, AJAY BAKHSHI, ANDREW ARNOLD, KATHERINE A. SIMINOVITCH, AND THOMAS A. WALDMANN

1. Introduction

The immunoglobulin (Ig) genes ultimately responsible for the generation of antibody diversity and thus the uniqueness or idiotype of each individual molecule produced are organized in a subsegmental, discontinuous fashion in their germ-line form.[1-4] As we will explore, the design of these coding gene subsegments and even the probable mechanisms for their DNA assemblage have been remarkably conserved over evolutionary time.[5-9] This elaborate system utilizes movable gene subsegments, flexibility at the sites of their recombination, and somatic mutation to maximize the number of unique antibody molecules that can be generated from a necessarily limited amount of germline material. While the somatic process of gene recombination creates an amazing diversity of products, these rearrangements have also proven to be rather error-prone. Multiple, alternative chances and choices for assembling an Ig gene appear to compensate for these abortive attempts. We will show that the assemblage of Ig gene subsegments occurs in a sequential fashion during early B-cell development and helps ensure that the final B cell makes but a single Ig molecule. This hierarchy of Ig gene recombination events, mandatory during B-cell development, has proved of great importance in assessing the clonality and stage of differentiation of a variety of human neoplasms. Following the rearrangements that generate the antibody diversity and idiotypes necessary for immune regulation, the Ig gene loci may at times undergo an additional recombination. As we will see, this latter rearrangement is one between chromosomes and results in the translocation of a cellular oncogene to an Ig gene locus within certain human B-cell malignancies.

STANLEY J. KORSMEYER, AJAY BAKHSHI, ANDREW ARNOLD, KATHERINE A. SIMINOVITCH, AND THOMAS A. WALDMANN • Metabolism Branch, National Cancer Institute, Bethesda, Maryland 20205.

2. Evolutionary Conservation of Ig Gene Organization and Assembly

Humans possess multiple separate variable regions, an alternate set of joining regions, and but one constant region for each Ig class or subclass of both light- and heavy-chain genes. The final heavy-chain variable-region polypeptide contains internal information, corresponding to the third hypervariable region (or complementarity-determining region, CDR3) which is contributed in part by additional diversity (D_H) gene segments.[9–11] The three human Ig gene families are located on separate chromosomes with the κ gene complex at 2p11, λ genes at 22q11, and the heavy-chain genes at chromosome 14q32.[12–14] The precise recombinatorial machinery responsible for the assemblage of an intact heavy-chain variable region $(V_H/D_H/J_H)$ and light-chain variable region $(V_\kappa/J_\kappa$ or $V_\lambda/J_\lambda)$ is also likely to be highly conserved. Each of the germ-line V, J, and D_H subsegments is flanked by a heptanucleotide (which is an inverted repeat or palindrome of CAC_T^AGTG). This heptanucleotide is found on the 3′ side of each V segment, 5′ side of each J segment, and on both sides of the D_H segment.[15–17] Flanking each heptanucleotide of a V_H, J_H, J_κ, and V_λ is a spacer of 22 or 23 nucleotides and then a stretch of nine conserved base pairs. This interestingly corresponds to a complementary nonanucleotide that is separated by 11 or 12 bp from a heptanucleotide flanking germ-line D_H, V_κ, and J_λ segments. Thus, it appears that a heptanucleotide and nonanucleotide possessing an internal 11-bp spacer always pairs with a matched set of sequences containing the 22-bp spacer.[10] The fact that the heptanucleotides and nonanucleotides flank all of these subsegments and are found in all species examined suggests that they are active participants in bringing V_L/J_L and $V_H/D_H/J_H$ regions together.

In addition, in certain B-cell neoplasms the Ig gene loci parrticipate in a novel type of recombination which juxtaposes pieces of separate chromosomes. These chromosomal translocations introduce a cellular oncogene, c-*myc*, into one of the Ig gene regions on chromosome 14, 2, or 22 within selected acute human B-cell malignancies.[18] This also represents an evolutionarily conserved recombinatorial event as mouse plasmacytomas also translocate c-*myc* into portions of their chromosomes bearing Ig genes.[19]

3. Human κ Light-Chain Genes

κ light chains comprise approximately 60% of human light-chain protein. The general design of this locus is presented in the schematic diagram in Fig. 1. The human κ gene locus is located on the short arm of chromsome 2 at band 2p11.[12] There are multiple different V_κ segments in man each of which is foreshortened, coding for only the first 95 amino acids of the final variable-region protein. Each of the regions appears to have its own associated leader or signal peptide sequence coding for a highly hydrophobic peptide which facilitates the transmembrane passage of this molecule. The precise number of germ-line V_κ segments has not been determined. Four distinct V_κ subgroups are known to exist from available protein sequence data. Subgroup II has a distinctly unique family of V_κ genes coding for it, whereas data from Bently and Rabbitts argue that the genes responsible for the V_κ I, III, and IV subgroups may cross-hybridize and perhaps belong to a single large family.[5,20] If so, the number of available germ-line V_κ genes in man (perhaps around 30 or less) may be considerably less than the estimated repertoire of V_κ segments in the

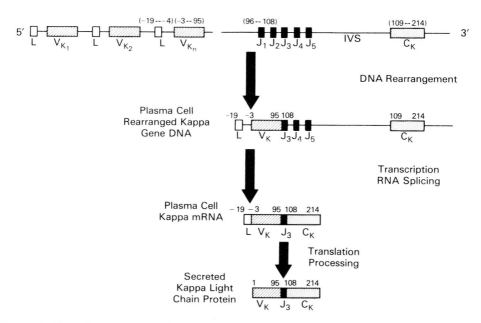

FIGURE 1. Schematic representation of the human κ gene locus, located on chromosome 2 at band 2p11. In its germ-line form there are multiple different variable regions (V_κ) each accompanied by a leader (L) sequence. Man has five functional joining (J_κ) segments but there is only one constant region (C_κ) per allele. A DNA rearrangement juxtaposes a single V_κ and J_κ segment. This rearranged gene is transcribed and the remaining intervening sequence (IVS) information is removed by RNA splicing.

mouse.[20] Man does have five fully functional joining (J_κ) segments which can presumably recombine with any of the available V_κ segments.[6] While there are identifiable allelic forms of κ chain based on the single amino acid marker, Inv, there is but one constant C_κ region per allele. The Inv marker, as it is located within the C_κ region, is unlikely to significantly alter the structure of the molecule or contribute to the unique difference of idiotype. At some point during the differentiation of a B-cell precursor into a κ-producing B cell, a process of DNA rearrangement occurs which juxtaposes one of the many V_κ regions with a particular joining J_κ segment (Fig. 1). This rearranged allele is transcribed and the remaining intervening sequences removed by RNA splicing. The final mRNA is translated into a complete light-chain product that includes the 19-amino-acid leader peptide responsible for the transmembrane passage of this secreted protein; the leader sequence is subsequently removed, presumably by enzymatic cleavage.

4. Human λ Light-Chain Genes

Man frequently utilizes his λ light-chain genes, being present in approximately 40% of Ig molecules, whereas the mouse uses λ less than 5% of the time. Based on amino acid sequences the V_λ gene repertoire will prove to be much greater in man than the markedly contracted system in the mouse. In contrast to the κ gene locus, the λ gene locus has multiple duplicated C_λ regions each of which may have its own J_λ segment.[7] These λ genes are arranged in tandem along the long arm of chromosome 22 at band 22q11 (Fig. 2). Nucleic acid sequencing of the first three constant regions in this locus revealed that they represented genes encoding the C_λ regions bearing the amino acid markers Mcg, Ke$^-$Oz$^-$, and Ke$^-$Oz$^+$, respectively (Fig. 2).[7] These distinctive C_λ isotypes were previously identified by serological and amino acid analysis of human λ light-chain proteins. This human λ gene locus has proven to be rather polymorphic in the normal population as depicted by a series of restriction fragment length polymorphisms.[21] As is evident in Fig. 2 this genetic polymorphism is detected by variations in the length of the center EcoRI fragment. Taub et al.[21] revealed that in its simplest form this fragment is but 8 kb in size and contains the two constant λ regions, Ke$^-$Oz$^-$ and Ke$^-$Oz$^+$. There are, however, multiple allelic forms of this center fragment which can be either 8, 13, 18, or 23 kb in size (Fig. 2). Curiously, the increment in each enlargement of this EcoRI fragment is approximately 5 kb. In fact, this internally duplicated 5-kb fragment actually contains a single C_λ region such that while the 8-kb allele has but two C_λ regions, the 23-kb alternative has five. The presence of this repeated unit suggests that the duplication event might have arisen by an unequal crossing over at meiosis. The variable amplification of the C_λ genes in this locus means that the actual number of C_λ genes in man can vary between 6 and 9 per haploid genome depending on whether the 8-, 13-, 18-, or 23-kb allele is inherited. As a J_λ region may prove to be associated with each C_λ region, this gene duplication may provide an advantage to the organism by increasing antibody diversity. In addition, this EcoRI-defined restriction fragment length polymorphism also serves as an allelic marker located directly at the DNA level of chromosome 22. Such markers may facilitate the mapping of inherited diseases to specific chromosomes in man. In summary, the light-chain gene classes are much more balanced in their expression in man than for example in the mouse. In addition, the respective contribution of κ and λ genes to antibody diversity has been accomplished in a strikingly different evolutionary fashion. The κ genes utilize a tandem strip of multiple alternative J segments, while the λ gene locus has expanded, and may still be amplifying, $J_\lambda C_\lambda$ units.

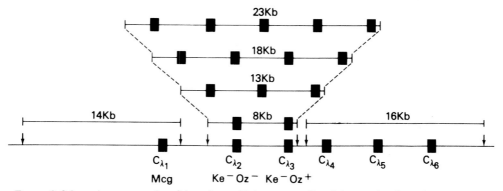

FIGURE 2. Schematic representation of the polymorphic human germline C_λ gene regions located on chromosome 22 at 22q11. In its simplest form, six C_λ regions are found on EcoRI-generated restriction endonuclease fragments of 14, 8, and 16 kb. There are multiple allelic forms of the center EcoRI fragment which can be 8, 13, 18, or 23 kb. This incremental enlargement of the center fragment actually increases the number of C_λ regions present. Mcg, Ke, and Oz represent amino acid markers that distinguish the separate C_λ regions.

5. Human Heavy-Chain Genes

The heavy-chain gene locus is similar to that of light chains but has the additional complexity of having a third genetic component of the variable-region protein, the so-called D_H or diversity segment.[9] Early nucleic acid sequences of germline variable (V_H) and joining (J_H) gene segments indicated that they did not encode a central portion of the variable heavy-chain protein which fell within the third hypervariable region (CDR3). As mentioned earlier, the spacer between the heptanucleotide and nonanucleotide recombinatorial signals was 22 bp for both the 3' side of the V_H segments and the 5' side of the J_H segments. This was inconsistent with the previously noted rule for association of an 11- with a 22-bp spacer in V/J recombination of light-chain genes. These observations predicted the existence of the third gene subsegment for the heavy-chain variable protein. This genetic element has been found in both mice and humans and consists of a short coding segment flanked on both 5' and 3' sides with the predicted 11-bp spacer separating the recombinatorial sequences. These elements have been termed *diversity segments (D$_H$)* and there appear to be closely related families of D_H segments which are tandemly arranged within the genome (Fig. 3A).[9-11] Siebenlist, Leder, and co-workers have now identified at least three such distinct families of D_H segments in man located within approximately 35 kb of DNA on chromosome 14. Of note is the remarkably even spacing of these D_H segments within the genome and the considerable amount of homology shared by the flanking sequence surrounding these elements. These findings suggest that the multiple D_H segments have arisen by a relatively recent duplication of a basic subunit.[9]

There are six active joining (J_H) gene segments in man located 5' to the switch and constant μ (C_μ) regions (Fig. 3A).[8] Additionally, three pseudo-J_H sequences exist within this area as does a germ-line D_H region which is between $J_\psi 1$ and $J_H 1$ (Fig. 3B).[8] The J_H region of man is thus more complex than that of the mouse and this appears to be attributable to recent duplication events. Over 90% of the variable-region protein sequences available for this portion of the molecule can be accounted for by the six functional J_H regions. The three nonfunctional pseudo-J_H regions have lost their 3' donor splice sites necessary for proper RNA splicing to join the J_H and C_μ information. In addition, their internal sequences have apparently drifted and no longer encode recognizable J_H-region protein sequences. Surprisingly, however, these three pseudo-J_H regions have retained rather authentic heptanucleotide aned nonanucleotide recombinatorial signals and the proper 22-bp spacers.[8] This indicates that they may well be utilized in D/J recombinations that would not result in a functional variable-region protein (aberrant rearrangements). The conservation of the recombinatorial signals in fact suggests that such aberrant rearrangements may themselves serve a purpose that is selectively retained!

The major portion of the variable-region protein is contributed by the intact germline gene subsegment, the variable (V_H) region.[22] The V_H regions encode approximately the first 99 amino acids of the variable portion of the molecule which contains the first and second hypervariable regions (CDR1 and CDR2). There are four V_H subgroups in man predicted from amino acid sequences and corresponding V_H gene families have been identified. The precise number and exact location of the V_H regions are as yet uncertain. Some of these germline V_H segments have been shown to be pseudogenes, so that the number of functional V_H elements may well be less than the total.[22] No further subcompartmentalization of the variable regions has been identified within germline DNA.[23] Thus, while

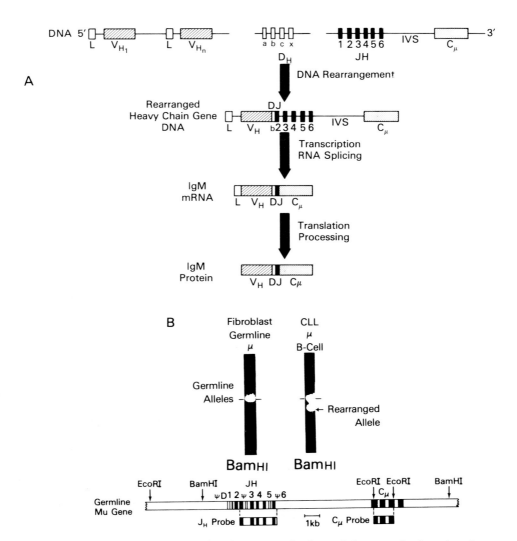

FIGURE 3. (A) Schematic representation of the human germ-line heavy-chain gene region located on chromosome 14 at 14q32. Multiple variable regions (V_H) each have their own associated leader sequences (L) and
there are six functional joining (J_H) segments separated by an intervening sequence (IVS) from a single con-
stant-μ (C_μ) region. In addition, there are several families of diversity (D_H) segments which are the middle
component of the $V_H/D_H/J_H$ recombinations formed by the first DNA rearrangement. (B) Map of the germ-
line heavy-chain gene region indicating a J_H probe and C_μ probe which can be used to identify a rearranged
heavy-chain gene in the *Bam*HI-digested DNA of a μ-producing monoclonal B cell from a patient with chronic
lymphocytic leukemia (CLL).

the D_H segment and its site of juncture with V_H and J_H segments corresponds neatly to the CDR3 region, there are no identified further gene subsegments or recombinational signals which can account for the presence of the CDR1 and CDR2 regions. Curiously, however, homology has been noted between a hypervariable II sequence and a human D_H gene subsegment.[24] This might reflect a common evolutionary origin of the D_H gene and an internal portion of the germ-line V_H gene; alternatively, it may be that the long stretch of tandemly arranged diversity (D_H) elements are capable of influencing internal portions of germline V_H regions through other mechanisms such as gene conversion.

6. Sequential Rearrangement of Human Ig Genes

An examination of the B-cell precursor series of man reveals evidence for serial stages of Ig gene recombination during ontogeny. The previously termed "non-T, non-B" type of acute lymphocytic leukemia has been shown to represent monoclonal expansions of human B-cell precursors.[25] All of these cells had rearrangements of their heavy-chain genes. Approximately one-half of these cases display only rearranged heavy-chain genes but have retained light-chain genes in their germ-line configuration (Figs. 3 and 4). There is also a sequential expression of B-cell-associated surface antigens in which those sets of cells with heavy-chain gene rearrangements alone are the least mature, displaying ony the earliest antigens.[26] A close examination of these heavy-chain gene rearrangements indicated that all had undergone recombination at the J_H gene subsegments. Such rearrangements can be either D_H/J_H intermediate forms of rearrangement or attempts at $V_H/D_H/J_H$ recombinations. Of note, there were no instances in which the D_H gene segments were recombined and the J_H regions remained germ line. This is consistent with the thesis that D_H/J_H recombinations would precede V_H/D_H joining.[27] However, Siebenlist, Leder, and coworkers (unpublished data) have identified a V_H/D_H recombinant on an allele which also displays a separate D_H/J_H joining. This establishes that V_H recombination to a D_H segment that has not recombined with a J_H segment can occur, as well as joining of V_H segments secondarily to preexisting D_H/J_H recombinations. If these H-chain recombinations of $V_H/D_H/J_H$ are effective, cytoplasmic μ chain may be present.[28] Alternatively, such recombinations can be ineffective or aberrant with no production of μ chain. This system of gene subsegment assemblage is extraordinarily flexible, but appears also to be rather error-prone.[29] Up to 80% of these B-cell precursors do not produce cytoplasmic Ig and many may represent cells that possess only aberrantly rearranged heavy-chain genes.[26] Within this group may be a set of cells that are ostensibly trapped in the B-cell precursor series because their ineffective rearrangements have eliminated necessary germline gene subsegments required for the assemblage of an effective heavy-chain gene (Fig. 4). Predictable examples of such genetically trapped cells would be cells that had aberrantly rearranged D_H segments to the J_H region that is farthest downstream (J_H6) on both heavy-chain gene chromsome 14s. Such cells would lack any remaining germ-line J_H segments necessary for recombinations. Another example of cells incapable of maturing to Ig-bearing B cells would be those with aberrant $V_H/D_H/J_H$ recombinations on both heavy-chain alleles. Such cells may well have deleted all of their internal D_H gene families and be unable to assemble a valid gene (Figs. 3A and 4).

Also within the B-cell precursor leukemias of man are cells that have progressed to

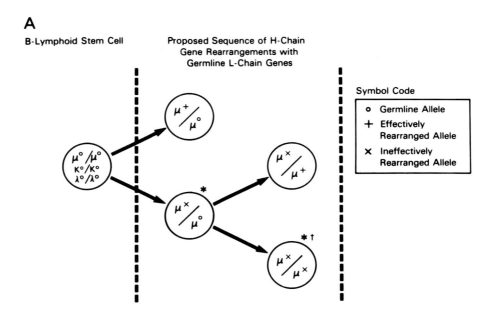

FIGURE 4. (A) Hypothetical sequence of heavy-chain gene rearrangements in B-cell precursors in which an uncommitted B-lymphoid stem cell would have all of its Ig genes in the germ-line form ($\mu°$ $\kappa°$ $\lambda°$). Rearrangement would begin with the heavy-chain genes and if effective (μ^+) a μ-producing cell capable of further maturation would result. Many rearrangements are ineffective ($\mu^\times$) and result in cells incapable of heavy-chain production regardless of whether their light chains subsequently rearrange (*). This would include a subset of cells trapped within the B-cell precursor series (†) because they have eliminated all germ-line J_H or D_H segments necessary for further recombinations of their genes. (B) Proposed sequence of light-chain rearrangements within human B-cell precursors which had rearranged heavy-chain genes. Light-chain gene rearrangements begin with κ genes and if ineffective ($\kappa^\times$), λ rearrangements could follow. Cells with effectively rearranged κ^+ or λ^+ could become mature B cells (‡) if prior heavy-chain rearrangements were also effective. Cells with only ineffective rearrangements (*) would remain within the B-cell precursor series as they would lack light-chain production. Similarly, a population of B-cell precursors which had exhausted all light-chain recombinational opportunities might exist (†).

light-chain gene recombination.[25] Their patterns of κ and λ light-chain gene recombination predict a model in which κ light-chain genes rearrange before λ in man.[25] As noted, humans utilize both light-chain classes, expressing κ approximately 60% of the time and λ, 40%. Despite this, an examination of mature human B-cell lines and leukemias revealed that κ producers retained germ line λ genes whereas λ-producing B cells had no germline genes remaining, having either rearranged or deleted them (Fig. 5).[30] This loss of germline κ genes in λ-producing B cells proved to be a normal developmental event and not a phenomenon secondary to transformation. Specifically, over 95% of the collective κ genes in the λ-bearing B cells of peripheral blood from a normal individual were no longer in their germline form.[31] The majority of these κ genes were deleted (60%) while the remainder were present but in a rearranged state. In addition, the incidence of κ gene deletion was higher in older established λ B-cell lines than in fresh cell lines or normal cells, indicating that the deletion of κ genes may constitute a secondary event that follows a V/J recombi-

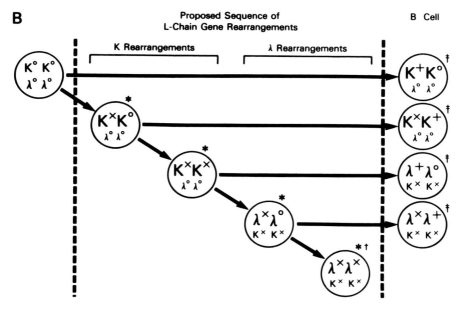

FIGURE 4. (Continued)

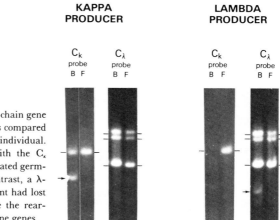

FIGURE 5. A representative example of light-chain gene analysis on κ- and λ-producing B cells (B) as compared to a matching fibroblast (F) from the same individual. A rearranged κ gene was demonstrable with the C_κ probe while the C_λ probe revealed the anticipated germline λ gene in a κ-producing B cell. In contrast, a λ-producing B cell with a λ gene rearrangement had lost both copies of its C_κ gene. Arrows indicate the rearranged genes; hashmarks indicate the germline genes.

nation.[31] Such findings in normal and transformed mature B cells predicted a series of intermediate light-chain gene configurations within B-cell precursors as diagrammed in Fig. 4. This included the occasional loss of germline κ genes in cells that had not rearranged their λ genes. Such potential patterns of light-chain gene rearrangement were indeed observed within the B-cell precursor leukemias. Overall, each of the seven B-cell precursors in which κ genes had been recombined retained germline λ genes, whereas the four with λ recombinations had no remaining germline κ genes.[26]

Thus, despite the nearly equal usage of the two light-chain isotypes in man, there appears to be an order to their rearrangement in which κ precedes λ. Due to the appreciable use of both light-chain classes in man, their ordered rearrangement cannot be explained as a purely statistical event. If this order were determined only by chance, then λ recombinations should frequently be observed in κ-producing B cells and λ-bearing B cells should at times retain germline κ genes. However, the observed order of κ before λ recombination in man might be based on different inherent rates of recombination for the κ and λ genes. If, for example, aberrant recombinations around the J_κ region occurred more readily than λ rearrangements, then any cell that ultimately produced λ light chain would nearly always have rearranged its κ genes. A greater frequency of κ over λ rearrangements might result not only from a difference in the number of $V_\kappa J_\kappa$ vs. $V_\lambda J_\lambda$ recombination sites, but also from an inherent difference in their recombinational affinities. Alternatively, it is also possible that the recombination of κ genes before λ is a strictly regulated system that requires κ gene recombination before λ genes can be rearranged. One could imagine a negative control element located near the κ gene that prevented λ recombination. This hypothesis would hold that this element would have to be inactivated by an attempted κ gene rearrangement before λ rearrangement would be allowed to proceed.

Neither the mechanism nor the exact advantage of a hierarchial system which proceeds from heavy-chain gene rearrangements to light chain and from κ to λ within the light-chain genes is certain. If, however, Ig gene rearrangement occurs at a time of rapid cell division, such a staggered cascade of rearrangements might well enhance antibody diversity. For example, if a B-cell progenitor cell that rearranged its heavy-chain genes effectively underwent cell division, its numerous progeny would each be capable of independent light-chain selection. Similarly, cell divisions during light-chain rearrangements might also increase the number of unique κ and λ chains associated with the original heavy chain. By the same token, it has been proposed that aberrant rearrangements precede effective recombinations and that the latter halt the recombinatorial process.[33] If cell division were occurring during this process, then even the initial aberrant rearrangement of Ig heavy- or light-chain genes might also serve the same purpose of increasing the number of antibody specificities generated from an initial B-lymphoid stem cell. Such a hierarchial system of aberrant and effective rearrangements may also help ensure that an individual B cell make but a single allele of a selected isotype (Fig. 4).[30-33]

7. Human Heavy-Chain Gene Order and Class Switch

During the development of a B cell it initially expresses only surface IgM, but subsequently may simultaneously produce IgM and IgD, and later is capable of switching to the production of another isotype of IgG, IgA, or IgE. When such switches in the constant heavy-chain isotype occur, however, the same assembled variable region and its consequent idiotype appears to be retained. This phenomenon has been shown to result from a second type of DNA rearrangement, the heavy-chain class switch, which moves a more distally located constant region into closer proximity with the previously assembled $V_H/D_H/J_H$ segments (Fig. 6).[34-37] These recombinatorial events appear to be mediated through switch sites that are located at the 5' side of each constant region. These switch (S) regions are comprised of tandemly arranged units of 5-bp repetitive elements of GAGCT and GGGGT.[35] These switch regions may span several thousand base pairs 5' to each of the constant regions. Analysis of heavy-chain genes in mature B cells and plasmacytomas that have switched from IgM production, has revealed that the exact site of recombination has occurred within the S_μ and the S site of the ultimately expressed constant region (Fig. 6).[36] This recombination is presumably facilitated by the striking homology of the repeated units comprising switch regions. While the precise location of recombination can vary, the consensus sequence of YAGGTTA has been noted near such recombination points and may be involved in focusing the point of recombination.[37] While the sequence homology of the various isotype-associated switch regions is remarkably similar, their functional homology as measured by their affinity for one another by heteroduplex analysis does vary. For example, the human S_μ and S_α appear more homologous to each other than either does to various S_γ regions.[38,39] The presence of such differences leaves open the possibility that class-specific mechanisms might exist which help direct the isotype selected.

The establishment of the heavy-chain gene order has also provided insights into the mechanisms of expression for the different classes. While the precise gene order and relative spacing for the entire heavy-chain gene cluster are as yet not totally determined, considerable information does exist (Fig. 6). The close proximity of the C_μ and C_δ regions in man, as was found in the mouse, appears to allow the simultaneous production of IgM and IgD.[8,40,41] RNA transcripts including the same recombined $V_H/D_H/J_H$ segments could either terminate after the C_μ or C_δ region and subsequently undergo a differential processing at alternative RNA splice sites to produce a mature μ mRNA or δ mRNA. In contrast,

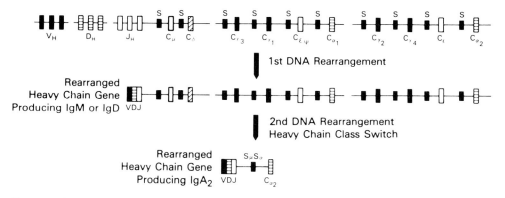

FIGURE 6. Schematic representation of the human germline C_H-region gene order. Following the first DNA rearrangement assembling $V_H/D_H/J_H$ segments, a cell can produce IgM and IgD. A second DNA rearrangement involving the highly homologous switch sites (S) results in the production of one of the distally located isotypes as is demonstrated here for an IgA2-producing cell.

the C_γ, C_ϵ, and C_α regions are located considerably more distally and have undergone a switching event between the S_μ region and their respective S sites in IgG-, IgE-, or IgA-producing mature human B cells.

Analysis of cosmid clones containing germline genes for human heavy-chain constant regions has indicated that the evolutionary expansion of heavy-chain genes in man involves a relatively large distal (3′) duplication (Fig. 6).[42] This event appears to have duplicated two C_γs, a C_ϵ, and a C_α unit. The first C_ϵ region is a pseudogene lacking the C_H1 and C_H2 domains.[43] Man is known to express both a $C_\alpha1$ and a $C_\alpha2$ gene as well as four C_γ genes. In addition, there appears to be a pseudogamma gene within this locus.[44] The gene order of these human constant regions is of considerable interest when considering some humoral immunodeficiency syndromes. It is curious that a number of patients with IgA deficiency, associated with several different disease states, have also been noted to have reduced or absent IgE, IgG2, and IgG4. These underproduced heavy-chain isotypes happen to be the most distally located genes in this cluster (Fig. 6). All such cases examined to date do have these constant-region genes present in their germ-line DNA. However, their 3′ location raises the possibility that there might be a defect in the capacity to switch to or express these distal constant regions.

The heavy-chain class switch itself does not change the antibody specificity generated by the first DNA rearrangement which generates the $V_H/D_H/J_H$ recombination. It has, however, been proposed that the change to IgG or IgA heavy-chain isotypes is associated with a higher incidence of somatic mutation within the variable region. Of certain immense importance to the organism, however, is the functional diversity created by this switching process. By introducing new constant regions to the previously established antibody specificity, numerous different final effector functions can be associated with a given variable region.

8. Summary of Mechanisms in the Generation of Antibody Diversity

At least four types of genetic mechanisms contribute to the generation of the total repertoire of unique antibody specificities or individual idiotypes that can be produced. These different mechanisms include (1) a large number of germline gene subsegments that encode portions of the final variable-region peptide, (2) random recombination of these various gene subsegments to create multiple different assortments, (3) a flexibility at the recombination sites, and (4) mutation that results in changes of amino acids within the variable-region protein. Both heavy- and light-chain variable-region peptides result from the presumably random assemblage of multiple alternative gene subsegments belonging to separate gene families of heavy, κ and λ genes. For example, in the case of the heavy-chain genes: if each individual D_H segment were capable of 3′ recombination with any of six functional J_H segments and 5′ recombination with any of a large number of available V_H regions, then considerable diversity could result from such recombinational shuffling alone. In addition, the flexible frame of recombination at the juncture sites of $V_H/D_H/J_H$ and V_L/J_L segments generates different amino acid codons at these junctional locations; this has been termed *junctional diversity*.[45] An analysis of the heavy-chain gene recombinations has revealed additional amino acid changes about the D_H recombination points not accounted for in the germline genes. These additional nucleotides (N) may reflect the existence of an exonuclease and add-on mechanism that contributes further unique nucleotides at the juncture sites of $V_H/D_H/J_H$ rearrangements.[27]

Another process capable of enhancing diversity beyond what is present as germ-line information is somatic mutation. Clear examples of somatic mutation affecting the variable-region proteins of both heavy and light chains are now available.[46–49] Such mutations have been noted throughout the variable regions, including their flanking introns, and are thus not solely focused at the sites of CDRs. In fact, the exact importance of somatic mutation versus other potential mechanisms such as gene conversion in accounting for the variability in CDR1 and CDR2 is as yet unresolved. While the precise number of functional V_H and D_H segments is unknown, it is clear that recombinatorial joining of the three heavy-chain subsegments, together with the contributions of junctional diversity and later somatic mutation, should be able to create well over 10^5 different heavy-chain variable-region proteins. Similar genetic mechanisms operate for both types of light-chain genes, κ and λ. If each different heavy- and light-chain gene product which could be produced could associate with each other, a further multiplication of antibody specificities would result. These genetic mechanisms provide the organism with the capacity to somatically generate the requisite 10^6 to 10^9 different antibodies of the immune response.

In addition to the above mechanisms that generate variation in antigen-binding specificity, further events in these loci expand the functional diversity of the system. The second DNA rearrangement of the heavy-chain locus that accomplishes the class switch allows the same assembled $V_H/D_H/J_H$ and its resultant specificity to be recombined with the multiple different effector functions contributed by the separate constant-region isotypes of C_γ, C_α, and C_ϵ. Similarly, the optional sites of poly(A) addition following the C_μ and C_δ region, coupled with alternative patterns for RNA splicing, allow the same antibody specificity to be simultaneously expressed on both IgM and IgD molecules. This same mechanism of differential RNA processing also allows either a secreted or a membrane terminus to be alternatively attached to each of the heavy-chain isotypes.[50,51] This process, once again, enables two functionally distinct peptides with different effector functions to be created for a single antibody specificity.

9. Further Rearrangements within the Ig Gene Locus; Burkitt's Lymphoma

Chromosomal translocation represents an additional DNA recombination that may occur near the various Ig loci within certain acute human B-cell malignancies. This is a rearrangement that involves the juxtaposition of information originally located on separate chromosomes. Certain chromosomal translocations are indeed specifically associated with histologically distinct neoplasms.[52] One such translocation is frequently found in Burkitt's lymphoma and occasionally in other acute human B-cell malignancies. This chromosomal aberration t(8;14) usually involves a reciprocal translocation of chromosome 14 at band q32 and chromosome 8 at band q24 (Fig. 7). It was of considerable interest that somatic cell genetic studies placed the human heavy-chain genes on chromsome 14, and later refinements in chromosomal *in situ* hybridization allowed Kirsch and his co-workers to pinpoint this locus to 14q32.[14,53] This potential association of Burkitt's lymphoma translocations with Ig gene loci was strengthened when several cells with variant forms of translocation

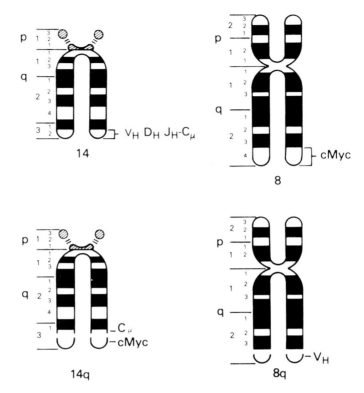

FIGURE 7. Schematic presentation of the normal and reciprocally translocated chromosomes in Burkitt's lymphoma t(8;14) translocation. The normal chromosome 14 possesses the effectively rearranged $V_H/D_H/J_H$ responsible for the cell's IgM production. The normal chromosome 8 retains a germ-line copy of c-*myc*. The $14q^+$ chromosome has received a portion of chromosome 8 bearing c-*myc* at band 14q32 and usually retains the C_μ region on that chromosome. The $8q^-$ chromosome at the breakpoint 8q24 has reciprocally received a portion of chromosome 14 which often includes V_H gene segments.

involving chromosomes 2p11 and 22q11 were discovered.[54] These sites subsequently proved to be the location of the κ and λ Ig genes, respectively.[12,13] Thus, one side of this chromosomal recombination seemed to occur at or near the Ig gene loci which are actively transcribed and involved in the phenotypic identity of a B cell. Considerable attention focused on what the other chromosomal segment, 8q24, that was uniformly involved with either 14q32, 2p11, or 22q11 translocations, might be contributing. As these translocations were found in some malignant human B cells but not in normal human B cells or even Epstein–Barr virus-transformed B-cell lines, the possibility that the locus at 8q24 was contributing to the malignant phenotype was entertained. Within recent years a candidate set of cancer-related genes have been identified within higher eukaryotic organisms. These so-called cellular oncogenes (c-*onc*) represent the normal cellular homologs of the transforming principles identified in a number of retroviruses (v-*onc*).[55] These c-*onc* genes are highly conserved throughout evolution, are probably the source of the transforming v-*onc* sequences present in viruses, and presumably play important roles in normal cellular growth and differentiation. In fact, one such c-*onc* gene, known as c-*myc*, was known to be activated by the nearby integration of avian leukosis virus in bursal lymphomas of the chicken.[56] The finding by Taub, Kirsch, and their co-workers, by *in situ* hybridization, that the human c-*myc* gene was located at 8q24 was of profound importance (Fig. 7).[18] Not only was it at the exact band involved in the Burkitt's translocation, but examination of DNA from such cells showed that it was actually rearranged in a number of instances. Further studies by Erickson and co-workers have revealed important aspects about this event.[57] They prepared a series of cross-species somatic cell hybrids between Burkitt's lymphoma cells and mouse plasmacytomas which variably retained different human chromosomes. Using these hybrids they have been able to show that the normal chromosome 14 is the chromosome associated with the production of heavy-chain Ig in these cells and thus contains the effectively recombined $V_H/D_H/J_H$ and C_μ region producing IgM (Fig. 7). In contrast, the $14q^+$ translocated chromosome has the aberrantly rearranged Ig gene and has also had c-*myc* present on it in all cases analyzed to date. The $8q^-$ chromosome has reciprocally received various portions of the Ig gene locus, frequently having some V_H genes present there. The remaining normal chromosome 8 has a germ-line copy of the c-*myc* gene present (Fig. 7). Further studies by Nishikura, Croce, and co-workers have indicated that the translocated c-*myc* on the $14q^+$ chromosome and not the normal c-*myc* left on chromosome 8 is selectively transcribed when it is placed into a mouse plasmacytoma. Interestingly, this translocated c-*myc* is not expressed when the $14q^+$ chromosome is placed into a fibroblast, indicating that there may be some tissue restriction to its expression.[58] This further focuses attention on the importance of introducing the c-*myc* gene into a position near the Ig genes. As Ig genes are actively transcribed at this stage of B-cell differentiation, it is possible that mechanisms which augment Ig transcription in such cells may also positively influence the transcription of c-*myc*. In this regard, Gillies, Tonegawa, and co-workers have discovered an apparent enhancer sequence located within the heavy-chain gene locus between J_H and S_μ areas.[59] This area is capable of augmenting the production of extraneous genes linked to it if they are introduced into a plasmacytoma target cell. It is tantalizing to speculate that this Ig-region enhancer might play a role in augmenting the production of an associated, translocated c-*myc* gene. In this regard, we questioned what would happen to the expression of c-*myc* in a B-cell stage lymphoma bearing a classic t(8;14) translocation that could be induced to differentiate toward the plasma cell stage. Following exposure to a phorbol ester this B cell became more plasmacytoid, increasing its secretion of IgM with an antecedent increase in the transcription of C_μ that was predominantly the secreted, μ_s, as oppose to the membrane, μ_m, mRNA form If c-*myc* were pivotally responsible for maintaining the arrested state of maturation, one would envisage that the transcription of c-*myc* might decrease as the cell underwent the process of differentiation. In fact, however, c-*myc* transcription was minimally increased as was Ig gene transcription during differentiation, supporting the hypothesis that these genes might be coordinately regulated in this setting.[60]

The precise recombinational breakpoint on the $14q^+$ chromosome between the heavy-chain gene locus and the c-*myc* gene locus can vary considerably. Studies by Taub, Battey, Leder, and co-workers[18] have revealed that c-*myc* can be introduced into the human Ig gene region in either orientation and is frequently in the opposite orientation of the C_μ region, with c-*myc* transcription consequently originating off the opposite strand from C_μ.

The translocated c-*myc* gene may contain all three of its original exons including the first nontranslated exon or may only move the second and third structural coding exons to chromosome 14. They have found that the precise breakpoint on chromosome 14 may be as close as the S_μ area proximal to C_μ or can be a considerable distance removed. Even if the gene is not in direct proximity to C_μ, it may be that the translocation even results in a change in the environment of the c-*myc* locus which is the most important shared feature of this phenomenon. The precise importance of this oncogene shuffling awaits the identification of the function of the c-*myc* product and its effect on normal B cells.

10. Ig Gene Rearrangements in Human B-Lymphoid Neoplasms

The analysis of Ig gene rearrangements has proven to be of marked value in determining the cellular lineage and clonality of a variety of controversial human lymphoid malignancies. Rearrangement of both heavy- and light-chain genes is mandatory within mature B cells and occurs early during differentiation in a sequential order in man as we have previously discussed.[25] In contrast, most hemopoietic cells of non-B-cell origin retain their Ig genes in the germ-line form. This includes monocytic, histiocytic, myeloid, and promyelocytic cell lines and leukemias, which display germline heavy- and light-chain genes.[26] In addition, all human T-cell malignancies we have studied uniformly retained germline light-chain genes and most (23/25) also retained germline heavy-chain genes. These findings would indicate that any antigen-specific receptor present on these T cells was not the product of Ig genes as they have classically been utilized in B cells. Specifically, we do not find uniform rearrangements or deletions of the J_H, D_H, C_H, J_κ and C_κ, or J_λ and C_λ segments. Therefore, the detection of rearranged heavy- and light-chain genes within a lymphoid neoplasm also serves as a B-cell-lineage specific marker.[61]

We have utilized this difference in Ig gene configurations in the B-cell series versus non-B cells to examine a variety of human malignancies of controversial cellular origin. As discussed above, all cases of the "non-T, non-B" type of acute lymphocytic leukemia in reality represent a developmental series of B-cell precursors that revealed evidence for the sequential rearrangement of Ig genes in man.[25,26] Similarly, the lymphoid blast crisis phases of chronic myelogenous leukemia (CML) lacked definitive cell surface antigens that would allow them to be clearly classified as of either T-cell or B-cell origin. When their Ig genes were examined, they displayed heavy-chain gene rearrangements and some cases had progressed on to light-chain gene rearrangement.[62] These findings were strong evidence for placing the cells of CML lymphoid blast crisis in a B-cell precursor category. In addition, serial studies of a single patient during multiple phases of his disease revealed that two separate lymphoid blast crisis episodes represented monoclonal expansions of malignant cells at distinctly different stages of genetic maturation. Both crises displayed identical heavy-chain gene rearrangements, but one had progressed to λ light-chain gene recombination while the other had germline light-chain genes. Thus, the clonally affected B cells in CML are capable of differentiation and sequential Ig gene rearrangements. The discovery of effectively rearranged and transcribed Ig genes, characteristic of a mature B-cell stage of development, also definitively assigned the cellular origin of hairy cell leukemia. Quite provocatively, however, this genotypic B-cell malignancy appears to represent a unique stage of B-cell differentiation that expresses a T-cell activation antigen (Tac) that is the membrane receptor for T-cell growth factor.[63]

A polyclonal population of normal B cells possesses numerous different Ig gene rearrangements, and collectively none of its Ig gene rearrangements are detectable because they are below the threshold of sensitivity for a Southern blot. In contrast, a monoclonal expansion represents the progeny of a single cell that will display a unique, identifiable DNA rearrangement. This serves as a sensitive and specific marker capable of identifying even minority populations (5%) of clonal B cells within tissues of mixed cellularity.[61] This genetic marker of Ig rearrangement has enabled us to assign a diagnosis of lymphoma to a malignancy of totally uncertain cell type. We have also demonstrated the presence of monoclonal B cells in several malignant lymph nodes in which T cells actually predominated and mistaken diagnoses of T-cell lymphomas had been made. In addition, we have detected the presence of a clonal B-cell subpopulation within the progressively enlarging lymph nodes of an immunodeficient patient (Fig. 8). The histopathological impression of this lymph node was that of an atypical hyperplasia and not a follicular lymphoma. Whether the clonal B-cell subpopulation present in this lymph node is benign and still under regulation or represents the early detection of a malignancy will require serial examinations to resolve. The detected DNA rearrangements do, however, provide the necessary genetic marker unique to these clonal cells that will enable us to follow their natural history.[61]

It is frequently impossible to detect a small percentage of malignant cells within a given tissue because of the lack of sensitive, truly tumor-specific markers. If an initial mature B-cell malignancy secretes a monoclonal Ig, an anti-idiotype antibody can be produced which marks that tumor with the necessary specificity.[64] As we have seen, however, the individual idiotype that is produced is the product of a specific DNA rearrangement of

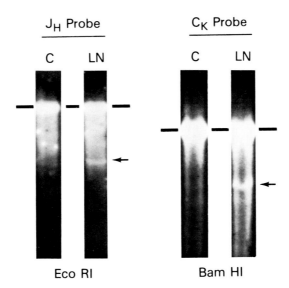

FIGURE 8. Southern analysis revealing the presence of a monoclonal B-cell subpopulation bearing a clonally rearranged heavy-chain gene (J_H probe on EcoRI-digested DNA) and a clonally rearranged κ gene (C_κ probe on BamHI-digested DNA) as denoted by the arrows. This clonal subpopulation of B cells was present within the hyperplastic lymph nodes (LN) of an immunodeficient patient as compared to a control source of cells (C). The clonal rearrangement (arrow) was considerably less prevalent than the germline genes (dash marks) contributed by other cells in this node.

heavy- and light-chain Ig gene subsegments. Therefore, the detection of an Ig gene rearrangement pattern specific to an individual tumor has the requisite specificity to identify that cell and its progeny. In addition, it does not require the laborious preparation of an anti-idiotype antibody and can also be performed on B-cell precursors which fail to express their clonally rearranged genes. Such DNA rearrangements serve as rather sensitive tumor-specific markers that should enhance the ability to identify persistent tumor following therapy and facilitate the early detection of recurrences within a given tissue.

11. Summary

Thus, the molecular description of the somatic assembly process for Ig genes has provided tremendous insights into the generation of total antibody diversity as well as the creation of a unique idiotype for individual antibody molecules. In addition, a sequential process of Ig gene rearrangements has been defined in humans which begins with the heavy-chain genes and then proceeds to light chains in an order of κ before λ. These insights have proven of tremendous value in establishing the cellular origin as well as the stage of differentiation of a number of controversial lymphoid malignancies. The unique pattern of Ig gene rearrangements in each B-cell-lineage neoplasm is serving as a tumor-specific marker which promises to improve our capacity to detect such malignancies at an early stage and follow the progeny of such cells over time. Finally, recent observations within Burkitt's lymphoma are providing potential insights into the mechanisms of transformation itself. Within this select set of human B-cell malignancies the Ig gene regions are participating in a further recombination, this one interchromosomal, which actually introduces a cellular oncogene into this locus. Therefore, the molecular genetic dissection of the Ig genes has provided not only a wealth of information concerning the generation of antibody diversity, but is beginning to provide insights into immunopathological states as well.

References

1. Dreyer, W. J., and Bennett, J. C., 1965, The molecular basis of antibody formation: A paradox, *Proc. Natl. Acad. Sci. USA* **54**:864–869.
2. Hozumi, N., and Tonegawa, S., 1976, Evidence for somatic rearrangement of immunoglobulin genes coding for variable and constant regions, *Proc. Natl. Acad. Sci. USA* **73**:3628–3632.
3. Brack, C., Hirama, M., Lenhard-Schuller, R., and Tonegawa, S., 1978, A complete imunoglobulin gene is created by somatic recombination, *Cell* **15**:1–14.
4. Seidman, J. G., and Leder, P., 1978, The arrangement and rearrangement of antibody genes, *Nature* **276**:790–795.
5. Hieter, P. A., Max, E. E., Seidman, J. G., Maizel, J. V., Jr., and Leder, P., 1980, Cloned human and mouse kappa immunoglobulin constant and J region genes conserve homology in functional segments, *Cell* **22**:197–207.
6. Hieter, P. A., Maizel, J. V., Jr., and Leder, P., 1982, Evolution of human immunoglobulin κ J region genes, *J. Biol. Chem.* **257**:1516–1522.
7. Hieter, P. A., Hollis, G. F., Korsmeyer, S. J., Waldmann, T. A., and Leder, P., 1981, Clustered arrangement of immunoglobulin λ constant region genes in man, *Nature* **294**:536–540.
8. Ravetch, J. V., Siebenlist, U., Korsmeyer, S., Waldmann, T., and Leder, P., 1981, Structure of the human immunoglobulin μ locus: Characterization of embryonic and rearranged J and D genes, *Cell* **27**:583–591.

9. Siebenlist, U., Ravetch, J. V., Korsmeyer, S. J., Waldmann, T. A., and Leder, P., 1981, Human immunoglobulin D segments encoded in tandem multigenic families, *Nature* **294**:631–635.

10. Early, P., Huang, H., Davis, M., Calame, K., and Hood, L., 1980, An immunoglobulin heavy chain variable region gene is generated from three segments of DNA: V_H, D and J_H, *Cell* **19**:981–992.

11. Sakano, H., Kurosawa, Y., Weigert, M., and Tonegawa, S., 1981, Identification and nucleotide sequence of a diversity DNA segment (D) of immunoglobulin heavy-chain genes, *Nature* **290**:562–565.

12. Malcolm, S., Barton, P., Murphy, C., Ferguson-Smith, M. A., Bentley, D. L., and Rabbitts, T. H., 1982, Localization of human immunoglobulin κ light chain variable region genes to the short arm of chromosome 2 by *in situ* hybridization, *Proc. Natl. Acad. Sci. USA* **79**:4957–4961.

13. McBride, O. W., Hieter, P. A., Hollis, G. F., Swan, D., Otey, M. C., and Leder, P., 1982, Chromosomal location of human kappa and lambda immunoglobulin light chain constant region genes, *J. Exp. Med.* **155**:1480–1490.

14. Kirsch, I. R., Morton, C. C., Nakahara, K., and Leder, P., 1982, Human immunoglobulin heavy chain genes map to a region of translocation in malignant B lymphocytes, *Science* **216**:301–303.

15. Seidman, J. G., Max, E. E., and Leder, P., 1979, A κ-immunoglobulin gene is formed by site-specific recombination without further somatic mutation, *Nature* **280**:370–375.

16. Max, E. E., Seidman, J. G., and Leder, P., 1979, Sequences of five potential recombination sites encoded close to an immunoglobulin κ constant region gene, *Proc. Natl. Acad. Sci. USA* **76**:3450–3454.

17. Sakano, H., Huppi, K., Heinrich, G., and Tonegawa, S., 1979, Sequences at the somatic recombination sites of immunoglobulin light-chain genes, *Nature* **280**:288–294.

18. Taub, R., Kirsch, I., Morton, C., Lenoir, G., Swan, D., Tronick, S., Aaronson, S., and Leder, P., 1982, Translocation of the c-*myc* gene into the immunoglobulin heavy chain locus in human Burkitt's lymphoma and murine plasmacytoma cells, *Proc. Natl. Acad. Sci. USA* **79**:7837–7841.

19. Ohno, S., Babonits, M., Wiener, F., Spira, J., Klein, G., and Potter, M., 1979, Nonrandom chromosome changes involving the Ig gene-carrying chromosomes 12 and 6 in pristane-induced mouse plasmacytomas, *Cell* **18**:1001–1007.

20. Bently, D. L., and Rabbitts, T. H., 1981, Human $V_κ$ immunoglobulin gene number: Implications for the origin of antibody diversity, *Cell* **24**:613–623.

21. Taub, R. A., Hollis, G. F., Hieter, P. A., Korsmeyer, S. J., Waldmann, T. A., and Leder, P., 1983, The variable amplification of immunoglobulin lambda light chain genes in human populations, *Nature* **304**:172–174.

22. Matthyssens, G., and Rabbitts, T. H., 1980, Structure and multiplicity of genes for the human immunoglobulin heavy chain variable region, *Proc. Natl. Acad. Sci. USA* **77**:6561–6565.

23. Rechavi, G., Bienz, B., Ram, D., Ben-Neriah, Y., Cohen, J. B., Zakut, R., and Givol, D., 1982, Organization and evolution of immunoglobulin V_H gene subgroups, *Proc. Natl. Acad. Sci. USA* **79**:4405–4409.

24. Wu, T. T., and Kabat, E. A., 1982, Fourteen nucleotides in the second complementarity determining region of a human heavy-chain variable region gene are identical with a sequence in a human D minigene, *Proc. Natl. Acad. Sci. USA* **79**:5031–5032.

25. Korsmeyer, S. J., Hieter, P. A., Ravetch, J. V., Poplack, D. G., Waldmann, T. A., and Leder, P., 1981, Developmental hierarchy of immunoglobulin gene rearrangements in human leukemic pre-B-cells, *Proc. Natl. Acad. Sci. USA* **78**:7096–7100.

26. Korsmeyer, S. J., Arnold, A., Bakhshi, A., Ravetch, J. V., Siebenlist, U., Hieter, P. A., Sharrow, S. O., LeBien, T. W., Kersey, J. H., Poplack, D. G., Leder, P., and Waldmann, T. A., 1983, Immunoglobulin gene rearrangement and cell surface antigen expression in acute lymphocytic leukemias of T-cell and B-cell precursor origins, *J. Clin. Invest.* **71**:301–313.

27. Alt, F. W., and Baltimore, D., 1982, Joining of immunoglobulin heavy chain gene segments: Implications from a chromosome with evidence of three D-J_H fusions, *Proc. Natl. Acad. Sci. USA* **79**:4118–4122.

28. Siden, E., Alt, F. W., Shinefeld, L., Sato, V., and Baltimore, D., 1981, Synthesis of immunoglobulin μ chain gene products precedes synthesis of light chains during B-lymphocyte development, *Proc. Natl. Acad. Sci. USA* **78**:1823–1827.

29. Leder, P., Max, E. E., Seidman, J. G., Kwan, S.-P., Scharff, M., Nau, M., and Norman, B., 1980, Recombination events that activate, diversify, and delete immunoglobulin genes, *Cold Spring Harbor Symp. Quant. Biol.* **45**:859–865.

30. Hieter, P. A., Korsmeyer, S. J., Waldmann, T. A., and Leder, P., 1981, Human immunoglobulin κ light-chain genes are deleted or rearranged in λ-producing B cells, *Nature* **290**:368–372.

31. Korsmeyer, S. J., Hieter, P. A., Sharrow, S. O., Goldman, C. K., Leder, P., and Waldmann, T. A., 1982, Normal human B-cells display ordered light-chain gene rearrangements and deletions, *J. Exp. Med.* **156:**975–985.

32. Coleclough, C., Perry, R. P., Karjalainen, K., and Weigert, M., 1981, Aberrant rearrangements contribute significantly to the allelic exclusion of immunoglobulin gene expression, *Nature* **290:**372–378.

33. Alt, F. W., Enea, V., Bothwell, A. L. M., and Baltimore, D., 1980, Activity of multiple light chain genes in murine myeloma cells producing a single, functional light chain, *Cell* **21:**1–12.

34. Davis, M. M., Kim, S. K., and Hood, L. E., 1980, DNA sequences mediating class switching in α-immunoglobulins, *Science* **209:**1360–1365.

35. Kataoka, T., Miyata, T., and Honjo, T., 1981, Repetitive sequences in class-switch recombination regions of immunoglobulin heavy chain genes, *Cell* **23:**357–368.

36. Obata, M., Kataoka, T., Nakai, S., Yamagishi, H., Takahashi, N., Yamawaki-Kataoka, Y., Nikaido, T., Shimizu, A., and Honjo, T.,1981, Structure of a rearranged γ1 chain gene and its implication to immunoglobulin class-switch mechanism, *Proc. Natl. Acad. Sci. USA* **78:**2437–2441.

37. Marcu, K. B., Lang, R. B., Stanton, L. W., and Harris, L. J., 1982, A model for the molecular requirements of immunoglobulin heavy chain class switching, *Nature (London)* **298:**87–89.

38. Ravetch, J. V., Kirsch, I. R., and Leder, P., 1980, Evolutionary approach to the question of immunoglobulin heavy chain switching: Evidence from cloned human and mouse genes, *Proc. Natl. Acad. Sci. USA* **77:**6734–6738.

39. Rabbitts, T. H., Forster, A., and Milstein, C. P., 1981, Human immunoglobulin heavy chain genes: Evolutionary comparisons of C_μ, C_δ, and C_γ, genes and associated switch sequences, *Nucleic Acids Res.* **9:**4509–4524.

40. Knap, M. R., Liu, C.-P., Newell, N., Ward, R. B., Tucker, P. W., Strober, S., and Blattner, F., 1982, Simultaneous expression of immunoglobulin μ and heavy chains by a cloned B-cell lymphoma: A single copy of the V_H gene is shared by two adjacent C_H genes, *Proc. Natl. Acad. Sci. USA* **79:**2996–3000.

41. Moore, K. W., Rogers, J., Hunkapiller, T., Early, P., Nottenburg, C., Weissman, I., Bazin, H., Wall, R., and Hood, L., 1981, Expression of IgD may use both DNA rearrangement and RNA splicing mechanisms, *Proc. Natl. Acad. Sci. USA* **78:**1800–1804.

42. Flanagan, J. G., and Rabbitts, T. H., 1982, Arrangement of human immunoglobulin heavy chain constant region genes implies evolutionary duplication of a segment containing γ, ϵ, α genes, *Nature* **300:**709–713.

43. Max, E. E., Battey, J., Ney, R., Kirsch, I. R., and Leder, P., 1982, Duplication and deletion in the human immunoglobulin ϵ genes, *Cell* **29:**691–699.

44. Takahashi, N., Ueda, S., Obata, M., Nikaido, T., Nakai, S., and Honjo, T., 1982, Structure of human immunoglobulin gamma genes: Implications for evolution of a gene family, *Cell* **29:**671–679.

45. Max, E. E., Seidman, J. G., Miller, H., and Leder, P., 1980, Variation in the crossover point of kappa immunoglobulin gene V–J recombination: Evidence from a cryptic gene, *Cell* **21:**793–799.

46. Bothwell, A. L. M., Paskind, M., Reth, M., Imanishi-Kari, T., Rajewsky, K., and Baltimore, D., 1981, Heavy chain variable region contribution to the NP[b] family of antibodies: Somatic mutation evident in a γ2a variable region, *Cell* **24:**625–637.

47. Gearhart, P. J., Johnson, N. D., Douglas, R., and Hood, L., 1981, IgG antibodies to phosphorylcholine exhibit more diversity than their IgM counterparts, *Nature* **291:**29–34.

48. Pech, M., Hochtl, J., Schnell, H., and Zachau, H. G., 1981, Differences between germ-line and rearranged immunoglobulin V_κ coding sequences suggest a localized mutation mechainsim, *Nature* **291:**668–670.

49. Selsing, E., and Storb, U., 1981, Somatic mutation of immunoglobulin light-chain variable-region genes, *Cell* **25:**47–58.

50. Early, P., Rogers, J., Davis, M., Calame, K., Bond, M., Wall, R., and Hood, L., 1980, Two mRNAs can be produced from a single immunoglobulin μ gene by alternative RNA processing pathways, *Cell* **20:**313–319.

51. Cushley, W., Coupar, B. E. H., Mickelson, C. A., and Williamson, A. R., 1982, A common mechanism for the synthesis of membrane and secreted immunoglobulin α, γ, and μ chains, *Nature* **298:**77–79.

52. Rowley, J. D., 1980, Chromosome abnormalities in cancer, *Cancer Genet. Cytogenet.* **2:**175–198.

53. Croce, C. M., Shadner, M., Martinis, J., Cicurel, L., D'Ancona, G. G., Dolby, T. W., and Koprowski, H., 1979, Chromosomal location of the genes for human immunoglobulin heavy chains, *Proc. Natl. Acad. Sci. USA* **76:**3416–3420.

54. Lenoir, G. M., Preud'homme, J. L., Bernheim, A., and Berger, R., 1982, Correlations between immuno-globulin light chain expression and variant translocation in Burkitt's lymphoma, *Nature* **298**:474–476.
55. Bishop, J. M., 1983, Cancer genes come of age, *Cell* **32**:1018–1020.
56. Hayward, W. S., Neel, B. G., and Astrin, S. M., 1981, Activation of a cellular *onc* gene by promoter insertion in ALV-induced lymphoid leukosis, *Nature* **290**:475–480.
57. Erickson, J., Finan, J., Nowell, P. C., and Croce, C. M., 1982, Translocation of immunoglobulin V_H genes in Burkitt lymphoma, *Proc. Natl. Acad. Sci. USA* **79**:5611–5615.
58. Nishikura, K., Ar-Rushdi, A., Erickson, J., Watt, R., Rouevco, G. and Croce, C. M., 1983, Differential expression of the normal and of the translocated human c-*myc* oncogenes in B cells, *Proc. Natl. Acad. Sci. USA* **80**:4822–4826.
59. Gillies, S. D., Morrison, S. L., Oi, V. T., and Tonegawa, S., 1983, A tissue specific transcription enhancer element is located in the major intron of a rearranged immunoglobulin heavy-chain gene, *Cell* **33**:717–728.
60. Benjamin, D., Magrath, I. T., Triche, T. J., Schroff, R. W., Jensen, J. P., and Korsmeyer, S. J., 1984, Induction of plasmacytoid differentiation by phorbol ester in B-cell lymphoma cell lines bearing 8;14 trans-locations, *Proc. Natl. Acad. Sci. USA* (in press).
61. Arnold, A., Cossman, J., Bakhshi, A., Jaffe, E., Waldmann, T. A., and Korsmeyer, S. J., 1983, Immu-noglobulin gene rearrangements as unique clonal markers in human lymphoid neoplasms, *N. Engl. J. Med.* **309**:1593–1599.
62. Bakhshi, A., Minowada, J., Arnold, A., Cossman, J., Jensen, J. P., Whang-Peng, J., Waldmann, T. A., and Korsmeyer, S. J., 1983, Lymphoid blast crises of chronic myelogenous leukemia represent stages in the development of B-cell precursors, *N. Engl. J. Med.* **309**:826–831.
63. Korsmeyer, S. J., Greene, W. C., Cossman, J., Hsu, S.-M., Jensen, J. P., Neckers, L. M., Marshall, S. L., Bakhshi, A., Depper, J. M., Leonard, W. J., Jaffe, E. S., and Waldmann, T. A., 1983, Rearrangement and expression of immunoglobulin genes and expression of Tac antigen in hairy cell leukemia, *Proc. Natl. Acad. Sci. USA* **80**:4522–4526.
64. Miller, R. A., Maloney, D. G., Warnke, R., and Levy, R., 1982, Treatment of B-cell lymphoma with monoclonal anti-idiotype antibody, *N. Engl. J. Med.* **306**:517–522.

6

Analysis of the GAT B Repertoire

MICHEL FOUGEREAU, JOSÉ ROCCA-SERRA, CLAUDINE SCHIFF, AND CÉCILE TONNELLE

1. Introduction: The GAT Polypeptide and the Immune Response

Synthetic polypeptides[1] were first used as structurally well-defined models to understand the antigenicity of proteins, for which the exact nature of any given epitope was and still remains far from clear, except in a very few cases.[2,3] They subsequently proved decisive tools to discover genes which regulate the immune response in the guinea pig[4] and the mouse.[5] Among synthetic polypeptides, the $(Glu^{60}Ala^{30}Tyr^{10})_n$ random terpolymer, known as "GAT," has been extensively used. This polymer, with molecular weights usually ranging between 30,000 and 100,000, is recognized by the immune system mostly through conformational epitopes,[6] and contains a high amount of α-helix. Genetic control of the immune response to GAT has been largely documented in the mouse, allowing definition of responder and nonresponder strains,[7] the later being of the $H\text{-}2^b$, $H\text{-}2^q$, and $H\text{-}2^s$ haplotypes. As "nonresponder" (NR) strains could be forced to make anti-GAT antibodies provided the synthetic polypeptide was coupled to a carrier, such as methylated BSA,[8] the absence of response in NR strains was not due to a deficient repertoire at the B-cell level. In fact, a more detailed analysis of anti-GAT antibodies produced by both responder and "nonresponder" strains indicated that the repertoires looked very similar with respect to idiotypic specificities identified on GAT-specific antibodies.[9]

2. Idiotypic Specificities of the GAT System

2.1. Definition of the Main Idiotypic Specificities

Most of the murine anti-GAT antibodies (i.e., up to 70%) express a common set of idiotypic specificities, termed CGAT, and initially defined by a guinea pig anti-idiotypic

MICHEL FOUGEREAU, JOSÉ ROCCA-SERRA, CLAUDINE SCHIFF, AND CÉCILE TONNELLE • Centre d'Immunologie INSERM-CNRS de Marseille-Luminy, 13288 Marseille Cedex 9, France.

antiserum raised against D1.LP anti-GAT antibodies.[9,10] The CGAT public idiotopes were identified in all 40 mouse strains tested, and also in nine rat strains, whatever their *MHC* and *Igh* genotypes.[10] Furthermore, these cross-reactive idiotypes were induced following immunization with a variety of polymers, provided they contained glutamic acid and tyrosine. Production and analysis of GAT-specific monoclonal antibodies made it possible to define the CGAT family in more precise terms,[11,12] and to describe within the CGAT⁻ anti-GAT antibodies a family of idiotypic specificities also expressed in anti-GA antibodies, and for that reason termed GA-1 idiotypes.[13] Antibodies expressing this public idiotypic specificity are primarily associated with the recognition of Glu-Ala determinants. These antibodies, when produced after immunization with the GAT polymer, represent, on the average, 10% of total polyclonal anti-GAT antibodies. A similar proportion was found whenever monoclonal antibodies were analyzed.[14] All strains of mice that were tested expressed the GA-1 idiotype, with the exception of CE/J.[13]

Anti-GAT antibodies from mice bearing either the Igh-1^e or the Igh-1^b allotype were shown to express another set of common idiotypic specificities, designated Gte.[15] These specificities are expressed on CGAT-bearing molecules,[12] and could be mapped within the *Igh-V* region, close to *Igh-Np* genes.[16] More recently, another idiotype, termed GA-2, was identified in all strains of mice.[17] All Ga-1$^+$ antibodies also expressed the GA-2 specificities whereas the GA-2 hybridomas can express all, part, or none of the GA-1 specificities.

Using a rabbit antiserum,[18,19] similar public idiotypic specificities were identified on anti-GAT antibodies of all strains of mice, but also on those of rats and guinea pigs.[19,20] A detailed analysis of the GAT-specific idiotypic specificities defined four classes of specificities[21]:

1. A highly conserved idiotypic specificity (h.c. GAT), found in mouse, rat, and guinea pig antibodies
2. The pGAT public idiotypic specificities, which may be considered very similar if not identical with the CGAT idiotype, and which were identified in all mouse strains tested, either at the conventional polyclonal level[21] or in monoclonal anti-GAT antibodies from BALB/c, DBA/2, or (C57BL/6 × DBA/2)F₁ mice[22]
3. Strain-restricted (s.r.) idiotypic specificities, only expressed in a number of mouse strains, such as the s.r. GAT-1 specificities, which were found only on anti-GAT antibodies derived from mice with Igh-1^a, Igh-1^c, and Igh-1^e allotypic markers[21]
4. Individual, or private idiotypic specificities[12,22] identified on one given anti-GAT monoclonal antibody, or occasionally also found on a very few other GAT-specific monoclonal antibodies.

2.2. Anti-GAT Antibody Polypeptide Chains, Antibody Combining Site, and Idiotypic Specificities

In direct line with the original definition of idiotypy,[23] it was shown that idiotype-anti-idiotype reactions could be inhibited by the hapten recognized by the idiotype,[24] suggesting that at least some idiotopes must be very close to the antibody combining site, if not completely contained within it. It was also shown that some idiotopes clearly lie outside of the combining site,[25] so that the most general case is best described by the presence of two types of idiotopes, one closely associated to the antibody combining site, the other not.[26]

Inhibition of the idiotype–anti-idiotype binding by the antigen has been obtained in the GAT system for the pGAT and h.c. GAT specificities, but not for the s.r. specificities.[27] This would suggest that the two former may be site-associated whereas the latter rather constitutes a framework marker. The GAT antigen, however, is a large molecule (in this experiment 39,000 daltons), so that steric hindrance might be misleading. Peptides having a molecular weight of about 3000 daltons and isolated after cleavage of GAT with mercurylpapain were also able to inhibit the idiotype–anti-idiotype binding under the same conditions as those reported for the native antigen.[27] This observation therefore strengthened the conclusions that at least some of the pGAT and h.c. GAT idiotopes were site-associated.

Using chain recombination experiments it was shown that the public pGAT and the individual i_1-GAT idiotopes required the presence of both the heavy and the light chains of the idiotype in order to be expressed.[27] This observation is in agreement with the situation described for most idiotypic systems,[28–31] although in some cases, either the H or the L chain may play a major role.[32]

2.3. The "Minimum Model" for the GAT System

Anti-GAT antibodies may be more simply classified into three discrete groups depending on whether they express one public idiotypic specificity, CGAT or pGAT, the other, GA-1, or none. The idiotypic formulas are thus: $CGAT^+$, $GA\text{-}1^-$; $CGAT^-$, $GA\text{-}1^+$; $CGAT^-$, $GA\text{-}1^-$, as summarized in Fig. 1. It should be noticed that anti-GAT, $CGAT^+$ antibodies primarily recognize the GT determinants, whereas anti-GAT, $GA\text{-}1^+$ antibodies, which can also be induced by a poly-GA copolymer, may be regarded as GA-specific. This feature strengthens the relationship between antigenic recognition and idiotopes, and seems in line with the inhibition experiments described above, suggesting that the CGAT determinants are, at least partly, site-associated.

The structural bases for the major public idiotypes were analyzed using a collection of monoclonal anti-GAT antibodies derived from BALB/c,[22] DBA/2, or (C57BL/6 ×

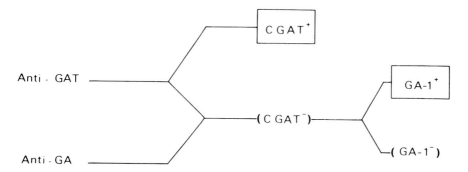

FIGURE 1. Three main classes of GAT-specific antibodies, as defined by public idiotypic specificities.

DBA/2)F$_1$ hybrids,[12,33] representing a sampling of the three populations depicted in Fig. 1. The NH$_2$-terminal amino acid sequences were determined for 17 monoclonal H–L pairs.[33–36] Sequences of the heavy chains are given in Fig. 2. The four BALB/c sequences were identical up to the last residue determined, i.e., residue 43. Interestingly, 66% of the polyclonal antibody heavy chains, which were isolated from BALB.B mice, possessed the same sequence, related to the V$_H$II subgroup,[37] as opposed to the remaining chains, that could be assigned to the V$_H$III subgroup. Monoclonal heavy chains derived from (BALB/c × DBA/2)F$_1$ hybrids or DBA/2 mice were very similar to the major sequence present in BALB/c mice, which already suggests that a small number of V$_H$ germ-line genes must be operating to generate GAT-specific antibodies which express the CGAT idiotypic specificities. More surprising was the finding that anti-GAT (F9 series) or anti-GA (F27 series) antibodies expressing the GA-1 public specificities used a heavy chain which clearly was very close to that previously defined, suggesting that the same V$_H$ gene might be used to generate both types of antibodies.[33,34] By contrast, a C57BL/6 GAT-specific sequence (F17) appeared distinct, although related.[36] The last group of V$_H$ sequences, corresponding to antibodies that express neither the CGAT nor the GA-1 specificities, was found to be much more heterogeneous, although most chains were related to the V$_H$III subgroup.

NH$_2$-terminal amino acid sequences of the corresponding light (κ) chains were also determined up to residue 43 (Fig. 3) (38 in Kabat's numbering[37]). Again, the four CGAT$^+$ BALB/c sequences, corresponding to the V$_\kappa$1 subgroup,[38] were found to be extremely conserved, two chains being completely identical. Light chains derived from other strains or hybrids had sequences which were very close to that of the BALB/c antibodies, but the presence of identical amino acid substitutions at positions 27b and 34 (Ile/Leu and Tyr/His, respectively) is strongly suggestive that a second V$_\kappa$ germ-line gene, which is possibly allelic in nature, must be operating.

In sharp contrast with the conservation of the V$_H$ structures, the V$_\kappa$ sequences identified for the anti-GAT or anti-GA antibodies that express the GA-1 specificities differed markedly from the CGAT κ chains. They were closely related to one another and may be considered to be encoded by a common "V$_\kappa$-GA-1" germ-line gene.

Finally, light chains from anti-GAT antibodies that express neither specificities had sequences that profoundly differed from the two previous sets.

On these bases, the "minimum model" which may account for the generation of anti-GAT and anti-GA antibodies is summarized in Fig. 4. The central message is that the two sets of antibodies use the same V$_H$ repertoire, associated with discrete V$_\kappa$ genes.

3. Analysis of the V$_H$ Repertoire in the CGAT (or pGAT) Idiotypes

3.1. Structural Data

The amino acid sequence covering residues 1–120 of five anti-GAT monoclonal heavy chains, and thus encompassing the V$_H$, D$_H$, and J$_H$ regions, was determined,[36,39] using a combination of NH$_2$-terminal amino acid sequencing and mRNA nucleotide sequencing, as adapted[40] from the chain terminator method.[41] These sequences are reported in Fig. 5. The four chains of the G series were derived from BALB/c mice. Two of them, G5 Bb 2.2 and G8 Ca 1.7, were completely identical, including the D gene-encoded region. These

Antibodies	Strain	CGAT	GA-1	Sequence (CDR1; positions 10, 20, 30, 40)
				E V Q L Q Q S G A E L V K P G A S V K L S C T A S G F N I K D T Y M H W V K Q R P E Q
G5 Bb 2.2	BALB/c	+		————————————
G7 Ab 2.9	"	+		————————————
G8 Ad. 3.8	"	+		————————————
G8 Ca 1.7	"	+		————————————
Polyclonal	"	+	66%	————————————
			33%	D—VE—GG—Q—G—A—TF—Y—
H51 5 2	BALB/cxDBA/2	+	-	———IY—G—
H51 129 2	"	+	-	DI—T—L—
H56 406 48	DBA/2	+	-	———T—D—
F17 170 2	C57BL/6	+	-	Q—P—K—YTFTSYW—GR
F27 105 12	DBA/2	-	+	—L—I–
F27 243 4	"	-	+	X—P—
F9 102 2	"	-	+	—XXE—
G6 Bd 2.6	BALB/c	±	-	D—E—PG—N–SQ–LS–T—VT–YS–TMA–AWNWIR–F–G
F27 127 12	DBA/2	-	-	D—E—PD—SQ–LS–T—VT–YS–TXG–A
H51 31 6	BALB/cxDBA/2	-	-	—K–VE—GG—Q—G–T—A—TFS–YG–V—S—GK
H51 54 33	"	-	-	—VE—GG—Q–VG–L—ATG—KF–TYA—V–S–G
H51 81 5	"	-	-	D—VE—GG—Q—G–R—S—TFS–FG—
H51 85 2	"	-	-	—P—M—S—YTFXXYV–Y—L–

FIGURE 2. NH_2-terminal amino acid sequences of anti-GAT antibody heavy chains, covering a sampling of the three main groups as defined relative to public idiotypic specificities.

Sequence reference (positions 10, 20, 27abcde, 30):

D V V M T Q T P L S L P V S L G D Q A S I S C R S S Q S I V H S N G N T Y L Y W Y L Q

Antibodies	Strain	CGAT	GA-1	Sequence
G5 Bb 2.2	BALB/c	+		(—)
G7 Ab 2.9	"	+		— N — X —
G8 Ad 3.8	"	+		— I — E —
G8 Ca 1.7	"	+		(—)
H51 5 2	BALB/cxDBA/2	+	-	— L — H —
H51 129 2	"	+	-	— L — H — F—
H56 406 48	DBA/2	+	-	— L — L — K — H —
F17 170 2	B6xD2	+	-	— L — H —
Polyclonal	BALB	+	-	— L —
F27 105 12	DBA/2	-	+	—I__AAP_V__TP_ESV____KNLL_T
F27 243 4	"	-	+	—I__AAP_I__TP_ESV_M___KNLL
F9 102 2	"	-	+	—I__EAAK_V__TP_ESVX__KA_KNLL_____F_
G6 Bd 2.6	BALB/c	±	-	____S Y___E
H51 31 6	BALB/cxDBA/2	-	-	—I__S_S_S__A__EKVTM___KIL___LLN_STXKNYLAWY
H51 54 33	"	-	-	—I__S_S_SW_A__V_EKVTM__K_X__LLYX_NQKNYLA
H51 81 5	"	-	-	—I__S_S__AM_V_QKVTR__R___XLN_SNQKNYLAWY
H51 85 2	"	-	-	—I__AAS_N__T_TS_____K_LL____I
F27 127 12	DBA/2	-	-	_I__S_S_S____V_EKVTMN_K_T__LLY_ANQKNSLAWY

FIGURE 3. NH₂-terminal amino acid sequences of anti-GAT antibody light chains.

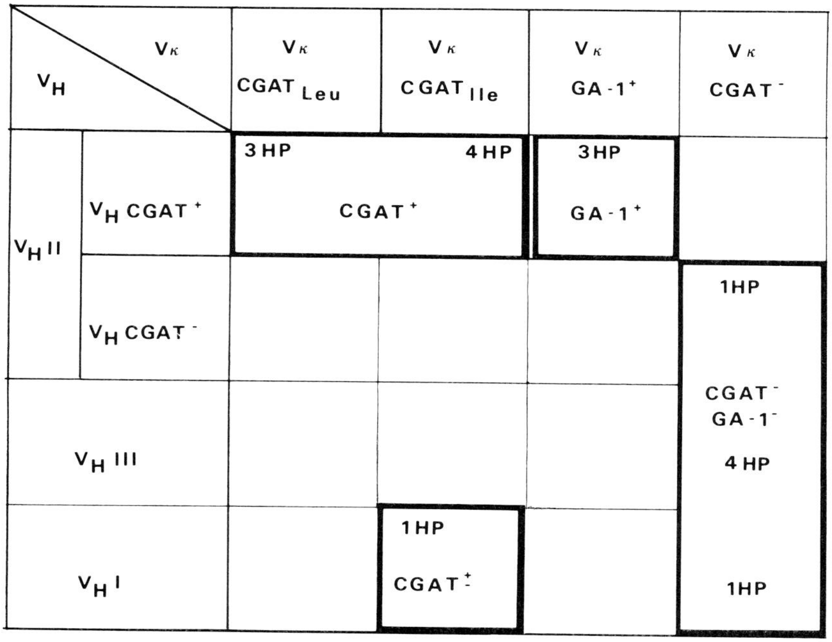

V_H \ V_κ	V_κ CGAT$_{Leu}$	V_κ CGAT$_{Ile}$	V_κ GA-1$^+$	V_κ CGAT$^-$
V_H II — V_H CGAT$^+$	3HP CGAT$^+$	4HP CGAT$^+$	3HP GA-1$^+$	
V_H II — V_H CGAT$^-$				1HP
V_H III				CGAT$^-$ GA-1$^-$ 4HP
V_H I		1HP CGAT$^\pm$		1HP

FIGURE 4. Germline genes expressed in the GAT and GA systems.

```
                    10                  20                  30                  40
G5 Bb  2.2   E V Q L Q Q S G A E L V K P G A S V K L S C T A S G F N I K D T Y M H W V K Q R
G8 Ca  1.7   ————————————————————————————————————————————————————————————————————
G7 Ab  2.9   ————————————————————————————————————————————————————————————————————
G8 Ad  3.8   ————————————————————————————————————————————————————————————————————
F17 170 2    Q———————P———————————————————————— K ———— Y T F T S Y W ——————————

                       50                  60                  70
             P E Q G L E W I G R I D P A N G N T K Y D P K F Q G K A T I T A D T S S N T A Y
             ————————————————————— X —S — G ——————— X —————————— S A ——
             ————————————————————— K ———————————————— T ————
             —G R ———————————————— N S _G ———— S E —— K S ———— L —V— K P_S ————

             80              90              100             110
             L Q L S S L T S E D T A V Y Y C A R G W L R R D A M D Y W G Q G T S V T V S S A    J H 4
             ———————————— G ——————————— T —— X F ———————————————————————    J H 4
             ———————————————————————————————————————————————————————————    J H 4
             ——F———————————————————————— T T V G R[] ——————————————— T L ———————    J H 2
             M———————————————S——————————— S E Y G N F [ ] ——————————— T L ———————    J H 2
```

FIGURE 5. Amino acid sequence of the complete variable regions (encompassing the *V-D-J*-encoded segments) of five anti-GAT monoclonal heavy chains derived from BALB/c (G series) and C57BL/6 (F17) mice.

two monoclonal antibodies express, in addition to the common pGAT idiotypes, identical individual i_1-GAT idiotypic specificities, and were derived from separate fusions. The D region contained an undecamer that was identical with a sequence contained in a *D.SP2* germ-line gene.[42] The two BALB/c remaining sequences were identical up to residue 54 (although silent nucleotide differences were detected at codons 23, 28, and 38), whereas a few amino acid differences in the second hypervariable and third framework regions were identified. All three heavy chains that used a *D.SP2* gene expressed J_H4, whereas the fourth one, which contained a *D.FL16*-related sequence, had a J_H2. Interestingly, the D.FL16 J_H2 combination was also found in the heavy chain (F17) that was derived from a (C57BL/6 × DBA/2)F_1 hybrid mouse. This heavy chain expressed the Igh[b] allotype of the C57BL/6 strain. The *F17* V_H gene-encoded sequence differed at 25% of the positions of the BALB/c counterparts.

3.2. Estimate of the Number of V_H CGAT Germline Genes

The high homology that was observed between the four BALB/c V_H sequences is suggestive that all four chains may be derived from the same germ-line gene, whose sequence is very close if not identical to that of the G5 Bb 2.2/G8 Ca 1.7 prototype. A cDNA library was constructed in pBR 322 from the G8 Ca 1.7 mRNA enriched for the H-coding fractions, and a CGAT-V_H clone was isolated, characterized, and sequenced.[43] A specific V_H probe was derived from this clone, and annealed to *Eco*RI and *Bgl*II restriction fragments of liver (i.e., unrearranged) DNA extracted from BALB/c, DBA/2, and C57BL/6 mice. The Southern hybridization patterns obtained at high stringency conditions (Fig. 6) clearly speak in favor of a very small number of related V_H genes. Interestingly, patterns obtained for the C57BL/6 and the BALB/c strains differed significantly. In fact, as the C57BL/6 and the BALB/c GAT-specific V_H sequences were only 75% homologous, it seems very likely that the cross-hybridization which is being detected does not involve the C57 V_H gene directly related to the reported sequence of the F17 hybridoma heavy chain. Whether the cross-hybridizing materials indeed contain genes which are used by the C57BL/6 strain to make anti-GAT antibodies remains to be proved. In a similar situation, a probe containing the coding sequence of a C57BL/6 anti-(4-hydroxy-3-nitrophenyl)acetyl (NP[b]) V_H region hybridized with BALB/c genomic DNA clones, the sequence of which did not resemble that of the actually expressed genes in the BALB/c context.[44]

4. Analysis of the V_κ Repertoire in the CGAT (or pGAT) Idiotypes

4.1. Structural Data

A similar approach, using protein and mRNA sequencing, was also applied to GAT-specific light chains. Eight complete V_κ sequences of various strain origins have been determined (C. Tonnelle *et al.*, 1983). All these sequences, whatever their origin, pertained to the $V_\kappa1$ subgroup.[38] On the basis of multiple identical amino acid substitutions, it was possible to distinguish at least two groups of sequences, and possibly a third one (Fig. 7).

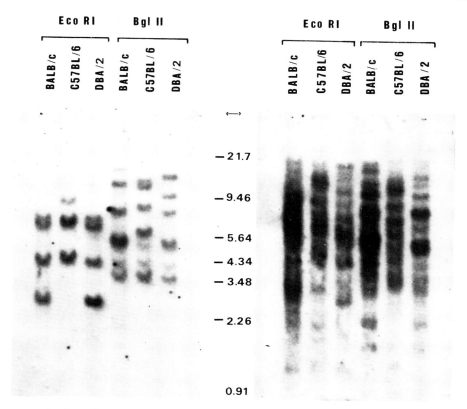

FIGURE 6. Southern blots of liver DNA *Eco*RI and *Bgl*II fragments using (left) stringent and (right) nonstringent conditions as revealed with the specific *G8 Ca 1.7 V$_{II}$* probe (Ref. 43), covering codons 4–81.

The two main groups differed by multiple alternate repeats at positions 27b (Ile/Leu), 34 (Tyr/His), and 50 (Arg/Lys). One of these groups, composed of four BALB/c light chains of the G series, was, in addition, extremely close to the 2205 κ sequence which was reported for a myeloma protein of NZB origin.[45] The second major group was composed of F17 (C57BL/6 × DBA/2), H56 (DBA/2), and H51 (BALB/c × DBA/2) hybridoma-derived chains. These chains all expressed, in addition to the alternative characteristic amino acids at positions mentioned above, a leucyl residue at position 83. These two groups are likely to represent two discrete germ-line genes, but it cannot be determined whether these two genes may be considered alleles, as the exact origin of the F17 and H51 chains cannot be determined. Nonetheless, the strong homology observed between the BALB/c V$_κ$ chains of the first group with an NZB sequence, and that observed between a DBA/2 GAT-specific (H56) and a BALB/c myeloma κ chain suggests that DBA/2, BALB/c, NZB (and, possibly, C57BL/6) mice possess the same potential repertoire, although each strain may use different V$_κ$ subsets to produce anti-GAT antibodies. Finally, one chain, of BALB/c origin (G8 Ad 3.8), was very close to the SAMM chain[46] sequenced only as far

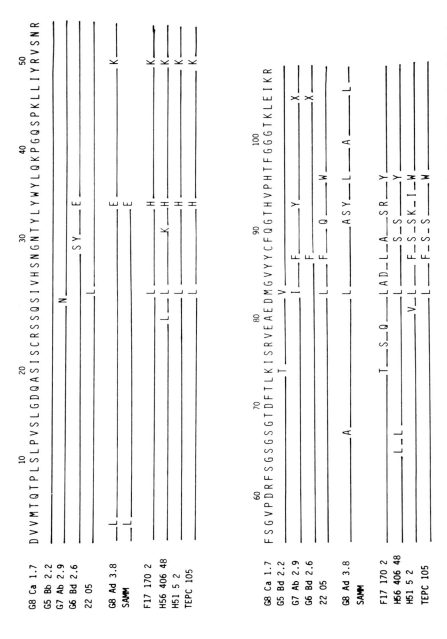

FIGURE 7. Amino acid sequence of light GAT-specific, CGAT monoclonal V_κ chains, as compared with the NZB myeloma light chain 2205,[45] BALB/c TEPC105,[45] and partial sequence of the BALB/c SAMM light chain.[46]

as residue 35, and might be encoded by a separate gene, with characteristic leucyl and glutamyl residues at positions 3 and 34, respectively.

4.2. Estimate of the Number of V_κ CGAT Genes at the Germline Level

Analysis of the CGAT-related V_κ repertoire was investigated at the germ-line level using hybridization of liver DNA restriction fragments with a V_κ probe that was isolated from a GAT-specific cDNA clone (C. Schiff et al., 1983). It was observed (Fig. 8) that both the EcoRI and the BamHI DNA fragment hybridization patterns, using highly stringent conditions, were very similar whenever they were derived from any of three strains (BALB/c, DBA/2, and C57BL/6). This is in contrast with the discrete strain patterns that were observed for the V_H hybridizations. Very few bands were detected, which again supports the hypothesis that only a very small number of germ-line genes must be involved in the CGAT expression.

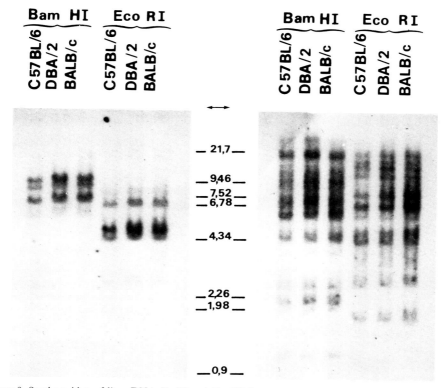

FIGURE 8. Southern blots of liver DNA EcoRI and BamHI fragments using (left) stringent and (right) nonstringent conditions as revealed with a specific G8 Ca 1.7 cDNA V_κ probe covering the leader and the V_κ cooling region to codon 80.

5. Structural Basis for Idiotypy in the GAT System

As already pointed out in this review,[1-3] precise structural definition of an antigenic determinant in proteins remains an unresolved question, except in a very few cases, as that of lysozyme.[3] Idiotopes follow the same lines. As most antigenic (idiotypic) determinants seem to be conformational in nature,[1] primary structure *correlates* of epitopes and/or idiotopes remain no more than *correlates*. This approach does not provide any answer as to the three-dimensional structure which is involved in the recognition by the antibody combining site, especially if one considers that in most cases, idiotope expression is largely dependent on H–L interactions. In a few cases, structural correlates of idiotypy seem to provide a simple view of the system. This is the case, for instance, for some idiotopes, public or private, of the dextran or galactan systems (see Chapter 7 this volume). One or two amino acid substitutions are sufficient to cause loss of expression of an entire set of determinants. This is also reminiscent of simple allotopes such as the d or e allotypic specificities expressed on the constant region of the rabbit heavy chain.[47,48] The precise "geometry" of the corresponding three-dimensional determinants remains, however, unknown in all cases. In the GAT system, we tried to define structural correlates of the public CGAT (or pGAT) and private i_1-GAT idiotopes. Two GAT-specific monoclonal antibodies, G5 Bb 2.2 and G8 Ca 1.7, which shared, in addition to the public pGAT idiotopes, identical i_1-GAT individual idiotypic specificities had identical heavy chains, including the D region, whereas their light chains differed by two amino acid substitution at positions 74 and 83. The remaining BALB/c monoclonal antibodies analyzed did not express the i_1-GAT specificities, and differed from the other two by a few amino acid substitutions, present on both the H and the L chains. No one had the same D region as that of G5 Bb 2.2.

More puzzling appears the situation observed for the public pGAT (or CGAT) specificities. The CGAT specificities are found on a family of anti-GAT antibodies which apparently uses a small number of V-region genes, various D–J combinations—so far $D.SP2-J_H4$ and $D.FL16-J_H2$—and various J_κ, leading to the expression of H and L chains that contain an appreciable number of amino acid substitutions, which appear mostly concentrated in the second half of the variable regions. The most intriguing observations concern the F17 and the G6 heavy chains. As reported and discussed above, the F17 H-variable region is largely different from its BALB/c counterparts (75% homology for the V_H-encoded section; D and J different). The F17 light chain also contains extensive differences localized at the end of the third framework and within the third hypervariable regions. The F17 antibody expresses, however, the pGAT/CGAT specificities, as do the antibodies of the G series derived from BALB/c, as tested with polyclonal anti-idiotypic antibodies.[22] An obvious proposal would be that the major contribution to the pGAT idiotopes is made by the light chain, which is highly conserved at least as far as the middle of the third framework region (see Fig. 5). Since, however, the pGAT determinants require the presence of both homologous H and L chains in order to be expressed, some stretches of the heavy chain must play a critical role in H–L interactions and/or in the direct expression of some idiotopes.

The G6 monoclonal antibody seems to express only part of the public pGAT idiotypic set.[27] The NH$_2$-terminal sequence of its heavy chain is very different from the pGAT$^+$ BALB/c counterparts. As the mRNA sequence has not been determined so far, it is not known whether the second part of the V_H region is also different. A definitive answer

Fougereau, M., 1983, Structural bases for public idiotypic specificities of monoclonal antibodies directed against poly (Glu^{60}Ala^{30}Tyr^{10}) and poly (Glu^{60}Ala^{40}) random copolymers, *Proc. Natl. Acad. Sci. USA* **80**:3040–3044.

34. Tonnelle, C., Pierres, M., Ju, S. T., Moinier, D., and Fougereau, M., 1981, NH$_2$-terminal aminoacid sequences of poly (Glu^{60}Ala^{30}Tyr^{10}) (GAT) and poly (Glu^{60}Ala^{40}) (GA) monoclonal antibody heavy chains, *Mol. Immunol.* **18**:979–984.

35. Rocca-Serra, J., Mazié, J.-C., Moinier, D., Leclercq, L., Sommé, G., Thèze, J., and Fougereau, M., 1982, The limited diversity of the mouse γ-chains anti-GAT repertoire does not seem to be noticeably amplified upon class switch, *J. Immunol.* **129**:2554–2558.

36. Rocca-Serra, J., Tonnelle, C., and Fougereau, M., 1983, Two monoclonal antibodies against different antigens use the same V$_H$ germ-line gene, *Nature* **304**:353–355.

37. Kabat, E. A., Wu, T. T., Bilofsky, H., Reid-Miller, M., and Perry, H., 1983, *Sequences of Proteins of Immunological Interest,* U.S. Department of Health and Human Services.

38. Potter, M., Newell, J. B., Rudikoff, S., and Haber, E., 1982, Classification of mouse V$_κ$ groups based on the partial amino acid sequence to the first invariant tryptophan: Impact of 14 new sequences from IgG myeloma, *Mol. Immunol.* **19**:1619–1630.

39. Rocca-Serra, J., Matthes, H. W., Kaartinen, M., Milstein, C., Thèze, J., and Fougereau, M., 1983, Analysis of antibody diversity: V–D–J mRNA nucleotide sequence of four anti-GAT monoclonal antibodies. A paucigene system using alternate D-J recombinations to generate functionally similar hypervariable regions, *EMBO J.* **2**:867–872.

40. Hamlyn, P. H., Brownlee, G. G., Cheng, C. C., Gait, M. J., and Milstein, C., 1978, Complete sequence of constant and 3′ non-coding regions of an immunoglobulin mRNA using the dideoxynucleotide method of RNA sequencing, *Cell* **15**:1067–1075.

41. Sanger, F., Nicklen, S., and Carlson, A. R., 1977, DNA sequencing with chain-terminating inhibitors, *Proc. Natl. Acad. Sci. USA* **74**:5463–5467.

42. Kurosawa, Y., and Tonegawa, S., 1982, Organization, structure and assembly of immunoglobulin heavy chain diversity DNA segments, *J. Exp. Med.* **155**:201–218.

43. Schiff, C., Milili, M., and Fougereau, M., 1983, Immunoglobulin diversity: Analysis of the germ-line V$_H$ gene repertoire of the murine anti-GAT response, *Nucleic Acids Res.* **11**:4007–4017.

44. Loh, D. Y., Bothwell, A. L. M., White-Scharf, M. E., Imanishi-Kari, T., and Baltimore, D., 1983, Molecular basis of a mouse strain-specific anti-hapten response, *Cell* **33**:85–93.

45. Lazure, C., Tung-Hum, W., and Gibson, D. M., 1981, Sequence diversity within a subgroup of mouse immunoglobulin kappa chains controlled by the Ig$_κ$-Ef2 locus, *J. Exp. Med.* **154**:146–155.

46. Morse, H. C., III, Goode, J. H., and Rudikoff, S., 1977, Murine plasma cells secreting more than one class of immunoglobulin heavy chain. IV. Sequence differences between chain of SAMM 368 IgG2b and IgA, *J. Immunol.* **119**:361–363.

47. Prahl, J. W., Mandy, W. J., and Todd, C. W., 1969, The molecular determinants of the A11 and A12 allotypic specificities in rabbit immunoglobulin, *Biochemistry* **8**:4935–4940.

48. Appella, E., Chersi, A., Mage, R. G., and Dubiski, S., 1971, Structural basis of the A14 and A15 allotypic specificities in rabbit immunoglobulin G, *Proc. Natl. Acad. Sci. USA* **68**:1341–1345.

49. Franèk, F., and Nezlin, R. S., 1963, Recovery of antibody combining activity by interaction of different peptide chains isolated from purified horse antitoxins, *Folia Microbiol. (Prague)* **8**:128–130.

50. Edelman, G. M., Olins, D. E., Gally, J. A., and Zinder, N., 1963, Reconstitution of immunoglobulin activity by interaction of polypeptide chains of antibodies, *Proc. Natl. Acad. Sci. USA* **50**:753–761.

51. Fougereau, M. Olins, D. E., and Edelman, G. M., 1964, Reconstitution of antiphage antibodies from L and H polypeptide chains and the formation of interspecies molecular hybrids, *J. Exp. Med.* **120**:349–358.

52. Metzger, H., Wofsy, L., and Singer, S. J., 1964, The participation of A and B polypeptide chains in the active sites of antibody molecules, *Proc. Natl. Acad. Sci. USA* **51**:612–618.

53. Amzel, L. M., Poljak, R., Saul, F., Varga, J., and Richards, F., 1974, The three dimensional structure of a combining region–ligand complex of immunoglobulin NEW at 3.5 Å resolution, *Proc. Natl. Acad. Sci. USA* **71**:1427–1430.

54. Brack, C., Hirama, M., Lenhard-Schuller, R., and Tonegawa, S., 1978, A complete immunoglobulin gene is created by somatic recombination, *Cell* **15**:1–14.

55. Sakano, H., Hüppi, K., Heinrich, G., and Tonegawa, S., 1979, Sequences at the somatic recombination sites of immunoglobulin light chain genes, *Nature* **280**:288–294.

56. Seidman, J. G., Max, E. E., and Leder, P., 1979, A κ immunoglobulin gene is formed by site-specific recombinations without further somatic mutation, *Nature* **280:**370–375.

57. Early, P., Huang, H., Davis, M., Calame, K., and Hood, L., 1980, An immunoglobulin heavy chain variable region gene is generated from three segments of DNA: V_H, D and J_H, *Cell* **19:**981–992.

58. Bothwell, A. L. M., Paskind, M., Reth, M., Imanishi-Kari, T., Rajewsky, K., and Baltimore, D., 1981, Heavy chain variable region contribution to the NP^b family of antibodies: Somatic mutations evident in a γ2a variable region, *Cell* **24:**625–637.

59. de Préval, C., and Fougereau, M., 1976, Specific interaction between V_H and V_L regions of human monoclonal immunoglobulins, *J. Mol. Biol.* **102:**657–678.

60. Hilschmann, N., and Craig, L. C., 1965, Amino acid sequence studies with Bence–Jones proteins, *Proc. Natl. Acad. Sci. USA* **53:**1403–1409.

61. Dryer, W. Y., and Bennett, J. C., 1965, The molecular basis of antibody formation: A paradox, *Proc. Natl. Acad. Sci. USA* **54:**864–869.

7

Structural Correlates of Idiotypes Expressed on Galactan-Binding Antibodies

STUART RUDIKOFF

1. Introduction

Antigenic determinants located on the variable region of the immunoglobulins (now commonly referred to as idiotypes) were originally described in humans in 1955[1] and in rabbits in 1963.[2] These markers have proven to be extremely valuable in the study of immunoglobulin genetics, diversity, and structure–function relationships. More recently, interest in idiotypes has expanded with the proposal of Jerne[3] suggesting that the determinants expressed on a given antibody population (Ab1) are recognized by a second set of antibodies (Ab2 or anti-idiotype) which may in turn be recognized by additional sets of antibodies (Ab3, Ab4, etc.) forming a network which is postulated to be intimately involved in the regulation of immune responses.

Considering the widespread interest and use of idiotypic markers, it is surprising how little is known about the structural basis of these determinants (reviewed in Ref. 4). One of the major problems inherent in the analysis of idiotypes is their apparent complexity. First, part of this difficulty is introduced by the very reagents employed in the identification of these markers. Anti-idiotype can be generated in heterologous, allogeneic, or syngeneic species. Each of these antisera may recognize different determinants on the same molecule or different aspects of the same determinant. Similarly, multiple antisera prepared in the same manner (or monoclonal antibodies) may display quite different specificities. Thus, the pattern of idiotypic reactivity displayed by a given antibody (or group of related antibodies) may be highly dependent on the particular set of reagents employed in the characterization.

STUART RUDIKOFF • Laboratory of Genetics, National Cancer Institute, Bethesda, Maryland 20205.

Second, idiotypes may be determined by amino acids located on the light (L) chain, the heavy (H) chain, or as frequently seems to be the case, by an interaction of both chains. It is therefore apparent that a delineation of the structural basis of given idiotypes requires a defined serological analysis in conjunction with complete L- and H-chain variable (V)-region sequences from structurally related molecules, some positive, and others negative, for the identified serological determinants.

The general approach taken to define the structural basis of idiotypes has been to assemble a group of monoclonal antibodies generated to the same haptenic determinant and perform serological and structural analyses as described above. To date, very few systems have been analyzed in sufficient detail to permit a precise definition of structural correlates to idiotypes. One such system under investigation in our laboratory consists of antibodies to $\beta(1,6)$-D-galactan moieties. $\beta(1,6)$-D-galactans are naturally occurring carbohydrates found in substances as diverse as lung extracts, tree gums, and hardwood shavings (commonly used in animal bedding).[5] In the remainder of this chapter I shall describe the characterization of a number of monoclonal antibodies reacting with the $\beta(1,6)$-galactan haptenic determinant and the structural basis of idiotypes expressed on these molecules.

2. Antibodies to $\beta(1,6)$-Galactans

In 1971 Sher and Tarikas described an IgA myeloma protein (J539) which precipitated with p-azophenyl-β-D-galactoside-bovine γ-globulin.[6] Subsequently, seven additional IgA myeloma proteins with the same binding specificity were identified in Michael Potter's myeloma collection at the NIH[5] (Table I). A number of these myeloma proteins have been characterized in considerable detail in terms of idiotypy,[7] binding specificity,[8,9] primary[10,11] and three-dimensional structure.[12] More recently, a series of hybridoma proteins (Table I) have been generated by fusion of spleen cells from galactan-immunized BALB/c mice with the nonsecreting Sp2/0 cell line.[13] Complete V-region structures have been determined for four of the myeloma and eight of the hybridoma proteins which, in conjunction with idiotypic serological analysis, provide the opportunity to assess the molecular basis of idiotypes expressed on these molecules.

TABLE I
Antibodies to $\beta(1,6)$-D-Galactan

Myelomas		Hybridomas		
X44	IgA,κ	HyGal	1	IgM,κ
X24	IgA,κ	HyGal	2	IgM,κ
T601	IgA,κ	HyGal	3	IgM,κ
J539	IgA,κ	HyGal	4	IgM,κ
JPC1	IgA,κ	HyGal	6	IgM,κ
CBPC4	IgA,κ	HyGal	10	IgM,κ
SAPC10	IgA,κ	HyGal	11	IgM,κ
		HyGal	12	IgM,κ

3. V-Region Sequences of Galactan-Binding Antibodies

Complete κ-chain V-region sequences have been determined for 16 of the galactan-binding antibodies[11,13] and 12 of these are presented in Fig. 1. κ light chains are encoded by two genes, one corresponding to the V_κ segment (usually amino acids 1–95) and one corresponding to the J_κ segment (amino acids 96–108).[14,15] The κ chains from the antigalactan proteins are all highly homologous and unusual in that 15/16 have an Ile at position 96 which is normally the first residue encoded by the J_κ gene. Ile is not encoded at this position in any of the germ-line J_κ genes nor can this amino acid be readily generated by alterations in the frame of recombination between V_κ and J_κ. It has therefore been proposed[11] that the antigalactan V_κ segments are actually one amino acid longer than normal and that the first codon of the J_κ gene is usually not employed. X44 is the single exception in which the Trp substitution at position 96 is, in fact, encoded by the first codon of the J_κ gene. Within the V_κ region 12 of these L chains are identical in sequence. A single substitution is found in HyGal 6, two identical substitutions in HyGal 7 and 9 (not shown), and 5 substitutions in J539. The sequence variation between amino acids 97 and 108 reflects the potential use of all four functional J_κ genes.

As is the case in the L chains, the H chains from these proteins (Fig. 2) demonstrate highly homologous sequences.[16] The immunoglobulin H chain is encoded by three gene segments, V_H, D, and J_H.[17,18] The V_H gene encodes amino acids 1–95; D, a portion of the third complementarity-determining region (CDR3); and J, amino acids 101–113. The V_H segments of proteins HyGal 1, 2, 3, 4, X44, and T601 are identical in sequence from position 1–94 and correspond exactly to the translated sequence of a germ-line V_H gene sequenced by Ollo et al.[19] HyGal 6 differs from the prototype sequence at three positions, HyGal 10 at three positions, HyGal 11, 12 at one position, X24 at four positions, and J539 at four positions. HyGal 11 and 12 are identical in sequence in both their L and H chains and are presumably derived from the same original clone. Three J_H segments are found in the antigalactan heavy chains with J_H2 and J_H3 being employed six and five times respectively and J_H1 occurring once in T601. Most of the sequence variation found in these H chains is concentrated in the CDR3 region and results from alterations in recombination between V_H–D and D–J_H as well as the use of different D genes. This region of the molecule is particularly interesting in that the number of amino acids encoded by the D gene appears to vary from two to six among these proteins, yet the overall length in CDR3 remains invariant as a result of the addition of extra amino acids on the NH_2 and COOH sides of D, presumably by repair enzymes (see Ref. 16 for a detailed discussion). As will be seen, the sequence variation observed in CDR3 correlates with most of the idiotypes expressed on these molecules.

4. Idiotype Analysis of Galactan-Binding Antibodies

Allogeneic antisera raised in A/He and SJL/J mice have been used extensively to characterize the galactan-binding antibodies.[7] Idiotypic antisera have been prepared to each of the hybridoma and myeloma proteins presented in Fig. 2 and assayed by solid-phase radioimmunoassay.[20] Two types of analyses have been performed with these

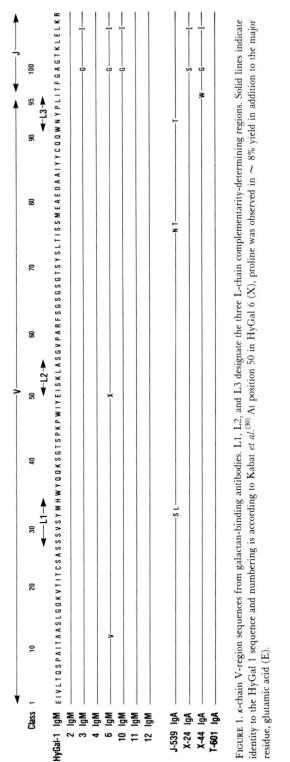

FIGURE 1. κ-chain V-region sequences from galactan-binding antibodies. L1, L2, and L3 designate the three L-chain complementarity-determining regions. Solid lines indicate identity to the HyGal 1 sequence and numbering is according to Kabat *et al.*[30] At position 50 in HyGal 6 (X), proline was observed in ∼ 8% yield in addition to the major residue, glutamic acid (E).

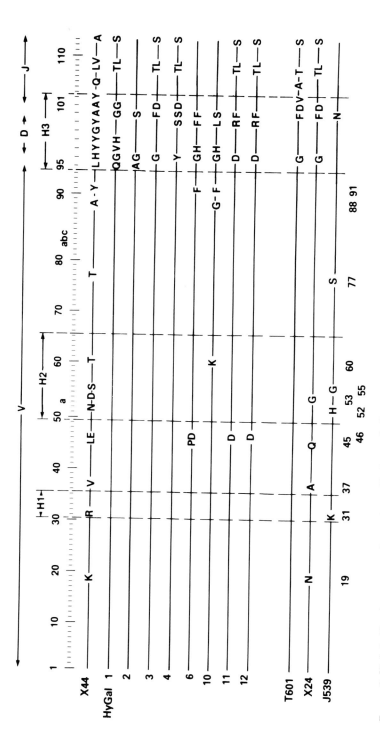

FIGURE 2. H-chain V-region sequences from galactan-binding antibodies. H1, H2, and H3 designate the three H-chain complementarity-determining regions. Solid lines indicate identity to the X44 sequence. At positions where substitutions occur the variant amino acid is given as well as the prototype found in X44. Numbering is according to Kabat et al.[30]

reagents. In the first, the immunizing protein is labeled with ^{125}I and the sera tested for competition of binding by other antigalactan hybridoma and myeloma proteins or sera from mice immunized with $\beta(1,6)$-galactan-containing polysaccharides. In the second form of the assay the ^{125}I-labeled target is not the immunizing protein but one of the other galactan-binding proteins previously found to also react with the particular antisera. Inhibitors are then tested as in the first assay. Results of competition assays using the immunogen as target are presented in Table II. Antisera to hybridoma proteins HyGal 1, 2, 4 and myeloma proteins X44, X24, J539 were essentially specific for the immunizing proteins using the arbitrarily assigned cutoff of 20× the weight of the immunogen for significant inhibition. Antisera to HyGal 3 cross-reacted with HyGal 2, T601, and X24 with the latter two inhibiting almost as well as the immunogen. Interestingly, antisera to T601 do not react with HyGal 2, but show strong cross-reactivity with X44. Antisera to HyGal 6 reacted equally well with HyGal 10 but none of the other proteins and antisera to HyGal 10 showed an identical reactivity pattern. Antisera to HyGal 12 reacted with all of the IgM

TABLE II

Idiotype Expression by Galactan-Binding Antibodies[a]

	Idiotypic systems[b]										
	HG1	HG2	HG3	HG4	HG6	HG10	HG12	T601	X44	X24	J539
Inhibitors											
Hybridomas											
HG1	[13]	>	>	>	>	>	>	>	>	>	>
HG2	>	[11]	[100]	>	>	>	[100]	>	>	>	>
HG3	300	>	[5]	>	>	>	[20]	[35]	>	>	>
HG4	>	>	700	[50]	>	>	[30]	>	>	>	>
HG6	>	>	>	>	[10]	[10]	[20]	>	>	>	>
HG10	>	>	>	>	[12]	[9]	[20]	>	>	>	>
HG12	>	>	250	>	>	500	[20]	>	>	>	>
Myelomas											
T601	>	>	[5]	>	>	>	>	[15]	>	>	>
X44	>	>	>	>	>	>	>	[150]	[6]	>	>
X24	>	>	[10]	>	>	>	>	[50]	>	[10]	>
J539	>	>	>	>	>	>	>	>	>	>	[3]

[a]Antisera to specified hybridoma or myeloma proteins were tested for competition of binding of radiolabeled immunogen. Values given represent number of ng required for 50% inhibition. > indicates 50% inhibition was not achieved at concentrations of 1000 ng or greater. Enclosed values represent significant inhibition arbitrarily defined as requiring less than 20 times the amount of homologous protein.

[b]Idiotypic antisera were prepared to the hybridoma and myeloma proteins indicated and tested with inhibitors listed in column at left.

hybridoma proteins, with the exception of HyGal 1, to approximately the same extent, but did not react with any of the IgA myeloma proteins. Two additional systems have been analyzed in which the ^{125}I-labeled target was not the immunogen (data not shown). When antisera to T601 were tested using [^{125}I]-X24 as the target, inhibition was obtained with X24, T601, and X44. Antisera to X44 with [^{125}I]-J539 as the target were inhibited by both X44 and J539.

The expression of a number of the myeloma idiotypes in immune sera has been tested in two pools, each consisting of sera from five mice taken 7 to 8 days following immunization (Table III).[21] As can be seen, the idiotype recognized by antisera to T601 with X24 as the target is well represented while the X44:J539, X24:X24, T601:T601 systems are moderately inhibited and the X44:X44 and J539:J539 systems show no inhibition. Thus, as might be expected from the cross-inhibition of hybridoma and myeloma proteins in Table II, several of the idiotypes expressed on these proteins are readily detected in the corresponding immune response.

5. Localization of Idiotypes

Since complete L- and H-chain sequences (Figs. 1 and 2) are available for eight hybridoma and four myeloma proteins, a comparison of these structures can define portions of the molecule involved in the formation of idiotypic determinants.[16] Regions of sequence identity in two or more proteins which are serologically distinguishable are presumed not to be involved in the generation of antigenic structures. Conversely, regions of sequence differences become candidates for these markers. Sequence differences fall into two general categories: (1) those unique to a given protein which may be responsible for individual idiotypes; (2) those shared by two or more proteins which thus distinguish subsets within the group and are candidates for cross-reacting or shared idiotypes. These two types of determinants are clearly not mutually exclusive as many homogeneous proteins express both individual and cross-reacting idiotypes. The following discussion of idiotype localization will be limited to the 12 galactan-binding antibodies for which complete sequences are available.

TABLE III
Expression of Antigalactan Idiotypes in Immune Sera

Antiserum: target	Reciprocal of serum dilution giving 50% inhibition	
	Pool 1	Pool 2
X24: Gal-KLH	355.0	833.0
T601: X24	105.0	155.0
X44: J539	17.7	14.2
X24: X24	6.2	26.0
T601: T601	14.0	20.0
X44: X44	—	—
J539:J539	—	2.2

Examination of the L-chain sequences (Fig. 1) reveals that only HyGal 6 and J539 display amino acid substitutions in the V_κ region and X44 has a substitution at residue 96, the point of V_κ–J_κ recombination. The single replacement at residue 12 in HyGal 6 cannot be involved in an idiotypic determinant since antisera to HyGal 6 react equally well with HyGal 10 (Table II) which expresses Ala at this position as do all of the other L chains. The substitution of Trp for Ile at position 96 in X44 is also considered not to be involved in idiotypic determinants as the three-dimensional structure determined for the crystallized J539 protein[12] (D. Davies, personal communication) reveals that position 96 is buried in the interior of the molecule and the Ile-Trp substitution can be readily accommodated without perturbation of the structure. Since no pattern of cross-reactivity is found among proteins sharing the same J_κ region, this segment of the molecule can be eliminated as idiotype-determining. Thus, among the 12 proteins being analyzed only the J539 L chain can contribute amino acids generating idiotypic determinants and, therefore, in each of the other proteins these markers must correlate with amino acid substitutions in the H chain.

From the H-chain sequences (Fig. 2) it can be seen that the galactan-binding proteins are all highly homologous in the V_H segment (amino acids 1–94). Hybridoma proteins HyGal 1, 2, 3, 4 and myeloma proteins X44, T601 are identical in this region. Since none of the antisera to these proteins (Table II) cross-reacts throughout the group, the V_H segment can be eliminated as idiotype-determining in these molecules. Proteins HyGal 6, 11, and 12 share the same Asp substitution at position 46, yet antisera to HyGal 6 do not cross-react with HyGal 12 and antisera to HyGal 12 cross-react with proteins expressing Glu at position 46. Thus, Asp-46 is not an idiotype-determining residue. The remaining V_H substitutions in the hybridoma proteins are found in HyGal 6 and 10. Since antisera to HyGal 6 react equally well with HyGal 10 (and conversely, antisera to HyGal 10 react equally well with HyGal 6), only the shared Phe-91 substitution could potentially be idiotype-determining. However, from the three-dimensional structure position 91 is in the L–H interface and would not be accessible as an antigenic determinant. Therefore, only in the myeloma proteins X24 and J539 could V_H substitutions contribute directly to idiotype determination. As was the case for the J_L segment, no pattern of cross-reactivity was observed among proteins sharing J_H segments, eliminating this region as idiotype-determining. It can thus be concluded that, except for myeloma proteins X24 and J539, the idiotypes expressed on each of the other galactan-binding proteins must be generated by the considerable sequence variation located in CDR3. A hypothetical model of the J539 myeloma proteins (Fig. 3),[22] as well as the J539 X-ray structure (D. R. Davies, personal communication), indicate that the CDR3 region in the antigalactan proteins is an external loop exposed to solvent. This segment is therefore in a position where one would predict antigen (idiotype)-determining amino acids to be located.

6. Structural Correlates of Idiotypes

Having localized the majority of idiotypes expressed by the galactan-binding antibodies to the H-chain CDR3 region, it is now possible to examine the CDR3 sequences and assign amino acids correlating with these antigenic markers.[16] It should be emphasized that, although the amino acids which generate these determinants can be precisely identified in many instances, it is by no means implied that these amino acids are necessarily the

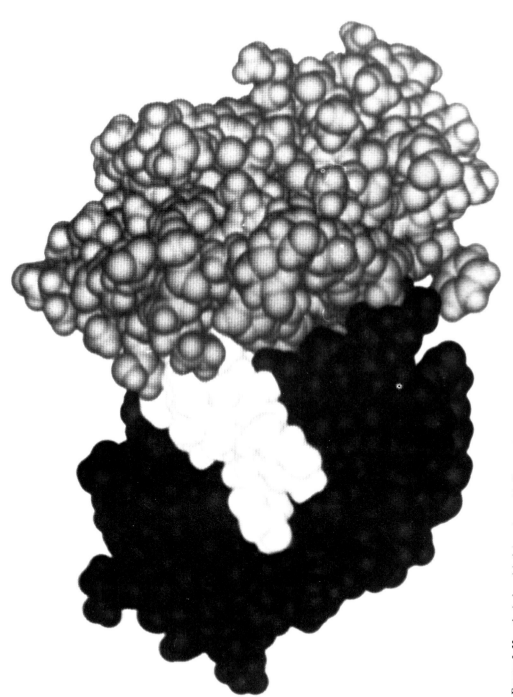

FIGURE 3. Hypothetical model of the galactan-binding myeloma protein, J539. Coloring is as follows: L chain, black; H chain, gray; H-chain CDR3 region, white.

actual antigenic determinants being recognized. Idiotypes may be very complex in nature and formed by the interaction of amino acids in CDR3 or by the interaction of these residues with other portions of the molecule which may either vary in sequence or be constant. In the subsequent analysis the serological characterizations in Table III will be compared to the CDR3 sequences (Fig. 4) to define idiotype-related amino acids.

From Table III it can be seen that HyGal 1 is serologically unique. The CDR3 sequence of HyGal 1 is the most divergent of the group and five amino acids can be identified which, either alone or in combinations, produce the HyGal 1 determinant.

Antisera to HyGal 2 were specific for the immunogen. The HyGal 2 CDR3 sequence is identical to that of proteins HyGal 3, T601, and X24 for positions 96–100 and differs only at residues 95 and 100a from other members of the group. Therefore, either Ala-95 or Ser-100a (or an interaction of the two) generates the HyGal 2 idiotype. It is unlikely that these amino acids "mask" the shared 96–100 sequence as antisera to HyGal 3 cross-react with HyGal 2 apparently via the 96–100 region. Therefore, the unique substitutions must be dominant idiotype-determining amino acids.

Antisera to HyGal 3 define a subset of cross-reacting molecules including HyGal 2, T601, and X24. These antisera appear directed predominantly against the "core" 96–100 sequence which characterizes this group. HyGal 2 which has substitutions on both sides of the "core" sequence inhibits less well, indicating that either these positions are part of the HyGal 3 determinant or that the substitutions cause a perturbation of the antigenic structure. HyGal 4 and 12 were found to weakly inhibit and share portions of the core sequence. The complexity of some of these idiotypes is pointed out by this result in that other proteins such as X44 and J539 which, based on their sequences in this region, might be expected to inhibit as well as HyGal 4 and 12, are negative. Interestingly, antisera to T601 show a

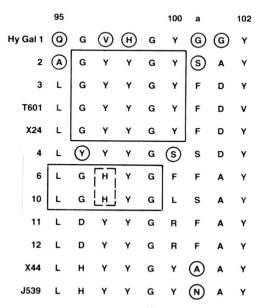

FIGURE 4. H-chain CDR3 sequences from galactan-binding antibodies. Circled and boxed amino acids designate residues likely involved in the generation of idiotypic determinants.

different pattern of reactivity as HyGal 2 does not inhibit this system. HyGal 3 and X24 are both good inhibitors and X44 reacts to a lesser extent. Thus, the same protein sequence is being "seen" differently by antisera to HyGal 3 and T601. The failure of HyGal 2 to inhibit the T601 system indicates that either position 95 or 100a is important to the determinant recognized by these sera. This same CDR3 sequence must also be the antigenic determinant in the cross-reacting system in which antisera to T601 are assayed using [125I]-X24 at the target. This system is also inhibited by T601, X24, and X44.

Antisera to HyGal 4 were found to react only with the immunogen. HyGal 4 has unique amino acids at positions 96 and 100 and either, or an interaction of the two, must generate this determinant.

HyGal 6 and 10 were indistinguishable by antisera raised against either protein. These molecules have a common sequence from positions 95 to 99 and are distinguishable from other members of the group by His-97. This amino acid would therefore be considered "dominant" in the determination of this cross-reacting idiotype.

Idiotypic antisera to HyGal 12 showed the broadest reactivity of any of the serological reagents. Among the IgM hybridomas only HyGal 1 failed to inhibit this reaction. All of the IgM proteins, with the exception of HyGal 1, share only the sequence Tyr-98, Gly-99. However, IgA myeloma proteins with the same sequence do not inhibit. If the Tyr-98, Gly-99 sequence is, in fact, idiotype-determining, the C_H1 region must effect expression of the marker either by being a part of the determinant or by steric hindrance in the case of the α C_H1. A similar result has been described for a monoclonal antibody to phosphocholine.[23]

Antisera to X44 were specific for the immunogen. X44 differs from J539 by a single Ala-Asn substitution at position 100a defining this residue as idiotype-determining and providing an example in which a single substitution apparently completely alters an antigenic determinant. Interestingly, in the cross-reacting system in which antisera to X44 were assayed with [125I]-J539 as target, inhibition was obtained with both X44 and J539. These proteins are distinguished by the shared His-96 substitution which likely produces the determinant recognized by a subset of antibodies present in the antisera.

Protein X24, which has a CDR3 sequence identical to that found in HyGal 3 and T601, inhibits antisera to both of these proteins. However, antiserum to X24 is not inhibited by either of these proteins, indicating that this reagent is directed against a determinant not located in CDR3. X24 has four substitutions in the V_H segment (Fig. 2) and we have previously suggested that this idiotype correlates with Gly-53 found in CDR2.[21] Furthermore, the specificity of this antiserum appears to be different from that of a monoclonal antibody to X24 which was found to react moderately well with X44 and weakly with several of the other galactan-binding antibodies.[20]

Antisera to J539 were also specific for the immunogen. This protein has a number of substitutions in both V_H and V_L (Figs. 1 and 2), making an assignment of a structural correlate to the J539 idiotype impossible at this time.

7. Conclusions and Comments

The above analysis has permitted a delineation at the molecular level of amino acids involved in the generation of both individual and cross-reacting idiotyopic determinants. At present, these studies probably represent the limits to which the structural basis of idiotypy can be defined. The CDR3 region of the antigalactan H chains, in which nearly all of the described idiotype-generating amino acids are located, is an exposed loop on the surface of the molecule as might be expected for a region presumed to be involved in antigenic structures. However, although possible, it does not necessarily follow that these amino acids are, in all cases, the actual antigenic determinants being recognized by anti-idiotypic reagent. It is suggested from the serological systems that some determinants probably involve the interaction of amino acids in CDR3, but it is also possible that actual antigenic sites arise from interactions between amino acids in CDR3 and others located elsewhere in the molecule. Thus, the complexity of the antigenic structure being recognized is unknown.

The precise structural requirements for the generation of idiotypes are emphasized by the antigalactan proteins. A change of one or two amino acids between proteins results in a complete alteration of determinants in many cases. Thus, while some proteins are approximately 99% homologous over their V regions, they appear unrelated by serological analysis. It must be cautioned that the conclusions concerning idiotypes are restricted to the particular reagents being employed and that entirely different correlates are likely to be found with other antisera or monoclonal antibodies. Furthermore, the observation that the same protein sequence can be "seen" differently, as is the case with antisera to HyGal 3 and T601, suggests an additional dimension of complexity in idiotypic relationships. It is, therefore, probably not too surprising that we are just beginning to achieve an understanding of the molecular basis of idiotypy (see Ref. 4).

To date, it has been possible to reasonably define structural correlates of idiotypes in only a limited number of other systems. Two idiotypes have been localized to the L chains of inulin-binding myeloma proteins.[24] One of these correlated with three possible substitutions,[25] and the second with amino acids in CDR2.[26] The most extensive existing data on idiotype structure have been derived from studies of myeloma and hybridoma proteins which bind the haptenic determinant $\alpha(1,3)$-dextran[27−29] (Fulton et al., this volume). Two classes of marker have been identified, one a cross-reacting determinant located in the H-chain CDR2 and the second a series of unique determinants which are localized to CDR3. The individual idiotypes in CDR3 correlate with substitutions in the D region which are limited to two amino acids. Antibodies sharing D-region sequences show cross-reactivity with heterologous antisera, yet surprisingly, proteins which have unrelated D sequences were found to cross-react with a monoclonal antibody. The basis for this latter reactivity is unclear. Additionally, it should be noted that these assignments have been made assuming that all of the L chains, which are λ type, are identical although this has not been established experimentally.

As we now begin to generate an understanding of the structural basis of idiotypes in systems such as $\alpha(1,3)$-dextran- and $\beta(1,6)$-galactan-binding antibodies, it becomes interesting to speculate on the possible role of these markers in biological systems such as immune networks as proposed by Jerne.[3] The idiotypes recognized in the antigalactan proteins are all detected by homologous antisera and are directed toward the most variable portion of the molecule, the region including D and the two recombination events V_H–D and D–J_H. Thus, as was found among these proteins, a large number of idiotypes are potentially generated in a given immune response. If the markers recognized by autologous anti-idiotype in a network *in vivo* were similar in nature, and if this antigenic diversity is an accurate reflection of the immune response, then a corresponding large number of anti-idiotypes would be necessary for regulation. These insights into the structure of idiotypic determinants therefore raise provocative questions concerning the nature of markers that might be recognized in regulatory systems and additionally point out the need for additional analyses to test the generality of these observations.

References

1. Slater, R. J., Ward, S. M., and Kunkel, H. G., 1955, Immunological relationships among the myeloma proteins, *J. Exp. Med.* **101**:85–108.
2. Oudin, J., and Michel, M., 1963, Une nouvelle forme d'allotypie des globulins du sérum de lapin apparement lié à la fonction et à la spécificité anticorps, *C. R. Acad. Sci. Ser. D* **257**:805–808.
3. Jerne, N., 1974, Toward a network theory of the immune system, *Ann. Immunol. (Inst. Pasteur)* **125C**:373–389.
4. Rudikoff, S., 1983, Immunoglobulin structure-function correlates: Antigen binding and idiotypes, *Contemp. Top. Mol. Immunol.* **9**:169–209.
5. Potter, M., 1977, Antigen-binding myeloma proteins of mice, *Adv. Immunol.* **25**:141–211.
6. Sher, A., and Tarikas, H., 1971, Hapten binding studies on mouse IgM myeloma proteins with antibody activity, *J. Immunol.* **106**:1227–1233.
7. Mushinski, E. B., and Potter, M., 1977, Idiotypes on galactan binding myeloma proteins and anti-galactan antibodies in mice, *J. Immunol.* **119**:1888–1893.
8. Jolley, M. E., Rudikoff, S., Potter, M., and Glaudemans, C. P. J., 1973, Spectral changes on binding of oligosaccharides to murine immunoglobulin A myeloma proteins, *Biochemistry* **12**:3039–3044.
9. Jolley, M. E., Glaudemans, C. P. J., Rudikoff, S., and Potter, M., 1974, Structural requirements for the binding of derivatives of D-galactose to two homogeneous murine immunoglobulins, *Biochemistry* **13**:3179–3184.
10. Rao, D. N., Rudikoff, S., Krutzsch, H., and Potter, M., 1979, Structural evidence for independent joning region gene in immunoglobulin heavy chains from anti-galactan myeloma proteins and its potential role in generating diversity in complementarity determining regions, *Proc. Natl. Acad. Sci. USA* **76**:2890–2894.
11. Rudikoff, S., Rao, D. N., Glaudemans, C. P. J., and Potter, M., 1980, κ chain joining segments and structural diversity of antibody combining sites, *Proc. Natl. Acad. Sci. USA* **77**:4270–4274.
12. Navia, M. A., Segal, D. M., Padlan, E. A., Davies, D. R., Rao, D. N., Rudikoff, S., and Potter, M., 1979, Crystal structure at 4.5 Å resolution of the galactan-binding mouse J539 immunoglobulin Fab, *Proc. Natl. Acad. Sci. USA* **76**:4071–4074.
13. Pawlita, M., Potter, M., and Rudikoff, S., 1982, κ-chain restriction in anti-galactan antibodies, *J. Immunol.* **129**:615–618.
14. Max, E. E., Seidman, J. G., and Leder, P., 1979, Sequences of five recombination sites encoded close to an immunoglobulin κ constant region gene, *Proc. Natl. Acad. Sci. USA* **76**:3450–3454.
15. Sakano, H., Huppi, K., Heinrich, G., and Tonegawa, S., 1979, Sequences at the somatic recombination sites of immunoglobulin light chain genes, *Nature* **280**:288–294.
16. Rudikoff, S., Pawlita, M., Pumphrey, J., Mushinski, E., and Potter, M., 1983, Galactan binding antibodies; Diversity and structure of idiotypes, *J. Exp. Med.* **158**:1385–1400.
17. Early, P., Huang, H., Davis, M., Calame, K., and Hood, L., 1980, An immunoglobulin heavy chain variable gene is generated from three segments of DNA: V$_H$, D and J$_H$, *Cell* **19**:981–992.
18. Sakano, H., Maki, R., Kurosawa, Y., Roeder, W., and Tonegawa, S., 1980, Two types of somatic recombination are necessary for the generation of complete immunolgobulin heavy chain genes, *Nature* **286**:676–683.
19. Ollo, R., Auffray, C., Sikorar, J. L., and Rougeon, F., 1981, Mouse heavy chain variable regions: Nucleotide sequence of a germline V$_H$ gene segment, *Nucleic Acids Res.* **9**:4099–4109.
20. Pawlita, M., Mushinski, E., Feldmann, R. J., and Potter, M., 1981, A monoclonal antibody that defines an idiotope with two subsites in galactan-binding myeloma proteins, *J. Exp. Med.* **154**:1946–1956.
21. Potter, M., Mushinski, E. B., Rudikoff, S., Glaudemans, C. P. J., Padlan, E. A., and Davies, D. R., 1979, Structural and genetic basis of idiotypy in the galactan-binding myeloma proteins, *Ann. Immunol. (Inst. Pasteur)* **130C**:263–271.

22. Feldmann, R., Potter, M., and Glaudemans, C. P. J., 1981, A hypothetical space-filling model of the galactan-binding myeloma immunoglobulin J539, *Mol. Immunol.* **18**:683–689.
23. Morahan, G., Berek, C., and Miller, J. F. A. P., 1983, An idiotypic determinant formed by both immunoglobulin constant and variable regions, *Nature* **301**:720–722.
24. Lieberman, R., Vrana, M., Humphrey, W., Chien, C. C., and Potter, M., 1977, Idiotypes of inulin binding myeloma proteins localized to variable region light and heavy chains: Genetic significance, *J. Exp. Med.* **146**:1294–1304.
25. Vrana, M., Rudikoff, S., and Potter, M., 1979, The structural basis of a hapten-inhibitable κ-chain idiotype, *J. Immunol.* **122**:1905–1910.
26. Johnson, N., Slankard, J., Paul, L., and Hood, L., 1982, The complete V domain amino acid sequences of two myeloma inulin binding proteins, *J. Immunol.* **128**:302–307.
27. Schilling, J., Clevinger, B., Davie, J. M., and Hood, L., 1980, Amino acid sequence of homogeneous antibodies to dextran and DNA rearrangements in heavy chain V-region gene segments, *Nature* **283**:35–40.
28. Clevinger, B., Schilling, J., Hood, L., and Davie, J. M., 1980, Structural correlates of cross-reactive and individual idiotypic determinants on murine antibodies to α(1,3) dextran, *J. Exp. Med.* **151**:1059–1070.
29. Clevinger, B., Thomas, J., Davie, J. M., Schilling, J., Bond, M., and Hood, L., 1981, Antidextran antibodies; sequences and idiotypes, in: *Immunoglobulin Idiotypes and Their Expression: ICN–UCLA Symposium on Molecular and Cellular Biology,* Volume 20 (C. Janeway, E. E. Sercarz, H. Wigzell, and C. F. Fox, eds.), Academic Press, New York, pp. 159–168.
30. Kabat, E. A., Wu, T. T., and Bilofsky, H., 1979, Sequence of Immunoglobulin Chains, National Institutes of Health Publication 80-2008.

PART II
SEROLOGIC AND STRUCTURAL
CORRELATES OF IDIOTYPES

8

Idiotypic Markers and the Three-Dimensional Structure of Immunoglobulins

ROBERTO J. POLJAK

1. Introduction

A discussion of the structural correlates of idiotypic markers is a difficult task at the present state of our knowledge of the three-dimensional structure of immunoglobulins and of the amino acid sequence definition of idiotypic markers. Only a few three-dimensional immunoglobulin structures have been determined at high resolution (reviewed in Refs. 1–3), and none of these are from immunoglobulin molecules that possess the major idiotypic markers associated with some immune responses.[4] In addition, the characterization of idiotypic markers by protein sequencing or by DNA sequencing has not progressed enough to give suitably general examples that could facilitate the conformational analysis of idiotypic markers. Another conceptual difficulty arises from the fact that idiotypes are defined operationally, often by serological reactions whose complexity escapes accurate structural description. Here we enter the area of protein–protein interactions for which we have few adequate examples that have been studied with the structural detail that would be necessary for the present analysis. In these interactions the contacting residues could be capable of assuming several conformational states one of which will be selected for the formation of a stable complex.

   At the present state of our knowledge it is not possible to predict the tertiary structure of a protein from its amino acid sequence. Even a simpler task, that of predicting the effect of mutations or amino acid side-chain replacements on the conformation of a known three-dimensional structure, is difficult and must be submitted to experimental analysis for verification. As an example of this situation we can consider the case of the mutant hemoglobin

ROBERTO J. POLJAK • Département d'Immunologie, Institut Pasteur, 75724 Paris Cedex 15, France.

Zurich[5] in which a histidine residue (63) of the β chain is replaced by an arginine. This single substitution alters the properties of hemoglobin, in particular its ability to discriminate between the ligands oxygen and carbon monoxide, rendering the molecule more susceptible to "poisoning" by reaction with carbon monoxide. The structural correlation of this clinical condition necessitated in addition to amino acid sequence determination a detailed *de novo* analysis by X-ray crystallography[5] to determine the altered hemoglobin structure and the role of the replaced side chain in the physiological behavior of hemoglobin Zurich.

Bearing in mind the limitations mentioned above we will attempt to discuss a few topics that are of interest in considering the correlations between idiotypic markers and the three-dimensional structure of immunoglobulins.

2. The Km Antigenic Markers of Immunoglobulins: A Structural Model

Several proteins whose detailed three-dimensional structure is known have been studied from the point of view of their antigenicity. Among these are myoglobin,[6] lysozyme,[7] and several other proteins and viruses (reviewed in Ref. 8). This topic has enjoyed a recent revival due to its practical and theoretical interest.[9]

Serological reactions have been widely used in immunology as an analytical tool to characterize immunoglobulin molecules. The correlation between genetics, molecular structure, and serological studies has led to a classification of antigenic markers present in immunoglobulins as isotypic, allotypic, and idiotypic. Their meaning is familiar to readers of this volume so that they do not need to be defined here.

Antigenic allotypic markers in immunoglobulin molecules have been analyzed by genetic and molecular studies, resulting in amino acid sequence correlations which are of the type that one would like to obtain with idiotypic markers. Here we will review the molecular structure of the Km (or Inv) allotypes of human immunoglobulin κ light chains as an example of well-defined antigenic markers that are under the control of alleles of a single gene. This system can be taken as a suitable model for the analysis of correlations between antigenic markers and three-dimensional structure.

Three antigenic markers of human κ chains, designated Km(1), Km(2), and Km(3), have been described.[10] They are recognized by serological reagents anti-Km(1,2), anti-Km(1), and anti-Km(3) (see Table I). Most human κ chains having the serological type Km(1) also express the Km(2) antigenic marker. The relation between antigenic markers and amino acid sequences[10] is given in Table I. It can be seen that a positive reaction for

TABLE I
Km Phenotypes

Km markers	Sequence positions	
	153	191
1, 2, −3	Ala	Leu
1, −2, −3	Val	Leu
−1, −2, 3	Ala	Val

Km(3) correlates with the occurrence of a Val residue at position 191, whereas a positive reaction with anti-Km(1,2) or anti-Km(1) reagents corresponds to a Leu residue at position 191. The difference between Km(1) and Km(1,2) is given by amino acid replacement at position 153 as shown in Table I. Consequently, there are two "determinants" that are necessary for the discrimination among the Km markers: the Leu 191 side chain [without which Km(3) is detected] and the Ala/Val 153.

In human λ light chains, subisotypic serological markers designated as Kern (Gly/Ser, residue 152) and Oz (Lys/Arg, residue 190) occur at similar positions in the three-dimensional structure, at a distance of about 12 Å[11,12] (see Fig. 1).

In the case of the κ chains, two epitopes distant in primary sequence but brought to close proximity (about 12 to 15 Å) by three-dimensional folding contribute to a unique antigenic determinant. Several conclusions can be drawn from this example: (1) the antigenic markers occur at an exposed region of the three-dimensional structure; (2) the antibodies that react specifically with the Km(1,2) κ chains must simultaneously recognize positions 153–191; in fact, it seems logical to think that there is a "readout" of the whole area between these positions in the formation of the protein–protein, antigen–antibody complex; (3) a change from Val to Ala at position 153 does not alter the Km(1)-positive character of the κ chain, a fact that can be explained by the smaller side-chain volume of Ala relative to Val.

The example of the Km markers is chosen to illustrate the correlations that can be made between three-dimensional structure, amino acid sequence, and antigenicity and also the complexity and ambiguity that can arise in serological typing or in typing with monoclonal antibodies even in a relatively simple, well-defined case.

3. Immunoglobulin Genes and the Conformation of the Combining Site

It has been shown that the joining of V and J gene segments generates diversity in the amino acid sequences of the variable (V) regions of the light (L) and heavy (H) chains of immunoglobulin molecules.[13–19] This section describes a correlation of the amino acid sequence diversity generated by this process and the three-dimensional structure of antibodies.

The antigen-combining sites and the antibody–ligand interactions of two immunoglobulins, M603 and New, have been studied and characterized by high-resolution X-ray diffraction.[12,20,21] The finding that somatic recombination processes add to the diversity coded by mouse immunoglobulin genes[13,19] prompted us to examine the structural significance of the diversity generated by these processes and its possible role in the antigen-binding function of antibodies.

The variable (V_L) regions of murine immunoglobulin κ L chains are coded by multiple variable-region genes and by four different "joining" (J_κ) gene segments.[14,15] The joining of these coding segments can generate amino acid sequence diversity at position 96 in the third hypervariable region of V_κ. The mouse immunoglobulin H chains are also coded by multiple V_H genes and several J_H segments and, in addition, by diversity or D segments.[16,19] Thus, the nature of amino acid side chains at the third complementarity-determining region will be affected by recombinational events between V_H, D, and J_H gene segments. In the case of some antibodies, a direct joining between V_H and J_H could take

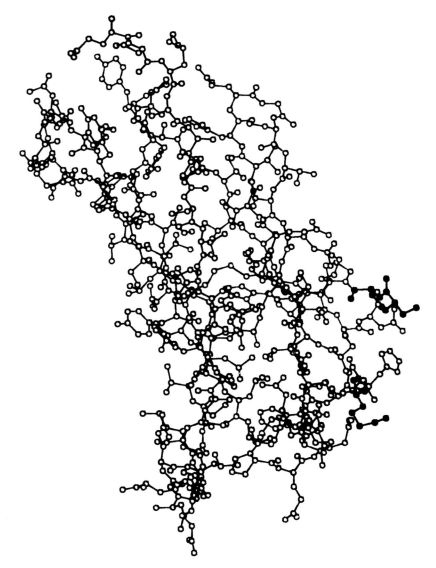

FIGURE 1. View of the C_L region of IgG New. The amino acid side chains filled in black, Ser 152 (above) and Lys 190 (below) correspond to the serological markers Kern and Oz, respectively.

place, without insertion of a D-segment sequence. This will result in a shallower combining site. We can analyze the possible antigen-binding role of sequence variations at the joining point between V_L and J_L in mouse κ chains and in the joining region between V_H, D, and J_H. For this purpose we use the high-resolution structure of Fab New[21] as a basic three-dimensional model.

Residue 96, which is subject to extensive variation by the mechanism of recombination between V_κ and J_κ gene segments, corresponds to Arg 95 in V_L New (see Fig. 2). This

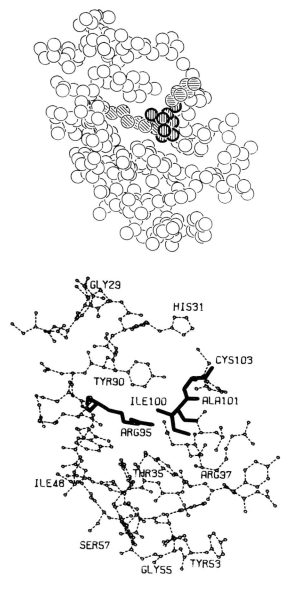

FIGURE 2. View of the combining site of IgG New. The top figure gives a partial space-filling representation (atomic radii about 0.8 Å), the bottom figure is a skeletal model in the same orientation. The residues which can be modified by a recombinational event between V_L and J_L gene segments (Arg 95 in V_L New) are indicated by diagonal shading. Of the residues which depend on the insertion of a D segment or that can be modified by recombinational events between V_H, D, and J_H, Ile 100 and Ala 101 are indicated by vertical and horizontal shading, respectively.

residue occupies a central position at the combining site and any variation in the nature of its amino acid side chain could be important in determining antigen complementarity. Variations in other positions of J_κ sequences are further removed and do not contribute directly to antigen–antibody contacts. Recombinational variations resulting in antigen-binding diversity occur in the region corresponding to V_H residues 99–101 in Fab New (Fig. 2). This is in fact the region encompassed by the D segments and the joining point between D and J_H. Residues 99 and 101 occupy a central position at the combining site of IgG New, opposite V_L residue 96 (Arg 95 in Fig. 2). Thus, although binding of ligands and antigens is not a function of these residues alone, they could make an important contribution to variations at the combining site.

Further support for this conclusion can be found in a study[22] of the combining site of M603 and related phosphocholine-binding mouse myeloma proteins. In these proteins, H-chain residues Tyr 33, Glu 35, Arg 52, and Glu 59, all outside the D segment, closely interact with phosphorylcholine. Trp 102 and the residue at position 96 in th L chain also participate in contacts with the ligand. Since position 102 is in the J_H segment, the amino acid residue at this position will vary depending on the recombinational event between V_H, D, and J_H. M167 differs from other antiphosphocholine myeloma proteins in having Gly, not Trp, at position 102, and together with M511, an Asp residue at position 100 in the D segment. These amino acid sequence variations are reflected in a lower binding affinity for phosphorylcholine but a higher affinity for free choline in murine myeloma proteins M167 and M511 as compared to other phosphorylcholine-binding proteins.[23] The residue at position 96 in V_L contributes to binding contacts with phosphocholine[22]; hence, it can be expected that variations at this position will also affect antigen specificity or binding affinity.

We conclude that the amino acid variations generated by the process of recombination between V_L and J_L, and between V_H, D, and J_H generate structural diversity at a central part of the combining site. This diversity is important in determining the stereochemistry of the combining site and the specificity and affinity of antigen–antibody interactions.

Finally, as can be seen in Fig. 2 (and more quantitatively in Table IV of Ref. 21) V_L residue Arg 95 (96 in κ chains) and V_H residues 98 and 99 make close contacts (interatomic distances close to the sum of van der Waals radii for C, N, and O). Arg 95 also makes close contacts with V_H Trp 47. In addition, V_H Ala 101 makes close contacts with V_L Tyr 90 and V_L His 31. Thus, residues which are subject to variation by the process of somatic recombination between V_L and J_L and between V_H, D, and J_H participate in close V_H–V_L contacts which can determine the preferential association of H and L chains.[21,24] This observation suggests that the genetic mechanism that controls the recombination of different DNA segments also selects H and L chain pairing and the resulting antibody specificity.

4. Idiotypic Determinants and the Antibody Combining Site

The analysis above, concerning the genetic determination of the structure of the antibody combining site, can be extended to idiotypic markers. In doing so, it will be assumed that true idiotypic markers occur only in the hypervariable regions, which express amino acid sequences and antigenic determinants unique to every monoclonal protein. This is only a simplifying assumption since, for example, a mutational variation (a point mutation) could give rise to an idiotypic antigenic marker outside the hypervariable regions, much like the variations that determine the Km allotypes of human κ chains discussed in a preceding section. Other "idiotypic" markers which will not be located in the hypervariable region could arise as a result of the operational definition of an idiotype, e.g., from antigenic markers belonging to a set of rarely expressed genes. An idiotypic marker has recently been reported in phosphocholine-binding murine antibodies in whch the C_H region of the heavy chain contributes to the idiotype.[25] In the following discussion we will arbitrarily disregard cases in which idiotypes are not part of hypervariable regions. With this bias, idiotypic markers will be close to the antigen-combining site of antibodies. However, not all antigen-contacting residues are in an accessible conformation such that they can be recognized as idiotype or idiotypic markers of an antibody. Conversely, not all idiotypic markers will correspond to amino acid positions that are directly involved in antigen recognition contacts. It is interesting to note here that the complementarity-determining regions correspond to segments of polypeptide chains that exhibit motion, i.e., different conformational states that could be recognized in several different ways by different anti-idiotypic antibodies. Also, the inhibition of anti-idiotypic reactions by hapten binding could be due to conformational changes at the combining site and in the surrounding region arising from the binding of the hapten, rather than by a competition between the hapten and the anti-idiotypic antibody for the combining site.

The light and the heavy chains of an antibody molecule are both potential contributors to its idiotypic markers. From the discussion of the Km markers in a preceding section it is easy to visualize that markers expressed by one chain may not be reactive with an anti-idiotypic reagent if this chain is paired with a different light or heavy chain. Flexibility at the combining-site residues will give rise to different conformations depending on the partner (H or L) polypeptide chain.

From the example of the Km allotypes of human κ chains we can conclude that an anti-idiotypic antiserum or anti-idiotypic antibody could be recognizing a unique combination of idiotypes contributed by each chain, since parts of the hypervariable regions of both chains are sufficiently close in space to provide a suitable substrate. Alternatively, each chain (H or L) could by itself provide the recognized idiotypes. Heavy chains exhibit more variation at a larger exposed area to provide a preferential substrate for anti-idiotypic reactions. In summary, from a consideration of the three-dimensional structure of immunoglobulins, idiotypic markers could arise from a very large number of possibilities.

The recombination of the genetic segments V_L, J_L, V_H, D, and J_H introduces further complexity in this analysis. Just as for the individual heavy or light chain, some of these segments by themselves or by their particular associations will give rise to unique idiotypic markers. For example, the D segment of heavy chains is in a most favorable structural position to provide idiotypic markers by itself (see Fig. 2). Since those markers can be associated with different V_H and V_L segments, a given idiotype or a cross-reacting antigenic determinant carried by different antibodies can be associated with different antigen-binding specificities as originally observed by Oudin and Cazenave[26] and in many other laboratories since then. It follows that a regulatory network,[27] composed of antibodies that cross-stimulate or repress each other by mutual interactions involving idiotypic markers, should lead to a polyclonal stimulation since there will be markers present in D segments, or in V_H, V_L segments associated with different antigen-binding specificities. Such type of stimulation would not be very different in principle from that observed with Fc fragments or subfragments[28] since both would lead to a polyclonal response. Similar conclusions were expressed by Takemori *et al.*[29] in their study of idiotypy in the anti-NP system in C57BL/6 mice. Furthermore, we agree with their conclusions concerning "internal images" of antigens since it is very difficult to envisage how an anti-idiotypic antibody could constitute the structural image of an immunizing antigen, or how an anti-anti-idiotypic reagent[30] could exactly reproduce the structure of the idiotypic antibody.

References

1. Davies, D. R., Padlan, E. A., and Segal, D., 1975, Three-dimensional structure of immunoglobulins, *Annu. Rev. Biochem.* **44:**639–667.
2. Kabat, E. A., Wu, T. T., Bilofsky, H., Reid-Miller, M., and Perry, H., 1983, *Sequences of Proteins of Immunologicial Interest,* U.S. Department of Health and Human Services, NIH, Bethesda.
3. Poljak, R. J., 1978, Correlations between three-dimensional structure and function of immunoglobulins, *CRC Crit. Rev. Biochem.* **5:**45–84.
4. Eichmann, K., 1975, Genetic control of antibody specificity in the mouse, *Immunogenetics* **2:**491–506.
5. Phillips, S. E. V., Hall, D., and Perutz, M. F., 1981, Structure of deoxyhemoglobin Zurich (His E7(63β)→Arg), *J. Mol. Biol.* **150:**137–141.
6. Atassi, M. Z., 1979, The antigenic structure of myoglobin and initial consequences of its precise determination, *CRC Crit. Rev. Biochem.* **6:**337–369.
7. Arnon, R., 1977, Immunochemistry of lysozyme, in: *Immunochemistry of Enzymes and Their Antibodies* (M. R. J. Salton, ed.), Wiley, New York, pp. 1–28.
8. Van Regenmortel, M. H. V., 1982, *Serology and Immunochemistry of Plant Viruses,* Academic Press, New York.
9. Lerner, R. A., 1982, Tapping the immunological repertoire to produce antibodies of predetermined specificity, *Nature* **299:**592–596.
10. Milstein, C. P., Steinberg, A. G., McLaughlin, C. L., and Solomon, A., 1974, Amino acid sequence change associated with genetic marker Inv(2) of human immunoglobulin, *Nature* **248:**160–161.
11. Schiffer, M., Girling, R. L., Ely, K. R., and Edmundson, A. B., 1973, Structure of a λ-type Bence–Jones protein at 3.5 Å resolution, *Biochemistry* **12:**4620–4631.
12. Poljak, R. J., Amzel, L. M., Avey, H. P., Chen, B. L., Phizackerley, R. P., and Saul, F., 1973, Three-dimensional structure of the Fab' fragment of a human immunoglobulin at 2.8 Å resolution, *Proc. Natl. Acad. Sci. USA* **70:**3305–3310.
13. Brack, C., Hirama, M., Lenhard-Schuller, R., and Tonegawa, S., 1978, A complete immunoglobulin gene is created by somatic recombination, *Cell* **15:**1–14.
14. Sakano, H., Huppi, K., Heinrich, G., and Tonegawa, S., 1979, Sequences at the somatic recombination sites of immunoglobulin light-chain genes, *Nature* **280:**288–294.
15. Max, E. E., Seidman, J. G., and Leder, P., 1979, Sequence of five potential recombination sites encoded close to an immunoglobulin constant region gene, *Proc., Natl. Acad. Sci. USA* **76:**3450–3454.
16. Early, P., Huang, H., Davis, M., Calame, K., and Hood, L., 1980, An immunoglobulin heavy chain variable region gene is generated from three segments of DNA:V_H, D_H and J_H, *Cell* **19:**981–992.
17. Sakano, H., Maki, R., Kurosawa, Y., Roeder, W., and Tonegawa, S., 1980, Two types of somatic recombination are necessary for the generation of complete heavy chain genes, *Nature* **286:**676–683.
18. Gough, N. M., and Bernard, O., 1981, Sequences of the joining region genes for immunoglobulin heavy chains and their role in the generation of antibody diversity, *Proc. Natl. Acad. Sci. USA* **78:**509–513.
19. Alt, F. W., and Baltimore, D., 1982, Joining of immunoglobulin heavy chain gene segments: Implications from a chromosome with evidence of three D–J_H fusions, *Proc. Natl. Acad. Sci. USA* **79:**4118–4122.
20. Segal, D. M., Padlan, E., A., Cohen, G. H., Rudikoff, S., Potter, M., and Davies, D. R., 1974, The three-dimensional structure of a phosphorylcholine-binding mouse immunoglobulin Fab and the nature of the antigen binding site, *Proc. Natl. Acad. Sci. USA* **71:**4298–4302.
21. Saul, F. A., Amzel, L. M., and Poljak, R. J., 1978, Preliminary refinement and structural analysis of the Fab' fragment from human immunoglobulin New at 2.0 Å resolution, *J. Biol. Chem.* **25:**585–597.

22. Padlan, E. A., Davies, D. R., Rudikoff, S., and Potter, M., 1976, Structural basis for the specificity of phosphorylcholine-binding immunoglobulins, *Immunochemistry* **13**:945–949.
23. Leon, M. A., and Young, N. M., 1971, Specificity for phosphorylcholine of six murine myeloma proteins reactive with pneumococcus C polysaccharide and B-lipoprotein, *Biochemistry* **10**:1424–1429.
24. Stevens, F. J., Westholm, F. A., Solomon, A., and Schiffer, M., 1980, Self-association of human immunoglobulin kappa-I light chains: Role of the third hypervariable region, *Proc. Natl. Acad. Sci. USA* **77**:1144–1148.
25. Morahan, G., Berek, C., and Miller, J. F. A. P., 1983, An idiotypic determinant formed by both immunoglobulin constant and variable regions, *Nature* **301**:720–722.
26. Oudin, J., and Cazenave, P. A., 1971, Similar idiotypic specificities in immunoglobulin fractions with different antibody functions or even without detectable antibody function, *Proc. Natl. Acad. Sci. USA* **74**:4600–4604.
27. Jerne, N. K., 1974, Towards a network theory of the immune system, *Ann. Immunol. (Inst. Pasteur)* **125C**:1–9.
28. Berman, M. A., Spiegelberg, H. L., and Weigle, W. O., 1970, Lymphocyte stimulation with Fc fragments. I. Class, subclass and domain of active fragments, *J. Immunol.* **122**:89–96.
29. Takemori, T., Tesch, H., Reth, M., and Rajewsky, K., 1982, The immune response against anti-idiotope antibodies. I. Induction of idiotope-bearing antibodies and analysis of the idiotope repertoire, *Eur. J. Immunol.* **12**:1040–1046.
30. Margolies, M.N., Wysocki, L. J., and Sato, V. L., 1983, Immunoglobulin idiotype and anti-anti-idiotype utilize the same variable region genes irrespective of antigen specificity, *J. Immunol.* **130**:515–517.

9

Combining Site Specificity and Idiotypy

A Study of Antidigoxin and Antiarsonate Antibodies

Edgar Haber and Michael N. Margolies

1. Introduction

We are now rather close to understanding the mechanisms whereby antibody combining site diversity is generated. As this story has unfolded over the past several years, a number of unique genetic mechanisms have been uncovered and many of the issues that fueled controversy among laboratories have been resolved.

Antibodies are characterized by regions of conserved as well as variable amino acid sequence. Small portions of each molecule, highly variable in structure [the complementarity-determining regions (CDRs)], are arranged to form the surface that binds antigen. The amino acid sequences of the polypeptide chain segments that fold to form this region (approximately 60 amino acid residues) determine the nature of the antigen recognized. Three segments of the heavy and three of the light chain participate in forming the site.

How is the incredible sequence variability that characterizes the complementarity site determined? A number of mechanisms have been invoked. First, different heavy and light chains may assort, possibly in random permutations and combinations. Second, sequence variability is determined by several mechanisms. The variable region of the light chain, making up approximately its NH_2-terminal half, is the product of two genes: V_L, which occurs in several hundred copies, and J; four copies of mouse J_κ have been identified.[1-4] V_L and J_L may occur in any combination, providing a source of considerable variability. In

Edgar Haber • Cardiac Unit, Department of Medicine, Massachusetts General Hospital and Harvard Medical School, Boston, Massachusetts 02114.   Michael N. Margolies • Department of Surgery, Massachusetts General Hospital and Harvard Medical School, Boston, Massachusetts 02114.

addition, the region at their junction is subject to variation by virtue of nonhomologous somatic recombination. The heavy-chain variable region is the product of three genes: V_H, in several hundred copies; D, in 10 or more copies; and J_H, in four copies.[5,6] As in the light chain, any permutation and/or combination of these genes may occur and two sites of somatic recombination are present. These mechanisms alone can account for 10^7 different CDRs (see Tonegawa[7] for review). In addition, somatic point mutation[8] has been shown to occur at a high frequency in V, D, and J segments. Recently, Clarke et al. have demonstrated that gene conversion among sets of related variable-region genes is also a likely mechanism for generating diversity.[9] Thus, the number of possible antibodies may well exceed 10^{10}.

The antibody molecule is arranged into six rather discrete spatial domains. One such domain, which may be isolated following enzymatic cleavage,[10] has a size of 25,000 daltons and is capable of binding antigen with the same affinity as the intact antibody. A detailed analysis of the known crystal structures of immunoglobulins[11–13] suggests that the essential region of the combining site, containing the complementarity-determining residues that contact the antigen, as well as essential supporting amino acid residues, may comprise only 12,000 daltons.[14]

This brief summary of a great deal of work indicates that there is now substantial understanding of a number of aspects related to the structure and origin of the antibody combining site, yet two rather important questions remain unresolved. First, how are the primary and tertiary structure of the antibody combining site related to the selectivity and affinity for a particular ligand bound by that site? Second, with the potential for selection among 10^{10} different amino acid sequences, why are some structures so strongly favored that, within a given strain of inbred animals, they dominate the humoral immune response to a given antigen? In this chapter some insights into both issues will be offered, although final answers are not available. An analysis of the primary structures of a set of digoxin-specific antibodies will cast some light on the first question, while an examination of dominant and minor idiotypes generated in inbred mice in response to immunization with *p*-azophenylarsonate coupled to protein will bear on the second.

2. Digoxin-Specific Monoclonal Antibodies

Digoxin, in contrast to other haptens, is a relatively large organic molecule (Fig. 1), measuring $31 \times 8 \times 9$ Å, which allows it to nearly completely occupy a typical antibody combining site, $34 \times 12 \times 7$ Å.[15] Its molecular structure[16] and that of five analogs has been determined by x-ray crystallography. The molecule consists of a steroid backbone, a lactone ring, and three digitoxose sugars (Fig. 1). Of particular interest in immunological studies is the rigidity of the steroid ring which does not allow major conformational changes when functional groups are substituted. There are 64 available structural analogs that differ in substitutions on the steroid ring and in the number and identity of sugar residues, permitting an examination of fine antibody specificity.[17]

2.1. Clinical Interest of Digoxin-Specific Antibodies

The selection of digoxin as a subject for immunological study grew out of our interest in the reversal of clinical digitalis toxicity by digoxin-specific antibodies. Subsequently, it

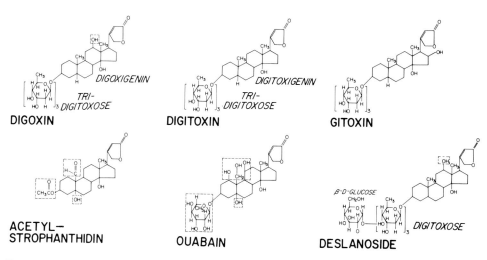

Figure 1. Structures of digoxin and related cardiac glycosides. Differences in steroid ring substitutions are indicated by broken lines.

became apparent that the molecule offered additional advantages as a vehicle for examining antibody combining site specificity and structure. The digitalis glycosides are of great value in the treatment of congestive heart failure and, consequently, are frequently used in clinical medicine. Unfortunately, they are characterized by a very close toxic–therapeutic ratio. Digitalis intoxication is one of the most frequent adverse drug reactions reported. There is no specific antidote, and the cardiac arrhythmias that are a feature of digitalis intoxication are commonly fatal. If an antibody specific to the digitalis glycosides were to have a higher affinity for the drug than the physiological receptor, it should be possible to transfer the ligand from the receptor to the antibody simply by mass action. For optimal effectiveness, diffusion distances should be minimal and the antibody present in high concentration in extracellular fluid in proximity to the receptor. It would also be desirable to remove the antibody–drug complex rapidly from the body. These goals can be satisfied by using Fab fragments instead of intact IgG.

The desirable properties of Fab in comparison to IgG are: more rapid equilibrium distribution in extracellular fluid; a greater volume of distribution; and elimination with a shorter half-life.[18] In addition, when injected intravenously, Fab is less immunogenic than IgG[18] and complement cannot be fixed because the relevant binding sites on the Fc have been lost.

Initial studies on the reversal of digoxin toxicity were carried out long before the advent of monoclonal antibodies. In order to obtain sufficient materials for clinical studies, sheep were immunized with digoxin–protein conjugates and high-affinity antibody was purified from antiserum utilizing affinity chromatography with immobilized ouabain. These antibodies bound digoxin and digitoxin with similar affinities. Fab was then isolated after papain cleavage.[19] Following demonstration of safety and effectiveness in animal studies, clinical investigations were initiated. At the time of this writing, more than 26 patients with life-threatening digitalis intoxication have been studied in a multicenter national trial.[20] Patients were admitted to the trial if they presented a life-threatening rhythm disturbance or hyperkalemia, and were resistant to conventional therapeutic approaches. The overdoses occurred either during the course of therapy ($N = 13$), or as a result of accidental or suicidal overdose. In each case, a dramatic reversal of the signs or symptoms of intoxication occurred. Twenty-one patients left the hospital well and without any sequelae. Five patients died, one because inadequate quantities of Fab were available, and the remaining four because irreversible brain or cardiac damage had occurred by the time Fab was administered.

The history of a recently reported patient is typical of the group.[21] She was a 34-year-old woman who took 20 mg of digitoxin, a massive overdose, with suicidal intent. She appeared to be well on admission to the hospital except for nausea, but soon lapsed into a series of life-threatening arrhythmias that included multiple ventricular fibrillations (treated with countershock), as well as asystole (treated with ventricular pacing). At the time the antibody Fab became available to the physicians treating her, she was in shock, was anuric, and exhibited dilated pupils. Her serum potassium was elevated, a grave prognostic sign in digitalis intoxication.[22] Within an hour after the intravenous administration of antibody Fab, her atrioventricular conduction had returned, and she was soon in normal sinus rhythm. No further dysrhythmias occurred. The patient was discharged from the hospital without sequelae several days later. Fig. 2 demonstrates the initial marked increase of serum digitoxin concentration in this patient as tissue-bound drug equilibrated with the antibody (antibody-bound drug is pharmacologically inactive), followed by rapid clearance of both drug and Fab. It should be noted that the half-life of digitoxin in man is normally 3.5 days, with hepatic metabolism of the drug being the major source of removal. It is apparent that excretion has been markedly accelerated by the antibody Fab, the half-life

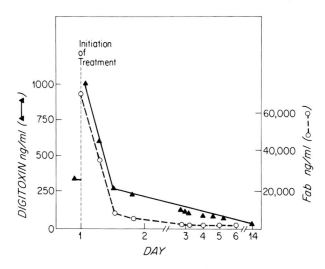

FIGURE 2. Blood levels of digitoxin and Fab fragments after intravenous administration of antibody Fab to a 34-year-old woman suffering a series of life-threatening arrhythmias as a result of a massive overdose (20 mg) of digitoxin. Within an hour of intravenous administration of antibody Fab, atrioventricular conduction had returned. (Reprinted from Haber, *Contributions of Chemical Biology to the Biomedical Sciences,* Academic Press.)

seemingly reduced to about 12 hr. Both antibody and Fab appeared in the urine largely within the first 24 hr after Fab administration.

More recently, one of the high-affinity antidigoxin monoclonal antibodies described in this chapter (antibody 26-10) and its Fab have been demonstrated to be equally effective in the reversal of lethal digoxin toxicity in cats,[23] and in guinea pigs,[24] suggesting that monoclonal antibodies may be a logical successor to polyclonal serum antibodies for human therapy. In addition, these hybridomas can replace polyclonal antisera in radioimmunoassays of serum digoxin levels.[25] The advantages of choosing monoclonal antibodies for clinical use include the certainty of supply of a defined reagent and the potential for selection of hybridomas of a given fine specificity.

It should be apparent that this approach could be applied to many other drugs or toxins. Of particular interest is the acceleration of excretion of a substance that is normally metabolized slowly. Fab is capable of altering the route of disposal from hepatic metabolism to renal excretion.[26]

2.2. Production of Digoxin-Specific Monoclonal Antibodies

The immunizing antigen was synthesized by covalently coupling digoxin through its terminal digitoxose moiety to human serum albumin utilizing periodate oxidation of the terminal digitoxose sugar.[27] Four strains of mice—BALB/c, SWR/J, RF/J, and A/J— were examined, but only A/J mice gave a significant positive primary response to digoxin.[25] The frequency of digoxin-specific precursor B cells in adult A/J mice was determined to be 1/35,000, which was similar to restricted frequencies determined in BALB/c mice for other haptens such as phosphorylcholine (PC) (1/50,000)[28] or p-azophenylarsonate (Ars) (1/65,000).[29] A/J mice were thus selected as the strain used in subsequent fusion experiment.

Immunizations were carried out intraperitoneally utilizing complete Freund's adjuvant followed by intravenous boosting. Somatic cell fusion was carried out by the general approach of Kohler and Milstein,[30] utilizing secreting cell lines in early experiments. Later, the nonsecreting line Sp2/0-Ag14[31] was used exclusively in order to avoid the problem of mixed-chain molecules for affinity and structure studies. The RIA used for screening culture media from fusion wells for antidigoxin antibody is based on that reported by Klinman et al.[32] using digoxin–hemocyanin as antigen. The hybridoma cultures were amplified in the ascites of (BALB/c × A/J) mice.

2.3. Characterization of Digoxin-Specific Monoclonal Antibodies

Digoxin-specific hybridoma proteins were purified from ascites by ion-exchange chromatography on DEAE–cellulose, or affinity chromatography on digoxin–BSA–Sepharose or ouabain–amine–Sepharose. Average intrinsic affinity constants (K_0) were determined for each subcloned antidigoxin hybridoma present in the culture media or after purification from ascites. An RIA utilizing [^{3}H]digoxin and dextran-coated charcoal to separate free [^{3}H]digoxin from antibody-bound digoxin was used. This method has been shown previously to yield affinity data comparable to those obtained by equilibrium dialysis using rabbit antiouabain antisera.[33] The specificity of each antidigoxin antibody for related cardiac glycosides was assessed by the inhibition of binding of antibody in the dextran-charcoal RIA.[33] Each of the compounds in Figure 1, in addition to digoxin, was tested with this method to determine the amount of the compound required to achieve 50% inhibition relative to that required for unlabeled digoxin. Amino acid sequence analyses of heavy and light chains and peptide fragments were done by Edman degradation in a modified Beckman spinning cup sequencer,[34,35] and PTH-amino acids analyzed by high-pressure liquid chromatography.[36,37]

More than 20 subcloned digoxin-specific monoclonal antibodies are now available for study. Of these, 11 have been examined in detail with respect to affinity, specificity, and partial amino acid sequence. The isotype and affinity of each monoclonal antibody are shown in Table I. All but three of the proteins are IgG1,κ in isotype, and the others are either IgG2a,κ or IgG2a,λ. The affinity for digoxin for all of the antibodies is very high, ranging from 1.1×10^9 to 1.7×10^{12} M^{-1}.

Figure 1 details the structures of the cardiac glycosides and aglycones used in fine specificity analysis. Structural differences that proved to have significant consequences with respect to antigenic recognition include: the presence or absence of sugar moieties (e.g., digitoxin vs. digitoxigenin); substitutions on the A and B rings (digoxin vs. ouabain or acetylstrophanthidin); a substitution on the C ring (12-OH) that differentiates digoxin from digitoxin; or substitution on the D ring (16-OH) that differentiates gitoxin from digitoxin. Two typical sets of binding curves, shown in Fig. 3, compare the binding of selected compounds to two different monoclonal antibodies. For hybridoma 40-160, note that the binding of digoxin, digitoxin, and deslanoside are indistinguishable. Thus, the presence or absence of 12-OH or the addition of β-D-glucose to the third digitoxose sugar appears to have no influence. Digoxigenin and digitoxigenin bind less well, indicating significant participation of the digitoxose sugars. Acetylstrophanthidin, ouabain, and gitoxin bind still less well. While several changes characterize the difference between digoxin and acetylstrophanthidin and ouabain (these include both alterations in the sugars and changes in substitutions on the A and B rings), gitoxin differs from digitoxin only in the absence of 12-OH and the presence of 16-OH. Since 12-OH is not involved in antigen recognition (no

TABLE I

Binding Affinities of Antidigoxin Hybridomas

Antidigoxin antibody	Isotype	K_0
Dig 26-10	γ_{2a},κ	6.9×10^9
Dig 35-20	γ_1,κ	1.9×10^9
Dig 40-020	γ_1,κ	1.7×10^9
Dig 40-040	γ_1,κ	3.0×10^{11}
Dig 40-060	γ_1,κ	6.2×10^9
Dig 40-090	γ_1,κ	3.8×10^{10}
Dig 40-100	γ_1,κ	6.4×10^9
Dig 40-120	γ_{2a},κ	2.6×10^{11}
Dig 40-140	γ_1,κ	1.1×10^9
Dig 40-160	γ_1,κ	2.6×10^{11}
Dig 45-20	γ_{2a},λ	1.7×10^{12}

TABLE II

Concentration of Inhibitor Relative to Digoxin Giving 50% Inhibition of [³H]-Digoxin Binding, Grouped by Inhibition Sets

		Digoxi-genin	Digitoxin	Digitoxigenin	Deslano-side	Gitoxin	Ouabain	Acetylstro-phanthidin
A	26-10	1.1	1.2	3.5	0.93	3.5	66	1.5
A₁	45-20	2.4	1.6	17.1	⟨n.d.⟩	24	10.6	12.8
B	35-20	0.85	3.0	2.5	0.88	20	350	110
C	40-160	3.7	1.1	10	0.91	29	140	32
D₁	40-020	7.7	95	>1000	0.91	(29)	>1000	>100
	40-090	9.6	80	>1000	0.98	40	>1000	>1000
	40-100	9.1	94	>1000	0.99	34	>1000	>1000
D₂	40-060	16	120	>1000	0.99	44	>1000	>1000
E₁	40-040	13	2.6	49	1.1	23	>1000	>100
	40-140	13	1.2	21	1.0	34	>1000	>100
E₂	40-10	20	1.4	120	1.0	27	>1000	440
F	45-10	16	9.1	196	⟨ n.d.⟩	47	>1000	>1000

difference between digoxin and digitoxin), a structure on the D ring, 16-OH, interferes with binding. Thus, in the case of antibody 40-160, it is likely that the antibody combining site contacts both the digitoxose sugars and the D ring of the steroid, two rather distant parts of the molecule, without being significantly influenced by structures between.

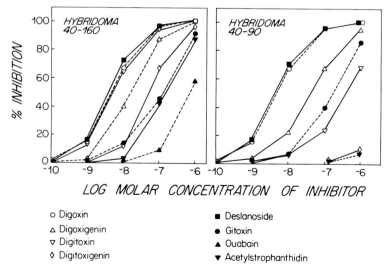

FIGURE 3. Inhibition of binding of two monoclonal antibodies (40-160; 40-090) to [³H]digoxin by various cardiac glycosides, using a dextran-coated charcoal radioimmunoassay.

The inhibition profile of hybridoma 40-090 in Fig. 3 is quite different from that of 40-160. Here, only deslanoside binds with affinity equal to that of digoxin, indicating that the terminal glucose sugar does not participate in antigen binding. In contrast to 40-160, removal of 12-OH causes a profound diminution in binding. As in 40-160, removal of the digitoxose sugars, or addition of substitutions on the A, B, and C rings significantly affects binding. Thus, for antibody 40-090, the A, B, and C rings of the steroid, as well as at least the first digitoxose sugar, contact the antibody combining site.

Similar studies were carried out with each of 12 monoclonal antibodies and the results are summarized in Table II. The table lists the concentrations of unlabeled inhibitor (as a multiple of the concentration of digoxin $= 1.0$) required to effect 50% inhibition of binding of [^{3}H]digoxin. The 12 monoclonal antibodies can be divided into nine sets by virtue of similar specificity profile; for example, 45-20 and 26-10, shown at the top, recognize all of the compounds with very similar affinities. Minor differences between these include a lesser binding of ouabain by 26-10 and diminished binding of digoxigenin and gitoxin by 45-20. Antibody 35-20 differs from 26-10 in that it recognizes all compounds tested equally except ouabain and acetylstrophanthidin. Hybridoma 26-10 does not differentiate among any of the compounds except ouabain. The difference in structure between ouabain and acetyl-strophanthidin is the presence of substitutions on the β surface of the ring in the former, which are not present in the latter. Thus, binding to one surface of the steroid A and B rings, as opposed to the other, differentiates the two specificities. In groups D_1 and D_2, the presence of the 12-OH and the presence of the digitoxose sugars are both important, as shown by the significant reduction of binding when either digitoxin or digoxigenin is compared to digoxin. In groups E_1 and E_2, neither 12-OH nor the sugars are of importance, though substitutions of any kind on the A and B rings eliminate measurable binding. Group F is similar, though there is somewhat more influence of sugars and 12-OH.

2.4. Amino Acid Sequence Studies

Partial amino acid sequence data from both the heavy and the light chains of the 12 monoclonal antibodies are shown in Figs. 4 and 5. Both light and heavy chains can be divided into at least five and six homology groups, respectively. Thus, because of several repeats in some of these sets, a limited number of V_H- and/or V_L-region genes may be selected among digoxin-specific antibodies (although this conclusion must be confirmed when fusion products from additional individual animals can be examined, since 8 of the 12 antibodies derive from the same fusion). It is of great interest that similar light chains can be associated with different heavy chains; 26-10, which has a unique heavy chain not homologous with any in this set, has a light chain similar to those utilized in antibodies 40-060, 40-090, and 40-100, confirming the hypothesis that permutations of light and heavy chains may play a role in the generation of antibody diversity. On the other hand, another homology group of heavy chain, 40-120, 40-040, 40-140, 40-160, and 35-20, are each associated with the same group of light chains that are very closely related to one another. This set of light chains differs from six other antidigoxin light chains sequenced, in that they are five residues shorter in CDR1. Of the third homology group of heavy chains in Fig. 4, three members, 40-090, 40-060, and 40-100, share the same homology group of light chains (sequence data are unavailable for 40-020). Thus, the majority of heavy-chain sets (possibly representing V_H gene families or even somatic mutants of the same V_H gene) associate with

```
                1        10        20        30      35a      40        50    52a      60
26-10          EVQLQQSGPELVKPGASVRMSCKSSGYIFTDFYMN·WVRQSHGKSLDYIGYISPYSGVTGYNQLF

40-120         DVQLQESGPGLVKPSQSLSLTCTVTGYSITSDYAWSWIRQFPGNKLEWMGYIT·YNGY
40-040
40-140                                                      R
40-160                                        Y
35-20                                      F_E_N                           S·-S-S

40-020         EVHLVESGGGLVKPGGSLKLSCVASGFTFSSYAM·SWVRQTPEKRLEWVGGIS·SGDGYTYYPDTVKGRFTI
40-060                                          T
40-090
40-100

45-020         EVQLVESGGDLVEPGGSLKLSCAA GFISNNYAM·EW  Q PG

40-150         DVKLVESGGGLVKPGGSLKLSCAASGFTFRSYM·AWVRQIPDKRLEWVATIS·ISDIYTYYPDNV

40-050         Blocked
```

FIGURE 4. Partial amino acid sequences of antidigoxin hybridoma heavy chains. A one-letter code is used.[81] Numbering is according to Kabat *et al.*[82] The sequences are arbitrarily divided into six homology sets. In each set the sequences are compared to the topmost member of the set. Lines indicate identity with the sequence above.

```
                  1        10        20     27abcde 30        40        50        60
26-10     DVVMTQTPLSLPVSLGDQASISCRSSQSLVHSNGNTYLNWYLQKAGQSPKLLIYKVSNRFSGVPD
40-060    ─────────────────────────────F──────────────────P──────────────────
40-090    ─────────────────────────────F──────────────────P──────────────────
40-100    ─────────────────────────────F──────────────────P──────────────│

40-150    DVVMTQT LQL  IGQPASISCKSSQ LLNSDGQ Y

40-040    DIKMTQSPSSMYASLGERVTITCKASQ·····DINSYLSWFQQKPGKSPKTLIY TK LVDG
40-160    ──────────────────────·····────────────────────────────
40-140    ──────────────────────·····─────────────────────────────────
40-120    ─────────L──────────I─·····────D─────────────────────R─R──────
35-20     ───────────────F──────·····────N─────────R──I──RANR───────

40-050    DIVLTQSPASLAVSLGQRATISCRASKSVST·SGYSHIHWYQQK

45-020    BLOCKED
```

FIGURE 5. Partial amino acid sequences of antidigoxin hybridoma light chains. The sequences are divided arbitrarily into five homology sets. For further details see legend to Fig. 4.

the same light-chain set, though exceptions occur. These findings can be compared to observations made with a set of phosphorylcholine-specific hybridomas[38] in which a single V_H gene product appears to be associated with one of three V_κ gene products. A second V_H gene product is only occasionally used.

V_H-region gene sets do not appear to determine antigen-binding specificity. Within each set, varied fine specificities for hapten are found. Even the second homology set of heavy chains in Fig. 4 (40-120, etc.) that is associated with a single homology set of light chains is characterized by at least four distinguishable sets of antigen-binding specificities (Table I). Of course, sequence analysis is as yet incomplete and these variable regions may well be associated with different D or J genes or, alternatively, somatic mutation may be decisive in altering specificity.

Each of these monoclonal antibodies, with the exception of 40-090 and 40-100, has been distinguished by possessing either a unique amino acid sequence, antigen specificity profile, or V_H gene based on Southern blots of hybridoma DNA (R. Near, personal communication). While 26-10 and 45-020 have similar, although not identical specificities, they have very different V_H and V_L sequences (see Fig. 4). Although 40-040 and 40-140 have identical partial V_L and identical V_H sequences, save one substitution at position 44 in V_H, they utilize different V_H genes based on DNA Southern blots using a J probe (R. Near, personal communication). The pair of antibodies 40-040 and 40-120 have identical partial V_H sequences. Southern blots suggest that the same V_H and J_H genes are used for both. Their affinities for digoxin are identical within experimental error (3.0×10^{11} and 2.6×10^{11}, Table II) and they fall into similar specificity groups (E_1 and E_2, Table I), differing only significantly in digitoxigenin binding. Yet, they differ at 6 amino acid residues out of 60 light-chain positions sequenced.

It is now apparent that a further understanding of the factors determining fine specificity must await the determination of the complete sequence of a number of closely related antibodies. The complete variable-domain sequence of antibody 26-10 has been determined[35] (J. Novotny and M. N. Margolies, unpublished data) (Fig. 6). The heavy-chain J region of 26-10 is unusual in that it is derived from the J_H4 gene by two somatic mutations (positions 111 and 113 in Fig. 6). The nearly complete variable-region sequence of the unrelated antidigoxin antibody 35-20 (not shown) has also been determined. Antibody 35-20 utilizes an entirely different V_H gene and D gene. The remarkable differences that are apparent throughout the variable region indicate the convergence of two very different structural solutions for binding the same ligand.

A rigorous approach to understanding fine specificity is the construction of a three-dimensional model of the antibody combining site. Antibody 26-10 has now been crystallized with and without digoxin in the combining site.[39] We eagerly await the uncovering of structural details.

3. Arsonate-Specific Monoclonal Antibodies

3.1. The Predominant Antiarsonate Idiotype in A/J Mice

A heritable idiotype (here designated Id^{CR}) dominates the immune response of A/J mice to Ars–protein conjugates.[40] Such idiotypes represent phenotypic markers which are

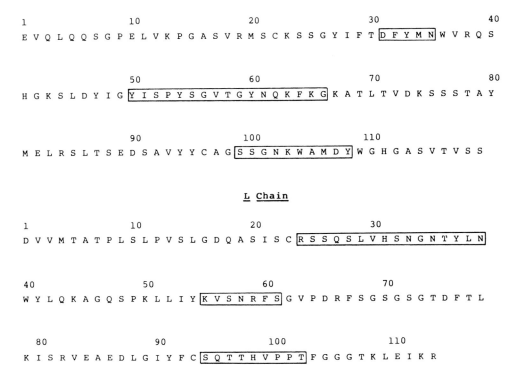

FIGURE 6. The complete variable-domain amino acid sequence of the antidigoxin hybridoma 26-10[35] (J. Novotny and M. N. Margolies, unpublished). Complementarity-determining regions are enclosed in boxes. Fab fragments of this hybridoma have been successfully crystallized.[39]

thought to be products of germ-line genes encoding antibody variable regions. Exogenously administered anti-idiotypic antisera cause suppresssion of the production of idiotype-bearing antibodies[41] consistent with the existence of a regulatory idiotype–anti-idiotype network.[42] If such a network is physiologically relevant, it is necessary to characterize the structural identity and diversity of a given idiotype at both the phenotypic (hybridoma) level and the germ-line genes from which they arise. We summarize here protein and gene structural studies on (1) the major Ars-associated idiotype (Id^{CR}) in A/J mice, and (2) a second idiotype family (Id$^{36-60}$) expressed in both A/J and BALB/c strains. Included in each of these idiotype sets are hybridomas in which idiotype and antigen binding are dissociated (Id$^+$Ars$^-$), due to differences in variable-region structure. The existence of such "variants" permits one to sort out, in a preliminary way, those structural features involved in antigen binding and those contributing to idiotypic determinants.

Earlier structural studies on pooled polyclonal A/J anti-Ars antibodies bearing Id^{CR} indicated that the same sequence was present in all V_H regions expressing Id^{CR},[43] an observation consistent with the predominant idiotype arising from a single or a few related germline V_H gene(s).[40] However, when Id^{CR}-bearing anti-Ars hybridoma products were examined, they proved to be heterogeneous in their reaction with conventional rabbit anti-idiotypic sera (raised against pooled Id^{CR+} antibodies), and also with antisera of more restricted specificity.[44] Monoclonal anti-idiotypic reagents may detect different idiotopes among Id^{CR+} hybridomas; some of these idiotopes may be shared or "overlapping."[45,46] Suppression induced by the monoclonal anti-idiotopes may be idiotope-specific. Although individual monoclonal antibodies bear distinct private idiotypes[47] which are present in small amounts in Ars-immune sera, this family of monoclonal antibodies was shown to possess common shared determinants.[44,48] The diversity among Id^{CR+} hybridoma proteins in their serological reactions and in suppression studies is reflected in the results of amino acid sequence analyses[44,49–51]; for both heavy and light chains, sequence differences occur in both framework and complementarity-determining regions. This is illustrated in Fig. 7 for V_H where each sequence is compared to that of hybridoma protein 36-65. All of the Ars-binding Id^{CR} proteins depicted result from independently derived hybridomas. Similar results have been found for the κ light chains.[51–53] The sequence results demonstrate that Id^{CR} constitutes a family of highly homologous (~95%), but nonidentical, variable regions.

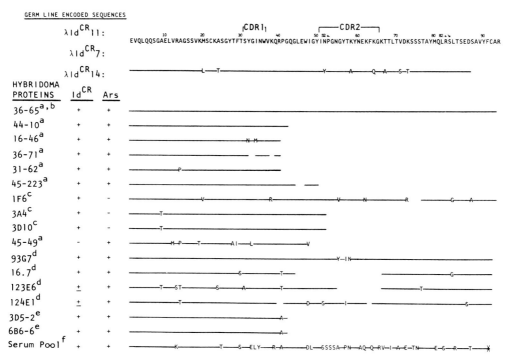

FIGURE 7. Comparison of the amino acid sequences encoded by A/J embryonic Id^{CR} V_H genes[54,55] with sequences determined for Id^{CR}-derived hybridoma proteins and the serum pool.[43,44,51,59,62,83–85] The amino acid sequence encoded by the $\lambda Id^{CR}11$ gene is shown at the top for reference. Horizontal lines indicate identity with that sequence. The DNA sequences of $\lambda Id^{CR}7$ and $\lambda Id^{CR}14$ are identical to each other but differ from $\lambda Id^{CR}11$ at eight amino acids in V_H. The Id^{CR+} hybridoma heavy-chain sequences appear to be derived from the germline gene $\lambda Id^{CR}11$. Substitutions found in $\lambda Id^{CR}7$ and $\lambda Id^{CR}14$ sequences have not been found in any hybridoma heavy chains.

The results of these protein structural studies made it necessary to determine whether this family of sequences reflected the presence of multiple germ-line genes, or originated by somatic diversification from a single germ-line gene. Siekevitz *et al.* cloned the expressed V_H gene from the Id^{CR+} hybridoma cell line 36-65.[54] In DNA hybridization studies involving a variety of mouse strains, they demonstrated that the presence or absence of a single structural gene was correlated directly with the presence or absence of the Id^{CR} phenotype. In all Ars-binding Id^{CR+} cell lines, the same germ-line V_H was rearranged with the J_H2 gene segment. Although three Id^{CR}-like genes were cloned from a single 6.4-kb band in EcoRI-digested A strain DNA, only one of these appears to produce the Id^{CR+} V_H family. In Fig. 7, the protein sequence encoded by the V_H Id^{CR} gene (λ phage $Id^{CR}11$) is identical to that of the DNA sequence of the rearranged hybridoma 36-65.[55] The two other genes shown in Fig. 7 ($\lambda Id^{CR}7$ and $\lambda Id^{CR}14$) encoded heavy-chain V regions differing from 36-65 by eight amino acids. As none of the 16 hybridoma V_H sequences shown in Fig. 7 exhibit these latter substitutions, it was concluded that all Id^{CR+} H chains were encoded by a single gene ($\lambda Id^{CR}11$). This sequence differs at multiple positions (32) from that previously reported for V_H from pooled serum Id^{CR+} antibodies.[43] It is unlikely that the V_H serum sequence arose from the Id^{CR} gene which gave rise to the hybridoma V_H regions; it is possible that this is due to errors inherent in sequencing complex mixtures of immunoglobulins.

Based on the DNA and protein structures summarized above, the large Id^{CR+} family includes V_H regions which have arisen by somatic mutation from a single germ-line V_H gene. These results exclude the possibility that Id^{CR} dominates the A/J anti-Ars response because of the presence of a large number of Id^{CR} V_H genes. The occurrence of a shared or "public" idiotype implies a conserved heritable V_H (and/or V_L) gene(s). The contribution of homologous D gene-encoded sequences may also be important (see below). The occurrence of private serological idiotypes among hybridomas with Id^{CR} is likely related to somatic mutations or somatic recombinations which introduce a variety of new structural epitopes that may be detected at low levels in most Ars-immune sera.[47]

The precise molecular identity of Id^{CR} is not known. However, structural analyses on anti-Ars hybridoma proteins that lack Id^{CR}, and on Id^{CR}-bearing hybridomas which do not bind arsonate, provide a few clues. Anti-Ars hybridomas lacking Id^{CR} demonstrate greater diversity in V-region sequence (Figs. 8 and 9) than the Id^{CR+} family[51] in both heavy and light chains, suggesting that multiple germ-line genes are recruited in the anti-Ars response when selection is not based on shared idiotype. [In addition, a second idiotype family (Id^{36-60}) was detected among Id^{CR-} antibodies,[56] and is discussed below.] All of the Id^{CR-} heavy chains belong to V-region subgroups different from those of the Id^{CR+} heavy chains except for antibody 45-49 (Fig. 8). In addition, the light chain of 45-49 is indistinguishable from the Id^{CR+}-associated sequence (Fig. 9). A similar molecule (91A3) has been described by Milner and Capra.[57] Siekevitz *et al.*[54] demonstrated that the 45-49 V_H gene is derived from the same germ-line gene that encodes the Id^{CR+} antibodies. None of the other Id^{CR-} cell lines proved related to the Id^{CR+} V probe. One explanation for these results is that antibody 45-49 has lost the predominant idiotype because of somatic mutation in V_H, although it still retains Ars binding. Such Ars-binding molecules are presumably no longer subject to regulation by anti-idiotype. Recent data, however, suggest a second, although not mutually exclusive, possible explanation for the lack of idiotype in 45-49. Id^{CR+} heavy chains appear to utilize a D gene core sequence (see Fig. 10) corresponding to a combination of the D genes $FL16.2$ and $SP2.3$ reported for BALB/c mice by Kurosawa and

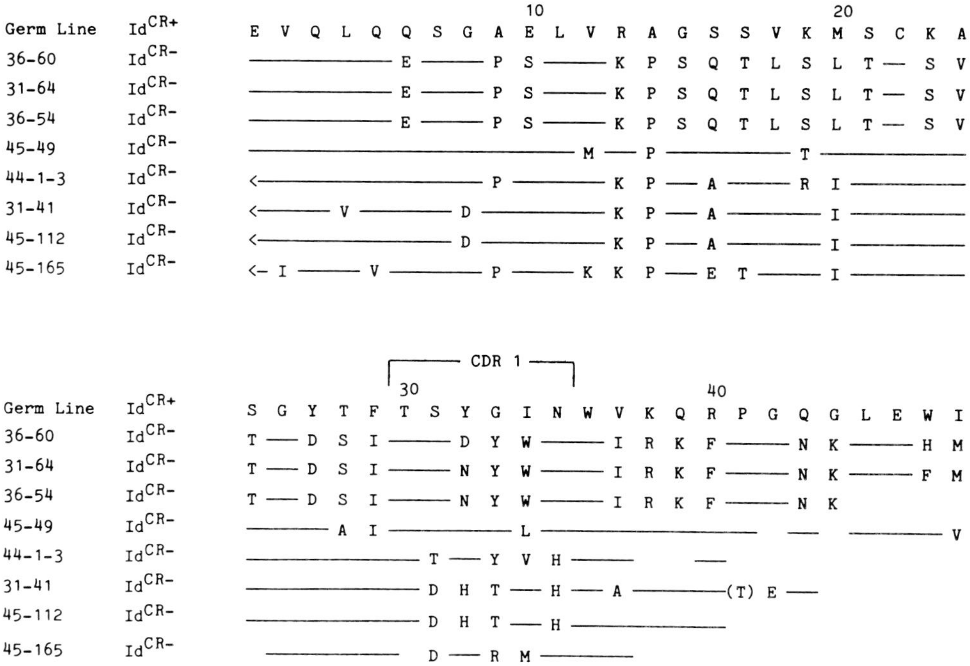

```
                              10                        20
Germ Line  Id^CR+  E V Q L Q Q S G A E L V R A G S S V K M S C K A
36-60      Id^CR-  ——————————— E ——————— P S ———— K P S Q T L S L T — S V
31-64      Id^CR-  ——————————— E ——————— P S ———— K P S Q T L S L T — S V
36-54      Id^CR-  ——————————— E ——————— P S ———— K P S Q T L S L T — S V
45-49      Id^CR-  ——————————————————————— M — P ———————— T ——————————
44-1-3     Id^CR-  <—————————————— P ——————— K P — A ———— R I ——————————
31-41      Id^CR-  <——— V ——————— D ——————— K P — A ——————— I ——————
45-112     Id^CR-  <—————————— D ——————— K P — A ——————— I ——————
45-165     Id^CR-  <— I ——— V ——————— P ——— K K P — E T ———— I ——————


                          ┌——— CDR 1 ———┐
                          30             40
Germ Line  Id^CR+  S G Y T F T S Y G I N W V K Q R P G Q G L E W I
36-60      Id^CR-  T — D S I ——— D Y W ——— I R K F ——— N K ——— H M
31-64      Id^CR-  T — D S I ——— N Y W ——— I R K F ——— N K ——— F M
36-54      Id^CR-  T — D S I ——— N Y W ——— I R K F ——— N K
45-49      Id^CR-  ——— A I ——————— L —————————— —— ———————— V
44-1-3     Id^CR-  ——————— T — Y V H ———   —
31-41      Id^CR-  ——————— D H T — H — A ————(T) E —
45-112     Id^CR-  ——————— D H T — H —————
45-165     Id^CR-  ——————— D — R M —————
```

FIGURE 8. Amino acid sequences of murine A/J anti-Ars Id^{CR-} monoclonal antibody heavy chains.[51,56] They are compared to the Id^{CR+} germ-line V_H sequence (hybridoma 36-65) (see Fig. 7). The < indicates an NH$_2$-terminal pyrrolidone carboxylic acid residue; the sequence of these chains was obtained following digestion with pyroglutamyl aminopeptidase.

Tonegawa,[58] with scattered variations possibly due to somatic mutation.[59,60] The amino acid sequence corresponding to the D gene core for the 36-65 H chain shown in Fig. 10 is Y-Y-G-G-S-Y. In contrast, the Id^{CR} 45-49 heavy chain exhibits the sequence F-D-I-Y-M-Y (M. N. Margolies and M. Gefter, unpublished results) which does not appear related to known D gene sequences in the BALB/c strain.[58] Therefore, the lack of Id^{CR} for 45-49 could be due to recombination with a different D gene, rather than to alterations in V_H, since (1) 45-49 V_H is derived from the germline Id^{CR+} gene; (2) its light chain is thus far indistinguishable from Id^{CR+} light chains (see Fig. 8); and (3) the 45-49 heavy chain uses an unmutated $J_H 2$ segment. Further structural data are needed before it can be established whether or not major Id^{CR} determinants are contributed to by D gene-encoded residues.

Idiotype-bearing Ars-nonbinding A/J hybridomas may be produced by manipulations other than conventional immunization with Ars–protein conjugates. Three such Id^{CR+}Ars$^-$ hybridoma proteins (3D10, 1F6, 3A4) were produced by immunization of A/J mice with a monoclonal rat ani-idiotypic antibody.[61] The availability of antigen-nonbinding, idiotype-bearing monoclonal antibodies provides a unique approach for detecting putative network effects. In Figs. 11 and 12 are displayed partial V_H and V_L amino acid sequences of these three hybridoma proteins, along with two other Id^{CR+}Ars$^-$ molecules derived by dif-

```
                                        10                        20
Consensus  Id^CR+    D I Q M T Q T T S S L S A S L G D R V T I S C R
36-60      Id^CR-    — V V ——————— P L T ——— V T I — Q P A S ——————— K
31-64      Id^CR-    — V V ——————— P L T ——— V I I — Q P A S ——————— K
36-54      Id^CR-    — V V ——————— P L T ——— V T I — Q P A S ——————— K
31-41      Id^CR-    E N V L ——— S P A I M ——— P — E K ——— M T ——
45-112     Id^CR-    ————————— S P ————————— E ——— S L T ——
45-165     Id^CR-    ——— V — S — S P ——— A V — A — E K ——— M ——— K
45-49      Id^CR-    ——————————————————————————————————————————
44-1-3     Id^CR-    Blocked


                                   ┌———————— CDR 1 ————————┐
                             30         34 a  b  c  d  e  f          40
Consensus  Id^CR+    A S Q D I S N Y L N — — — — — — W Y Q Q K P D G
36-60      Id^CR-    S ——— R L L D S D G K T Y L N — — L L — R — G Q
31-64      Id^CR-    S ——— S L L D S D G K T Y L S — — L L — R — G Q
36-54      Id^CR-    S ——— S L L D S D G K T Y L N — — L ——
31-41      Id^CR-    ——— S S V S S Y F — — — — — — ——
45-112     Id^CR-    ——— E ——— G ——— S — — — — — — — L ——
45-165     Id^CR-    S ——— S L L — S R T R K N Y L T ——————— G Q
45-49      Id^CR-    —————————— — — — — — — —
```

FIGURE 9. Amino acid sequences of murine A/J anti-Ars Id^CR− monoclonal antibody light chains.[51,56] They are compared to a reference Id^CR+ light-chain sequence.[51]

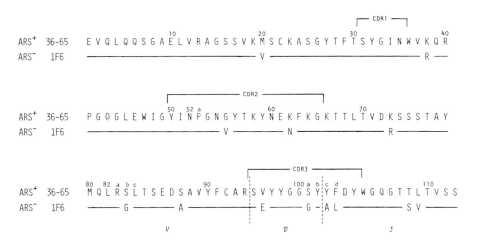

FIGURE 10. Amino acid sequences of Id^CR+ A/J hybridoma heavy chains. The sequence of heavy-chain 36-65 is identical to the germline gene sequence for Id^CR[54,55] in its V_H-encoded portion (residues 1–94). The Id^CR+ hybridoma 1F6 does not bind Ars and was produced following immunization with anti-idiotype.[61] Portions of the sequence encoded by the V_H, D, and J_H genes are divided by vertical broken lines. The precise limits of D gene-encoded residues with respect to those resulting from junctional diversity are unknown.

HEAVY CHAINS

						CDR1			CDR2	

```
                            10              20              30          40                50
ARS+  GERMLINE  E V Q L Q Q S G A E L V R A G S S V K M S C K A S G Y T F T S Y G I N W V K Q R P G Q G L E W I G Y I N P G N G Y
ARS-  3D10      ——————————————T————————————————————————————————————————————————————————————————————————————————————————
ARS-  1F6       ——————————————————————————V——————————————————————————————————————R————————————————————————————————V—————
ARS-  3A4       ——————————————T——————————————————————————————————————————————————————————————————————————————————————————
ARS-  3D7-10-D2-9 ————————————————————————————————————————————————————————————————————————————————————————————————————————
ARS-  332E7-2   ——————————————————————————————————————————————————————————————————————————————————————————————————————————
```

FIGURE 11. Amino acid sequences of heavy chains of murine A/J hybridoma proteins bearing a predominant cross-reacting idiotype Id[CR(59,62)]. Sequences of the heavy chains of five Ars-nonbinding hybridomas are compared to the V_H germline gene sequence of the Ars-binding hybridoma 36–65 shown at the top.[54,55] Hybridomas 3D10, 1F6, and 3A4 were produced by immunization with monoclonal anti-idiotype.[61] The IgM hybridoma 3D7-10-D2-9 is a result of fusion following LPS stimulation, and hybridoma 332E7-2 is an Ars-nonbinding protein resulting from fusion following immunization with arsonate linked to *Brucella abortus*.

LIGHT CHAINS

					10		CDR1	20			30				40		CDR2- 50

CONSENSUS D I Q M T Q T T S S L S A S L G D R V T I S C R A S Q D I S N Y L N W Y Q Q K P D G T V K L L I Y Y T S

3D10 ———————— S ——

1F6 ——— N ————————————————————————————————

3A4 ———————— S ——

3D7–10–D2–9 — V ———— S Q K F M — T – V ————— S V T – K ———— N V G T N V A ———— G Q S P – A ———— S A –

332E7–2 — L ———— S P ——— M – V ————— T – S – T – K ——— G ——— S N I G — L ——— G K – F – T –

FIGURE 12. Amino acid sequences of light chains of murine A/J hybridoma proteins bearing a predominant cross-reacting idiotype (see legend to Fig. 11 for further details).

ferent methods (discussed below). For both V_H and V_L, the $Id^{CR+}Ars^-$ antibodies 3D10, 1F6, and 3A4 are nearly identical to the $Id^{CR+}Ars^+$ sequences.[62] These data, combined with the results of DNA hybridization studies,[54,55,63] demonstrate that $Id^{CR+}Ars^-$ and $Id^{CR+}Ars^+$ hybridoma proteins are derived from the same germline V_H gene. The marked homology among the V_L sequences also indicates that both sets are derived from similar or identical V_L germline genes. The lack of binding of Ars in these molecules may be due to heavy-chain amino acid substitutions (see below)., Structural studies on two other idiotype-bearing Ars-nonbinding molecules, produced by a different strategy, are also displayed in Figs. 11 and 12. Hybridoma 3D7-10-D2-9 was isolated from a fusion with LPS-stimulated A/J splenocytes from an unimmunized donor (D. Wechsler and V. Sato, unpublished results). Hybridoma 332E7-2 was the result of fusion with spleen cells from a CAL-20 mouse immunized with Ars coupled to *Brucella abortus*. Each of these two IgM antibodies has the Id^{CR+} germ-line V_H sequence (Fig. 11), while their light chains are vastly different from usual $Id^{CR+}Ars^+$-associated light chains and from each other. It is not known whether the lack of Ars-binding in these two antibodies is due to "incorrect" L-chain pairing, or to changes elsewhere in the H-chain V region. The structural data on 3D7-10-D2-9 and 332E7-2 indicate that Id^{CR} determinants are largely related to the heavy chain, as each of these molecules has light chains markedly different from those ordinarily associated with $Id^{CR+}Ars^+$ molecules.

The assignment of idiotypic determinants with respect to the relative contributions of the heavy and light chains is dependent on the particular serological reagents used to detect idiotypy. Using rabbit anti-idiotypic antisera, both chains appear necessary,[46,64] although in all instances the appropriate heavy-chain donor is dominant. Several monoclonal anti-idiotypic reagents of murine or rat origin, including those that are hapten-inhibitable, are capable of reacting with determinants on isolated heavy chains purified by conventional methods,[46] or by Western blotting.[65]

In an effort to further localize the structural elements related to idiotypy and to antigen binding, the complete V_H-region amino acid sequence of antibody 1F6 ($Id^{CR+}Ars^-$) was determined. In Fig. 10, 1F6 is compared to the germline V_H sequence (residues 1–94) represented by the $Id^{CR+}Ars^+$ antibody 36-65.[54,55] The heavy chain of the Ars-nonbinding antibody 1F6 differs from the V_H germ-line sequence at seven positions. Utilizing a nucleic acid probe specific for Id^{CR+} H chains, Siekevitz et al.[54] and L. Wysocki (unpublished data) demonstrated that the $Id^{CR+}Ars^-$ hybridomas utilized the same V_H gene. Thus, *1F6* V_H arises from the Id^{CR+} germline V_H by somatic mutation at least seven amino acid residues, each of which may be accounted for by a single nucleotide base change. As noted above, both 36-65 and 1F6 (see Fig. 10) employ the same D gene core sequence except for a single mutation at position 100a. (It is not known whether the amino acid substitution at position 96 arises as a result of V–J_H joining diversity.) While both the $Id^{CR+}Ars^+$ antibody 36-65 and the $Id^{CR+}Ars^-$ antibody 1F6 utilize the same V_H and D genes (and likely the same V_L genes), 36-65 utilizes the J_H2 gene while the 1F6 sequence corresponds to J_H4[66] with a somatic mutation at position 100D. The amino acid sequences confirm the observation of Siekevitz et al.[54] that one V_H germ-line gene rearranges with the J_H2 segment in all $Id^{CR+}Ars^+$ hybridoma cell lines, but in $Id^{CR+}Ars^-$ cells, rearrangement occurs to any of the four J_H regions.[63] As Id^{CR} may be expressed irrespective of the J_H segment used, it is unlikely that J_H-encoded amino acids contribute to this public idiotype (unless one argues that residues shared among all J_H regions contribute to Id^{CR} in concert with other V-region residues).

Since all Id^{CR+} Ars-binding hybridomas thus far examined utilize the J_H2 segment, but Id^{CR+} hybridomas which do not bind arsonate utilize *any* of the four J_H segments, it is possible that in some instances (as for 1F6 in Fig. 10), the loss of Ars binding is due to structural differences in the J_H segment used, or $D-J_H$ junctional changes. Indeed, Cook et al.[67] have shown that a single amino acid difference, in the J_H segment in a mutant protein derived from the anti-PC myeloma S107, markedly alters antigen binding. However, examination of the sequences of $Id^{CR+}Ars^+$ 36-65 and $Id^{CR+}Ars^-$ 1F6 in Fig. 10, also suggests that substitutions elsewhere in V_H could result in lack of Ars binding. As noted above, the partial sequence of the 1F6 light chain (J. Smith and M. N. Margolies, unpublished results) is thus far identical to $Id^{CR+}Ars^+$ sequences.[52,53] In this connection, Rudikoff et al.[68] have described another variant myeloma derived from S107 which has preserved idiotype, but lost antigen binding owing to a single interchange in the heavy-chain CDR1. They emphasize that structure–function relationships are unlikely to be revealed in systems where positive selection by antigen is employed. However, negative selection for antigen-nonbinding mutants, as used in the PC system,[67,68] permits analysis of antibodies with major alterations in binding. A similar opportunity is provided in the Ars system, by the production of antigen-nonbinding, idiotype-bearing hybridomas described above, through manipulations of the spleen cell fusion donor that do not involve conventional immunization with antigen. The existence of such antigen-nonbinding molecules with preserved idiotype, and the occurrence of an Ars-binding antibody (45-49) derived from the Id^{CR+}-associated V_H genes which lack idiotypic reactivity, are further reminders that "idiotopes" and "paratopes" are not synonymous; the variable-region amino acids contributing to idiotypic determinants and those residues involved in antigen contact need not occupy the same topographical sites.[13]

3.2. The Id^{36-60} Idiotype Family

In addition to the predominant Id^{CR} antibody family, structural and serological analysis identified a second idiotype family, designated Id^{36-60}, in A/J mice.[51,56] Among eight randomly selected Id^{CR-} monoclonal antibodies, three (36-60, 31-64, 36-54) proved more than 95% homologous to each other in both V_H and V_L partial sequence (Figs. 8 and 9). The V_H and V_L sequences of the Id^{36-60} anti-Ars antibody family (see also Figs. 13 and 14) are markedly different from those of Id^{CR+}, differing in length within the CDRs, consistent with Id^{36-60} arising from genes other than those encoding Id^{CR}. A rabbit anti-idiotypic antiserum, produced by immunization with hybridoma 36-60, reacted only with the three homologous monoclonal antibodies 36-60, 31-64, and 36-54 (Figs. 8 and 9), but not with any other Id^{CR-} nor Id^{CR+} hybridoma protein. Id^{36-60} is expressed at a level of 10–20% in A/J Ars-immune sera, relative to the levels of Id^{CR},[56,69] but unlike Id^{CR}, it represents a major component in BALB/c sera. In A/J sera, Id^{CR} and Id^{36-60} are nonoverlapping sets. Moreover, each idiotype is suppressed independently of the other, thus providing independent markers for examining network regulation of the anti-Ars response.[56] In earlier studies, Nisonoff and co-workers[70] described a population of minor idiotypes in A/J mice in addition to Id^{CR}. One of these proved related to a BALB/c idiotype designated CRI_c[71,72] which is similar to Id^{36-60}. Id^{36-60} is defined by antisera raised against a monoclonal antibody (36-60) of known sequence. The homologous Id^{36-60} antibodies are derived from a single

V_H gene in both A/J and BALB/c mice (see below). The idiotype CRI_c was defined by an antiserum raised against serum anti-Ars antibodies and could include other minor idiotypic families.[73]

On the basis of the early structural and serological data, Marshak-Rothstein et al.[56] predicted that the Id^{36-60} family is the product of one, or a few closely related, germ-line genes shared by the BALB/c and A/J mouse strains. Recent structural data at the protein and DNA level confirmed that this idiotype family in fact arises from a single V_H gene in each strain which differ at only two nucleotides.[69] In addition, the complete V_L structures are also closely related.[59,74]

The complete heavy-chain variable-region sequence of the A/J hybridoma 36-60[75] and that of the BALB/c hybridoma 1210.7 are shown in Fig. 13, along with partial sequences of other A/J Id^{36-60} proteins. The 36-60 and 1210.7 heavy chains differ from each other at only four positions (32, 47, 84, 93) in V_H, suggesting that they are related to identical or highly homologous germline V_H genes. The D regions of each protein (positions 98–99) are identical and correspond to a part of the BALB/c D gene *FL16.1*.[58] In addition, the $J_H 3$-region sequences[66] utilized in both antibodies are also identical. The results of these amino acid sequence analyses are consistent with the results of Southern blot data,[69] in which all Id^{36-60} hybridoma DNA demonstrate identical rearrangements, utilizing one germline V_H, D, and $J_H 3$ segment in all strains expressing Id^{36-60}. Although most strains possess five genes markedly similar to the V_H^{36-60} germline gene, only one V_H gene is utilized in Id^{36-60} hybridomas. Near et al.[69] have cloned and sequenced the V_H genes for Id^{36-60} in both A/J and BALB/c mouse strains. The Id^{36-60} germline V_H DNA sequences from A/J and BALB/c are identical except for two nucleotide differences at amino acid position 32 (Asp in A/J, Gly in BALB/c) and at position 84 (Ser/Thr). Two other A/J proteins show somatic mutations at position 32 (Asp→Asn). As protein 36-54 is IgM, the occurrence of somatic mutation here is unusual, since data from PC-binding monoclonal antibodies[76] suggest that somatic mutation occurs following immunoglobulin class switching. The amino acid sequence of the 36-60 V_H[75] is in complete agreement with the DNA sequence of the rearranged hybridoma V_H 36-60 gene.[69] The rearranged V_H 36-60 gene has three mutations relative to the A/J germline sequence; two of these are expressed at positions 47 (Tyr→His) and 93 (Ala→Thr). The third nucleotide change, at position 15, is silent. The amino acid sequence of the BALB/c V_H 1210.7 does not exhibit somatic mutation, i.e., it is identical to the BALB/c DNA germline V_H sequence. Thus, the four amino acid differences between proteins 36-60 and 1210.7 shown in Fig. 13 are accounted for by germline differences between the two strains at positions 32 and 84, and by somatic mutations away from the A/J V_H gene sequence in the 36-60 heavy-chain V region at positions 47 and 93. The A/J protein 31-64 also demonstrates somatic mutation (Tyr→Phe) at position 47. As the V_H 36-60 germline sequence and the $J_H 3$ sequence[66] are known, the D region must encode only two amino acids (Leu-Arg) at positions 98–99 in both the 36-60 and 1210.7 antibodies (Fig. 13).

The complete light-chain variable-region sequences[74] for 36-60 and 1210.7 are shown in Fig. 14 along with other partial sequences from the same Id^{36-60} family. The A/J 36-60 and BALB/c 1210.7 light chains differ by only two amino acids, at position 27a in CDR1 and a framework difference at position 72. The difference (Arg/Ser) at position 27a is also found in two other A/J V_L sequences, 31-64 and 36-54. The striking homology among the Id^{36-60} V_L sequences suggests that they are derived from the same, or

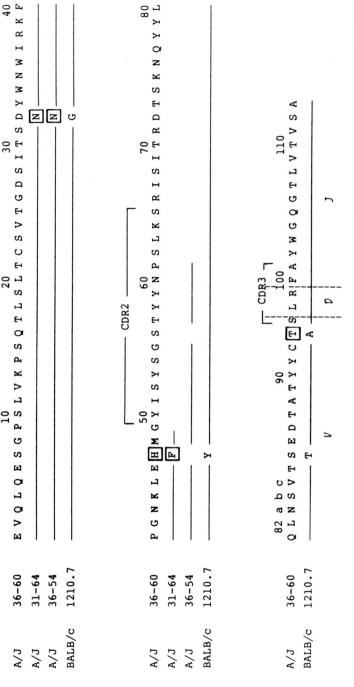

FIGURE 13. Amino acid sequences of anti-Ars hybridoma heavy chains bearing a minor idiotype (Id[36-60]) shared by the A/J and BALB/c strains[56,75] (E. Juszczak and M. N. Margolies, unpublished data). The amino acid residues enclosed in boxes are those which differ in A/J proteins from the sequence encoded by the A/J Id[36-60] germline V_H gene.[69] The A/J and BALB/c Id[36-60] germline V_H sequences differ at two nucleotides (amino acid residues 32 and 84). The BALB/c heavy-chain 1210.7 is the unmutated product of the BALB/c germline V_H gene. Portions of the sequence encoded by V_H, D, and J_H genes are divided by vertical broken lines. Numbering of residues and designation of CDRs are according to Kabat *et al.*[82]

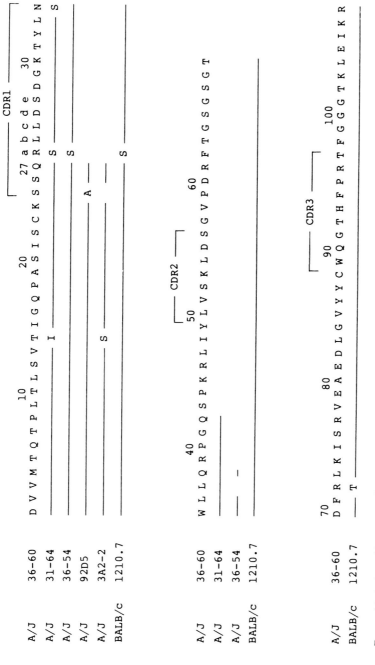

FIGURE 14. Amino acid sequences of anti-Ars hybridoma light chains bearing a minor idiotype (Id^{36-60}). Partial sequences of hybridomas 36-60, 31-64, 36-54, and 1210.7 were reported previously.[56,59] The complete sequences of the A/J 36-60 and BALB/c 1210.7 chains are the unpublished work of E. Juszczak, R. Near, and M. N. Margolies. The sequence of 92D5 was reported by Estess et al.[50] The sequence of 3A2-2 was reported by Alkan et al.[85]

very similar, germline gene(s), analogous to results described above for the heavy chains. The affinity of the BALB/c hybridoma protein 1210.7 for antigen is low compared to that of 36-60.[69,77] The L-chain differences (see Fig. 14) between these two proteins include a framework difference unlikely to contribute to alterations in binding (position 72), and a CDR1 substitution (Ser at position 27a) that is seen in the A/J Ars-binding V_L of 31-64 and 36-54 which have affinities comparable to 36-60; therefore, the "defect" in the 1210.7 binding site likely arises from the amino acid differences at positions 32 and/or 93 in the heavy chain (Fig. 13). As noted above, Rudikoff et al.[68] have correlated single amino acid differences in heavy-chain CDR with marked alterations in binding behavior among PC-binding mutant antibodies. The BALB/c germline Id^{36-60} V_H gene encodes a heavy chain (1210.7) associated with weak Ars affinity, yet this idiotype is dominant in the anti-Ars response of that strain. (The affinity for the antigen of the putative protein encoded directly by the A/J germ-line Id^{36-60} V_H gene is not known.) In the PC system, an increase in affinity is associated with somatic mutation away from the germline sequence.[8] It is likely that an examination of additional BALB/c Id^{36-60} hybridomas will reveal somatic mutants with higher affinity for Ars.

3.3. Relationship between the Structure of Digoxin and Arsonate-Specific Monoclonal Antibodies

Anti-Ars hybridomas bearing Id^{36-60}, and a subset of antidigoxin hybridomas (40-120, 40-040, 40-140, 40-160, and 35-20) (Figs. 4 and 5), belong to the V_H1 subgroup and are 80–85% homologous to each other (Fig. 15). Most mouse strains possess five genes which are highly homologous, only one of which[69] encodes the V_H of Id^{36-60}. One of these other germline genes from A/J mice (denoted "anti-X" in Fig. 15) has been partially sequenced by R. Near (unpublished results). The protein sequence corresponding to this gene, as well as those for the A/J and BALB/c Id^{36-60} germline genes, are compared to the sequences of the anti-Ars Id^{36-60} hybridoma proteins, the A/J antidigoxin hybridomas 35-20, 40-120, 40-040, and the anti-DNP myelomas MOPC315 and MOPC460. The homology between the "anti-X" V_H germ-line gene and the antidigoxin V_H sequences varies from 86 to 92%. The set of five different antidigoxin hybridomas (40-120, 40-040, 40-140, 40-160, and 35-20 in Figs. 4 and 5) belonging to the V_H1 subgroup is encoded by a minimum of two germ-line genes based on Southern blots of restriction enzyme digests of rearranged DNA using a J probe (R. Near, unpublished results). Some of the variability among the highly homologous set of germline genes in A/J and BALB/c shown in Fig. 15 could be explained by invoking gene conversion.[69] The difference between the BALB/c V_H Id^{36-60} germline gene and that from A/J at position 32 could be accounted for by the codon GGT from an A/J Id^{36-60} family member replacing the A/J Id^{36-60} germline codon GAT, thus giving rise to the BALB/c germ-line V_H Id^{36-60} sequence. The "anti-X" A/J germ line gene sequence at position 32 (Fig. 15) shows GGT and could represent such a family member. Similarly, a comparison among the set of A/J and BALB/c sequences in Fig. 15 raises the possibility of analogous gene conversion events occurring during somatic diversification to explain the distribution of residues at position 23, for example.

Although the antidigoxin hybridoma 35-20 V_H is closely related to V_H Id^{36-60}, the

```
                              10                  20                  30                  40
                          E V Q L Q E S G P S L V K P S Q T L S L T C S V T G D S I T S D Y · W N W I R K F P
A/J anti-Ars germ line    ─────────────────────────────────────────────────────────────────────────────
A/J anti-Ars 36-60        ──────────────────────────────────────────────────────────────── ·
BALB/c anti-Ars germ line ──────────────────────────────────────────────────── G ───── · 
BALB/c anti-Ars 1210.7    ──────────────────────────────────────────────────── G ───── ·
BALB/c anti-DNP MOPC 460  ─────────────────────────────────────────────── N G ───── M
A/J anti-X germ line      D ─────────── S ─────────────── T ──── Y ──── G ─ S ─ Y ──── Q
A/J anti-Dig 35-20        D ─────────── S ──── G ───────── T ─ Y ─ F ─ Y ─ E ─ A ──── Q
A/J anti-Dig 40-120       D ─────────── S ──── G ───────── T ──── Y ──── A ──── Q
A/J anti-Dig 40-040       D ─────────── S ──── G ───────── T ──── Y ──── A ──── Q
BALB/c anti-DNP MOPC 315  D ─────────── S ──── G ───────── T ──── Y ──── G ─ F ──── Q

                              50                  60                  70                  80
                          G N K L E Y M G Y I S Y S G S T Y Y N P S L K S R I S I T R D T S K N Q Y Y L Q L N S
A/J Ars germ line         ───────────────────────────────────────────────────────────────────────────────────
A/J anti-Ars 36-60        ──────── H ─────────────────────────────────────────────────────────────────────────
BALB/c anti-Ars germ line ───────────────────────────────────────────────────────────────────────────────────
BALB/c Anti-Ars 1210.7    ───────────────────────────────────────────────────────────────────────────────────
A/J anti-X germ line      R ─────── W ─────── H ──────── N ───────────────────── F F ──────────────── D ─
A/J anti-Dig 35-20        ──────── W ─────────────────── N ───────────────────── F F ──────────────── D ─
A/J anti-Dig 40-120       ──────── W ──── T ─ N ─ Y ─────────────────────────────────────────────────
A/J anti-Dig 40-040       ──────── W ──── T ─ N ─ Y ─────────────────────────────────────────────────
BALB/c anti-DNP MOPC 315  W L ─ F ─ K ─ D ──── B ─ G B ──────── N ─ V ──────── E ──── F F ─ K ─ D ─
```

FIGURE 15. Partial amino acid sequences of V_H1 heavy chains from A/J and BALB/c mice from murine antibodies which bind Ars, digoxin, and DNP. The sequences are compared to the Id$^{36-60}$ protein sequence encoded by the A/J germ-line gene[69] shown at the top. The A/J anti-Ars hybridoma 36-60 differs from that germ-line sequence at two amino acids. The third line represents the V_H protein sequence encoded by the Id$^{36-60}$ BALB/c germ-line gene. It differs from the A/J sequence at two nucleotides, corresponding to amino acids 32 and 84 (cf. Fig. 13). The amino acid sequence of the Id$^{36-60}$ BALB/c hybridoma 1210.7 is identical to this germ-line sequence. The protein sequences of the BALB/c myeloma anti-DNP proteins MOPC460 and 315[82] are included for comparison. The A/J "anti-X" germ-line gene is one of five genes highly homologous to Id$^{36-60}$ in the A/J strain which encodes proteins very similar to a subset of antidigoxin hybridoma proteins, here represented by hybridomas 35-20, 40-120, 40-040 (see Fig. 4). The complete V_H sequences of 1210.7 and 36-60 are given in Fig. 13.

former does not possess the 36-60 idiotype, nor does it bind Ars. This difference could be due to the fact that the 35-20 set of hybridomas employs different light chains than do the 36-60 proteins (cf. Figs. 5 and 14). In addition, the homology between D and J_H regions of these two sets is not known. However, idiotype "connectance" has been demonstrated[78] between the anti-DNP MOPC460 idiotype and the anti-Ars Id$^{36-60}$ which share similar V_H1 sequences (Fig. 15). Thus, the V_H1 gene family consists of highly homologous V_H regions encoding antibodies of markedly different antigen specificity. Even among the closely related subset of antidigoxin hybridomas (Fig. 4, 35-20 group), the members each display different patterns of fine specificity for antigen. The homologies in the V_H1 proteins are detectable not only at the level of DNA hybridization and amino acid sequence, but also, not surprisingly, at the level of serological idiotypic cross-reactivity. In light of the diversity in anti-idiotypic reagents, the definition of the idiotopes involved in the reaction with a given anti-idiotypic reagent, or those involved in antigen binding, will require determination of complete V-domain sequences of the members of this group. The definition of the structural correlates of idiotypy and antigen binding will most likely be revealed using antibodies selected for study because of loss of idiotypy, or loss of antigen binding.

4. A Look into the Future

One might now ask whether the systematic exploration of variable-region sequences of antibodies of defined specificity will ever lead to a detailed understanding of structure–function relationships in the antibody combining site. Some rather interesting insights have already been obtained from spontaneous mutants occurring in the PC system (see above). We have described here sequence variations in antidigoxin and anti-Ars monoclonal antibodies that are likely responsible for alterations in antigen binding and in idiotypy (see Sections 2.3, 2.4, 3.1, and 3.2). These molecules, and those reported for the PC system, were selected for study by screening products of somatic cell fusion or mutant myelomas. Perhaps a more directed approach than waiting for the desired mutations to appear is required. As discussed above, the digoxin-specific antibody 26-10 of known amino acid sequence is presently being studied by X-ray crystallography,[39] and we shall soon know the precise relationship between the atoms of the ligand and the antibody combining site. Yet it is too much to expect that an entire set of digoxin- and Ars-specific antibodies can be examined by X-ray crystallography, since this method depends primarily on luck to produce suitable crystals and their isomorphous derivatives, and secondarily, on long and arduous effort. Since it appears that a member of the V_H germ-line gene family of 35-20 is available, it may be possible to utilize it as a probe to isolate the rearranged gene from the hybridoma. The techniques for inserting such cloned germ-line genes into myeloma cell cultures and expressing the resulting immunoglobulin efficiently have now been developed.[79,80] It is only a short step to applying site-directed mutagenesis of the cloned gene. When this is accomplished, one can ask direct and critical questions concerning the role of each amino acid side chain in the antibody combining site or idiotope. It should also be possible to learn the rules for combining site construction, so that antibody specificity may be dictated and refined at will.

ACKNOWLEDGMENTS. This work was supported by NIH Grants HL–19259 and CA–24432. We are grateful to Malcolm Gefter, Richard Near, Lawrence Wysocki, Vicki Sato, and Meredith Mudgett-Hunter for making their unpublished results available to us.

References

1. Brack, C., Hirama, M., Lenhard-Schuller, R., and Tonegawa, S., 1978, A complete immunoglobulin gene is created by somatic recombination, *Cell* **15**:1–14.
2. Sakano, H., Kurosawa, Y., Weigert, M., and Tonegawa, S., 1981, Identification and nucleotide sequence of a diversity DNA segment (D) of immunoglobulin heavy-chain genes, *Nature* **290**:562–565.
3. Seidman, J. G., Leder, A., Nau, M., Norman, B., and Leder, P., 1978, Antibody diversity: The structure of cloned immunoglobulin genes suggests a mechanism for generating new sequences, *Science* **202**:11–17.
4. Seidman, J. G., Max, E. E., and Leder, P., 1979, A kappa-immunoglobulin gene is formed by site-specific recombination without further somatic mutation, *Nature* **280**:370–375.
5. Early, P., Huang, H., Davis, M., Calame, K., and Hood, L., 1980, An immunoglobulin heavy chain variable region gene is generated from three segments of DNA: V_H, D, and J_H, *Cell* **19**:981–992.
6. Weigert, M., Gatmaitan, L., Loh, E., Schilling, J., and Hood, L., 1978, Rearrangement of genetic information may produce immunoglobulin diversity, *Nature* **276**:785–790.
7. Tonegawa, S., 1983, Somatic generation of antibody diversity, *Nature* **302**:575–581.
8. Gearhart, P. J., 1983, Effect of somatic mutation on antibody affinity, *Ann. N.Y. Acad. Sci.* **418**:171–176.
9. Clarke, S. H., Claflin, J. L., and Rudikoff, S., 1982, Polymorphisms in immunoglobulin heavy chains suggesting gene conversion, *Proc. Natl. Acad. Sci. USA* **79**:3280–3284.
10. Hochman, J., Inbar, D., and Givol, D., 1976, An active antibody fragment (Fv) composed of the variable portions of heavy and light chains, *Biochemistry* **12**:1130–1135.
11. Marquart, M., Deisenhofer, J., Huber, R., and Palm, W., 1980, Crystallographic refinement and atomic models of the intact immunoglobulin molecule Kol and its antigen-binding fragment at 3.0 Å and 1.0 Å resolution, *J. Mol. Biol.* **141**:369–391.
12. Segal, D. M., Padlan, E. A., Cohen, G. H., Rudikoff, S., Potter, M., and Davies, D. R., 1974, The three-dimensional structure of phosphorylcholine-binding mouse immunoglobulin Fab and the nature of the antigen binding site, *Proc. Natl. Acad. Sci. USA* **71**:4298–4302.
13. Saul, F. A., Amzel, L. M., and Poljak, R. J., 1978, Preliminary refinement and structural analysis of the Fab fragment from human immunoglobulin New at 2.0 Å resolution, *J. Biol. Chem.* **253**:585–595.
14. Novotny, J., Bruccoleri, R., Newell, J., Murphy, D., Haber, E., and Karplus, M., 1983, Molecular anatomy of the antibody combining site, *J. Biol. Chem.* **258**:14433–14437.
15. Kabat, E. A., 1966, The nature of an antigenic determinant, *J. Immunol.* **97**:1–11.
16. Go, K., Kartha, G., and Chen, J. P., 1980, Structure of digoxin, *Acta Crystallogr. Sect. B* **36**:1811–1819.
17. Fieser, L. F., and Fieser, M., 1959, *Steroids,* Reinhold, New York, p. 727.
18. Smith, T. W., Lloyd, B. L., Spicer, N., and Haber, E., 1979, Immunogenicity and kinetics of distribution and elimination of sheep digoxin-specific IgG and Fab fragments in the rabbit and baboon, *Clin. Exp. Immunol.* **36**:384–396.
19. Curd, J., Smith, T. W., Jaton, J. C., and Haber, E., 1971, The isolation of digoxin-specific antibody and its use in reversing the effects of digoxin, *Proc. Natl. Acad. Sci. USA* **68**:2401–2406.
20. Smith, T. W., Butler, V. P., Jr., Haber, E., Fozzard, H., Marcus, F. I., Bremner, W. F., Schulman, I. C., and Phillips, A., 1982, Treatment of life-threatening digitalis intoxication with digoxin-specific Fab antibody fragments: Experience in 26 cases, *N. Engl. J. Med.* **307**:1357–1362.
21. Aeberhard, P., Butler, V. P., Smith, T. W., Haber, E., Tse Eng, D., Brau, J., Chalom, A., Glatt, B., Thebaut, J. F., Delangenhagen, B., and Morin, B., 1980, Le traitement d'une intoxication digitalique massive (20 mg de digitoxine) par les anticorps anti-digoxine fractionnes (Fab), *Arch. Mal. Coeur Vaiss.* **73**:1471–1478.
22. Bismuth, C., Gaultier, M., Conso, F., and Efthymiou, M. L., 1973, Hyperkalemia in acute digitalis poisoning: Prognostic significance and therapeutic implications, *Clin. Toxicol.* **6**:153–162.

23. Margolies, M. N., Mudgett-Hunter, M., Smith, T. W., Novotny, J., and Haber, E., 1981, Monoclonal antibodies to the cardiac glycoside digoxin, in: *Monoclonal Antibodies and T Cell Hybridomas* (G. Hammerling, U. Hammerling, and J. F. Kearney, eds.), Elsevier/North-Holland, Amsterdam, pp. 367–374.

24. Lechat, P., Mudgett-Hunter, M., Margolies, M. N., Haber, E., and Smith, T. W., 1984, Reversal of lethal digoxin toxicity in guinea pigs using monoclonal antibodies and Fab fragments, *J. Phys. Exp. Ther.* (in press).

25. Mudgett-Hunter, M., Margolies, M. N., Ju, A., and Haber, E., 1982, High-affinity monoclonal antibodies to the cardiac glycoside digoxin, *J. Immunol.* **129**:1165–1172.

26. Ochs, H. R., and Smith, T. W., 1977, Reversal of advanced digitoxin toxicity and modification of pharmacokinetics by specific antibodies and Fab fragments, *J. Clin. Invest.* **60**:1303–1313.

27. Smith, T. W., Butler, V. P., and Haber, E., 1970, Characterization of antibodies of high affinity and specificity to the digitalis glycoside digoxin, *Biochemistry* **9**:331–337.

28. Sigal, N. H., Gearhart, P. J., and Klinman, N. R., 1975, The frequency of phosphorylcholine-specific B cells in conventional and germ free Balb/C mice, *J. Immunol.* **114**:1354–1358.

29. Sigal, N., 1977, The frequency of *p*-azophenylarsonate and dimethylamino-propthalene sulfonyl-specific B cells in neonatal and adult Balb/C mice, *J. Immunol.* **119**:1129–1133.

30. Kohler, G., and Milstein, C., 1975, Continuous cultures of fused cells secreting antibody of predefined specificity, *Nature* **256**:494–497.

31. Shulman, M., Wilde, C. D., and Kohler, G., 1978, A better cell line for making hybridomas secreting specific antibodies, *Nature* **276**:269–270.

32. Klinman, N. R., Pickard, A. R., Sigal, N. H., Gearhart, P. J., Metcalf, E. S., and Pierce, S. K., 1976, Assessing B cell diversification by antigen receptor and precursor cell analysis, *Ann. Immunol. (Paris)* **127C**:489–502.

33. Smith, T. W., 1972, Ouabain specific antibodies and immunochemical properties and reversal of Na-K-ATPase inhibition, *J. Clin. Invest.* **51**:1583–1593.

34. Brauer, A. W., Margolies, M. N., and Haber, E., 1975, The application of 0.1 M Quadrol to the microsequence of proteins and the sequence of tryptic peptides, *Biochemistry* **14**:3029–3035.

35. Novotny, J., and Margolies, M. N., 1983, Amino acid sequence of light chain variable region from a mouse anti-digoxin hybridoma antibody, *Biochemistry* **22**:1153–1158.

36. Margolies, M. N., and Brauer, A. W., 1978, Protein microsequencing using high pressure liquid chromatography of phenylthiohydantoin amino acids, *J. Chromatogr.* **148**:429–439.

37. Margolies, M. N., Brauer, A. W., Oman, C. L., Klapper, D. G., and Horn, M. J., 1982, Improved automatic conversion for use with a liquid-phase sequencer, in: *Proceedings of IVth International Conference on Methods in Protein Sequence Analysis* (M. Elzinga, ed.), Humana Press, Clifton, N.J., pp. 189–203.

38. Clarke, S. H., Claflin, J. L., Potter, M., and Rudikoff, S., 1982, Polymorphisms in anti-phosphocholine antibodies reflecting evolution of immunoglobulin gene families, *J. Exp. Med.* **157**:98–113.

39. Rose, D. R., Seaton, B. A., Petsko, G. A., Novotny, J., Margolies, M. N., Locke, E., and Haber, E., 1983, Crystallization of the Fab fragment of a monoclonal anti-digoxin antibody and its complex with digoxin, *J. Mol. Biol.* **164**:203–206.

40. Kuettner, M. G., Wang, A. L., and Nisonoff, A., 1972, Quantitative investigations of idiotypic antibodies. VI. Idiotypic specificity as a potential genetic marker for the variable regions of mouse immunoglobulin polypeptide chains, *J. Exp. Med.* **135**:579–595.

41. Pawlak, L. L., Hart, D. A., and Nisonoff, A., 1973, Requirements for prolonged suppression of an idiotypic specificity in adult mice, *J. Exp. Med.* **137**:1442–1458.

42. Jerne, N. K., 1974, Towards a network theory of the immune system, *Ann. Immunol. (Inst. Pasteur)* **125C**:373–389.

43. Capra, J. D., and Nisonoff, A., 1979, Structural studies on induced antibodies with defined idiotypic specificities. VII. The complete amino acid sequence of the heavy chain variable region of anti-*p*-azophenylarsonate antibodies from A/J mice bearing a cross-reactive idiotype, *J. Immunol.* **123**:279–284.

44. Marshak-Rothstein, A., Siekevitz, M., Margolies, M. N., Mudgett-Hunter, M., and Gefter, M. L., 1980, Hybridoma proteins expressing the predominant idiotype of the antiphenylarsonate response of the A/J mouse, *Proc. Natl. Acad. Sci. USA* **77**:1120–1124.

45. Marshak-Rothstein, A., Margolies, M. N., Riblet, R., and Gefter, M. L., 1981, Specificity of idiotype suppression in the A/J anti-azophenylarsonate system, in: *Immunoglobulin Idiotypes* (C. Janeway, E. E. Sercarz, and H. Wigzell, eds.), Academic Press, New York, pp. 739–749.

46. Rothstein, T. L., Margolies, M. N., Gefter, M. L., and Marshak-Rothstein, A., 1983, Fine specificity of idiotype suppression in the A/J anti-azophenylarsonate response, *J. Exp. Med.* **157**:795–800.

47. Marshak-Rothstein, A., Benedetto, J. D., Kirsch, R. L., and Gefter, M. L., 1980, Unique determinants associated with hybridoma proteins expressing a cross-reactive idiotype: Frequency among individual immune sera, *J. Immunol.* **125**:1987–1992.

48. Nelles, M. J., Gill-Pazaris, L. A., and Nisonoff, A., 1981, Monoclonal anti-idiotypic antibodies reactive with a highly conserved determinant on A/J serum anti-p-azophenylarsonate antibodies, *J. Exp. Med.* **154**:1752–1763.

49. Estess, P., Nisonoff, A., and Capra, J. D., 1979, Structural studies on induced antibodies with defined idiotypic specificities. VIII. NH$_2$-terminal amino acid sequence analysis of the heavy and light chain variable regions of monoclonal anti-*p*-azophenylarsonate antibodies from A/J mice differing with respect to a cross-reactive idiotype, *Mol. Immunol.* **16**:1111–1116.

50. Estess, P., Lamoyi, E., Nisonoff, A., and Capra, J. D., 1980, Structural studies on induced antibodies with defined idiotype specificities. IX. Framework differences in the heavy- and light-chain-variable regions of monoclonal anti-*p*-azophenylarsonate antibodies from A/J mice differing with respect to a cross-reactive idiotype, *J. Exp. Med.* **151**:863–875.

51. Margolies, M. N., Marshak-Rothstein, A., and Gefter, M. L., 1981, Structural diversity among anti-*p*-azophenylarsonate monoclonal antibodies from A/J mice: Comparison of Id$^-$ and Id$^+$ sequences, *Mol. Immunol.* **18**:1065–1077.

52. Siegelman, M., and Capra, J. D., 1981, Complete amino acid sequence of light chain variable regions derived from five monoclonal anti-*p*-azophenylarsonate antibodies differing with respect to a cross-reactive idiotype, *Proc. Natl. Acad. Sci. USA* **78**:7679–7683.

53. Ball, R. K., Chang, J. Y., Alkan, S. S., and Braun, D. G., 1983, The complete amino acid sequence of the light chain variable region of two monoclonal anti-*p*-azobenzene-arsonate antibodies bearing the cross-reactive idiotype, *Mol. Immunol.* **20**:197–201.

54. Siekevitz, M., Gefter, M. L., Brodeur, P., Riblet, R., and Marshak-Rothstein, A., 1982, The genetic basis of antibody production: The dominant anti-arsonate idiotype response of the strain A mouse, *Eur. J. Immunol.* **12**:1023–1032.

55. Siekevitz, M., Huang, S. Y., and Gefter, M. L., 1983, The genetic basis of antibody production: One variable region heavy chain gene encodes all molecules bearing the dominant anti-arsonate idiotype in the strain A mouse, *Eur. J. Immunol.* **13**:123–132.

56. Marshak-Rothstein, A., Margolies, M. N., Benedetto, J. D., and Gefter, M. L., 1981, Two structurally distinct and independently regulated families associated with the A/J response to azophenylarsonate, *Eur. J. Immunol.* **11**:565–572.

57. Milner, E. C. B., and Capra, J. D., 1982, V$_H$ families in the antibody response to *p*-azophenylarsonate: Correlation between serology and amino acid sequence, *J. Immunol.* **129**:193–199.

58. Kurosawa, Y., and Tonegawa, S., 1982, Organization, structure and assembly of immunoglobulin heavy chain diversity DNA segments, *J. Exp. Med.* **155**:201–218.

59. Margolies, M. N., Juszczak, E. C., Near, R., Marshak-Rothstein, A., Rothstein, T. L., Sato, V. L., Siekevitz, M., Smith, J. A., Wysocki, L. J., and Gefter, M. L., 1983, Structural correlates of idiotypy in the arsonate system, *Ann. N.Y. Acad. Sci.* **418**:48–64.

60. Capra, J. D., Slaughter, C., Milner, E. C. B., Estess, P., and Tucker, P. W., 1982, The cross-reactive idiotype of A strain mice, serological and structural analysis, *Immunol. Today* **3**:332–339.

61. Wysocki, L. J., and Sato, V. L., 1981, The strain A anti-*p*-azophenylarsonate major cross-reactive idiotypic family includes members with no reactivity towards *p*-azophenylarsonate, *Eur. J. Immunol.* **11**:832–839.

62. Margolies, M. N., Wysocki, L. J., and Sato, V. L., 1983, Immunoglobulin idiotype and anti-anti-idiotype utilize the same variable region genes irrespective of antigen specificity, *J. Immunol.* **130**:515–517.

63. Gefter, M. L., Margolies, M. N., Near, R., and Wysocki, L. J., 1984, Analysis of the anti-azo-benzene-arsonate response at the molecular level, *Ann. Inst. Pasteur* **135**:17–30.

64. Milner, E. C. B., and Capra, J. D., 1983, Structural analysis of monoclonal anti-arsonate antibodies: Idiotypic specificities are determined by the heavy chain, *Mol. Immunol.* **20**:39–46.

65. Cannon, L. E., and Woodland, R. T., 1983, Rapid and sensitive procedure for assigning idiotype determinants to heavy or light chains: Application to idiotype associated with the major cross-reactive idiotype of A/J antiphenylarsonate antibody, *Molec. Immunol.* **20**:1283–1288.

66. Sakano, H., Maki, R., Kurosawa, Y., Roeder, W., and Tonegawa, S., 1980, Two types of somatic recom-

bination necessary for the generation of complete immunogloublin heavy-chain genes, *Nature* **286:**676–683.

67. Cook, W. D., Rudikoff, S., Giusti, A., and Scharff, M. D., 1982, Somatic mutation in a cultured mouse myeloma cell affects antigen binding, *Proc. Natl. Acad. Sci. USA* **79:**1240–1244.

68. Rudikoff, S., Giusti, A. M., Cook, W. D., and Scharff, M. D., 1982, Single amino acid substitution altering antigen-binding specificity, *Proc. Natl. Acad. Sci. USA* **79:**1979–1983.

69. Near, R. I., Juszczak, E. C., Huang, S. Y., Sicari, S. A., Margolies, M. N., and Gefter, M. L., 1984, Expression and rearrangement of homologous immunoglobulin V_H genes in two mouse strains, *Proc. Natl. Acad. Sci. USA* **81:**2167–2171.

70. Gill-Pazaris, L. A., Brown, A. R., and Nisonoff, A., 1979, The nature of idiotypes associated with anti-p-azophenylarsonate antibodies in A/J mice, *Ann. Immunol. (Inst. Pasteur)* **130C:**199–213.

71. Brown, A. R., and Nisonoff, A., 1981, An intrastrain cross-reactive idiotype associated with anti-*p*-azophenylarsonate antibodies of Balb/C mice, *J. Immunol.* **126:**1263–1267.

72. Brown, A. R., Lamoyi, E., and Nisonoff, A., 1981, Relationship of idiotypes of the anti-*p*-azophenylarsonate antibodies of A/J and Balb/C mice, *J. Immunol.* **126:**1268–1273.

73. Brown, A. R., 1983, Idiotypic heterogeneity of the cross-reactive idiotype associated with the anti-*p*-azophenylarsonate antibodies of Balb/C mice, *J. Immunol.* **131:**423–428.

74. Juszczak, E. C., Near, R., and Margolies, M. N., 1984, in preparation.

75. Juszczak, E. C., and Margolies, M. N., 1983, Amino acid sequence of the heavy chain variable region from the A/J mouse anti-arsonate monoclonal antibody 36-60 bearing a minor idiotype, *Biochemistry* **22:**4291–4296.

76. Gearhart, P. J., Johnson, N. D., Douglas, R., and Hood, L., 1981, IgG antibodies to phosphorylcholine exhibit more diversity than their IgM counterparts, *Nature* **291:**29–34.

77. Rothstein, T. L., and Gefter, M. L., 1983, Affinity analysis of idiotype-positive and idiotype-negative arsonate-binding hybridoma proteins and Ars-immune sera, *Mol. Immunol.* **20:**161–168.

78. Lewis, G. K., Kaymakcalan, Z., Yao, J., and Goodman, J. W., 1983, Idiotype connectance between anti-arsonate and anti-dinitrophenyl responses in Balb/C mice, *Ann. N.Y. Acad. Sci.* **418:**282–289.

79. Frederick, W. A., and Baltimore, D., 1982, Joining of immunoglobulin heavy chain gene segments: Implications from a chromosome with evidence of 3 D–J_H fusions, *Proc. Natl. Acad. Sci. USA* **79:**4118–4122.

80. Oi, V. T., Morrison, S. L., Herzenberg, L. A., and Berg, P., 1983, Immunoglobulin gene expression in transformed lymphoid cells, *Proc. Natl. Acad. Sci. USA* **89:**825–829.

81. IUPAC–IUB Commission on Biochemical Nomenclature, 1968, *J. Biol. Chem.* **243:**3557–3559.

82. Kabat, E. A., Wu, T. T., and Bilofsky, H., 1979, Sequences of immunoglobulin chains: Tabulation and analyses of amino acid sequences of precursors, V-regions, C-regions, J-chains and BP-microglobulins, NIH Publication 80-2008.

83. Siegelman, M., Slaughter, C., McCumber, L., Estess, P., and Capra, J. D., 1981, Primary structural studies of monoclonal A/J anti-arsonate antibodies differing with respect to a cross-reactive idiotype, in: *Immunoglobulin Idiotypes* (C. Janeway, E. E. Sercarz, and H. Wigzell, eds.), Academic Press, New York, pp. 135–158.

84. Sims, J., Rabbitts, T. H., Estess, P., Slaughter, C., Tucker, P. W., and Capra, J. D., 1982, Somatic mutation in genes for the variable portions of the immunoglobulin heavy chain, *Science* **216:**309–310.

85. Alkan, S. S., Knecht, R., and Braun, D. G., 1980, The cross-reactive idiotype of anti-4-azobenzene-arsonate hybridoma-derived antibodies in A/J mice constitutes multiple heavy chains, *Z. Physiol. Chem.* **361:**191–195.

10

The Murine Antibody Response to Phosphocholine

Idiotypes, Structures, and Binding Sites

J. Latham Claflin, Jacqueline Wolfe,
Anne Maddalena, and Susan Hudak

1. Introduction and Historical Background

Idiotypic determinants on immunoglobulin molecules serve two very useful purposes—one to the scientist who studies them, the other to the animal that expresses them. For the researcher they provide an invaluable probe for studies of antibody variability, for mapping V_H and V_L genes, and for examining the evolution of immunoglobulin genes. In the animal they serve as targets through which idiotypically specific, regulatory cells or molecules modulate immune responses in a highly selected manner. The work in our laboratory has used idiotypy in the former sense, that is, as a tool to investigate the diversity of an antibody response and, because this particular response is preserved in mice, to study the evolution of immunoglobulin genes. In this chapter we will briefly review the events in our laboratory that led to a dissection of the antibody response to phosphocholine (PC), a process in which idiotypes play a crucial role. We will not attempt a review of the literature in the field since the PC system has attracted many talented investigators. Detailed descriptions of much of that work can be found in other chapters of this volume or in reviews.[1-3]

The power of the PC system as a model for studying antibody diversity is due largely to the findings of three different groups of investigators. In 1970, Potter and Lieberman showed that, among a large collection of myeloma proteins produced by Michael Potter and Melvin Cohn, five with specificity for PC expressed the same individual antigenic specificity or idiotype.[4] This group of five myeloma proteins became known as the T15

J. Latham Claflin, Jacqueline Wolfe, Anne Maddalena, and Susan Hudak • Department of Microbiology and Immunology, The University of Michigan Medical School, Ann Arbor, Michigan 48109.

group. Almost simultaneously, Leon and Young demonstrated that the members of the T15 group shared the same binding site characteristics for PC and a group of PC analogs.[5] Two other PC-binding myelomas, M603 and M167, which had unique idiotypic determinants,[4] also possessed unique binding characteristics. Shortly thereafter, Cosenza and Kohler,[6] and independently Sher and Cohn,[7] found that idiotypic determinants common to the T15 group of myeloma proteins also existed on induced antibodies of the same specificity. Thus, by 1972 prototype anti-PC antibodies with distinct idiotypes and definable binding sites had been characterized. Many laboratories were attracted to this antibody system, and in a brief time it became one of the premier systems for analyzing an antibody repertoire and evaluating mechanisms of antibody diversity. An additional factor which led a number of us to select this system was the fact that the antigen PC is a natural component of the cell wall in a number of diverse microorganisms such as *Streptococcus, Morganella, Aspergillus,* and *Ascaris.*[8] Indeed, we now know from the work of Briles *et al.*[9,10] that anti-PC antibodies are biologically relevant antibodies which are protective against infection by the virulent, PC-containing microbe, *Streptococcus pneumoniae.* The introduction of hybridoma technology by Köhler and Milstein[11] as a means of obtaining monoclonal antibodies of one's own choice, the analysis of the three-dimensional structure of one PC-binding myeloma protein, M603,[12] and the fact that molecular biologists chose anti-PC antibodies as the first set of antigen-binding antibodies to explore in depth at the DNA level[13,14] were additional contributing factors which led to the rapid dissection of the anti-PC antibody system. As a consequence, we now have an almost complete picture of the structure of anti-PC antibodies and the germline genes that encode them. A summary of this information is provided in Fig. 1 (see Section 5.2).

At the outset of our effort in the PC system in 1972, only rudimentary information about the anti-PC response was available—PC-binding myelomas were described, the shared idiotype had been found in the T15 group, and we knew that T15 Id$^+$ antibodies dominated the anti-PC response in BALB/c. We (Joseph Davie and J.L.C.) became interested in the PC system because it offered an excellent opportunity for studying the regulation of the IgM to IgG switch at the cellular level. Although this effort led to one of the first demonstrations of idiotypic determinants on the immunoglobulin receptor of B lymphocytes,[15] it became difficult to study the switch process because, unlike the DNP system,[16] the receptors maintained their dominant μ^+ status during the response. Few γ^+ PC-reactive B cells were seen. We were also unaware of the importance of the IgG3 subclass in the response to carbohydrate antigens and, like everyone else, we had no specific antisera to that subclass. At the same time we were using Ids as clonal markers, we were also exploring the possibility that fine specificity of hapten binding would be a suitable marker. In what turned out to be a portentous result, Claflin and Davie discovered that all mice, *regardless* of genetic background, displayed the same T15-like, hapten inhibition profile for PC and two close analogs, glycerophosphocholine and choline (Fig. 2).[17,18] The finding was remarkable because such a conservation in binding sites, i.e., antibodies, had not been demonstrated before and portentous because this result dictated our research effort for the next 10 years. As it turned out we were lucky; T15-type antibodies dominate the anti-PC response in most strains, they yield high-quality PFC, and, in spite of structural diversity among them, their site for hapten appears remarkably constant even among different strains of mice.

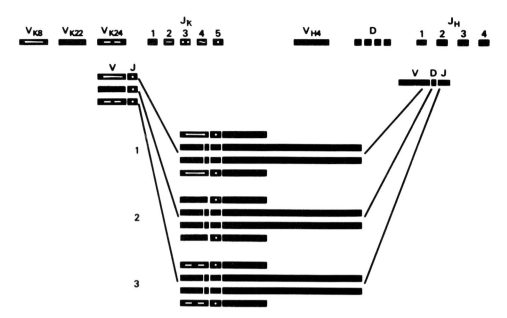

FIGURE 1. Schematic illustration of the germ-line component of anti-PC antibodies in mice. Molecules 1, 2, and 3 represent the prototypic antibodies for the M603, the T15, and the M511 families, respectively. Structural diversity arises through somatic mutations in the V region, use of different D, and mutations, insertions, and deletions at the $VJ(V_\kappa)$ and at the VDJ (V_H) boundaries to generate three families of structurally similar but nonidentical molecules.[60]

2. Conservation in the Response to PC

2.1. Idiotypic Studies

The fine-specificity analysis of anti-PC PFC described above in its simplest form suggested that the anti-PC response in mice was (1) dominated by antibodies having a single type of binding site, and (2) conserved not only within all members of a strain but also among strains of widely different genetic backgrounds. One prediction was that the antibodies should be idiotypically related. However, when an A/J anti-T15 antiserum was used to test this possibility, a paradox arose. A large portion of the anti-PC antibody within a strain did express the idiotype; however, this occurred only in Igh^a strains.[19] Why were mice of the other Igh haplotypes Id negative? One possibility was that the binding sites among mice were preserved, i.e., used the same V_H and V_L, but the A/J anti-T15 was an allospecific anti-Id. In other words, there was polymorphism among T15-type antibodies and the A/J antiserum was detecting one allelic set.

To test this possibility and circumvent the problem of alloantisera, a procedure was devised to obtain binding site-specific antibodies from a heterologous (rabbit) antiserum to T15. The procedure represented a novel approach to obtaining anti-Id antibodies, and yielded an antiserum called anti-T15$_s$ (originally anti-H8$_s$) which was indeed specific for

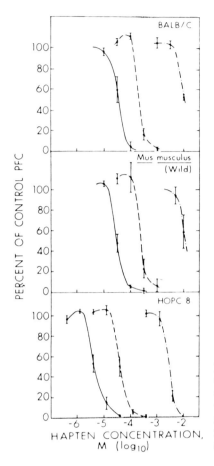

FIGURE 2. PFC inhibition profiles obtained with BALB/c and wild *Mus musculus* spleen cells and H8 tumor cells. Spleen cells were obtained 3–5 days after the second of two i.v. injections of 10^8 *S. pneumoniae*. H8 tumor cells were obtained from ascites fluid. The results represent the mean ± S.E. of eight (mice) or three (H8) separate assays: inhibition with PC (———), glycerophosphocholine (– – –), and choline (· – · –).[18]

the binding site of T15.[20] Thus, the reaction between T15 and anti-T15$_s$ was completely inhibited by PC. When the anti-PC antibodies from the different strains were retested with this anti-T15$_s$, all were shown to be positive (Table I). The concentration of T15$_s$-positive antibodies ranged from as little as 12% in DBA/2 to nearly 100% in BALB/c mice. Now by two rather different criteria binding sites had been shown to be indistinguishable among more than 17 different inbred strains of mice as well as wild *Mus musculus*.[19]

This study was extended to determine whether idiotypic determinants characteristic of the combining regions of the available PC-binding myeloma proteins were also present in anti-PC immune sera or purified antibodies (Table I).[21] M511$_s$ idiotypic determinants were readily detected in all strains with the exception of BALB/c, which consistently expressed low levels of this idiotype. Negligible amounts of Ids with M603$_s$, M167$_s$, and W3207$_s$ characteristics were observed even though our assay was capable of measuring as little as 0.1–0.5 µg/ml. One additional antiserum to M603, which was rendered specific by conventional absorption procedures, did react with anti-PC antibodies in the majority of mouse strains examined; BALB/c was again a low responder. Summation of the T15,

TABLE I
Idiotype Composition of Anti-PC Antibodies

			Idiotypic determinant[a,b]										
			T15$_s$		M511$_s$		M603$_s$		M603$_{ns}$		W3207$_s$		M167$_s$	
Strain	Igh	Ig (µg/ml)[c]	µg/ml	%	µg/ml	%	µg/ml	%	µg/ml	%	µg/ml	%	µg/ml	%
BALB/cJ	a	55	52	95	5	9	<0.05	0	<0.05	0	<0.05	0	<0.01	0
C58/J	a	600	218	35	162	27	<0.05	0	<0.05	0	<0.05	0	<0.01	0
C57BL/6J	b	55	16	29	21	38	<0.05	0	14	25	<0.05	0	<0.01	0
DBA/2J	c	580	70	12	244	42	<0.05	0	ND		<0.05	0	<0.01	0
AKR/J	d	65	55	84	7	11	<0.05	0	2	3	<0.05	0	<0.01	0
A/J	e	36	11	30	14	38	<0.05	0	10	27	<0.05	0	<0.01	0
CE/J	f	250	69	28	75	30	<0.05	0	25	10	<0.05	0	<0.01	0

[a]The concentration of anti-PC antibody (% of Ig) giving 50% inhibition of binding of ^{125}I-labeled myeloma protein to the corresponding anti-idiotypic antibody was compared to a standard curve obtained with the appropriate myeloma protein. The error for each determination is ±15% of the calculated concentration.
[b]The subscripts n and ns refer to site-specific and non-site-specific idiotypes, respectively.
[c]Ig concentration of purified antibody.

M511, and M603 Ids accounted for 60–100% of the anti-PC antibody in each of these strains. Thus, antibodies bearing binding sites and/or idiotypic determinants of three different myeloma proteins were regularly expressed in genetically different inbred strains of mice and in every instance comprised the majority of the response to PC.

2.2. Structural Studies

In order to put these results into a meaningful framework, information on the structure of the induced antibodies was needed. Partial and some complete sequences of the H and L chains of the myeloma proteins were available.[22] These data showed that three distinct V_L regions were used—$V_\kappa 22$ for members of the T15 group, $V_\kappa 24$ for M511 and M167, and $V_\kappa 8$ for M603 and W3207—and one to three V_H, all very similar to $V_H 4$, were used.[1] Sequencing of purified anti-PC antibodies seemed impractical because the antibodies, though idiotypically restricted, were undoubtedly heterogeneous and also because insufficient amounts of purified material could be obtained. The hybridoma technology which eliminated these problems was still a year away. Isoelectric focusing (IEF) of native immunoglobulins had been perfected and proven valuable for discriminating structurally similar IgG antibodies. Unfortunately, the antigen we used to induce an anti-PC response, *S. pneumoniae* strain R36A, stimulated predominantly IgM antibodies and the IEF procedure was inadequate for distinguishing among various IgM proteins. However, we had an indication from our idiotypic studies that three different antibodies, or sets of antibodies, were present and, if the myeloma proteins were appropriate prototypes, each of these antibodies should express a different L chain. We had also demonstrated by the IEF technique that we could distinguish easily between the three different myeloma type L chains.[23] Therefore, as a first assessment of the structural heterogeneity in anti-PC antibodies, we isolated L chains from purified serum antibodies of all 17 inbred strains tested previously and examined them by IEF.[24] The resulting IEF patterns from eight representative strains are shown in Fig. 3 and compared with the three different L chains seen in PC-binding myeloma proteins. The L chains of even a monoclonal antibody appear as a set of closely grouped bands rather than as a single band due to postsynthetic modifications of the polypeptide chain. The L-chain banding patterns of most mouse anti-PC antibodies were complex; however, it is evident that sets of bands corresponding in position to those of T15, M603, and M511 are present in each strain except BALB/c. Careful analysis of these data, in fact, demonstrated only these three L-chain types among the 17 inbred strains and one other which was expressed in only two strains, CE and C58. This fourth L-chain type has not been identified. BALB/c anti-PC antibodies, even at different times after immunization, contained L chains which were almost exclusively those of T15. To test whether there was a direct association between idiotype and L-chain type, anti-PC antibodies were fractionated with anti-T15$_s$, anti-M511$_s$, and anti-M603$_{ns}$, and examined for their L-chain type by IEF. Results obtained with BALB/c, C57BL/6, AKR, and CE, which were selected for detailed study, showed that in each instance adsorption with an anti-Id antibody removed immunoglobulin whose L chains cofocused with the L chains of the prototypic Id. In BALB/c, fractionation with anti-M511$_s$ and anti-M603$_{ns}$ yielded little activity.[21]

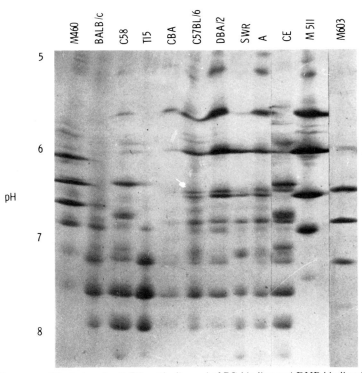

FIGURE 3. IEF patterns of L chains of anti-PC antibodies and of PC-binding and DNP-binding (M460) myeloma proteins. IEF was carried out in a thin-layer polyacrylamide slab gel in pH 5–9.5 ampholytes.[24]

```
       1          10          20          30
A/J    E V K L V Z S G G G L V Q P G G S L R L S C A T S G F T F S B F Y M Z (W)
                                                 Z

T15    ─────────────────────────────────────────── A ───────────────────────────
M603   ─────────────────────────────────────────── A ───────────────────────────
M167   ───── V ─────────────────────────────────── A ───────────────────────────
M511   ─────────────────────────────────────────── A ───────────────────────────


       1          10          20          30
A/J    D I V M T Q S P T F L A V T A S K K V T I S C T A S Z S L (Y) S S K (H)
             M       S P S S L S       T A G Z K     T M     K S     Z   L     B K G (B)
             I       B Z L S B P       S S G Z S     S L     S     K     L         B G

T15    D I V M T Q S P T F L A V T A S K K V T I S C T A S Z S L   Y   S S K   H
M603   ─────────────── S S L S ─ S ─ G Z R ─── M S ─ K S ─────── L   B ─ G   B
M167   ───── I ── B Z L S B P ── S G Z S ─ S I T ─ R S ─ K ─────── L   Y K B   G
M511   ───── I ── B Z L S K P ── S G Z S ─ S I T ─ R S ─ K ─────── L   Y K B   G
```

FIGURE 4. Heavy (upper) and light (lower) chains of A/J anti-PC antibodies.[25] Sequences of T15, M603, M511, and M167 are shown for comparison.[22] Amino acids in parentheses were tentatively identified.

Because the anti-idiotypic antibodies used in these studies recognized only particular H–L combinations in myeloma proteins, these data demonstrated that (1) the correlation between myeloma idiotype and L-chain type could be extended to induced anti-PC antibodies, (2) the response in an individual strain was largely restricted to three (in two cases four) major Ids, and (3) the response between strains of mice was remarkably similar, in fact, so similar that we felt it was probably conserved at the genetic level.[21]

To directly test this idea that equivalent sets of antibodies were preserved in mice, Stuart Rudikoff, in collaboration with our laboratory, sequenced anti-PC antibodies obtained from pooled sera of immunized A/J mice.[25] This strain was chosen because it was genetically quite different from BALB/c. By idiotypic and L-chain IEF analyses, the antibody preparation contained approximately equal amounts of antibodies bearing T15$_s$, M511$_s$, and M603 idiotypic determinants. The results of these studies (Fig. 4) were even more striking than we anticipated. The H-chain sequence in both the first framework (positions 1–29) and the first CDR (positions 30–35) was essentially identical to the BALB/c H chains from the PC-binding myeloma proteins. The L-chain sequences, although complicated by the simultaneous sequencing of multiple chains, gave essentially the same results. Three different L chains could be identified and these corresponded closely to those of the prototype myeloma proteins T15, M603, and M511.

This crucial test of amino acid sequencing made two points. In the first place it demonstrated that antibodies were conserved in mice. Other laboratories, particularly those studying a cross-reactive Id (CRI) on antiarsonate antibodies, had shown that antibodies within a strain were structurally quite similar; antibodies between CRI-positive strains had not been compared.[26] On the other hand, two groups of human myeloma proteins had been compared both idiotypically and structurally.[27,28] Striking structural similarities could be found. The similarity is remarkable considering that they came from an outbred population. Subsequent investigations into other idiotypic systems have revealed conservation of antibodies within a species.[29] Formal proof of conservation still needs to be made at the DNA level.

The second point brought out by these studies was the clonal nature of the response to PC in mice. We had found evidence for a minimum of three clones in the response (or four in C58 and CE). We now know that these clones were structurally similar to T15, M511, and M603. Since the response was so highly conserved in mice and apparently uniform among members of a strain, we felt that there were three to four responding clones in the response and that the information for the structural genes was encoded in the germ line.[21] A role for somatic mutation in determining the origin of the three clonotypes was not indicated by the data.

3. Heterogeneity in the Response to PC

Even though we felt convinced of the germ-line basis of the anti-PC response, we actually had insufficient data to determine how diverse the repertoire was. Our studies to this point had used the PC-containing microbe *S. pneumoniae* strain R36A as the antigen, and this antigen stimulates principally IgM antibodies. Appropriate techniques did not exist which would allow us to readily detect heterogeneity of IgM in the serum pool. Gearhart *et al.*,[30,31] from an analysis of anti-PC-positive splenic foci with xenogeneic and allo-

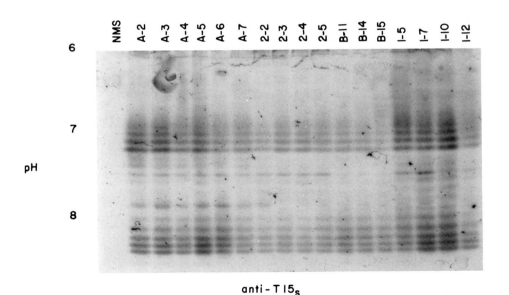

Figure 5. T15 idiotype-specific IEF profiles in serum of individual BALB/c mice immunized with PC-KLH. Sera of mice from four separate experiments were isofocused and the gel reacted with ^{125}I-labeled anti-T15$_s$. Samples were obtained 5–8 days after a second injection of PC-KLH either 1 (Expt. B), 2 (Expt. A and 1), or 5 (Expt. 2) weeks after the primary injection.[34]

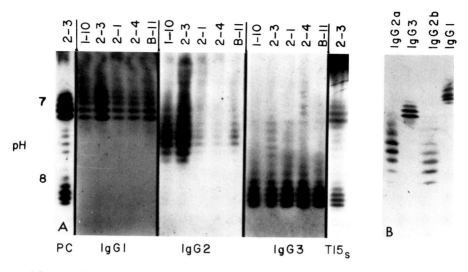

FIGURE 6. Immunoglobulin class analysis of PC-specific antibodies from individual BALB/c. (A) Immune sera (see Fig. 5) were isofocused in quintuplicate sets and reacted with radioiodinated PC-RNase, anti-T15$_s$, or class-specific antibodies. (B) Purified myeloma proteins were isofocused, fixed, and stained with Coomassie blue; IgG1 is M21, IgG2a is LPC-1, IgG2b is M195, and IgG3 is J606.[34]

geneic anti-T15, had suggested that a small percentage of the T15 response was heterogeneous. We wanted an alternative means of detecting V-region heterogeneity within a group of idiotypically related antibodies. Gearhart et al.[31] had been able to generate an IgG response when PC–protein conjugates rather than S. pneumonia organisms were used as antigens. Kreth and Williamson[32] and Keck et al.[33] had demonstrated that IEF, followed by an overlay with radioactive antigen, could readily detect heterogeneity among antibodies of a single specificity without the need to purify the specific antibody.

We took advantage of these observations and developed a technique which would allow us to separate a heterogeneous mixture of IgG anti-PC antibodies (IEF) and then to analyze them in situ for isotype and Id.[34,35] Using this procedure one can identify PC-specific antibodies of one subclass and one Id in an individual sample of serum, or one can compare simultaneously these same properties in a group of sera.

The first set of samples we examined were from BALB/c. As mentioned above, this strain had the peculiar habit of making a T15 Id and T15 L-chain-dominant response to R36A.[6,24] This trait also occurred following immunization with a PC–protein conjugate,[30] but in addition to an IgM response (20–100 μg/ml), the mice also produced an IgG response (80–300 μg/ml).[31,34] By IEF analysis 65 BALB/c examined all produced an identical spectrotype pattern of antibodies possessing T15 idiotypic determinants. Examples are shown in Figure 5. (Only on occasion did we observe T15 Id$^+$ bands outside this redundant pattern. These are discussed below.) The time that elapsed between primary and secondary immunization had no effect on this banding pattern. Three major sets of bands were seen but they represented the expression of T15 Id$^+$ antibodies in each of the three murine IgG subclasses: IgG1, IgG2 (a + b), and IgG3 (Fig. 6). Since the banding pattern of T15 Id$^+$ antibodies within each isotype resembled myeloma proteins so closely (Fig. 6), we felt that the response in each BALB/c mouse could be derived from a single V_H–V_L pair which occurred in IgM, in each of the IgG subclasses, and in IgA. It was possible that each class could have its own set of V_H genes associated with it,[35] but the more straightforward explanation was that one V_H gene paired with each C_H gene as a consequence of class switching[37] and that this occurred during the ontogeny of a B-cell clone.

One of our concerns with this approach was whether we would be able to detect somatic mutations which were expressed in some progeny cells. IEF has its limitations since only substitutions affecting the charge of a molecule will generate a new pattern. Moreover, a sufficient but unknown number of charge substitutions would probably have to occur before this new pattern would occupy a position in the IEF gel that was discernibly different from the parent pattern. Nevertheless, there was evidence that we would detect somatic variants of a germ-line clone,[38] although many would be missed. Since variant

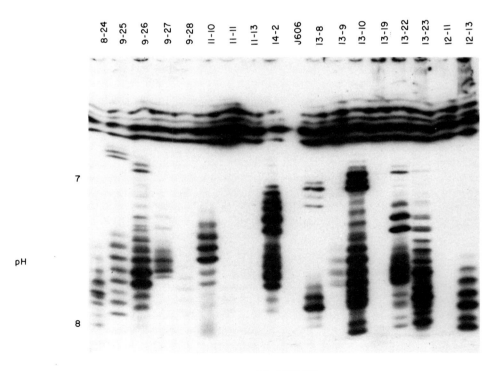

PC-RNASE

FIGURE 7. PC-specific IEF profiles in serum of individual BALB/c mice immunized with *M. morganii*. Continuous bands at pH 6.0–6.2 are not PC-specific. The majority of these antibodies bear M603 IdX determinants. Samples were tertiary day 12 bleedings for Expts. 8 and 9, and secondary day 11 bleedings for Expts. 10–14.[35]

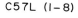

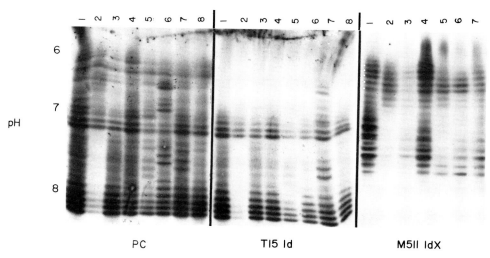

FIGURE 8. M511 and T15 idiotype-specific IEF profiles of purified anti-PC antibodies from individual C57L mice immunized with PC-KLH. Focused antibodies were developed with radioiodinated anti-κ (left panel), C57 anti-T15 (middle panel, see Table III), or C70 anti-M511 (right panel, see Table IV). Samples obtained as pools of serum from day 11, primary plus days 5 and 7, secondary.[41]

IEF patterns or clonotypes were detected infrequently and not to the exclusion of the dominant pattern, we tentatively concluded that the dominant T15 Id$^+$ response in BALB/c was essentially encoded directly in the germ line and that the evolutionary process had successfully selected out a V_H and V_L gene pair which was optimally suited to bind PC. This could be expected since PC is found on a number of different microorganisms, some of which are pathogens, e.g., *Aspergillus* sp., *S. pneumoniae,* and *Ascaris* sp.

When the examination of T15 Id$^+$ antibodies was extended to 15 additional strains, all (save those of the *Igh^j* haplotype) exhibited the same type of restricted response. Three sets of myeloma-type IEF bands were observed in each immunized mouse of 15 strains, and these three sets could be assigned to the IgG1, IgG2, and IgG3 isotypes as they had before.[39] Thus, the argument for a germ-line basis of the T15 response proposed for BALB/c held for these strains as well. In CBA, C3H, and PL mice, all *Igh^j* strains, three major band groups were present in each IgG isotype, suggesting that three different clonotypes were responsible for the diversity. Whether this diversity is derived from multiple V, J, or D is not known.[40]

The *in situ* identification of Id$^+$, anti-PC IgG antibodies was extended by Williams[35] and Wolfe[41] to an analysis of M603 and M511 Id$^+$ antibodies, respectively. The results were surprising in both cases. Examples of typical IEF gels are shown in Figs. 7 and 8. Unlike T15 Id$^+$ antibodies, anti-PC antibodies bearing these idiotypic determinants were regularly heterogeneous in all strains. A minimum of 15 different antibodies expressing M603 determinants were observed in BALB/c and A/J.[35] More than six different M511 Id$^+$ antibodies were seen in C57L and SEC mice.[41] We found these results puzzling. It was clear that the heterogeneity was real and not an artifact; hybridoma antibodies now bear that out. It was also clear that idiotypically related antibodies to other specificities, such as $\alpha(1,3)$-dextran and phenyloxazolone, were just as heterogeneous as the M511 and M603 Id$^+$ anti-PC antibodies. Either extensive somatic mutations were regularly occurring or more than one V_H and one V_L were being utilized in each case. The demonstration of somatic mutations in V_λ[44] and $V_\kappa 21$[45] and the recent finding that V genes exist as families of related genes made both viable possibilities. Detailed consideration of this issue required monoclonal antibody-producing cell lines, something that hybridoma technology ultimately provided.

4. Diversity among T15 Id$^+$ Antibodies

One curious phenomenon that these studies on IgG anti-PC brought out was the apparent uniqueness of the T15 response in most inbred strains. Every other idiotypic system, including M511 and M603 Id$^+$ antibodies, showed definite though limited heterogeneity in IEF gels. Was monoclonality suggested by the redundant T15 Id$^+$ IEF pattern apparent or real? During the course of examining the T15 IEF pattern in literally hundreds of mice, we had noted the occasional appearance of T15 IEF bands outside the redundant pattern in IgG1, IgG2, and IgG3 (Fig. 8, middle panel). These occurred in both IgG1 and IgG3 subclasses at low frequency but were not rare (2–10%). During the course of examining wild mice we were surprised to find that they displayed a heterogeneous T15 IEF spectrotype. Even more surprising was the response of two lines congenic to BALB/c, BALB.B ($K^b I^b S^b D^b$) and BALB.G ($K^d I^d S^d D^b$). Virtually every mouse responded with multiple T15 Id$^+$ antibodies in both IgG1 and IgG3 isotypes but more so in the former. Thus, mice clearly have the potential to generate a rather diverse family of T15 Id$^+$ antibodies, but for unexplained reasons it is not normally expressed.[46]

Follow-up studies on the "abnormally" restricted T15 response in inbred mice have demonstrated that the *H-2* locus does not control the response pattern. In fact, breeding experiments have demonstrated no genetic control at all, but a strong maternal influence on the progeny's response profile. Exactly how this "trait" is transmitted from mother to offspring is not clear, but reciprocal foster-rearing studies have shown that transmission occurs after birth (L. Pease and L. Claflin, unpublished observations). Further research on this interesting phenomenon of Id regulation is under way. Even without these studies it is clear that this idiotypic system is already highly regulated within a short time after birth. Any attempts to evaluate Id networks using the T15 system as a model must take this into account.

5. Hybridoma Antibodies

The foregoing series of experiments on serum anti-PC antibodies had strongly implied that the murine response to PC was composed of three families of antibodies related to the myeloma proteins T15, M603, and M511. A simple interpretation of the data was that three different V_L paired with a single V_H to generate germline prototype antibodies.[25]

Somatic mutations in these rearranged germ-line genes would then be responsible for the creation of a family of functionally and idiotypically related antibodies. Two lines of evidence, however, were against this simple interpretation. First, complete amino acid sequences of the V_H from the BALB/c myeloma proteins showed that their V_H could differ by as many as 13 residues from one another.[1] This argued that more than one germline V_H gene contributed to diversity among anti-PC antibodies. Second, the evidence accumulating from molecular analysis of antibody genes suggested that very similar V_H could be generated from multiple germline gene (segments). V-region genes were shown to be encoded not by a single gene but by two (L) or three (H) gene segments.[47–49] Each of these gene segments was actually not a single entity but a family of highly homologous genes. V segments were generally found in clusters of 3–10 genes, J segments in a single cluster of five genes (four functional ones), and the D segments for H chains in three or more clusters, each of which was composed of a number of related segments. Thus, the possibility for generating considerable diversity in anti-PC antibodies from the germline was significant enough to account for much of the conserved diversity seen within an antibody family. Variation in the D alone generated six different V_H among antidextran antibodies; use of three different J segments paired with the same V segments had also been observed.[50]

In order to analyze the various genetic mechanisms responsible for generating antibody diversity, we utilized the hybridoma technique of Köhler and Milstein[11] to produce large amounts of antigen-induced homogeneous populations of cells and their antibodies. All were produced by fusion with the nonsecreting cell lines SP2/0 or X63-Ag8.653. Screening of growing hybrids was done with PC-containing antigens not used as immunogens, or with the H-chain-specific (V_H4) anti-idiotypic antiserum, anti-VHPC,[51] or with both. Secondarily, hybridomas were screened with antisera specific for T15, M603, and M511. We deliberately avoided trying to bias our selection toward PC-binding, Id$^+$ hybridomas. Nevertheless, more than 95% of the clones possessed these two characteristics. The myeloma-specific antisera deserve specific mention since they differed from the binding site anti-Id used previously. Each anti-Id was prepared by immunization with one, or sometimes with two or three, monoclonal antibodies expressing a single L-chain type. The resulting antisera were adsorbed by non-PC-binding antibodies, then with PC-binding antibodies expressing the other L-chain types. Such anti-Id reagents were Fab-specific, but only for myeloma proteins having the same L-chain type [e.g., anti-M603 bound M603 and W3207 (both $V_\kappa 8$), but not T15, H8 ($V_\kappa 22$), or M511 and M167 ($V_\kappa 24$)]. Since any one pair of myeloma proteins were not structurally identical, the antisera must detect shared or cross-reactive idiotypic determinants (IdX).

Table II summarizes the origin and characteristics of a partial list of the monoclonal anti-PC antibodies (HP) obtained by the aforementioned immunization and screening procedures. More detailed description of these antibodies (HP) can be found elsewhere.[52,53] As can be seen, the HP represent all the major serum isotypes except IgA and come from eight different strains. Idiotyping of the HP with the anti-IdX reagents consistently yielded the three major groups or families shown, regardless of strain. These Id families are nonoverlapping—no HP was found which expressed more than one IdX. IEF of the L chains showed that within a family, nearly all the L chains cofocused. The exceptions will be discussed separately.

TABLE II
Anti-PC Hybridoma and Myeloma Proteins

Monoclonal antibody[a]	Strain of origin	Immunogen	Ig class	*Igh*	Reference
The T15 family					
T15, H8	BALB/c	—	A	*a*	53
55.2D3	BALB/c	*S. pneumoniae*	M	*a*	53
167.4G5	BALB/c	PC–protein	G1	*a*	53
167.7C2	BALB/c	PC–protein	G3	*a*	53
59.6C5	BAB-14	*S. pneumoniae*	G3	*a/b*	53
99.1G3	C58	*S. pneumoniae*	M	*a*	53
C3	CBB-22	—	A	*b*	53, 60
293	C57BL/6N	PC–protein	M	*b*	53, 60
22.1A4	AKR	*S. pneumoniae*	M	*d*	53
140.7C6	CBA	PC–protein	M	*j*	53, 60
140.1C2	CBA	PC–protein	G2	*j*	53, 60
103.3C3	PL	*S. pneumoniae*	M	*j*	53
103.1C9	PL	*S. pneumoniae*	G2	*j*	53
The M511 family					
M511, M167	BALB/c	—	A	*a*	53
137.2D3	C57L	PC–protein	M	*a*	53
137.5G6, .7C9	C57L	PC–protein	G1	*a*	53
100.1C11	CBA	*S. pneumoniae*	M	*j*	53, 60
101.3C2	CBA	*S. pneumoniae*	M	*j*	53, 60
101.6G6	CBA	*S. pneumoniae*	M	*j*	53, 62
The M603 family					
M603, W3207	BALB/c	—	A	*a*	53
55.7C8, .6F3	BALB/c	*S. pneumoniae*	M	*a*	53
180.7C9	BALB.g	*P. morganii*	M	*a*	This chapter
180.2G6	BALB.g	*P. morganii*	G1	*a*	This chapter
180.2B2	BALB.g	*P. morganii*	G3	*a*	This chapter
131.3B8	BALB.g	PC–protein	G3	*a*	53
137.6F2	C57L	PC–protein	G2	*a*	53
100.6F9, .6G2	CBA	*S. pneumoniae*	M	*j*	53, 60

[a]Assignment to family based on two or more parameters, i.e., L-chain IEF, idiotype, and sequence.

These results greatly extended our previous results on serum anti-PC antibodies. As we had predicted, the monoclonal antibodies fell into three families and these three families were preserved among inbred strains. These data also implied an extensive germ-line commitment to the anti-PC response in mice. How diverse were the members of a family? This critical question was approached in three different ways—by idiotypy, by sequence analysis of representative HP, and by binding site studies. Sequence studies were performed as a collaboration by Steve Clarke, Stuart Rudikoff, and Mike Potter (NIH) who have had a long-standing interest in the structure of anti-PC antibodies. Idiotypic examination of each family was performed separately by A. Maddalena (T15 family), J. Wolfe and C. Andres (M511 family), and S. Hudak (M603 family). Binding site studies were performed by these same individuals.

5.1. Idiotypic Properties

As a first approximation of structural heterogeneity within a family, HP were tested against a variety of anti-IdX antisera prepared either in rabbits and guinea pigs or in mice. Many of these antisera have been described.[52,53] In each instance the antisera had no reactivity to C_κ or C_H isotype nor did they cross-react with members of more than one family.

5.1.1. T15 Family

Idiotypic analyses of members in the T15 family with three different anti-Id are shown in Table III.[54] These HP differ in two known parameters—polymorphism at the *Igh* and *Igk-PC* loci. This latter locus controls the phenotypic expression of two allelic forms of the T15 L chain, PC-A which is found in AKR, C58, RF, and PL, and PC-B which is found in all other strains.[55] The IdX detected by C57 anti-T15 is clearly present on each V_H4-$V_\kappa22$ antibody. The degree of expression of the IdX varied according to the L-chain phenotype. PC-A-containing antibodies express the T15 IdX much less well than do PC-B-containing antibodies. A similar observation was made with the A/J anti-T15 antiserum. A second level of heterogeneity revealed by the C57 anti-T15 IdX antiserum is seen when one compares CBA (*Igh^j*) and BALB/c (*Igh^a*) HP. At least a four- to five-fold

TABLE III

Expression of Idiotypic Determinants among Monoclonal Antibodies in the T15 Family^a

Monoclonal antibody	Strain	Ig class	*Igh*	*Igk-PC*	C57 vs. T15	A/J vs. T15	C74 vs. 103.1C9
					I_{50} levels (ng/ml)^b		
T15, H8	BALB/c	A	a	b	40–45	45–48	>1000
55.2D3	BALB/c	M			100	130	>1000
167.4G5	BALB/c	G1			38	41	>1000
167.7C2	BALB/c	G3			11	35	>1000
M6^c	BALB/c	M			150	>10,000	ND
G-14^c	BALB/c	G1			30	>10,000	ND
99.1G3	C58	M	a	a	1600	2,000	>1000
C3	CBB-22	A	b	b	40	42	>1000
293	C57BL	M			52	66	>1000
22.1A4	AKR	M	d	a	950	1,100	>1000
140.7C6	CBA	M	j	b	300	>10,000	>1000
140.1C2	CBA	G2			180	>10,000	>1000
103.3C3	PL	M	j	a	2700	>10,000	>1000
103.1C9	PL	G2			3000	>10,000	100

^a Data taken from Maddalena.[54]

^b The antisera listed in the first line were tested against the radiolabeled antibody (immunogen) in the second line. C and G indicate rabbit and guinea pig, respectively. Each monoclonal antibody listed in the table was tested by inhibition RIA for its ability to inhibit this reaction.

^c These HP have been described by Gearhart et al.[58] and were obtained from John Kearney (University of Alabama, Birmingham).

difference exists in their I_{50} values, suggesting a structural difference between T15 antibodies in these two strains.

The second antiserum, A/J anti-T15, recognizes an Id that is differentially expressed among T15 IdX^+ antibodies. First, like the C57 anti-T15, it distinguishes between PC-A- and PC-B-containing antibodies. Second, it distinguishes among HP from different *Igh* haplotypes (*a, b, d* versus. *j*). This effect correlates with previous studies which showed that T15 IdX^+ serum antibodies in BALB/c and other strains, but not in CBA, were A/ J Id^+. Using heterologous chain recombinants derived from A/J Id-positive and -negative HP, Maddalena et al.[56] have shown that the inability of CBA T15 HP to express the A/ J Id is totally dependent on the H chain. The third and most interesting characteristic of this antiserum is its ability to distinguish among T15 IdX^+ HP in BALB/c. These results clearly demonstrate that T15 antibodies within a strain are structurally heterogeneous. As pointed out by Gearhart et al.[30] it also verifies their earlier finding from studies of B-cell clones (splenic foci) that the "T15 repertoire" is heterogeneous.

The third Id, detected by C74 anti-103.1C9, illustrates an example of a private or clone-specific Id (IdI) in PL T15 IdX antibodies. An IgM from the same fusion and an IgM and an IgG2 from CBA, all T15 IdX^+, do not share the 103.1C9 IdI.

5.1.2. M511 Family

Idiotypic heterogeneity among members of the M511 family is depicted in Table IV.[57] The reference antiserum C70 anti-M511, when 137.7C9 or M511 (not shown) is used as the labeled ligand, detects all V_H4-$V_\kappa24$ molecules but to varying degrees. For example, even though M511 and M167 are both IgA, the latter consistently expresses the M511 IdX less well than the former. Structural studies of these two molecules show that they have similar but different sequences.[14] The other three antisera detect IdI, a feature which is common among members of this family. This parallels binding site studies which

TABLE IV

Expression of Public and Private Idiotypic Determinants among Monoclonal Antibodies in the M511 Family[a]

Monoclonal antibody	Strain	Ig class	I_{50} levels (ng/ml)[b]			
			C70 vs. 7C9	G52 vs. 5G6	G10 vs. M167	C77 vs. 6G6
M511	BALB/c	A	32	>1000	>5000	>1000
M167	BALB/c	A	100	>1000	30	>1000
137.5G6[c]	C57L	G1	7	9.5	>5000	>1000
137.7C9[c]	C57L	G1	15	8	>5000	>1000
137.2D3	C57L	M	45	>1000	>5000	>1000
101.3C2	CBA	M	36	>1000	>5000	>1000
101.6G6	CBA	M	87	>1000	5000	34

[a] Data taken in part from Wolfe.[57]
[b] See footnote *b* in Table III.
[c] These sister clones appear to be identical by the criterion of fine specificity as well.[57]

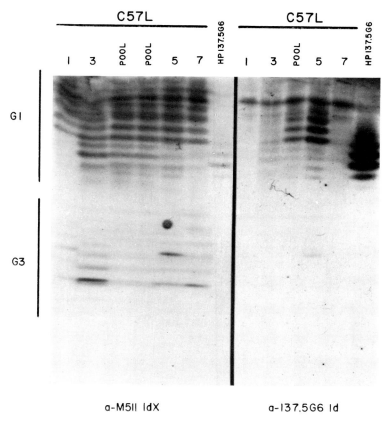

FIGURE 9. Expression of M511 IdX and HP5G6 IdI in PC-immune sera of C57L mice (Nos. 1, 3, 5, or 7) or pooled sera from C57L mice (Nos. 1–8). Twenty μl of serum or 1 μg HP5G6 was applied to the lanes indicated. Antibodies bearing M511 IdX and HP5G6 IdI determinants were visualized by overlay with [^{125}I]-C70 anti-M511 and [^{125}I]-G52 anti-HP5G6, respectively.[57]

show that no two M511 HP have the same hapten-binding profile for PC analogs (see below).

Can antibodies which are idiotypically related to 5G6, 6G6, and M167 be found in PC-immune sera? When appropriate strains were tested by conventional solid-phase radioimmunoassay, none expressed detectable levels of the IdI ($\leq$ 1–4 μg/ml).[57] The level of M511 IdX$^+$ antibodies ranged from 50 to 600 μg/ml. Therefore, antibodies expressing the various IdI appeared to represent less than 2–7% of the response. The search for serum antibodies related to 5G6 was pursued further by using the more sensitive *in situ* labeling procedure described in Section 3. Anti-PC antibodies from individual C57L mice and 5G6 protein were focused in two positions on a slab gel. The gel was split in half; one half was exposed to [^{125}I]-C70 anti-M511 and the other to [^{125}I]-G52 anti-5G6 (Fig. 9). The C70 antiserum reveals the M511 family of antibodies in these sera and the G52 reveals 5G6, as expected, but also a set of bands in the immune sera. This set of bands was present to variable degrees in the different sera but can be visualized with both C70 and G52. However, the antibodies expressing the 5G6 IdI do not cofocus with 5G6 itself and are more heterogeneous.

We conclude from these data that: (1) IdI can be expressed in immune sera although variably so, (2) the 5G6 IdI is expressed not just on 5G6 but on a set of antibodies, and (3) these 5G6 IdI$^+$ antibodies represent a subset of the M511 family. The results in Fig. 9 also demonstrate the limitations of IEF studies in analysis of structural diversity. By IEF, the set of 5G6 IdI$^+$ bands focus within the M511 IdX$^+$ antibodies. Thus, any estimate of the number of different antibody molecules based on IEF profile must be considered a minimum estimate of the true antibody diversity; the original estimate of about six grossly underestimates the real number of responding clones.

5.1.3. M603 Family

Because of our earlier results on serum anti-PC antibodies produced in response to *M. morganii,* we expected extensive diversity in the M603 family. This was borne out by our studies on idiotypy in this family. Antisera to M603, to W3207, or to a number of HP generally were individually specific. One example, C72a anti-100.6G2, is illustrated in Table V. An anti-IdX antiserum was obtained using two methods. The first used purified BALB/c anti-PC antibodies from *P. morganii* immune sera that contained only M603 L chains.[35] The second approach was to immunize rabbits in succession with different M603 HP. The resulting example is C72b which was obtained from rabbits immunized with 100.6G2, 100.6F9, and 55.7C8. This antiserum recognizes all V_H4–$V_\kappa 8$ anti-PC molecules although there are considerable differences in IdX expression among members of the family. Some of these differences are related to the immunoglobulin class, others must reflect structural heterogeneity within the V regions.

TABLE V
Expression of Public and Private Idiotypic Determinants among Monoclonal Antibodies in the M603 Family

Monoclonal antibody	Strain	Ig class	I_{50} levels (ng/ml)^a C72b vs. M603	C72a vs. 100.6G2
M603	BALB/c	A	1500	>5000
W3207	BALB/c	A	6000	>5000
55.7C8	BALB/c	M	650	2200
100.6F9	CBA	M	1000	5000
100.6G2	CBA	M	950	4
180.7C9	BALB.g	M	550	700
180.2G6	BALB.g	G1	700	>5000
180.2B2.1	BALB.g	G3	1100	2000

^{a}See footnote *b* in Table III.

5.2. Structural Properties

The diversity implied from IEF and idiotypic studies of serum and hybridoma antibodies is clearly much more extensive than that which could be encoded by three V_L and one V_H. The extent of this diversity and the genetic basis for it was established by sequencing both anti-PC antibodies and the genes that encode them.

Complete and partial variable-region amino acid sequencing of anti-PC antibodies from BALB/c[1−3,58,59] and CBA and C57BL/6[60] and DNA sequences of genes encoding BALB/c anti-PC antibodies[13,14] revealed the following (see Fig. 1). (1) Mice of each genotype used only three V_κ L chains and these were the same as those found in the myeloma proteins T15 ($V_\kappa 22$), M603 ($V_\kappa 8$), and M511 ($V_\kappa 24$) and in A/J serum anti-PC antibodies. (2) These three L chains were used in combination with a single V_H segment, encoded by a single V_H gene *(V1)*, to construct most anti-PC antibodies. (3) Where complete sequences of V_H and V_L segments were done, it was found that only one J_κ segment ($J_\kappa 5$) and one J_H segment ($J_H 1$) were used.[61] (4) Multiple, different D_H regions were used by each antibody family in each strain and there was no correlation with specificity.[60] (5) Somatic mutations can occur throughout the variable regions although they tend to cluster in and around the hypervariable regions.[58] (6) At least two antibodies out of 40 use a different V_H which is nevertheless homologous to *V1*. Thus, a second V_H can be used to produce an anti-PC antibody. One of these V_H appears to have arisen by gene conversion, suggesting an additional mechanism of generating V-region diversity.[62] The first four observations define the germ-line component of the anti-PC response and show that it is relatively simple. Anti-PC antibodies, regardless of which family they come from, use the same V_H, J_H, and probably J_κ gene segments. The existence of three families stems from the use of three nonhomologous V_κ gene segments. The last three observations explain how a large repertoire is generated from a small amount of genetic information.

6. Functional Diversity among Anti-PC Antibodies

Given the extensive repertoire that can be generated to PC, how does this translate into functional diversity? This problem is one of our primary areas of interest. The subject has been discussed in recent papers[2,52,53,60] and will be reviewed briefly.

Examination of the binding activity of our complete panel of HP (Table II) with a set of choline analogs yielded a "fingerprint" of the binding sites for hapten.[52,53] To our surprise every member of the T15 family gave the same binding pattern. The same result was obtained with all the M603 HP, although their binding profile differed from that of T15 HP. The M511 HP were the only ones to exhibit binding site variability and here the variability was extensive. Analysis of the three-dimensional model of M603[2,12] provides clues to how a "fixed" pocket arises. In the first place, PC occupies only a small portion of the binding site region in the antibody at the base of the pocket. Second, this region is lined by the principal contact residues for PC which are in V_H and, except in M167, these residues are preserved in all anti-PC antibodies. The region of greatest variability, the D segment, appears not to interact with PC. Third, V_L does interact with PC; the forces of interaction are weak but appear significant enough to affect specificity. One can speculate that these forces may act subtly in T15 and M603 HP but more dramatically in M511 HP. Heterologous chain recombination experiments between T15 and M603 H and L chains show that the fine specificity for hapten is determined by the L chain (S. Hudak and J. L. Claflin, 1984).

The need for two common pockets in anti-PC antibodies undoubtedly reflects the nature of PC-antigens in different environmental pathogens. As mentioned earlier, PC is ubiquitously distributed in nature in a variety of microorganisms, e.g., bacteria, fungi, and nematodes.[8] However, in each instance the structure, PC, is probably a constant; what it is coupled to in the organism, the carrier, is the variable. Thus, one can envision the evolution of antibodies with a conserved and a variable component in the binding site. The conserved component is the site among the CDRs at the base of the pocket which interacts with the hapten itself, the variable component would be the outer contours of the CDRs that come in contact with the cell wall components of the organisms immediately adjacent to where PC is attached. If one examines all the sequences of anti-PC antibodies and locates

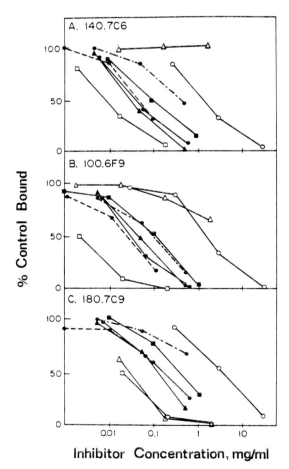

FIGURE 10. Specificities of PC-binding hybridoma antibodies to microbial antigens. Binding of [125I]-PC-RNase by the indicated antibodies (see Table II) was inhibited by soluble PC-containing extracts from *S. pneumoniae* (□—□), *M. morganii* (△—△), *Aspergillus niger* (●–·–●), *A. fumigatus* (●—●), *A. oryzae* (●---●), *Fusarium* sp. (▲—▲), *Trichoderma* sp. (■—■), and *Ascaris suum* (○—○).[54]

all mutations on the M603 three-dimensional structure (admittedly a hypothetical exercise), one finds that they congregate at the lip and outer surface of the binding site.

Do these substitutions affect binding to PC-carrier but not to PC? Maddalena[54] has screened our bank of monoclonal anti-PC antibodies for their ability to bind PC-antigens from a variety of microbes. Every HP, regardless of class, Id family, or whether they were immunized with *S. pneumoniae* organisms or PC-protein, gave the same inhibition pattern (Figs. 10A, B). These results were surprising from two standpoints. First, there was no evidence that the carrier microbe had any beneficial effect on binding activity. Second, it was puzzling that there were no negative effects created by different carriers. This meant that either our theory was wrong, the technique was insensitive, or the substitutions observed at the lip of the site were permissive. When HP from *M. morganii*-immunized mice were examined, a different picture emerged. All these HP showed a marked increase in their ability to bind a PC-antigen from *M. morganii* (Fig. 10C). The relative binding activity for other PC-antigens was unchanged. Recently, Rodwell *et al.*[63] have shown that, in HP derived from KLH-*p*-azophenylphosphocholine-immunized mice, two of five (that have been sequenced) have a higher affinity for phenylphosphocholine than for PC itself. In data published elsewhere we have found that anti-PC antibodies of the T15 family are more protective against infection with virulent *S. pneumoniae* organisms than are members of the M603 and M511 families.[64] Thus, carrier determinants can play a critical role. Sequence analysis of the anti-*M. morganii* HP in particular, coupled with model building exercises, may help to define those residues important to carrier binding and to position them in the binding region. We should then be in a position to directly test our hypothesis regarding two subregions in the binding site of anti-PC antibodies.

An additional and satisfying feature of these results is that they suggest a reason why three different V_κ genes are needed to construct anti-PC antibodies. Apparently, the PC antigens in various microorganisms are sufficiently different so that even with a mutational process and the availability of multiple D and J, more than one type of anti-PC antibody is needed.

7. Concluding Remarks

In the present chapter we have attempted to review those events in our laboratory which led to a dissection of antibody repertoire to the simple natural hapten, PC. Although we initially thought the response could be limited to just three conserved antibodies, subsequent idiotypic, protein and DNA structural studies from this and other laboratories revealed that the repertoire is essentially unlimited. However, the germ-line basis for the response is relatively simple. A single V_H gene segment (occasionally two), three V_L, one J_H, and one J_κ are the foundations for an anti-PC response; expansion through variation in and around D and through somatic mutations generates a vast repertoire of similar but distinct antibody molecules. This scheme is not unique to anti-PC antibodies; genetic analyses of antibodies to other simple haptens show that this is a common mechanism of generating diversity.[65,66]

In spite of the tremendous progress made in establishing genetic mechanisms for an antibody repertoire, there are still a number of questions that need answering. One of the most crucial is how *structural* diversity translates into *functional* diversity. Antibodies within a family can show many somatic substitutions and considerable variation in D, yet usually this has little or no demonstrable effect, either positive or negative, on antibody specificity.[2,53,60] Protein sequences and three-dimensional models of structurally similar but functionally distinct molecules need to be obtained. Examples from the M603 family which differ in their binding to *M. morganii* are already available and under investigation. Anti-$\alpha(1,3)$-dextran[67] and anti-$\beta(1,6)$-galactan[68] antibodies should also constitute appropriate examples. As a corollary to this research we need to test our hypothesis that variability in the binding site of anti-PC antibodies has evolved to accommodate PC in different microbial contexts. Will this explain the need for three different V_κ genes? One also hopes that from this work will emerge an understanding of how D functions in antibody diversity. The length of H-chain CDR3 in antibodies to $\alpha(1,3)$-dextran,[50] to $\beta(1,6)$-galactan,[2] and to PC in the T15 family[60] is invariant, implying that one role for the D segment is to maintain the proper length of this hypervariable region. What does this mean structurally and is this its only role?

Recent findings of unequal distribution of T15 Id$^+$ antibodies among B-cell subsets[69] raise completely new questions about the expression of V genes. What is the genetic and cellular basis for this restriction and how does it relate to the observations of apparent association between V regions (idiotypes), immunoglobulin isotypes, and antigen composition (carbohydrate versus protein)[36]? These are important and complex problems that will require an integrated research effort. There are also clinical applications since the unresponsiveness of infants to carbohydrate vaccines (e.g., for *S. pneumoniae, Hemophilus influenzae,* and *Neisseria meningitidis* infections) is inextricably associated with their concurrent inability to mount an IgG2 response.[70,71] Since the response to PC occurs in certain B-cell subsets and shows an isotype preference, and one can mount a response to it both in mouse and in man (B. Briles and B. Gray, personal communication), PC would be an excellent model antigen to use to explore this aspect of V gene expression. The fact that so much is known about the PC antibody response at the molecular level makes PC an optimal choice.

ACKNOWLEDGMENTS. The authors wish to thank the following journals for permission to use copyrighted figures: *Journal of Immunology* for Fig. 2, 5–8, *European Journal of Immunology* for Fig. 3, and *Journal of Experimental Medicine* for Fig. 4. We are indebted to Steve Clarke for permission to use a modification of the illustration in Fig. 1. We thank Emma Williams for preparing the manuscript. This work was supported by Grant AI-12533 from the National Institutes of Health.

References

1. Potter, M., 1977, Antigen-binding myeloma proteins of mice, *Adv. Immunol.* **25**:141–211.
2. Rudikoff, S., 1983, Immunoglobulin structure–function correlates: Antigen binding and idiotypes, in: *Contemporary Topics in Molecular Immunology,* Volume 9 (F. P. Imman and T. J. Kindt, eds.), Plenum Press, New York, pp. 169–209.
3. Huang, H., Crews, S., and Hood, L., 1981, Diversification of antibody genes through DNA rearrangements, *Adv. Exp. Med. Biol.* **137**:475–488.

4. Potter, M., and Lieberman, R., 1970, Common antigenic determinants in five of eight BALB/c IgA myeloma proteins that bind phosphorylcholine, *J. Exp. Med.* **132**:737–751.

5. Leon, M., and Young, N. M., 1971, Specificity of phosphorylcholine of six murine myeloma proteins reactive with *Pneumococcus* C polysaccharide and β-lipoprotein, *Biochemistry* **10**:1424–1429.

6. Cosenza, H., and Kohler, H., 1972, Specific inhibition of plaque formation to phosphorylcholine by antibody against antibody, *Science* **176**:1027–1029.

7. Sher, A., and Cohn, M., 1972, Inheritance of an idiotype associated with the immune response of inbred mice to phosphorylcholine, *Eur. J. Immunol.* **2**:319–323.

8. Potter, M., 1971, Antigen binding myeloma in mice, *Ann. N.Y. Acad. Sci.* **190**:306–321.

9. Briles, D. E., Nahm, M., Schroer, K., Davie, J., Baker, P., Kearney, J., and Barletta, R., 1981, Antiphosphocholine antibodies found in normal mouse serum are protective against intravenous infection with type 3 *Streptococcus pneumoniae, J. Exp. Med.* **153**:694–705.

10. Briles, D. E., Claflin, J. L., Schroer, K., and Forman, C., 1981, Mouse IgG3 antibodies are highly protective against infection with *Streptococcus pneumoniae, Nature* **294**:88–90.

11. Köhler, G., and Milstein, C., 1976, Derivation of specific antibody-producing tissue culture and tumor lines by cell fusion, *Eur. J. Immunol.* **6**:511–519.

12. Segal, D. M., Padlan, E. A., Cohen, G. H., Rudikoff, S., Potter, M., and Davies, D. R., 1974, The three-dimensional structure of a phosphorylcholine binding mouse immunoglobulin Fab and the nature of the antigen binding site, *Proc. Natl. Acad. Sci. USA* **71**:4298–4302.

13. Crews, S., Griffin, J., Huang, H., Calame, K., and Hood, L., 1982, A single V_H gene segment encodes the immune response to phosphorylcholine: Somatic mutation is correlated with the class of the antibody, *Cell* **25**:59–66.

14. Selsing, E., and Storb, U., 1981, Somatic mutation of immunoglobulin light chain variable region genes, *Cell* **25**:47–58.

15. Claflin, J. L., Lieberman, R., and Davie, J.M., 1974, Clonal nature of the immune response to phosphorylcholine. I. Specificity, class, and idiotype of phosphorylcholine-binding receptors on lymphoid cells, *J. Exp. Med.* **139**:58–73.

16. Davie, J. M., and Paul, W. E., 1972, Receptors on immunocompetent cells. V. Cellular correlates of the maturation of the immune response, *J. Exp. Med.* **135**:660–674.

17. Claflin, J. L., Lieberman, R., and Davie, J. M., 1974, Clonal nature of the immune response to phosphorylcholine. II. Idiotypic specificity and binding characteristics of antiphosphorylcholine antibodies, *J. Immunol.* **112**:1747–1756.

18. Claflin, J. L., and Davie, J. M., 1974, Clonal nature of the immune response to phosphorylcholine. III. Species-specific binding characteristics of rodent antiphosphorylcholine antibodies, *J. Immunol.* **113**:1678–1683.

19. Claflin, J. L., and Davie, J. M., 1974, Clonal nature of the immune response to phosphorylcholine. IV. Idiotypic uniformity of binding site associated antigenic determinants among mouse antiphosphorylcholine antibodies, *J. Exp. Med.* **140**:673–686.

20. Claflin, J. L., and Davie, J. M., 1975, Specific isolation and characterization of antibody directed against the binding site antigenic determinants, *J. Immunol.* **114**:70–75.

21. Claflin, J. L., and Rudikoff, S., 1977, Uniformity in a clonal repertoire: A case for a germ-line basis of antibody diversity, *Cold Spring Harbor Symp. Quant. Biol.* **41**:725–734.

22. Barstad, P., Rudikoff, S., Potter, M., Cohn, M., Konigsberg, W., and Hood, L., 1974, Immunoglobulin structure: Amino terminal sequences of mouse myeloma proteins that bind phosphorylcholine, *Science* **183**:962–964.

23. Claflin, J. L., Rudikoff, S., Potter, M., and Davie, J. M., 1975, Structural, functional, and idiotypic characteristics of a phosphorylcholine-binding IgA myeloma protein of C57BL/Ka allotype, *J. Exp. Med.* **141**:608–619.

24. Claflin, J. L., 1976, Uniformity in the clonal repertoire for the immune response to phosphorylcholine in mice, *Eur. J. Immunol.* **6**:669–674.

25. Rudikoff, S., and Claflin, J. L., 1975, Expression of equivalent clonotypes in BALB/c and A/J mice after immunization with phosphorylcholine, *J. Exp. Med.* **144**:1294–1304.

26. Pawlak, L. L., and Nisonoff, A., 1973, Distribution of a cross-reactive idiotypic specificity in inbred strains of mice, *J. Exp. Med.* **137**:855–869.

27. Capra, J. D., Kehoe, J. M., Williams, R. C., Feizi, T., and Kunkel, H. G., 1972, Light chain sequences of human IgM cold agglutinins, *Proc. Natl. Acad. Sci. USA* **69**:40–43.
28. Kunkel, H. G., Winchester, R. J., Joslin, F. G., and Capra, J. D., 1974, Similarities in the light chains of anti-γ-globulins showing cross-idiotypic specificities, *J. Exp. Med.* **139**:128–137.
29. Ju, S.-T., Benacerraf, B., and Dorf, M. E., 1978, Idiotypic analysis of antibodies to poly (Glu^{60}Ala^{30}Tyr^{10}): Intrastrain and interspecies idiotypic cross-reactions, *Proc. Natl. Acad. Sci. USA* **75**:6192–6196.
30. Gearhart, P.J., Sigal, N. H., and Klinman, N. R., 1977, The monoclonal antiphosphorylcholine antibody response in several murine strains: Genetic implications of a diverse repertoire, *J. Exp. Med.* **145**:876–891.
31. Gearhart, P. J., Sigal, N. H., and Klinman, N. R., 1975, Heterogeneity of the BALB/c antiphosphoryl-choline antibody response at the precursor cell level, *J. Exp. Med.* **141**:56–71.
32. Kreth, H. W., and Williamson, A. R., 1973, The extent of diversity of antihapten antibodies in inbred mice: Anti-NIP antibodies in CBA/H mice, *Eur. J. Immunol.* **3**:141–147.
33. Keck, K., Grossberg, A. L., and Pressman, D., 1973, Specific characterization of isoelectric focused immunoglobulins in polyacrylamide gel by reaction with ^{125}I-labeled protein antigen or antibodies, *Eur. J. Immunol.* **3**:99–102.
34. Claflin, J. L., and Cubberley, M., 1978, Clonal nature of the immune response to phosphocholine. VI. Molecular uniformity of a single idiotype among BALB/c mice, *J. Immunol.* **121**:1410–1415.
35. Williams, K., and Claflin, J. L., 1982, Clonotypes of antiphosphocholine antibodies induced with *Proteus morganii* (Potter). II. Heterogeneity, class and idiotypic analyses of the repertoires in BALB/c and A/HeJ mice, *J. Immunol.* **128**:600–607.
36. Slack, J., Der-Balian, G. P., Nahm, M., and Davie, J. M., 1980, Subclass restriction of murine antibodies. II. The IgG plaque-forming cell response to thymus-independent type 1 and type 2 antigens in normal mice and mice expressing an X-linked immunodeficiency, *J. Exp. Med.* **151**:853–862.
37. Parkhouse, R. M. E., and Cooper, M. D., 1977, A model for the differentiation of B lymphocytes with implications for the biological role of IgD, *Immunol. Rev.* **37**:105–126.
38. Cotton, R. G. H., Secher, D. S., and Milstein, C., 1973, Somatic mutation and the origin of antibody diversity: Clonal variability of the immunoglobulin produced by MOPC21 cells in culture, *Eur. J. Immunol.* **3**:135–140.
39. Claflin, J. L., and Cubberley, M., 1980, Clonal nature of the immune response to phosphocholine. VII. Evidence throughout inbred mice for molecular similarities among antibodies bearing the T15 idiotypes, *J. Immunol.* **125**:551–558.
40. Claflin, J. L., 1980, Clonal nature of the immune response to phosphocholine. VIII. Evidence that antibodies bearing T15 idiotypic determinants in *Igh^j* mice comprise a family of antibodies, *J. Immunol.* **125**:559–563.
41. Wolfe, J., and Claflin, J. L., 1980, Clonal nature of the immune response to phosphocholine. IX. Heterogeneity among antibodies bearing M511 idiotypic determinants, *J. Immunol.* **125**:2397–2401.
42. Hansburg, D., Briles, D. E., and Davie, J. M., 1976, Analysis of the diversity of murine antibodies to dextran B1355. I. Generation of a large, pauci-clonal response by a bacterial vaccine, *J. Immunol.* **117**:569–575.
43. Mäkelä, D., Kaartinen, M., Pelkonen, J. L. T., and Karjalainen, K., 1978, Inheritance of antibody specificity. V. Anti-2-phenyloxazoline in the mouse, *J. Exp. Med.* **148**:1644–1660.
44. Weigert, M. G., Cesari, I. M., Yankovitch, S. J., and Cohn, M., 1970, Variability in the lambda light chain sequences of mouse antibody, *Nature* **228**:1045–1047.
45. Weigert, M., Gatmaitan, L., Loh, E., Schilling, J., and Hood, L., 1978, Rearrangement of genetic information may produce immunoglobulin diversity, *Nature* **276**:785–790.
46. Pease, L. R., and Claflin, J. L., 1981, Clonal regulation in the response to phosphocholine. II. Heterogeneity among T15 idiotype positive antibodies in inbred and wild mice, *Eur. J. Immunol.* **11**:662–667.
47. Brack, C., Hirama, M., Lenhard-Schuller, R., and Tonegawa, S., 1978, A complete immunoglobulin gene is created by somatic recombination, *Cell* **15**:1–14.
48. Early, P., Huang, H., Davis, M., Calame, K., and Hood, L., 1980, An immunoglobulin heavy chain variable region gene is generated from three segments of DNA: V$_H$, D and J$_H$, *Cell* **19**:981–992.
49. Sakano, H., Maki, R., Kurosawa, Y., Roeder, W., and Tonegawa, S., 1980, Two types of somatic recombination are necessary for the generation of complete immunoglobulin heavy-chain genes, *Nature* **286**:676–683.

50. Schilling, J., Clevinger, B., Davie, J. M., and Hood, L., 1980, Amino acid sequence of homogeneous antibodies to dextran and DNA rearrangements in heavy chain V-region gene segments, *Nature* **283**:35–40.

51. Claflin, J. L., and Davie, J. M., 1975, Clonal nature of the immune response to phosphorylcholine. V. Cross-idiotypic specificity among heavy chains of murine anti-PC antibodies and PC-binding myeloma proteins, *J. Exp. Med.* **141**:1073–1083.

52. Claflin, J. L., Hudak, S., and Maddalena, A., 1981, Antiphosphocholine hybridoma antibodies. I. Direct evidence for three distinct families in the murine response, *J. Exp. Med.* **153**:352–364.

53. Andres, C. M., Maddalena, A., Hudak, S., Young, N. M., and Claflin, J. L., 1981, Antiphosphocholine hybridoma antibodies. II. Functional analysis of binding sites within three antibody families, *J. Exp. Med.* **154**:1584–1598.

54. Maddalena, A., 1983, The conservation of specificity in the T15 family of mouse antiphosphocholine antibodies, Ph.D. thesis, The University of Michigan.

55. Claflin, J. L., 1976, Genetic marker in the variable region of kappa chains of mouse antiphosphorylcholine antibodies, *Eur. J. Immunol.* **6**:666–668.

56. Maddalena, A., Hudak, S., and Claflin, J. L., 1984, Idiotypes of anti-PC antibodies: Structural correlates, *Ann. Immunol.* **135C**:117–122.

57. Wolfe, J., 1983, Sources of immunoglobulin diversity among murine antiphosphocholine antibodies in the M511 idiotype family, Ph.D. thesis, The University of Michigan.

58. Gearhart, P. J., Johnson, N. D., Douglas, R., and Hood, L., 1981, IgG antibodies to phosphorylcholine exhibit more diversity than their IgM counterparts, *Nature* **291**:29–34.

59. Kocher, H. P., Berek, C., and Jaton, J.-C., 1981, The immune response of BALB/c mice to phosphorylcholine is restricted to a limited number of V_H- and V_L-isotypes, *Mol. Immunol.* **18**:1027–1033.

60. Clarke, S. H., Claflin, J. L., Potter, M., and Rudikoff, S., 1982, Polymorphisms in antiphosphocholine antibodies reflecting evolution of immunoglobulin families, *J. Exp. Med.* **157**:98–113.

61. Rudikoff, S., Satow, Y., Padlan, E., Davies, D., and Potter, M., 1981, Kappa chain structure from a crystallized murine Fab': Role of jointing segment in hapten binding, *Mol. Immunol.* **18**:705–711.

62. Clarke, S., Claflin, J. L., and Rudikoff, S., 1982, Polymorphisms in immunoglobulin heavy chains suggesting gene conversion, *Proc. Natl. Acad. Sci. USA* **79**:3280–3284.

63. Rodwell, J. D., Gearhart, P. J., and Karush, F., 1983, Restriction in IgM expression. IV. Affinity analysis of monoclonal antiphosphorylcholine antibodies, *J. Immunol.* **130**:313–316.

64. Briles, D. E., Forman, C., Hudak, S., and Claflin, J. L., 1982, Anti-PC antibodies of the T15 idiotype are optimally protective against *Streptococcus pneumoniae*, *J. Exp. Med.* **156**:1177–1185.

65. Bothwell, A. L., Paskind, M., Reth, M., Imanishi-Kari, T., Rajewsky, R., and Baltimore, D., 1981, Heavy chain variable region contribution to the NP^b family of antibodies: Somatic mutation evident in a $\gamma 2a$ variable region, *Cell* **24**:625–637.

66. Siekewitz, M., Huang, S. Y., and Gefter, M. L., 1983, The genetic basis of antibody production: A single heavy chain variable region gene encodes all molecules bearing the dominant anti-arsonate idiotype in the strain A mouse, *Eur. J. Immunol.* **13**:123–132.

67. Newman, B., Sugii, S., Kabat, E. A., Torii, M., Clevinger, B. L., Schilling, J., Bond, M., Davie, J. M., and Hood, L., 1983, Combining site specificities of mouse hybridoma antibodies to dextran 1355S, *J. Exp. Med.* **157**:130–140.

68. Feldman, R. J., Potter, M., and Glaudemans, C. P. J., 1981, A hypothetical space-filling model of the V-region of the galactin-binding myeloma immunoglobulin J539, *Mol. Immunol.* **18**:683–698.

69. Wicker, L. S., Guelde, G., Scher, I., and Kenny, J. J., 1982, Antibodies from the Lyb5⁻ B cell subset predominate in the secondary IgG response to phosphocholine, *J. Immunol.* **129**:950–953.

70. Siber, G. R., Schur, P. H., Aisenberg, A. C., Weitzman, S. A., and Schiffman, G., 1980, Correlation between serum IgG-2 concentrations and the antibody response to bacterial polysaccharide antigens, *N. Engl. J. Med.* **303**:178–182.

71. Morell, A., Skvaril, F., Hitzig, W. H., and Barandun, S., 1972, IgG subclasses: Development of the serum concentrations in "normal" infants and children, *J. Pediatr.* **80**:960–964.

11

The Limiting Dilution Approach to the Analysis of the Idiotypic Repertoire

DANIÉLÉ PRIMI, DOMINIQUE JUY, AND
PIERRE-ANDRÉ CAZENAVE

1. Introduction

The expression of the variable gene repertoire can be studied using different strategies, but as each experimental protocol has its limitations, it follows that the final interpretation of the results obtained is always governed by the particular limitations of the strategy employed. Consequently, it is not surprising that many conflicting data have been reported in this field. For example, the available idiotypic repertoire can be studied using immunization with antigen, but this approach only provides information concerning the antigen-sensitive B-cell clones, and thus does not permit the evaluation of the complete representation of a given idiotope in the whole antibody pool. More representative data on the B-cell receptor repertoire can be obtained by the clonotype analysis of anti-idiotype-treated animals[1,2] but, in this case, different immunization protocols can also produce misleading results. An alternative way to obtain a quantitative description of the repertoire of both mature and precursor B cells is to polyclonally expand the B-cell pool and to study the frequency of B cells which are precursors for clones secreting immunoglobulin with a given paratope or idiotype.[3-5] This approach has the advantage of providing a complete description of the immune system with regard to the specific clones expressed within a B-cell subset. In addition, as the frequency of a given paratope or idiotope is determined in the absence of antigen, this analysis is preferable to others since it does not depend on a particular protocol of immunization but rather reflects the absolute frequency of competent B

DANIÉLÉ PRIMI, DOMINIQUE JUY, AND PIERRE-ANDRÉ CAZENAVE • Unité d'Immunochimie Analytique, Institut Pasteur, 75015 Paris, France.

cells in a steady state. For these reasons we have recently adapted this methodology for our studies on the expression of both the available and the potential idiotypic repertoire.

In this chapter we summarize the most relevant results obtained using this kind of analysis on the distribution of idiotypic specificities among mitogen-reactive B-cell subsets, on the association of various idiotopes with antibody paratopes, and on the role played by T cells and the maternal environment in the selection and maintenance of the V-region determinant repertoire. It should be stressed that the choice of the different idiotypic systems used in these studies was dictated by their particular stability for certain experiments.

Parts of this work have been reported elsewhere[6-8] and therefore we will describe here only the experimental protocols of our most recent unpublished data in detail.

2. The Distribution of Idiotypic Specificities on Mitogen-Reactive B-Cell Subsets

When we decided to quantify the expression of antibody variable (V) regions among mitogen-reactive precursor B cells, we were immediately confronted with the problem of uniform representation of the distribution of complementary elements (paratope or idiotope) among these B-cell subsets. Since polyclonal activation does not involve the variable region of immunoglobulins the triggering is not immunologically specific and therefore it has been proposed that the repertoire of antibody specificity is randomly distributed among the subsets of B-cell clones, defined by their reactivity to different mitogens.[9,10] Indeed, increased antibody synthesis specific for multideterminant antigens or haptens is always induced by various polyclonal B-cell activators (PBA). These observations, however, do not take into account the extreme degeneracy of the immune system or, in other words, the great lack of precision in the fit between antibody and antigen. Consequently, the question of whether different B-cell subpopulations, as defined by mitogen reactivity, selectively express identical clonotypes has not been answered as yet. We decided to address ourselves to this question by studying the expression of four idiotopes in the spleen cells of BALB/c mice activated by two mitogens, i.e., lipopolysaccharide (LPS) and Nocardia delipidated cell mitogen (NDCM).[11] Using the limiting dilution analysis of LPS- and NDCM-sensitive B lymphocytes we therefore determined the frequencies of clones secreting immunoglobulin molecules that bear the 66, 137, 395, or M460 idiotopes as well as of those specific for the β-galactosidase antigen. The 66, 137, and 395 idiotopes are present on the BALB/c monoclonal immunoglobulin 174, which reacts with β-galactosidase. Each of the three idiotopes is defined by a corresponding BALB/c monoclonal anti-idiotope antibody. None of these three determinants is normally expressed when BALB/c mice are immunized with β-galactosidase and therefore they can be classified as nonrecurrent idiotopes. In contrast, the M460 idiotope, defined by the monoclonal anti-M460 antibody F6(51), is present on a portion of antitrinitrophenyl (anti-TNP) antibodies produced by BALB/c mice after immunization with thymus-dependent (TD) or thymus-independent (TI) TNP antigens.[12] The frequencies of the idiotope-positive clonotypes obtained by LPS and NDCM could be directly compared since we have previously established that the frequencies of LPS- and NDCM-sensitive B cells are virtually identical (1/55 for LPS and 1/63 for NDCM).[6] The results of this analysis are collectively shown in Fig. 1. Thus, the number of β-galactosidase-specific precursor cells is equally distributed among the two subpopu-

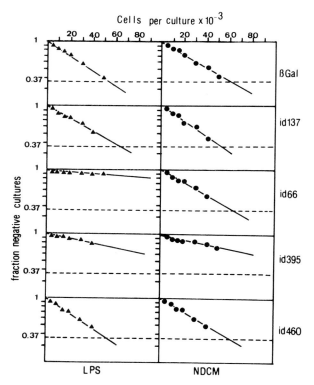

FIGURE 1. Spleen cells from BALB/c mice were treated with anti-Thy-1.2 and complement and cultured at the indicated concentrations with either LPS or NDCM in the presence of 3×10^6 rat thymocytes/ml. Results represent groups of 96 replicates assayed for the presence of anti-β-galactosidase antibodies or for the indicated idiotopes in the culture supernatants after 12 days. (From Ref. 6)

lations, therefore confirming the notion that the repertoire of antibody specificities seems to be repeated among B-cell subsets. The analysis of the frequency of idiotype-positive B-cell precursors, however, gave different results. Although the numbers of F6(51), 137, and 395 idiotype-positive precursors were found to be similar in both LPS- and NDCM-sensitive B-cell populations, the total numbers of 66 idiotope-positive cells varied dramatically depending on the mitogen added to the cultures. As we had previously detected the frequency of all clones stimulated by LPS or NDCM, we could correlate the frequencies of 66 idiotope-producing B cells to the total number of mitogen-reactive B cells and therefore obtain the frequencies of 66 idiotope-positive precursors within the pool of LPS- or NDCM-reactive B cells (Table I). Thus, 1 in 2000 NDCM-reactive B cells expresses the 66 idiotope whereas among the LPS B-cell pool the frequency of B lymphocytes secreting this idiotypic marker is almost negligible. Since we could also exclude the possibility that our results are due to a preferential *Igh-C* gene association of the 66 idiotope which would not be induced by LPS,[6] we must conclude that the *V* gene repertoire is not randomly distributed among mitogen-reactive B-cell subpopulations. These results therefore imply that the analysis of the idiotypic repertoire accomplished by mitogens is not necessarily

TABLE I
Absolute Frequencies of Anti-β-galactosidase and Idiotope-Secreting Clones among LPS- and NDCM-Reactive B Cells in Normal BALB/c Mice[a]

Mitogen	Ig-secreting clones/total B splenocytes	Anti-β-galactosidase clones	M460 Id⁺ clones	66 Id⁺ clones	137 Id⁺ clones	395 Id⁺ clones
LPS	1/30	1/2000	1/1800	<1/10,000	1/2000	<1/5000
NDCM	1/25	1/2400	1/2200	1/2400	1/2000	<1/5000

[a]From *J. Exp. Med.* **156**:181 (1982).

representative of the total repertoire of a given animal. Our studies also provided further important information. The 66, 137, and 395 determinants, as mentioned above, are not expressed at detectable levels in the anti-β-galactosidase antibody response of BALB/c mice immunized against β-galactosidase and therefore can be classified as private idiotopes. Our experiments, however, clearly establish that these specificities are not only part of the idiotypic repertoire of all BALB/c mice tested but also that they can be induced to expression on immunoglobulins devoid of anti-β-galactosidase activity with a frequency similar to that of a public idiotype, i.e., M460.

3. The Contribution of Individual Idiotopes to the Antibody–Antigen Binding Site

Having established the advantages and the limitations of the limiting dilution approach to the analysis of the idiotypic repertoire using B-cell mitogens we next pursued our studies by investigating the relationship between variable-region determinants and antigen specificity in anti-β-galactosidase antibodies. In the first section we demonstrated that a considerable number of idiotope-positive clonotypes devoid of anti-β-galactosidase activity could be detected and concluded that this might very well reflect the independent expression of V-region markers and paratopes. The existence of defined idiotopes on immunoglobulins without antibody activity has been fully documented for some time,[13–24] but, until now, it has been difficult to establish the possible existence of well-defined rules that govern the relationship between idiotopes and paratopes. Such studies have been hampered mainly by the difficulty selecting B-cell clones or hybridomas that are positive or negative for any possible combination of a number of well-defined sets of V regions. We were able to bypass this problem because, by knowing the absolute frequencies of each of the three idiotopes, i.e., 66, 137, and 395, we could design experimental protocols which allowed us to select and study individual clones of mitogen-reactive B cells positive for any combination of these determinants and to correlate these clones to anti-β-galactosidase activity. Briefly, the experimental design was as follows. On the basis of our previous frequency determination and in order to have less than one idiotype-positive clone per well, we set up large numbers of individual cultures each containing either LPS or NDCM. After 12 days of culturing, the supernatant of each well was individually tested for HA activity with SRBC, respectively coupled with 66, 137, or 395 antibodies or with the antigen β-galactosidase. The results based on the screening of 864 cultures of a typical analysis of this kind are shown in Table II and Fig. 2. These data can be summarized as follows. We could detect a large number of wells containing anti-β-galactosidase antibodies which did not bear any of the three idiotopes under study in both LPS- and NDCM-activated cultures. These results are not surprising since all these V-region determinants are not recurrently expressed in the BALB/c anti-β-galactosidase immune response.

Among those clones positive for one idiotypic determinant only, we constantly found with both LPS and NDCM that the 137 idiotope-positive wells were by far the most frequent. Since most of these wells did not contain anti-β-galactosidase activity we must conclude that the 137 determinant is indeed recurrently expressed in BALB/c animals, but in association with immunoglobulins specific for antigens other than β-galactosidase. The most surprising results, however, were those concerning the presence of one, two, or all three idiotopes in those wells containing anti-β-galactosidase activity. In both groups of culture containing LPS and NDCM in fact, only a minority of those clones positive for just one idiotope had reactivity against the antigen. In addition, similar results were obtained with culture supernatants positive for any combination of two idiotopes. These data, therefore, indicate the existence of complete independence of both idiotope expression

TABLE II

HA Activity of Supernatants of LPS- and NDCM-Activated Cultures[a,b]

β-Gal[c] SRBC	Agglutinated erythrocytes			No. of positive cultures activated with	
	137 SRBC	395 SRBC	66 SRBC	LPS	NDCM
+	+	+	+	23	26
+	+	−	−	40	10
+	−	+	−	4	3
+	−	−	+	3	4
+	+	+	−	3	1
+	+	−	+	0	5
+	−	+	+	1	3
+	−	−	−	119	139
−	−	−	−	547	544
−	+	−	−	97	80
−	−	+	−	9	12
−	−	−	+	10	21
−	+	+	−	3	4
−	+	−	+	2	9
−	−	+	+	3	1
−	+	+	+	0	2

[a]From *J. Exp. Med.* **156**:924 (1982).
[b]Cultures (864/group) contained 2×10^6 anti-Thy-1.2 and complement-treated BALB/c splenocytes and 50 μg/ml of LPS or NDCM. Supernatants were tested for HA activity on day 12.
[c]β-Galactosidase.

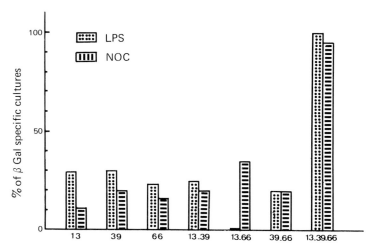

FIGURE 2. Percentage of anti-β-galactosidase clones among those cultures positive for one, two, or three idiotypic determinants. (From Ref. 7)

and antibody specificity in our system and should therefore caution us against considering idiotopes as clonal markers. The most striking result obtained, however, was the strong correlation between anti-β-galactosidase activity and the simultaneous presence of the three idiotopes observed in virtually all the cultures. As we had previously excluded the possibility that these findings could be accounted for by the presence of three clones, each positive for a single idiotope in a single well, our observation means that either these clones are all identical to the original 174 or that the spatial conformation of the three idiotopes designs the anti-β-galactosidase paratope. Although not mutually exclusive, these two hypotheses are different, inasmuch as the first implies that all the clones positive for the three idiotopes are identical whereas the second allows the existence of different clonotypes. These results also have some implications for our general understanding of network interactions. For several years the existence of idiotope-positive immunoglobulins without detectable antibody function has prompted considerable speculation. The antibody response of animals immunized with anti-idiotypic antibodies (Ab3 animals) has been particularly intriguing.[2,12,20,22,24–29] These responses can be characterized by antibodies idiotypically similar to Ab1, but they may not recognize the antigen originally used in the cascade. These molecules have been termed Ab3 and the current interpretation is that they recognize V-region determinants on Ab2 immunoglobulins. Although our data cannot completely exclude this interpretation, we would like to propose that the difference between Ab1 and Ab3α[30] antibodies might simply reside in the number of common V-region determinants they share which, as shown here, may greatly influence the antigen-binding site.

   Finally, we would like to conclude this section on a more practical note. As our experiments were designed to have less than one clone positive for each idiotope in each culture, we can formally exclude the presence of idiotope-induced antibodies (Ab3α)[30] in those cultures simultaneously reacting with three idiotopes and antigen. Thus, our approach could represent a useful tool for studying the directions of immunoglobulin interactions.

4. Selection of the Idiotypic Repertoire

It has by now been clearly demonstrated that a large number of B lymphocytes are constantly generated in the bone marrow and emigrate into the peripheral immune system where they either die or become members of the repertoire of the adult animal. This enormously high cell turnover raises the questions of how, when, and by which mechanism long-lived B cells are selected from the pool of continuously produced lymphocytes. The answers to these questions clearly require an analysis at the clonal level and we therefore approached these problems by following the B-cell precursor frequency of clones capable of interacting with the anti-M460 monoclonal idiotype, F6(51), in various B-cell populations. We chose the M460 system because, besides being well characterized, this idiotype is apparently equally distributed among mitogen-reactive B cells,[6] and therefore the results of the analysis of the M460-positive clonotypes induced by LPS can reasonably be extrapolated to the whole repertoire.

Previous studies have shown that the M460 idiotype can only be detected in the serum of mice possessing the Igh^a haplotype following immunization against dinitrophenylated antigens.[12] These conclusions, however, have recently been clouded by reports describing the detection of this idiotype as well as others in every strain of mice provided that T cells were removed,[31–35] therefore implying that regulatory mechanisms acting in the peripheral immune system play important roles in the selection of the B-cell receptor repertoire.[36–45] To obtain a more complete answer to this important issue we studied the frequency of precursors of clones reacting with F6(51) in various strains of mice. Fig. 3 collectively shows the results of this analysis. Two types of regression lines can be distinguished. The first is obtained with cells from all mice with the Igh^a allotypic haplotype (BALB/c, 129, B.C8) while the second is constantly observed when the cells of mice expressing different haplotypes are used. Thus, the frequencies of idiotope-positive precursor cells are in general agreement with the allotypic restriction of idiotype expression usually found in serum antibodies after anti-DNP immunizations.

We have to point out that our system does not allow us to discriminate between those clones which recognize the F6(51) antibodies from those that are recognized by it. As we found that the frequency of F6(51)-reacting clones is strictly restricted by the haplotype of the mice used, these results suggest either that we indeed detected only the former strain of molecules or that the expression of Ab3 molecules is submitted to the same genetic rules as epitope-induced immunoglobulins. This is one important issue that clearly deserves to be studied further.

The network hypothesis raises the possibility that the fate of newly arisen B cells might be determined by idiotypic interactions in the immune system into which these new lymphocytes migrate.[46–49] The repertoire of V regions expressed in newly arising B cells might therefore be considerably different from the repertoire expressed in the B-cell population after contact with the surrounding immune system. To test the veracity of this hypothesis we carried out limiting dilution analysis of F6(51)-binding cells using Ig⁻ bone marrow cells of BALB/c and DBA/2 animals. As can be seen in Fig. 4 the frequencies of F6(51)-reacting clones in bone marrow cells of DBA/2 and BALB/c mice maturing in cultures are very similar to those obtained with splenocytes. Similar results have also been independently obtained by Nishikawa et al.[50] We have to conclude, therefore, that LPS-reactive B cells reacting with F6(51) are neither positively nor negatively selected as they

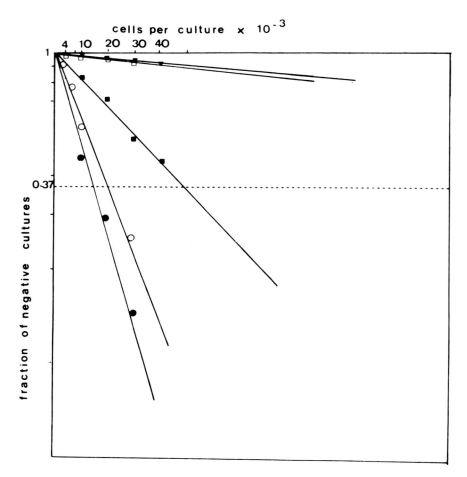

FIGURE 3. Spleen cells from (▼) DBA/2, (□) C57BL/6, (■) BALB/c, (○) 129, and (●) B.C8 were treated with anti-Thy-1.2 antibodies and complement and cultured at the indicated concentrations with 50 μg/ml of LPS. Results represent groups of 96 replicates tested for the presence of F6(51)-binding immunoglobulins in the supernatants after 12 days of culture. (From Ref. 8)

emerge from the bone marrow and migrate to the periphery in normal animals. Serological studies, however, have repeatedly shown that DBA/2 mice, which normally do not express the M460 idiotype, become capable of producing this molecule after anti-idiotypic immunization (reviewed in Ref. 35). The analysis of the F6(51)-binding clonotypes of splenocytes and bone marrow cells from F6(51)-immunized DBA/2 animals shown in Fig. 5 is consistent with these findings, as we found a highly significant increase in the frequency of these clones in spleen cells of such immunized animals. The most surprising result, however, was the significantly higher number of F6(51)-binding precursor cells observed in the Ig⁻ bone marrow cell population of these mice as compared to that obtained in the same population of untreated DBA/2 animals. Since we have previously excluded the possibility that these results could be due to recirculating memory cells,[8] our data imply either that

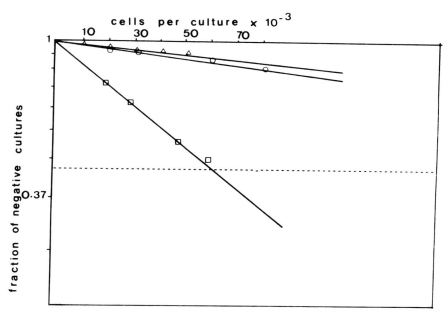

FIGURE 4. Spleen cells from (○) DBA/2 and the Ig⁻ population of the bone marrow from (△) DBA/2 or (□) BALB/c mice were treated with anti-Thy-1.2 and complement and cultured at the indicated concentrations in the presence of 50 μg/ml of LPS. The frequency determinations were carried out as described in Fig. 3. (From Ref. 8)

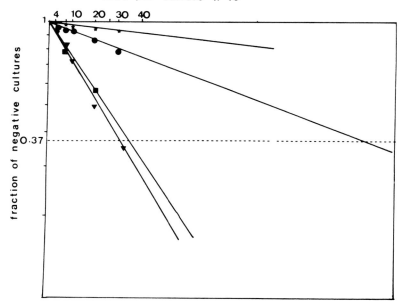

FIGURE 5. The frequencies of M460-positive splenocytes from F6(51)-treated DBA/2 which have been cultured in the absence (*) or in the presence (●) of 50 μg/ml of LPS were compared to those of Ig⁻ bone marrow cells cultured in the absence (■) or in the presence (▼) of LPS. The frequency analysis assay was carried out as described in Fig. 3. (From Ref. 8)

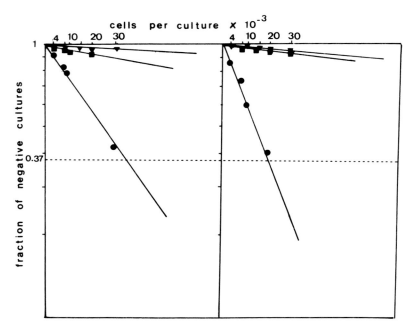

FIGURE 6. Frequency analysis of LPS-sensitive positive B splenocytes of C57BL/6 (▼) and BALB/c (●) nude mice as well as of C57BL/6 (■) normal animals carried out as described in Fig. 3. (From Ref. 8)

active immunization can profoundly alter the repertoire of idiotype-positive clonotypes, even at a very early stage of differentiation, or that our results are due to contaminant Ig$^+$ cells which escaped our cell purification.

The results presented so far indicate that the V-region repertoire expressed in peripheral B cells is similar if not identical to the repertoire of pre-B cells generated in the absence of any regulatory mechanism. However, bone marrow cultures may contain immature T cells which might differentiate *in vitro* and play a role in B-cell selection. To exclude this possibility and to obtain further information on the role played by T cells in clonotype selection, we determined the frequencies of F6(51)-binding B cells in the spleens of *Igh^a* and *Igh^b* athymic nude mice. As shown in Fig. 6, anti-Thy-1.2 and C' treated spleen cells from athymic nude mice with a BALB/c background contained 1–3 × 10^4 B-cell precursors of clones secreting F6(51)-binding immunoglobulin. In the spleen of *Igh^b* animals, however, the frequency of the same clonotype was too low to be determined. These results therefore seem to exclude conclusively a determinant T-cell role, not only in the maintenance but also in the establishment of the B-cell receptor repertoire.

5. The Maternal Influence on the B-Cell Repertoire Expression of the Progeny

As described in the preceding section, active anti-anti-idiotypic immunization can result in the profound alteration of the expression of the idiotypic repertoire apparently detectable already in bone marrow cells. This observation raises the possibility that the passive administration of preformed antibodies during the fetal life of an animal might similarly result in the expression of normally silent clones. This possibility seems very realistic since we often observed that the progeny of DBA/2 mothers which have been actively immunized during the gestation time with F6(51) anti-idiotypic antibodies contained high levels of F6(51)-binding molecules in their sera. To better understand this phenomenon and to better characterize the role played by the maternal environment in the selection of the idiotypic repertoire, we determined the frequencies of F6(51)-complementary clonotypes in the spleen and in the bone marrow of DBA/2 animals born from mothers actively immunized with F6(51) antibodies (Table III). It should be stressed that both the mothers and the progeny used in these experiments contained high levels of F6(51)-binding molecules in their sera. Surprisingly, however, the frequency of clonotypes reacting with the anti-idiotypic monoclonal antibodies in these animals was never, at any time tested, found to differ from that of mice born from nonimmunized mothers. Thus, passive immunization during fetal life does not seem to influence the recruitment of clonotypes in the peripheral immune system. It could be argued, however, that our results are due to the fact that in these experiments, the maternal environment was not permissive for the idiotype expression; therefore, we studied the question whether mice with the wrong haplotype (Igh^b) born from mothers with the permissive one (Igh^a) could indeed synthesize F6(51)-binding antibodies. Thus, BALB/c females were hyperimmunized with F6(51) antibodies and rendered pseudopregnant. C57BL/6 embryos at the blastocyst stage were then implanted in the uterus of these females and the progeny born from the implanted mothers tested for the frequency of F6(51)-binding cells. As shown in Table IV, the frequency of F6(51)-binding clones in the spleen of C57BL/6 mice born from BALB/c animals was essentially similar to that of normal C57BL/6 animals, i.e., too low to be detected.

Taken collectively, these results conclusively show that the maternal environment does not affect the generation of LPS-reactive cells and leaves the frequency of cells recognizing F6(51) untouched. These results contrast with previous observations demonstrating that

TABLE III

Influence of Maternal Antibodies on the Idiotypic Repertoire of the Progeny

Expt.	Mice	No.	Mother	Age	HA titer $\log_2$ in the sera with F6(51) SRBC	Frequency of F6(51)-binding cells in	
						Splenocytes	Bone marrow
1	DBA/2	1	Ab3[a]	3 weeks	> 12	ND[b]	—[c]
		2			> 12	ND	—
		3			> 12	ND	—
		4			> 12	ND	—
	BALB/c	5	Normal	4 weeks	0	$1/5.7 \times 10^4$	—
2	DBA/2	1	Ab3	6 weeks	2	ND	ND
		2			1	ND	ND
		3			4	ND	ND
	BALB/c	4	Normal		0	$1/3 \times 10^4$	$1/2.5 \times 10^4$

[a]Hyperimmunized with F6(51)-KLH.
[b]ND, not detectable.
[c]Not done.

TABLE IV
Influence of the Maternal Environment on the Idiotypic Repertoire of the Progeny

Mice	No.	Mother	Age	HA titer log$_2$ with F6(51) SRBC	Frequency of F6(51)-binding splenocytes
C57BL/6	1	Ab3^a BALB/c	3weeks	> 16	ND^b
	2			> 16	ND
	3			> 16	ND
BALB/c	4	Normal BALB/c	4weeks	0	$1/2.7 \times 10^4$
C57BL/6	5	Normal C57BL/6	4weeks	0	ND
BALB/c	6	Ab3 BALB/c	6weeks	> 12	$1/2 \times 10^4$

^{a}Hyperimmunized with F6(51)-KLH.
^{b}ND, not detectable.

the frequency of M460 idiotype-positive clones of the progeny of Ab2 mothers was lower as compared to normal animals.[5] One possible explanation for our negative results is that anti-idiotypic immunization results in the synthesis of both Ab1-like molecules and Ab3 antibodies and that these two immunoglobulin populations may have compensatory effects.

6. Conclusions

In this chapter we have summarized results concerning the B-cell repertoire obtained by the limiting dilution analysis of mitogen-reactive B cells. Although this methodology has the advantage of not being dependent on a particular protocol of immunization it is also based on the assumption that the V gene repertoire is randomly expressed among mitogen-reactive B-cell subsets. Our results have clearly demonstrated that this assumption is only valid for certain specificities while for others it appears that a preferential expression exists on certain B-cell subpopulations. The reason for this nonrandom distribution of specificities among mitogen-reactive B-cell subsets remains unclear at the present time; however, our findings should caution not only against considering the repertoire of mitogen-reactive B-cell subpopulations as completely representative for that of the entire B-cell pool, but they should also be taken into consideration when interpreting data obtained with conventional TD antigens.

The frequency analysis of F6(51)-binding precursor B cells led us to the possibility of studying the contribution of different idiotopes to the antigen-binding site of an antibody. These studies revealed that, although individual idiotopes can hardly be considered as clonal markers, a perfect correlation exists between the simultaneous expression of these three V-region determinants and β-galactosidase activity. At the present time we do not know whether this is a general phenomenon or is peculiar to our antibodies; however, our approach should facilitate the study of the relationship between epitopes and idiotopes in several other systems.

We especially devoted our attention to understanding the mechanism by which the receptor repertoire expressed in B cells is selected in the mature immune system. First, we asked the question whether the allotype linkage of idiotype expression is merely based on genetic constraints or whether regulatory mechanisms may also interfere. This question is particularly interesting as numerous conflicting reports on the available and potential idiotypic repertoire exist (reviewed in Ref. 51). We found allotypic restriction of idiotype expression not only at the B-cell precursor level in splenocytes but also when limiting dilution analyses were carried out using Ig⁻ bone marrow cells. In addition to this, the receptor repertoire of B cells generated from bone marrow pre-B cells *in vitro* was always found to be identical to the repertoire expressed in the B-cell population in the spleen of adult animals. As it is reasonable to assume that the receptor repertoire appearing *in vitro* reflects the set of antibody variable regions generated by *VDJ* recombination,[52] we must conclude that regulatory mechanisms acting at the periphery of the immune system do not play a fundamental role in the expression of the V-region repertoire. This conclusion is further substantiated by our experiments showing that the frequencies of F6(51) precursor B cells in the spleen of athymic nude mice were not basically different from those of normal animals.

Several published reports indicate the dramatic effect of the administration of anti-idiotypic antibodies in newborn animals or of the maternal environment on the receptor repertoire of the progeny B cells.[53–60] This evidence has lent support to the network hypothesis which suggests the possibility that the set of antibody variable regions present in the immune system into which newly arising B cells enter, will, through idiotypic interaction, determine whether a given B cell will multiply and become a component of the mature immune system or not.[46,47] Indeed, we constantly observed that mice born from anti-anti-idiotype-hyperimmunized mothers contained high levels of serum antibodies capable of reacting with the molecule used for maternal immunization. The analysis of the frequency of F6(51)-binding cells of animals born from Ab3 mothers, however, revealed that these mice have a number of clonotypes not sensibly different from mice born from normal untreated mothers. Thus, the high level of serum antibody detected in the progeny of immunized females is most likely due to passive maternal–fetal transmission of these molecules rather than to profound alteration of the idiotypic repertoire.

In conclusion, our results indicate that positive selection of the B-cell receptor repertoire does not occur during the migration of pre-B cells from the bone marrow to the periphery. More generally, our data, taken collectively, suggest that the receptor repertoire observed in adult animals reflects mainly the set of antibody variable regions generated by random combination of *V, D,* and *J* genes as they occur during early differentiation and that peripheral and external regulatory mechanisms do not seem to play a determinant role in the establishment of the idiotypic repertoire.

The impossibility of studying the B-cell repertoire in toto leads us to be cautious concerning the interpretation of our experiments, as they concern solely the LPS-reactive B-cell set. Whether this set functionally represents the pool of long-lived lymphocytes selected into the network of the functional immune system remains to be established.

ACKNOWLEDGMENT. We thank Dr. Charles Babinet for helping with the embryo transfer experiments.

References

1. Urbain, J., Wikler, M., Franssen, J. D., and Collignon, C., 1977, Idiotypic regulation of the immune system by the induction of antibodies against anti-idiotypic antibodies, *Proc. Natl. Acad. Sci. USA* **74**:5126–5130.

2. Cazenave, P.-A., 1977, Idiotypic–anti-idiotypic regulation of antibody synthesis in rabbits, *Proc. Natl. Acad. Sci. USA* **74:**5122–5125.

3. Anderson, J., Coutinho, A., and Melchers, F., 1977, Frequencies of mitogen-reactive B cells in the mouse. I. Distribution in different lymphoid organs from different inbred strains of mice at different ages, *J. Exp. Med.* **145:**1511–1519.

4. Anderson, J., Coutinho, A., and Melchers, F., 1977, Frequencies of mitogen-reactive B cells in the mouse. II. Frequencies of B cells producing antibodies which lyse sheep or horse erythrocytes, and trinitrophe nylated or nitroiodophenylated sheep erythrocytes, *J. Exp. Med.* **145:**1520–1530.

5. Barnabé, R. R., Coutinho, A., Martinez, C., and Cazenave, P.-A., 1981, Immune networks: Frequencies of antibody and idiotype producing B cell clones in various steady states, *J. Exp. Med.* **154:**552.

6. Primi, D., Mami, F., Le Guern, C., and Cazenave, P.-A., 1982, Mitogens-reactive B cell subpopulations selectively express different sets of V regions, *J. Exp. Med.* **156:**181.

7. Primi, D., Mami, F., Le Guern, C., and Cazenave, P.-A., 1982, The relationship between variable region determinants and antigen specificity on mitogen reactive B cell subsets, *J. Exp. Med.* **156:**924.

8. Juy, D., Primi, D., Sanchez, P., and Cazenave, P.-A., 1983, The selection and the maintenance of the V-region determinant repertoire is germ-line encoded and T cell independent, *Eur. J. Immunol.* **13:**326–331.

9. Gronowicz, E., and Coutinho, A., 1975, Functional analysis of B cell heterogeneity, *Transplant. Rev.* **24:**3.

10. Möller, G., 1976. The V gene repertoire as revealed by polyclonal B cell activators, *Ann. Immunol. (Paris)* **127C:**449.

11. Bona, C., Yano, A., Dimitriu, A., and Miller, R. G., 1978, Mitogenic analysis of murine B cell heterogeneity, *J. Exp. Med.* **148:**136.

12. Le Guern, C., Ben Aïssa, D., Juy, D., Mariamé, B., Buttin, G., and Cazenave, P.-A., 1979, Expression and induction of MOPC-460 idiotypes in different strains of mice, *Ann. Immunol. (Paris)* **30:**293.

13. Oudin, J., and Cazenave, P.-A., 1971, Similar idiotypic specificities in immunoglobulin fractions with different antibody functions or even without detectable antibody function, *Proc. Natl. Acad. Sci. USA* **68:**2616–2620.

14. Enghofer, E. M., Glaudemans, C. P. J., and Bosma, M. J., 1979, Immunoglobulins with different specificities have similar idiotypes, *Mol. Immunol.* **16:**1103–1110.

15. Hiernaux, J., and Bona, C. A., 1982, Shared idiotypes among monoclonal antibodies specific for different immuno dominant sugars of lipopolysaccharide of different gram-negative bacteria, *Proc. Natl. Acad. Sci. USA* **79:**1616–1620.

16. Ju, S.-T., Benacerraf, B., and Dorf, M. E., 1980, Genetic control of shared idiotype among antibodies directed to distinct specificities, *J. Exp. Med.* **152:**170–182.

17. Karol, R., Reichlin, M., and Noble, R. W., 1978, Idiotypic cross-reactivity between antibodies of different specificities, *J. Exp. Med.* **148:**1488–1497.

18. Kohno, Y., Boskower, I., Buckommayer, G., Minna, J. A., and Berzofsky, J. A., 1981, Shared among monoclonal antibodies to distinct determinants of sperm whole myoglobin, *J. Supramol. Struct. Cell. Biochem.* **5:**36.

19. Metzger, D. W., Miller, A., and Sercarz, K. M., 1980, Sharing of an idiotypic marker by monoclonal antibodies specific for distinct regions of hen lysozyme, *Nature* **287:**540–542.

20. Rajewsky, K., Reth, M., Takomori, T., and Kelsoe, G., 1981, A glimpse into the inner life of the immune system, in: *The Immune System,* Volume 2 (C. H. Steinberg, and I. Lefkovitz, eds.), Karger, Basel, pp. 1–11.

21. Takomori, T., Tesch, N., Reth, M., and Rajewsky, K., 1982, The immune response against anti-idiotype antibodies. Induction of idiotope-bearing antibodies and analysis of the idiotope repertoire, *Euro. J. Immunol.* **12:**1040–1046.

22. Wikler, M., Franssen, J.-D., Collignon, C., Leo, O., Mariamé, B., van de Walle, P., de Groote, D., and Urbain, J., 1979, Idiotypic regulation of the immune system: Common idiotypic specificities between idiotypes and antibodies raised against anti-idiotypic antibodies in rabbits, *J. Exp. Med.* **150:**184–195.

23. Wyaucki, I. J., and Sato, V.L., 1981, The strain A anti-fazophenylarsonate major crossreactive idiotypic family includes members with no reactivity toward *p*-azophenylarsonate, *Eur. J. Immunol.* **11:**832–839.

24. Dzierzak, E. A., and Janeway, C. A., Jr., 1981, Expression of an idiotype (Id-460) during in vivo antidinitrophenyl antibody responses. III. Detection of Id-460 in normal serum that does not bind dinitrophenyl, *J. Exp. Med.* **154:**1442–1454.

25. Bluestone, J. A., Epstein, S. L., Ozato, K., Sharrow, S. O., and Sachs, D., 1981, Anti-idiotypes to mono-

clonal anti-H-2 antibodies. II. Expression of anti-H-2^k idiotypes on antibodies induced by antiidiotype or H-2^k antigen, *J. Exp. Med.* **154**:1305–1318.

26. Bluestone, J. A., Krutzach, H. C., Auchincloss, H., Cazenave, P.-A., Kindt, T. J., and Sachs, D. H., 1982, Anti-idiotypes against anti-H-2 monoclonal antibodies: Structural analysis of the molecules induced by in vitro anti-idiotype treatment, *Proc. Natl. Acad. Sci. USA* **79**:7847–7851.

27. Bluestone, J. A., Metzger, J.-J., Knodo, M. C., Ozato, K., and Sachs, D. N., 1982, Anti-idiotypes to monoclonal anti-H-2 antibodies. I. Contribution of isolated heavy and light chains to idiotype expression, *Mol. Immunol.* **19**:515–524.

28. Leo, O., Slaoui, M., Mariamé, B., and Urbain, J., 1981, Internal images in the immune network, *J. Supramol. Struct. Cell. Biochem. Suppl.* **5**:84.

29. Rajewsky, K., Takemori, T., and Reth, M., 1981, Analysis and regulation of V gene expression by monoclonal antibodies, in: *Monoclonal Antibody and T. Cell Hybridoma: Perspective and Technical Advances* (G. J. Hämmerling, U. Hämmerling, and J. F. Kearney, eds.), Elsevier/North-Holland, Amsterdam, pp. 399–409.

30. Jerne, N. K., Roland, J., and Cazenave, P.-A., 1982, Recurrent idiotopes and internal images, *EMBO J.* **1**:243.

31. Benacerraf, B., 1980, Genetic control of the specificity of T lymphocytes and their regulatory products, in: *Progress in Immunology: Immunology 80,* Volume 4 (M. Fougereau and J. Dausset, eds.), Academic Press, New York, pp. 419–431.

32. Germain, R. N., Sy, S.-M., Rock, K., Dietz, M. H., Greene, M. I., Nisonoff, A., Weinberger, J. T., Ju, S.-T., Dorf, M. E., and Benacerraf, B., 1981, The role of idiotype and the MHC in suppressor T cell pathways, in: *Immunoglobulin Idiotypes: ICN–UCLA Symposia on Molecular and Cellular Biology,* Volume 20 (C. A. Janeway, Jr., E. K. Sercarz, and H. Wigzell, eds.), Academic Press, New York, pp. 709–723.

33. Bona, C., and Paul, W. E., 1979, Cellular basis of regulation of expression of idiotype. I. T-suppressor cells specific for MOPC 460 idiotype regulate the expression of cells secreting anti-TNP antibodies bearing 460 idiotype, *J. Exp. Med.* **149**:592–600.

34. Juy, D., Primi, D., Sanchez, P., and Cazenave, P.-A., 1982, Idiotype regulation: Evidence for the involvement of Igh-C-restricted T cells in the M-460 idiotype suppression pathway, *Eur. J. Immunol.* **12**:24–30.

35. Urbain, J., Wuilmart, C., and Cazenave, P.-A., 1981, Idiotypic regulation in immune networks, in: *Contemporary Topics in Molecular Immunology,* Vol. 8 (F. P. Inwan and W. J. Mandy, eds.), Plenum Press, New York, pp. 113–148.

36. Greene, M. T., Nelles, M. J., Sy, M.-S., and Nisonoff, A., 1982, Regulation of immunity to the azobenzenarsonate hapten, *Adv. Immunol.* **32**:253–300.

37. Janeway, C. A., Jr., Broughton, B., Dzierzak, E., Jones, B., Eardley, D. D., Durum, S., Yamauchi, K., Green, D. R., and Gershon, R. K., 1981, Studies of T lymphocyte function in B-cell deprived mice, in: *Immunoglobulin Idiotypes: ICN–UCLA Symposia on Molecular and Cellular Biology,* Volume 20 (C. A. Janeway, Jr., E. K. Sercarz, and H. Wigzell, eds.), Academic Press, New York, pp. 661–671.

38. Sercarz, E. K., and Metzger, D. W., 1980, Epitope-specific and idiotype specific cellular interactions in a model protein antigen system, *Springer Semin. Immunopathol.* **3**:145–170.

39. Tada, T., Okumura, K., Hoyakawa, K., Suzuki, G, Abo, R., and Kumagai, Y., 1981, Immunological circuitry governed by MHC and V$_H$ gene products, in: *Immunoglobulin Idiotypes: ICN–UCLA Symposia on Molecular and Cellular Biology,* Volume 20 (C. A. Janeway, Jr., E. K. Sercarz, and H. Wigzell, eds.), Academic Press, New York, pp. 563–572.

40. Rubinstein, E. J., Yeh, M., and Bona, C. A., 1982, Idiotype–anti-idiotype network. II. Activation of silent clones by treatment at birth with idiotypes is associated with the expansion of idiotype-specific helper T cells, J. *Exp. Med.* **156**:506–521.

41. Adorini, L., Harvey, M., and Sercarz, E.K., 1979, The fine specificity of regulatory T cells. IV. Idiotypic complementary and antigen-bridging interactions in the anti-lysozyme response, *Eur. J. Immunol.* **9**:906–909.

42. Bottomly, K., Janeway, C. A., Jr., Mathieson, P. J., and Mosier, D. E., 1980, Absence of an antigen-specific helper T cell required for the expression of the T 15 idiotype in mice treatment with anti-antibody, *Eur. J. Immunol.* **10**:159–163.

43. Cerny, J., and Caulfield, M. J., 1981, Modulation of specific antibody-forming cells in antigen-primed nude mice by the adaptive transfer of syngeneic anti-idiotypic T cells, *J. Immunol.* **126**:2262–2266.

44. Hetzelberger, D., and Eichmann, K., 1978, Recognition of idiotypes in lymphocyte interactions. I. Idiotypes selectivity in the cooperation between T and B lymphocytes, *Eur. J. Immunol.* **8**:846–852.

45. Woodland, R., and Cantor, N., 1978, Idiotype-specific T helper cells are required to induce idiotype-positive B memory cells to secrete antibody, *Eur. J. Immunol.* **8**:600–608.

46. Jerne, N. K., 1974, Towards a network theory of the immune system, *Ann. Immunol. (Paris)* **125C**:373–389.

47. Jerne, N.K., 1975, The immune system: A web of V domains, *Harvey Lect.* **70**:93–110.

48. Jerne, N. K., 1976, The immune system: A network of lymphocyte interactions, in: *The Immune System,* (F. Helcheb and K. Rajewsky, eds.), Springer-Verlag, Berlin, pp. 259–266.

49. Jerne, N. K., 1982, in: *Idiotypes: Antigens on the Inside* (I. Westen-Schnurr, ed.), Editiones Roche, Basel, pp. 12–15.

50. Nishikawa, S., Takemori, T., and Rajewsky, K., 1983, The expression of a set of antibody variable regions in LPS reactive B cells at various stages of ontogeny and its control by anti-idiotypic antibody, *Eur. J. Immunol* **13**:318–325.

51. Rajewsky, K., and Takemori, T., 1983, Genetic expression and function of idiotypes, *Annu. Rev. Immunol.* **1:** 1–18.

52. Sakano, H., Maki, R., Kurosawa, Y., Roder, W., and Tonegawa, S., 1980, Two types of somatic recombination are necessary for the generation of complete immunoglobulin heavy-chain genes, *Nature* **236**:676.

53. Accolla, R. S., Geschart, P. J., Signal, N. B., Cancro, M. P., and Klinman, N. R., 1977, Idiotype-specific monoclonal suppression of phosphorylcholine-responsive B cells, *Eur. J. Immunol.* **7**:876–881.

54. Augustin, A., and Cosenza, N., 1976, Expression of new idiotypes following neonatal idiotypic suppression of a dominant clone, *Eur. J. Immunol.* **6**:497–501.

55. Fung, J., and Köhler, N., 1980, Mechanism of neonatal idiotype suppression. II. Alterations in the T cell compartment suppress the maturation of B cell precursors, *J. Immunol.* **125**:2489–2495.

56. Hiernaux, J., Bona, C., and Baker, P. J., 1981, Neonatal treatment with low doses of anti-idiotypic antibody leads to the expression of a silent clone, *J. Exp. Med.* **153**:1004–1008.

57. Kearney, J. F., Barletta, R., Quen, Z. S., and Quintans, J., 1981, Monoclonal vs heterogeneous anti-H-8 antibodies in the analysis of the anti-phosphorylcholine response in BALB/c mice, *Eur. J. Immunol.* **11**:877–883.

58. Kim, B. S., and Hopkins, W. J., 1978, Tolerance rendered by neonatal treatment with anti-idiotypic antibodies. Induction and maintenance in athymic mice, *Cell. Immunol.* **35**:460–465.

59. Köhler, N., Kaplan, D. R., and Strayer, D. S., 1974, Clonal depletion in neonatal tolerance, *Science* **186**:643–644.

60. Wuller, I. J., Wuller, R., Springer, N., and Cosenza, N., 1977, Idiotype suppression by maternal influence, *Eur. J. Immunol.* **7**:591–597.

12

Antibody Diversity in the Response to Streptococcal Group A Carbohydrate

R. Jerrold Fulton, Moon H. Nahm, Neil S. Greenspan, and Joseph M. Davie

1. Introduction

In the past several years, a number of laboratories have used the murine antibody response to streptococcal group A carbohydrate (GAC) as a model system in which to study the development and regulation of humoral immunity. This system displays a number of features which are common to other antigen–antibody systems as well as unique features which make it particularly suitable to the study of antibody diversity. The scope of this chapter is to review the major characteristics of this antibody response and to discuss in more detail recent experiments from our laboratory which have exploited the anti-GAC response to ask questions concerning the rules which govern the pairing of heavy- and light-chain variable regions in the generation of antibody diversity. As with most other antibody systems which have been examined in detail, it has become increasingly apparent that the antibody response to GAC is assembled from a restricted set of heavy- and light-chain variable regions and constant regions. These observations have raised questions about the extent to which combinatorial diversity functions within the immune system and suggest the possibility that coordinated regulation results in the expression of V_L, V_H, and C_H gene products in restricted sets, irrespective of the constraints imposed by an antigen-specific system.

R. Jerrold Fulton, Moon H. Nahm, Neil S. Greenspan, and Jospeh M. Davie • Departments of Microbiology and Immunology and of Pathology, Washington University School of Medicine, St. Louis, Missouri 63110. *Present address for R. J. F.:* Department of Microbiology, University of Texas Health Science Center, Dallas, Texas 75235.

2. General Characteristics

The majority of the serum antibody produced in response to heat-killed group A streptococcal vaccine is directed toward the relatively simple hapten N-acetyl-D-glucosamine.[1,2] As with most other antibody responses, the primary antibody response to GAC is composed largely of IgM antibodies.[3] Hyperimmunization of mice with GAC vaccine leads to the production of high levels (> 10 mg/ml) of IgG antibodies depending on the mouse strain employed.[3,4] One of the most interesting features of the anti-GAC response, which is also common to other anticarbohydrate responses, is that virtually all of the IgG antibody is of the murine IgG3 subclass.[5–8] Light chains employed in the anti-GAC response are largely of the κ type.[5,9] Of over 50 monoclonal anti-GAC antibodies which have been examined in our laboratory, all are either IgM or IgG3 and only four contain λ light chains. Thus, diversity of 7 S antibodies and their constituent heavy and light chains can be assumed to be almost totally derived from variable-region differences. The antibody response to GAC has been shown to be thymus-dependent.[10,11] Environmental stimulation of the GAC response is virtually nonexistent in normal mice such that anti-GAC antibodies are undetectable in preimmune sera.[4,12] *In toto,* the characteristics discussed above indicate that the murine antibody response to GAC represents a fairly typical humoral immune response.

3. Diversity of Anti-GAC Antibodies

The antibody systems which have contributed most to our understanding of antibody diversity are those which display restricted heterogeneity among serum antibodies. A/J and BALB/cJ mice respond to GAC with serum antibodies of restricted electrophoretic mobility.[4,13] Spleen cells of one A/J mouse were cloned into irradiated recipients yielding the monoclonal antibody A5A which was subsequently used to produce anti-idiotypic antisera.[13] These anti-idiotypes, produced both in syngeneic mice and in guinea pigs, were shown to cross-react to varying degrees with anti-GAC antibodies from all A/J mice which were tested, but not with anti-GAC sera from several other inbred mouse strains.[13,14] Only strains DBA/2J and C57L/J produced significant amounts of antibodies which cross-reacted with anti-A5A sera.[14] Strain-specific idiotypes were also described in BALB/c and in SWR mice.[15,16] These studies provided strong evidence that the variable-region (V) genes encoding these antibodies were present in the germ line and were stably inherited. Particularly in the case of A/J mice, these studies gave the impression that virtually all members of the strain responded to GAC with a predominant antibody clonotype which was identical or very similar to antibody A5A. More recent studies have not supported this concept of the A/J anti-GAC response. Whereas the majority of A/J mice respond to GAC with a restricted set of serum antibodies [4,13] and antibody-forming cells,[3] there does not appear to be a single predominant clonotype which is shared by all A/J mice.[4,9,17] Cramer and Braun[4] observed restricted antibody responses in most BALB/c mice and approximately half of the A/J mice tested by isoelectric focusing (IEF) analysis of the serum antibody spectrotypes. Though these authors did observe A/J anti-GAC antibodies analogous to A5A, they made note of the "considerable pool size" of A/J anti-GAC antibodies. Similar analyses by Perlmutter *et al.*[17,18] and by Nahm *et al.*[9] have confirmed the fact that most A/J mice respond to GAC with a restricted set of serum antibodies and also emphasized the lack of a single predominant clonotype which is shared among individual mice. These characteristics of the A/J anti-GAC response were further corroborated by the production of monoclonal anti-GAC antibodies.[9] Nahm et al. compared the IEF spectrotypes of 17 monoclonal anti-GAC antibodies derived from six A/J mice. All of these antibodies displayed distinct IEF spectrotypes. Little, if any, of this diversity could be attributed to constant-region differences since all of the antibodies were IgG3,κ. Baked on a comparison of IEF spectrotypes of anti-GAC antibodies from A/J sera, Briles and Carroll[19] have estimated that the A/J strain is capable of producing approximately 200 different antibody clonotypes in response to GAC. Thus, the serum antibody response of A/J mice is somewhat unusual in that the response of individual mice is fairly restricted while the repertoire of the strain is quite diverse.

It is important to note that while IEF analysis suggests that significant diversity of anti-GAC antibodies exists in most strains of mice, it is not clear what this means in terms of V-region genes. In other words, is the diversity observed within a strain due to the usage of multiple heavy- and light-chain variable-region genes or simply a result of somatic mutation of a single, or very small number of V_H–V_L pairs? In this sense, the idiotypic analysis employed by Eichmann may provide a better indication of the similarity of antibodies or the genes which encode their V regions.

4. Diversity of Light Chains in Anti-GAC Antibodies

In an effort to further analyze the antibody diversity observed among anti-GAC antibodies, Perlmutter et al.[17] separated serum antibodies from SWR mice into their constituent heavy and light chains and subjected the light chains to IEF spectrotype analysis. These studies demonstrated that IgM and IgG anti-GAC antibodies expressed virtually identical sets of light chains as determined by IEF spectrotypes. This result is interesting in terms of the increased frequency of somatic mutation which has recently been observed in IgG as compared to IgM heavy-chain variable regions in other systems.[20,21] It is not clear whether these results indicate that light chains are not subject to the same somatic mutational mechanisms as heavy chains or simply that these mechanisms do not operate to the same extent in the anti-GAC antibodies as in antiphosphocholine antibodies. An unexpected result which derived from this study was the observation that a large number of SWR anti-GAC sera which displayed distinct IEF spectrotypes for intact antibodies displayed sharing of light-chain spectrotypes.[17]

Further examination of this phenomenon revealed that in spite of the apparent heterogeneity of 7 S antibodies observed among individual A/J mice, approximately half of the serum antibodies from most A/J mice contained κ light chains with an identical IEF spectrotype which was similar to the predominant spectrotype observed in SWR mice.[18] Thus, a single κ light chain, or restricted set of κ light chains, is predominantly expressed in the anti-GAC antibodies produced by most individual A/J mice and most members of the strain. In contrast to many other antibody systems, the diversity of light chains within the anti-GAC response appeared to be far less than the diversity of heavy chains.

These studies were extended by Nahm et al.[9] by the production of monoclonal anti-GAC antibodies. Again, approximately half of the monoclonal antibodies produced from A/J mice shared a common κ light chain, as determined by IEF analysis, termed the

$V_{\kappa}1^{GAC}$ light chain. The similarity of these light chains was further established by the production of a V_{κ}-directed anti-idiotype. With one exception, idiotypic cross-reactivity was perfectly correlated with the presence of the predominant light-chain IEF spectrotype. The one exception, antibody HGAC 11, was idiotypically cross-reactive but displayed a distinct IEF spectrotype. Further, all of the monoclonal antibodies which expressed the $V_{\kappa}1^{GAC}$ IEF spectrotype were idiotypically cross-reactive. Amino acid sequence analysis of the NH_2-terminal 70 residues of the HGAC 11 light chain and three HGAC light chains which express the $V_{\kappa}1^{GAC}$ IEF spectrotype has demonstrated that HGAC 11 is approximately 97% homologous to the other light chains (M. Bond and L. Hood, unpublished data). Thus, IEF analysis, in this case, appears to be a more sensitive measure of structural differences than idiotypic analysis. Conversely, it would seem that idiotypic analysis represents a more sensitive assay for structural relatedness than IEF. These results emphasize the fact that idiotypic cross-reactivity should not be interpreted as structural identity; however, they also emphasize the lack of quantitation of structural differences obtained by gross comparative techniques such as IEF spectrotype analysis.

5. Diversity of Heavy Chains in Anti-GAC Antibodies

Less information is available concerning heavy-chain diversity within the anti-GAC response. Serologic data obtained with anti-A5A reagents are rather difficult to interpret with regard to variability among heavy and light chains as separate entities. While A5A determinants were shown to be controlled by genes linked to the heavy-chain constant-region *(IgCH)* locus,[14] this does not prove heavy-chain association of the idiotype. Heavy-chain loci have been shown to influence the expression of light chains and light-chain determinants both in the anti-GAC response[18] (and discussed below) and in the anti-inulin response.[22] Furthermore, the chain specificity of the anti-A5A reagents used in the characterization of A/J anti-GAC antibodies is not clear.[13,14] Some anti-A5A sera recognized primarily heavy-chain determinants while others recognized V_{κ} determinants.[23] Nevertheless, the data obtained with anti-A5A indicate that the majority of A/J anti-GAC antibodies share idiotypic determinants and probably represent a related family of V_H regions.

This conclusion is supported by recent studies performed in our laboratory. Basta *et al.*[24] have recently reported the production of an antiserum which appears to recognize specific determinants in the V_H region of the myeloma protein J606. In collaboration with these authors, we have examined the cross-reactivity of this antiserum with approximately 50 anti-GAC monoclonal antibodies (N. Greenspan, unpublished data). Only one of these antibodies failed to react with the anti-J606 V_H reagent, indicating that the large majority of A/J anti-GAC V_H regions share at least some structural features. The V_H gene of monoclonal antibody HGAC 9 has recently been cloned and sequenced, and was shown to exhibit greater than 95% homology at the DNA level to the J606 V_H gene (R. Perlmutter and L. Hood, unpublished data). In the latter study, it was also clear that the HGAC 9 V_H gene was distinct from the A/J homolog of the BALB/c-derived J606 gene. Thus, it is clear that serologic cross-reactivity does not necessarily indicate that distinct antibodies are derived from the same *V*-region genes. This conclusion is stated with the caveat that the anti-J606 V_H antiserum probably recognizes framework-associated determinants whereas the majority of anti-idiotypes which have been used as probes of V-region structure are specific for combining-site determinants.

Preliminary efforts in our laboratory to characterize the heavy chains of anti-GAC antibodies by IEF spectrotype analysis have provided some interesting but incomplete results. We have performed heavy-chain focusing on five monoclonal anti-GAC antibodies from A/J mice. All of these antibodies display distinct IEF spectrotypes for the intact molecules; four bear the $V_{\kappa}1^{GAC}$ light chain and the fifth bears a distinct light chain by both IEF and idiotypic analysis. The isolated heavy chains of all of these antibodies were found to comigrate in IEF gels. This result was unexpected since the IEF heterogeneity observed among the $V_{\kappa}1^{GAC}$-bearing antibodies was assumed to be contributed by the heavy chains. Thus, these $V_{\kappa}1^{GAC}$-bearing antibodies display IEF heterogeneity which cannot be attributed to either chain. One explanation of these results is that either the heavy or the light chains, or both, contain sufficient differences in uncharged amino acids to allow distinct secondary and/or tertiary structures which alter the net charge of the intact antibodies. In conclusion, there is insufficient information to allow any firm statements concerning the diversity of heavy-chain variable regions employed in anti-GAC antibody response of A/J mice; however, preliminary evidence indicates that heavy-chain diversity may be less than was presumed on the basis of IEF analysis.

6. IgCH-Linked Effects on the Expression of Anti-GAC Light Chains

The studies of light-chain diversity performed by Perlmutter *et al.*[17,18] revealed strain-associated differences both in the light-chain spectrotypes which were expressed and in the heterogeneity of light-chain spectrotypes which were expressed in individual mice and strains of mice. Using allotype-congenic strains, it was demonstrated that the heavy-chain allotype *(IgCH)* locus was responsible for these interstrain differences in anti-GAC light-chain expression.[18] In other words, inbred strains with identical light genotypes expressed different light-chain variable regions among anti-GAC antibodies depending on the presence of a particular *IgCH* locus. Whether these effects on light-chain expression were actually mediated by immunoglobulin heavy-chain constant-region genes or by *IgCH*-linked genes is not clear. The possibility that V_H genes were responsible for these effects was supported by the observation that BAB-14 mice, which contain a portion of the BALB/c V_H locus,[25] expressed anti-GAC light chains more like BALB/c than did CB-20 mice which contain C57BL/ka V_H genes exclusively. Expression of a light chain, V_{κ}-11, among anti-inulin antibodies was also found to be influenced by *IgCH*-linked genes.[22] In this case, V_{κ}-11 expression was determined serologically with an antiserum which appeared to require association with BALB/c-derived V_H-5 for the expression of V_{κ}-11-specific determinants. Thus, it is likely that the *IgCH*-linked effect on V_{κ}-11 expression was also V_H rather than C_H mediated.

We have reexamined this phenomenon using the $V_{\kappa}1^{GAC}$ idiotypes discussed above as a marker for the expression of this light chain among anti-GAC antibodies. Two anti-idiotypes directed toward the $V_{\kappa}1^{GAC}$ light chain, anti-Id5 and anti-Id20, were used in these studies. Both of these antisera recognize $V_{\kappa}1^{GAC}$ framework-associated determinants independently of association with heavy chains.[9,12] Screening of anti-GAC antisera from inbred mouse strains representing most of the known IgCH allotypes revealed three patterns of $V_{\kappa}1^{GAC}$ expression.[26] The majority of strains tested expressed both idiotypes in a manner analogous to A/J and BALB/c mice with minor quantitative differences observed in the proportion of idiotype-positive anti-GAC antibodies.[26] C57BL/6J mice, $IgCH^b$, produced anti-GAC antibodies with reduced levels of Id5 and virtually undetectable levels of Id20. CE/J mice, $IgCH^f$, did not express detectable levels of either idiotype. These results indicate that the majority of inbred mouse strains use $V_\kappa 1^{GAC}$-related light chains in the production of anti-GAC antibodies.

To determine whether the $IgCH$ locus was responsible for the altered pattern of $V_\kappa 1^{GAC}$ idiotype expression observed in C57BL/6 mice, recombinant inbred and allotype-congenic mice between BALB/c and C57BL/6 were tested for production of the $V_\kappa 1^{GAC}$ idiotypes. Examination of serum antibodies from BALB/c × C57BL/6 recombinant mice demonstrated that the pattern of idiotype expression did not correlate with heavy-chain allotype.[26] CXBH and CXBI mice, $IgCH^b$, expressed the BALB/c idiotype pattern whereas CXBG, $IgCH^a$, expressed the C57BL/6 pattern. Interestingly, all three patterns of $V_\kappa 1^{GAC}$ expression discussed above were observed in the panel of recombinants. This result suggests that the lack of $V_\kappa 1^{GAC}$ idiotype expression seen in CE/J mice may result from regulation rather than the lack of a functional structural gene analogous to $V_\kappa 1^{GAC}$. To examine this question further, serum antibodies from allotype-congenic mice were tested for idiotype expression.[26] CB.20 mice ($IgCH^b$ on BALB/c background) expressed the C57BL/6 pattern, suggesting that the $IgCH$ locus did, in fact, control $V_\kappa 1^{GAC}$ expression; however, BC.8 mice ($IgCH^a$ on C57BL/6 background) expressed the same pattern of idiotype expression, indicating that the presence of a "permissive" $IgCH$ locus was not sufficient to control $V_\kappa 1^{GAC}$ expression. Serum antibodies from BAB-14 mice expressed the BALB/c idiotype pattern. Thus, the V_H, not the C_H, locus is important in determining the pattern of anti-GAC light-chain expression. Further, the relevant portion of the V_H locus is that portion which is distal to the crossover in BAB-14. These results are consistent with the conclusions of Perlmutter *et al.*[18] reached through the examination of anti-GAC light-chain IEF spectrotypes. The idiotype pattern observed with BC.8 mice also indicates that background genes (V_κ or regulatory) are involved in the expression of these light-chain idiotypes. Complete structural information is not yet available to allow a comparison of the anti-GAC light chains expressed by BALB/c and C57BL/6 mice; however, both IEF spectrotype analysis and serologic analysis of the isolated light chains from C57BL/6-derived anti-GAC monoclonal antibodies indicate that C57BL/6 mice do express light chains which appear identical to the $V_\kappa 1^{GAC}$ light chain.[26] This result is consistent with the experiments of others which have not demonstrated V_κ polymorphism between these mouse strains.[27-29] This finding may indicate the presence of a regulatory locus, not linked to $IgCH$, which influences the selection of heavy–light-chain pairs. In conclusion, the examination of light-chain diversity in the antibody response to GAC has provided some interesting insights into the regulation of heavy- and light-chain expression. Though clearly not definitive, these studies suggest that V_H and V_L genes may be expressed in coordinated sets. Whether these restricted sets merely represent the imposed constraints of an antigen-specific antibody response is not clear; however, the studies discussed below suggest that this is not the case.

7. Expression of the $V_\kappa 1^{GAC}$ Light Chain among the IgG Subclasses

The bulk of the antibody response of mice to GAC and many other carbohydrate antigens consists of IgM and IgG3 antibodies.[5-8] IgG subclass restriction of other antigen-specific and polyclonal antibody responses has been observed.[6,8,30-33] The reasons for IgG subclass restriction of an antibody response are not clear. Subclass restriction could result from the preferential stimulation of B-cell subpopulations by different antigens resulting in the preferential secretion of distinct IgG subclasses which are characteristic of distinct B-cell populations.[6,33] Alternatively, subclass restriction of antibody responses could result from restricted association of heavy- and/or light-chain variable regions with the IgG heavy-chain constant regions. Experiments from several laboratories have suggested that heavy-chain variable regions may, in fact, display restricted IgG subclass associations within the constraints of an antigen-specific antibody population.[34-36] In an attempt to examine the possible restriction of light-chain variable regions with IgG subclasses, we have measured the expression of the $V_\kappa 1^{GAC}$ light chain among normal serum immunoglobulins, devoid of anti-GAC antibodies, and among monoclonal antibodies which do not have specificity for GAC.[12] The anti-$V_\kappa 1^{GAC}$ antisera, anti-Id5 and anti-Id20, appear to be ideally suited for these measurements since both antisera recognize framework-associated determinants of $V_\kappa 1^{GAC}$.[9,12] Further, examination of *in vitro* heavy–light-chain recombinants demonstrated that reactivity of these antisera with this light chain does not appear to be affected by association with heavy chains containing V_H regions which do not bind GAC nor is it affected by association with C_H regions other than IgG3.[12] These results indicate that anti-Id5 and anti-Id20 should detect the $V_\kappa 1^{GAC}$ light chain in mouse immunoglobulins irrespective of antibody specificity or subclass.

To determine the distribution of $V_\kappa 1^{GAC}$ among the IgG subclasses in normal serum, IgG1, IgG2a, and IgG3 were purified from normal serum by affinity chromatography on anti-subclass-specific Sepharose columns. Each of these subclasses was recovered from the affinity columns with greater than 85% purity as determined by radioimmunoassay. The purified subclasses were tested for expression of $V_\kappa 1^{GAC}$ determinants by radioimmunoassay. Id20 was present at detectable levels only in the IgG3 fraction, whereas Id5 was present in both IgG2a and IgG3 fractions.[12] Neither idiotype was detected in the IgG1 fraction of normal serum. The percentage of idiotype-bearing IgG was 2- to 14-fold higher in IgG3 than in IgG2a for both idiotypes. As measured by Id20 expression, the $V_\kappa 1^{GAC}$ light chain was present in 0.6% of IgG3 and less than 0.05% of IgG2a or IgG1. Anti-Id5 reactivity showed a similar distribution, but was present in a much higher proportion of serum immunoglobulin, reacting with 3% of IgG3 and 1% of IgG2a. Thus, anti-Id5 appears to have a broader specificity than anti-Id20. The reasons for the quantitative differences in reactivity with serum immunoglobulins are not clear. Anti-Id5 does react strongly with serum IgG2a which is essentially negative for Id20 reactivity. The data discussed below indicate that anti-Id5 reacts with V_κ products which are structurally distinct from the $V_\kappa 1^{GAC}$ light chain. In summary, these experiments demonstrated that even in antibody populations devoid of anti-GAC antibody the $V_\kappa 1^{GAC}$ light chain associates preferentially with antibodies of the IgG3 subclass.

To further examine this preferential association between V_κ and C_H products, we have prepared approximately 20 monoclonal antibodies which were selected solely on the basis of Id5 expression (R. J. Fulton and J. M. Davie unpublished data). In every case, the antibodies are either IgG3 or IgG2a. Further, IEF spectrotype analysis of the isolated light chains from these antibodies has demonstrated that all light chains from IgG3 antibodies comigrate with the $V_\kappa 1^{GAC}$ light chain whereas all light chains from IgG2a antibodies display a distinct IEF spectrotype. Interestingly, the IgG2a-associated light chains comigrate with each other and three of the four examples were derived from different A/J mice.

These results indicate that the anti-Id5 reactivity observed with normal serum IgG2a was directed toward a light chain distinct from $V_\kappa 1^{GAC}$ and that anti-Id20 probably represents a more specific marker for $V_\kappa 1^{GAC}$. More importantly, however, these results reinforce our previous conclusion that the $V_\kappa 1^{GAC}$ light chain displays a profound IgG subclass preference and that this preference is probably not a result of antigen-specificity or unique antigenic stimulation by GAC vaccine.

The mechanism by which a light-chain variable region would be restricted in its association with heavy-chain constant regions is not known. Analysis of the light chains of serum anti-GAC and anti-inulin antibodies has previously indicated that the heavy-chain allotype locus can influence the expression of κ light chains.[18,22] It is possible that this phenomenon could be mediated by a regulatory locus linked to the *IgCH* locus. It is also possible that the heavy-chain influence on light-chain expression is mediated indirectly through a primary restriction on V_H–C_H association. As mentioned above, there is evidence that certain V_H regions are restricted to particular IgG subclasses. Scott and Fleischman[34] have recently demonstrated that two V_H-associated idiotypes found in IgG3 anti-DNP antibodies were not expressed in IgG1 anti-DNP antibodies. In addition, a V_H idiotype expressed by IgG1 anti-DNP antibodies was not expressed among IgG3 antibodies. Chang *et al.*[35,36] have also demonstrated subclass restriction of variable regions among serum antibodies to phosphocholine (PC). In these studies, serum antibodies to PC-KLH were divided into two fine-specificity groups based on hapten inhibition profiles. Group I antibodies were predominantly IgM, IgA, and IgG3, whereas group II antibodies were restricted to IgG1, IgG2a, and IgG2b.[35] Since heavy-chain gene rearrangement precedes light-chain gene rearrangement in the differentiating B cell,[37,38] it is possible that the rearranged V_H gene could direct V_κ rearrangement so that only V_κ genes from a distinct set were selected. Kubagawa *et al.*[39] have proposed the existence of a mechanism for coordinating heavy- and light-chain isotype expression based on their findings in human pre-B-cell leukemias. These authors observed that all of the pre-B leukemias they studied which had undergone a heavy-chain switch to IgG1 also expressed κ light chains. A functional V_κ–C_H restriction might also occur as a result of coordinate regulation of the immune response by isotype-specific and idiotype-specific T lymphocytes.[40-44] Whatever the mechanism through which V_H–V_L restriction occurred, it would significantly lower estimates of the total antibody repertoire which are based on simple compounding of the numbers of V_H and V_L genes. Nevertheless, it seems unlikely that such a restriction would severely affect the total antibody repertoire, particularly in light of the multigenic nature of both heavy- and light-chain variable regions.[45-47]

It is striking that every example of preferential association of immunoglobulin chains, whether V_H, V_L, or C_L, with an IgG subclass separates the IgG subclasses into IgG3 and non-IgG3. This is the same grouping of IgG subclasses which correlates with the functional and phenotypic subpopulations of B cells which have been observed in several experimental systems. These observations have prompted this laboratory and others to propose the existence of at least two major B-cell subpopulations which differ in their responses to mitogens and antigens,[6,33] expression of cell surface markers,[48-50] requirements for T-cell influences,[51,52] expression of different immunoglobulin subclasses,[6,33,53] and possibly in their expression of different immunoglobulin variable regions.

In conclusion, studies of the diversity of antibodies to GAC have provided interesting insights into the expression of immunoglobulin variable regions with the implication that this expression does not occur randomly. It will be important to determine how generalized the phenomenon of V_L–V_H–C_H restriction is within the immune system, and whether this phenomenon is associated with or independent of V_H and V_L subgroups and whether it is the result of regulation intrinsic or extrinsic to the B lymphocyte.

ACKNOWLEDGMENT. Supported by U.S. Public Health Service Grants AI-15926, AI-15353, CA-09118, and AI-07163.

References

1. Coligan, G. E., Schnute, W. C., and Kindt, T. J., 1975, Immunochemical and chemical studies on streptococcal group specific carbohydrates, *J. Immunol.* **114**:1654–1658.
2. Krause, R. M., 1970, The search for antibodies with molecular uniformity, *Adv. Immunol.* **12**:1–56.
3. Briles, D. E., and Davie, J. M., 1975, Clonal dominance. I. Restricted nature of the IgM antibody response to group A streptococcal carbohydrate in mice, *J. Exp. Med.* **141**:1291–1307.
4. Cramer, M., and Braun, D. G., 1974, Genetics of restricted antibodies to streptococcal group polysaccharides in mice. I. Strain differences of isoelectric focusing spectra of group A hyperimmune antisera, *J. Exp. Med.* **139**:1513–1528.
5. Perlmutter, R. M., Hansburg, D., Briles, D. E., Nicolotti, R. A., and Davie, J. M., 1978, Subclass restriction of murine anti-carbohydrate antibodies, *J. Immunol.* **121**:566–572.
6. Slack, J., Der-Balian, G. P., Nahm, M., and Davie, J. M., 1980, The IgG plaque-forming cell response to thymus-independent type 1 and type 2 antigens in normal mice and mice expressing an X-linked immunodeficiency, *J. Exp. Med.* **151**:853–862.
7. Der-Balian, G. P., Slack, J., Clevinger, B., Bazin, H., and Davie, J. M., 1980, Subclass restriction of murine antibodies. III. Antigens that stimulate IgG3 in mice stimulate IgG2c in rats, *J. Exp. Med.* **152**:209–218.
8. Yount, W. J., Dorner, M. M., Kunkel, H. G., and Kabat, E. A., 1968, Studies on human antibodies. VI. Selective variations in subgroup composition and genetic markers, *J. Exp. Med.* **127**:633–646.
9. Nahm, M., Clevinger, B. L., and Davie, J. M., 1982, Monoclonal antibodies to streptococcal group A carbohydrate. I. A dominant idiotypic determinant is located on V_κ, *J. Immunol.* **129**:1513–1518.
10. Braun, D., Kindred, B., and Jacobson, E., 1972, Streptococcal group A carbohydrate antibodies in mice: Evidence for strain differences in magnitude and restriction of the response, and for thymus-dependence, *Eur. J. Immunol.* **2**:138–143.
11. Briles, D. E., Nahm, M., Marion, T., Perlmutter, R., and Davie, J. M., 1982, Streptococcal group A carbohydrate has properties of both a thymus-independent (TI-2) and a thymus-dependent antigen, *J. Immunol.* **128**:2032–2035.
12. Fulton, R. J., Nahm, M., and Davie, J. M., 1983, Monoclonal antibodies to streptococcal group A carbohydrate. II. The $V_{\kappa_1}{}^{GAC}$ light chain is preferentially associated with serum IgG3, *J. Immunol.* **131**:1326–1331.
13. Eichmann, K., 1972, Idiotypic identity of antibodies to streptococcal carbohydrate in inbred mice, *Eur. J. Immunol.* **2**:301–307.
14. Eichmann, K, 1973, Idiotype expression and the inheritance of mouse antibody clones, *J. Exp. Med.* **137**:603–621.
15. Berek, C., Taylor, B. A., and Eichmann, K., 1976, Genetics of the idiotype of BALB/c myeloma S117: Multiple chromosomal loci for V_H genes encoding specificity for group A streptococcal carbohydrate, *J. Exp. Med.* **144**:1164–1174.
16. Briles, D. E., and Krause, R. M., 1974, Mouse strain-specific idiotypy and interstrain idiotypic cross-reactions, *J. Immunol.* **113**:522–530.
17. Perlmutter, R. M., Briles, D. E., and Davie, J. M., 1977, Complete sharing of light chain spectrotypes by murine IgM and IgG anti-streptococcal antibodies, *J. Immunol.* **118**:2161–2166.
18. Perlmutter, R. M., Briles, D. E., Greve, J. M., and Davie, J. M., 1978, Light chain diversity of murine anti-streptococcal antibodies: IgCH-linked effects on L chain expression, *J. Immunol.* **121**:149–158.

19. Briles, D. E., and Carroll, R. J., 1981, A simple method for estimating the probable numbers of different antibodies by examining the repeat frequencies of sequences or isoelectric focusing patterns, *Mol. Immunol.* **18**:29–38.

20. Gearhart, P. J., Johnson, N. D., Douglas, R., and Hood, L., 1981, IgG antibodies to phosphorylcholine exhibit more diversity than their IgM counterparts, *Nature* **291**:29–34.

21. Crews, S., Griffin, J., Huang, H., Calame, K., and Hood, L., 1981, A single V_H gene segment encodes the immune response to phosphorylcholine: Somatic mutation is correlated with the class of the antibody, *Cell* **25**:59–66.

22. Slack, J. H., Shapiro, M., and Potter, M., 1979, Serum expression of a Vκ structure, Vκ-11, associated with inulin antibodies controlled by gene(s) linked to the mouse IgCH complex, *J. Immunol.* **122**:230–239.

23. Krawinkel, U., Cramer, M., Berek, C., Hammerling, G., Black, S. J., Rajewsky, K., and Eichmann, K., 1976, On the structure of the T-cell receptor for antigen, *Cold Spring Harbor Symp. Quant. Biol.* **41**:285–294.

24. Basta, P., Kubagawa, H., Kearney, J. F., and Briles, D. E., 1983, Ten percent of normal B cells and plasma cells share a V_H determinant(s) (J606-GAC) with a distinct subset of murine V_HIII plasmacytomas, *J. Immunol.* **130**:2423–2428.

25. Fathman, C. G., Pisetsky, D. S., and Sachs, D. H., 1977, Genetic control of the immune response to nuclease. V. Genetic linkage and strain distribution of anti-nuclease idiotypes, *J. Exp. Med.* **145**:569–577.

26. Fulton, R. J., and Davie J. M., 1984, Influence of the immunoglobulin heavy chain loci on the expression of the $V\kappa_1{}^{GAC}$ light chain, *J. Immunol.* (in press).

27. Gibson, D., 1976, Genetic polymorphism of mouse immunoglobulin light chains revealed by isoelectric focusing, *J. Exp. Med.* **144**:298–303.

28. Gottlieb, P. D., 1974, Genetic correlation of a mouse light chain variable region marker with a thymocyte surface antigen, *J. Exp. Med.* **140**:1432–1437.

29. Claflin, J. L., 1976, Genetic marker in the variable region of kappa chains of mouse anti-phosphorylcholine antibodies, *Eur. J. Immunol.* **6**:666–668.

30. Devey, M. E., and Voak, D., 1974, A critical study of the IgG subclasses of the Rh anti-D antibodies formed in pregnancy and in immunized volunteers, *Immunology* **27**:1073–1079.

31. Robboy, S. J., Lewis, E. J., Schur, P. H., and Coleman, R. W., 1970, Circulating anticoagulants to factor VIII: Immunochemical studies and clinical response to factor VIII concentrates, *Am. J. Med.* **49**:742–752.

32. Vandvik, B., Natvig, J. B., and Norrby, E., 1977, IgG1 subclass restriction of oligoclonal measles virus-specific IgG antibodies in patients with subacute sclerosing panencephalitis and in a patient with multiple sclerosis, *Scand. J. Immunol.* **6**:651–657.

33. McKearn, J. P., Paslay, J. W., Slack, J., Baum, C., and Davie, J. M., 1982, B cell subsets and differential responses to mitogens, *Immunol. Rev.* **64**:5–23.

34. Scott, M. J., and Fleischman, J. B., 1982, Preferential idiotype–isotype associations in antibodies to dinitrophenyl antigens, *J. Immunol.* **128**:2622–2628.

35. Chang, S. P., Brown, M., and Rittenberg, M. B., 1982, Immunologic memory to phosphorylcholine. II. PC-KLH induces two antibody populations that dominate different isotypes, *J. Immunol.* **128**:702–706.

36. Chang, S. P., Brown, M., and Rittenberg, M. B., 1982, Immunologic memory to phosphorylcholine. III. IgM includes a fine specificity population distinct from TEPC 15, *J. Immunol.* **129**:1559–1562.

37. Maki, R., Kearney, J., Paige, C., and Tonegawa, S., 1980, Immunoglobulin gene rearrangement in immature B cells, *Science* **209**:1366–1369.

38. Perry, R. P., Kelly, D. E., Coleclough, C., and Kearney, J. F., 1981, Organization and expression of immunoglobulin genes in fetal liver hybridomas, *Proc. Natl. Acad. Sci. USA* **78**:247–251.

39. Kubagawa, H., Mayumi, M., Crist, W., and Cooper, M., 1983, Immunoglobulin heavy chain switching in pre-B leukemias, *Nature* **301**:340–342.

40. Kishimoto, T., and Ishizaka, K., 1973, Regulation of antibody response *in vitro*. V. Effect of carrier-specific helper cells on generation of hapten-specific memory cells of different immunoglobulin classes, *J. Immunol.* **111**:1–9.

41. Rosenberg, Y. J., 1982, Isotype-specific T cell regulation of immunoglobulin expression, *Immunol. Rev.* **67**:33–58.

42. Nisonoff, A., Ju, S.-T., and Owen, F. L., 1977, Studies of structure and immunosuppression of a cross-reactive idiotype in strain A mice, *Immunol. Rev.* **34**:89–118.

43. Krawinkel, V., Cramer, M., Melchers, I., Imanishi-Kari, T., and Rajewsky, K., 1978, Isolated hapten-binding receptors of sensitized lymphocytes. III. Evidence for idiotypic restriction of T-cell receptors, *J. Exp. Med.* **147**:1341–1347.

44. Eichmann, K., 1978, Expression and function of idiotypes on lymphocytes, *Adv. Immunol.* **26**:195–254.

45. Brack, C., Hirama, M., Lenhard-Schuller, R., and Tonegawa, S., 1978, A complete immunoglobulin gene is created by somatic recombination, *Cell* **15**:1–14.

46. Early, P., Huang, H., Davis, M., Calame, K., and Hood, L., 1980, An immunoglobulin heavy chain variable region gene is generated from three segments of DNA: V_H, D, and J_H, *Cell* **19**:981–992.

47. Kurosawa, Y., and Tonegawa, S., 1982, Organization, structure, and assembly of immunoglobulin heavy chain diversity DNA segments, *J. Exp. Med.* **155**:201–218.

48. Ahmed, A., Scher, I., Sharrow, S. O., Smith, A. H., Paul, W. E., Sachs, D. H., and Sell, K. W., 1977, B lymphocyte heterogeneity: Development and characterization of an alloantiserum which distinguishes B lymphocyte differentiation alloantigens, *J. Exp. Med.* **145**:101–110.

49. Huber, B., Gershon, R. R., and Cantor, H., 1977, Identification of a B-cell surface structure involved in antigen-dependent triggering: Absence of this structure on B-cells from CBA/N mutant mice, *J. Exp. Med.* **145**:10–24.

50. Huber, B., 1979, Antigenic marker on a functional subpopulation of B-cells controlled by the I-A subregion of the H-2 complex, *Proc. Natl. Acad. Sci. USA* **76**:3460–3463.

51. Asano, Y., and Hodes, R. J., 1982, T cell regulation of B cell activation: T cells independently regulate the responses mediated by distinct B cell subpopulations, *J. Exp. Med.* **155**:1267–1276.

52. Singer, A., Asano, Y., Shigeta, M., Hathcock, K. S., Ahmed, A., Fathman, G. G., and Hodes, R. J., 1982, Distinct B cell subpopulations differ in their genetic requirements for activation by T helper cells, *Immunol. Rev.* **64**:137–160.

53. Perlmutter, R. M., Nahm, M., Stein, K. E., Slack, J., Zitron, I., Paul, W. E., and Davie, J. M., 1979, Immunoglobulin subclass-specific immunodeficiency in mice with an X-linked B-lymphocyte defect, *J. Exp. Med.* **149**:993–998.

13

Idiotypes of *Ir* Gene-Controlled Anti-GAT Response

SHYR-TE JU

1. Introduction

In mice, the immune response to the synthetic polypeptide GAT, a random linear polymer, poly(L-Glu^{60},L-Ala^{30},L-Tyr^{10}), is under the control of immune response (Ir) genes localized in the *I* region of the major histocompatibility complex.[1] Mice bearing *H-2^{p,q,s}* haplotypes are nonresponders. This nonresponsiveness can be bypassed by immunization with GAT complexed with methylated bovine serum albumin (GAT-MBSA).[2] Prior injection of GAT into nonresponder strains induces a population of suppressor T cells that specifically suppress the anti-GAT response to a subsequent immunization with GAT-MBSA.[3] Furthermore, factors generated from GAT-specific suppressor T cells can specifically suppress the GAT-specific plaque-forming cell response to GAT-MBSA.[4] Subsequent studies demonstrated that these antigen-binding T-cell factors lack immunoglobulin constant-region determinants and possess MHC-coded determinants.[5] Because immunoglobulins presently comprise the only known system which exhibits antigen specificity and diversity among its members, it is possible that T-cell factors possess a structure equivalent to an immunoglobulin variable (V) region, associated with an MHC product, thus conferring T-cell receptors with antigen-specificity, diversity, and functional activity. This hypothesis, which has important implications for the nature of T-cell receptors if proven correct, prompted us to carry out systematic and extensive analyses on the idiotypes on anti-GAT antibodies. This effort has resulted in the identification of several related and distinct anti-GAT idiotypic families. More importantly, we have used well-characterized anti-idiotypic reagents to study the serological relationship between antigen-specific T-cell receptors and antibodies.[6-8] The purpose of this chapter is to review the immunochemical properties of murine anti-GAT idiotypic families. Each family will be discussed separately and focus

---

SHYR-TE JU • Department of Pathology, Harvard Medical School, Boston, Massachusetts 02115.

will be centered on the methods of identification as well as the common and the unique properties of each idiotypic family.

2. The Major Anti-GAT Idiotype

2.1. CGAT Idiotypic Family

Because GAT is a random polymer, its exact antigenic structures cannot be determined. However, its "functional" structures, i.e., antigenic determinants, can be defined based on serological cross-reactions.[9] For instance, anti-GAT antibodies cross-reactively bind to poly(Glu^{50},Tyr^{50}) (GT) and poly(Glu^{60},Ala^{40}) (GA) polymers. Conversely, anti-GT and anti-GA antibodies cross-reactively bind to GAT. Furthermore, the GT-reactive and GA-reactive antibodies in anti-GAT antibodies are largely, if not entirely, nonoverlapping populations.[9] These data indicate that there are at least two sets of antigenic determinants on GAT molecules, namely GT-related and GA-related determinants, that are not only accessible to antibody molecules but also functionally immunogenic in inducing the corresponding antibodies.

The presence of at least two different antigenic determinants on GAT did not cause any difficulty in the identification of the major anti-GAT idiotypes. This is because murine anti-GAT antibodies contain predominantly GT-specific (80–90%) antibodies.[9] Only 10–20% of anti-GAT antibodies are GA-specific. A major idiotype on the GT-reactive antibodies should be easily identified by the conventional inhibition assay for idiotype that preferentially detects the major idiotype on a population of antibodies.

Pooled, affinity-purified D1.LP anti-GAT antibodies were used to elicit anti-idiotypic antibodies in a guinea pig.[10] A major advantage in using pooled antibodies as idiotypic immunogen is that the levels of common idiotypic determinants remain relatively unchanged while the concentrations of private idiotypic determinants are greatly reduced to weak or nonimmunogenic levels. Therefore, the anti-idiotypic antiserum should contain largely antibodies to the common idiotypic specificities. Affinity-purified individual D1.LP anti-GAT antibodies not used in the immunization for anti-idiotypic antiserum were ^{125}I-labeled and then tested for the presence of common idiotype by a idiotype binding assay. This combination of idiotypic interactions preferentially detects common idiotypes. The individual preparation that exhibited the highest idiotype binding was chosen as the reference ligand.[10] In this example, 55% of the ligand was bound with excess anti-idiotypic antiserum. Approximately 50% of the bound ligand was GT-reactive (major) and 5%, GA-reactive (minor) antibodies.[10] This represents a contribution of 91 and 9% of the respective major and minor idiotypic antibodies to the 30% bound ligand. Normally, 30% idiotype binding is located at the linear range of idiotype–anti-idiotype interactions that can be efficiently blocked by a test sample bearing similar or identical idiotype. In this case, it is clear that a sample containing the major idiotype on GT-reactive antibodies can be identified because it causes strong inhibition of idiotype binding.

Individual anti-GAT antisera of 13 inbred strains were tested for the presence of this major idiotype. Unexpectedly, all inbred strains of mice regardless of their genetic origin produced anti-GAT antibodies having an idiotype either similar or identical to the major idiotype (Table I). Considering its common presence on anti-GAT antibodies, this major

TABLE I
Strain Distribution of CGAT Idiotype

Strain	Polymorphism			% inhibition of idiotype binding[a]		
	Igh	Ig1	H-2	Preimmune	Immune	Purified antibodies
BALB/c	a	b	d	8	96	98
C58/J	a	a	k	9	98	NT
C57BL/10	b	b	b	10	89	68
D1.LP	c	b	b	12	99	89
DBA/2	c	b	d	4	100	85
RF	c	a	k	10	96	79
AKR	d	a	k	2	94	76
A/J	e	b	a	5	100	95
CE/J	f	b	k	1	82	70
RIII	g	b	r	6	90	NT
SEA/GN	h	b	k	0	100	95
C3H.SW	j	b	b	5	92	84
NZW	n	b	z	10	100	88

[a]Ten μl of test samples were used to inhibit the binding of 10 ng of ^{125}I-labeled D1.LP anti-GAT antibodies to 0.2 μl of the guinea pig anti-idiotypic antiserum. In the absence of inhibitor, a net of 30 $\pm$ 2% was obtained. Immune sera were obtained 7 days after a secondary immunization with GAT at day 18. Purified anti-GAT antibodies were obtained by affinity chromatography over GAT-Sepharose 4B column. NT, not tested.

idiotype was termed CGAT idiotype.[11] To date, we have identified CGAT idiotype on the anti-GAT antibodies of more than 50 mouse strains. Thèze and colleagues have identified a similar common idiotype with a rabbit anti-idiotypic antiserum made against BALB/c anti-GAT antibodies.[12] The mice tested included those bearing different Ig-1 heavy-chain allotypes, different light-chain variable-region markers, and different *H-2* haplotypes.

In view of the ubiquitous nature of the CGAT idiotype, it is of paramount importance to establish the specificity of the idiotypic system. This can be demonstrated by (1) the inability of preimmune sera to inhibit idiotype binding, (2) the removal and recovery of the inhibitory activity of immune sera through specific immunoadsorption with GAT-Sepharose 4B column, and (3) the ability of specific antigen, i.e., GAT, to inhibit idiotype binding.[10]

The ubiquitous nature of the CGAT idiotype in inbred mouse strains prompted us to search for its presence in inbred strains of rats and other distantly related species.[11,13] The CGAT idiotype could not be detected in the anti-GAT antisera of guinea pigs and rabbits. Interestingly, 9 of 13 rat strains tested produced anti-GAT antibodies that were able to inhibit the CGAT idiotype binding. The shared idiotypic determinants on rat anti-GAT antibodies are similar rather than identical to the CGAT idiotypic determinants.[13] Furthermore, the production of this interspecies cross-reactive idiotype showed no apparent association with either rat *RT1* haplotypes or immunoglobulin H- and L-chain allotypic specificities.[13]

The conclusion that common idiotypic antibodies are coded for by structural germline and germline-derived *V* genes has been confirmed in several idiotypic systems.[14,15] In the CGAT idiotypic system, evidence that suggests that one V_H and one or two V_L germ-

line or germline-related genes are responsible for the generation of CGAT idiotypic antibodies has been obtained.[16] The presence of interstrain and interspecies cross-reactive idiotypes implies that (1) the diversification of CGAT V_H and C_H genes were independent
processes; (2) the CGAT V_H gene emerged before the diversification of C_H genes; (3) the
V_H gene encoding CGAT idiotype was conserved through murine evolution; and (4) despite
the strong tendency to conserve the CGAT V_H gene, certain permissible changes in the
gene occurred during evolution as demonstrated by (1) the similarity but not identity of
interspecies cross-reactive idiotype and (2) the presence of strain-specific idiotypic determinants on the CGAT$^+$ anti-GAT antibodies (see below).

2.2. Idiotypes of Nonresponder Strains

Immunization of nonresponder strains with GAT does not generate anti-GAT antibodies and, therefore, CGAT idiotype cannot be detected in the immune sera. Bypassing
this GAT nonresponsiveness by immunization with GAT-MBSA or GAT-fowl γ-globulin
conjugates leads to the production of both anti-GAT antibodies and CGAT idiotype.[9]
These data indicate that CGAT idiotypic clones are present in Ir-nonresponder strains and
that the Ir gene defect does not manifest itself at the B-cell level.

2.3. Antigenic Determinants Responsible for the Induction of the CGAT Idiotype

Based on the calculation in Section 2.1, it is argued that the CGAT idiotype resides
on the GT-reactive antibodies induced by the GT-related determinants on GAT molecules.
Subsequent studies demonstrated that this is indeed the case because GT-related determinants on GT, poly(Glu^{51},Lys^{34},Tyr^{15}) (GLT^{15}), and (Tyr,Glu)-D,L-Ala-Lys [(T,G)-A--L]
polymers also induce CGAT idiotypic antibodies (Table II).[17] A requirement for these
polymers to induce CGAT idiotypic antibodies is that the immunized strain must be a
responder toward that particular polymer.[17] For instance, all inbred strains are nonre-

TABLE II
Common Idiotype Induced by Antigenic Determinants on
Various Polypeptides

Polymer	No. of strains tested	Idiotype elicited[a]			
		CGAT	Gte	GA-1	GA-2
GAT	>50	+	+	+	+
GT	1	+	NT	−	NT
GLT^{15}	6	+	+	−	NT
(T,G)-A--L	4	+	+	−	−
GA	>16	−	−	+	+
GLA^{40}	14	−	−	+	+

[a]See text for the definition of idiotypes. NT, not tested.

sponders to GT, and upon immunization with GT, do not produce CGAT idiotypic antibodies. In contrast, a partially inbred strain, which is a responder to GT, produced CGAT idiotypic antibodies.[9] This observation provided strong evidence that GT-related antigenic determinants are sufficient for the induction of the CGAT idiotype. Furthermore, these polymers lack functional GA-related antigenic determinants. Thus, GA-related determinants on GAT molecules are not essential for the induction of the CGAT idiotype. In addition, anti-GA and anti-poly(Glu^{36},Lys^{24},Ala^{40}) (GLA^{40}) antisera from all mouse strains tested did not express CGAT idiotypic antibodies, although strongly cross-reactive GAT-binding activities were present in these sera.[11]

2.4. Immunochemical Properties of CGAT Idiotypic Antibodies

Two observations indicate that CGAT idiotypic determinants are closely associated with antibody combining sites that are specific to GT-related determinants.[10] First, GAT and GT but not GA inhibited CGAT idiotype binding. Second, guinea pig anti-idiotypic antiserum specifically inhibited the GAT-binding activity of CGAT idiotypic antibodies. Furthermore, the presence of active antibody combining sites is essential for the expression of CGAT idiotypic determinants. Purified heavy or light chains from CGAT$^+$ hybridoma antibodies expressed neither GAT-binding activity nor CGAT idiotype. Upon reconstitution into intact immunoglobulin molecules, both GAT-binding activity and CGAT idiotype were recovered. In addition, by using hybridoma variants we showed that inappropriate heavy or light chains cannot substitute for the corresponding CGAT$^+$ anti-GAT chains to reconstitute GAT-binding activity and CGAT idiotype.[17a]

2.5. Evidence for the Presence of CGAT Idiotypic Families

Although the idiotypic study on serum anti-GAT antibodies suggests that the germline V gene(s) responsible for generating CGAT idiotype is highly conserved, the actual extent of antibody diversity and the relationship of any such diversity to the germ-line V gene(s) are unknown. To determine the heterogeneity of B-cell clones producing CGAT idiotypic antibodies, we studied the idiotypic properties of a large number of GT-reactive hybridoma antibodies.[18,19] All of the GT-reactive hybridoma antibodies tested expressed the CGAT idiotype (Table III). If extensive diversity exists among individual hybridoma antibodies, each hybridoma antibody would be expected to possess individual antigenic determinants. Anti-idiotypic antisera were, therefore, made against individual hybridoma antibodies and were used to probe for the presence of these individual antigenic determinants or private idiotype. Indeed, nearly all of the hybridoma antibodies tested were found to have private idiotypic determinants (Table III). These observations indicate that the GT-reactive antibodies are extremely heterogeneous. In spite of such heterogeneity, these antibodies are related because they share CGAT idiotypic specificities. To account for such complex idiotypic relationships, we proposed that CGAT idiotypic determinants are encoded by germ-line V_H and V_L genes and that somatic diversification processes such as point mutation, VDJ (or VJ) rearrangement, and $D-D$ joining can operate on these genes to generate new idiotypic determinants while retaining the ability to bind GT-related epi-

TABLE III
Idiotypic Specificities on Hybridoma Antibodies

Origin and no. of hybridomas		Ig class	Specificity	Idiotype specificity[a]				
				CGAT	Gte	GA-1	GA-2	Private idiotype
DBA/2	(7)[b]	μ,κ	GT	+	−	−	−	+ (6/7)
B10	(3)	μ,κ	GT	+	+	−	−	NT
B6, B10	(8)	$\gamma1,\kappa$	GT	+	+	−	−	+ (5/5)
B6, B10	(2)	$\gamma3,\kappa$	GT	+	+	−	−	+ (1/1)
B6, B10	(4)	$\gamma1,\kappa$	GT	+	−	−	−	+ (2/2)
DBA/2	(1)	μ,κ	GA	−	−	+	+	+ (1/1)
DBA/2	(4)	$\gamma1,\kappa$	GA	−	−	+	+	+ (4/4)
DBA/2	(3)	$\gamma1,\kappa$	GA	−	−	−	−	+ (2/3)
CDF$_1$	(1)	μ,κ	GA	−	−	−	+	+ (1/1)

[a]See text for the definition of idiotypes. Private idiotype assays were established by binding of ^{125}I-labeled hybridoma antibodies to the anti-idiotypic antisera made against the same hybridoma antibodies. If this idiotype binding is inhibited only by the homologous hybridoma antibody but not by other hybridoma antibodies, it is designated as bearing a private idiotype. Values in parentheses indicate the frequency of expression of the private idiotype over the total idiotype systems tested. For example, 6/7 means 7 hybridoma idiotypic systems were tested and 5 of them exhibited private idiotypes not found on any other hybridoma antibodies. However, 2 hybridoma antibodies exhibited similar idiotypes that were not found on other hybridoma antibodies. NT, not tested.
[b]Values in parentheses are the number of individual hybridomas tested.

tope and express the CGAT idiotype. As a result, a family of CGAT idiotypic antibodies are generated and individual members of the family are characterized by having two sets of idiotypic specificities: one shared among members of the family and the other uniquely associated with the individual members. A similar conclusion was achieved by Leclercq *et al.* who reported that monoclonal anti-GAT antibodies with different fine antigen-binding specificities express the same common idiotype.[20]

3. The Minor Anti-GAT Idiotypes

3.1. GA-1 Idiotypic Family

As noted earlier, study of the idiotypes of GA-reactive antibodies was hindered by the low frequency of such antibodies in the D1.LP anti-GAT antibody population. However, in the course of studying the idiotypic properties of 15 hybridoma anti-GAT antibodies, we have noted one GA-reactive hybridoma antibody (F9-102.2) that did not express the CGAT idiotype but did bind to the anti-idiotypic antiserum made against pooled D1.LP antibodies (Table IV)[18] This observation indicates that at least two distinct groups of anti-idiotypic antibodies were present: one group that bound CGAT idiotypic determinants and the second group that bound the idiotypic determinants on the CGAT$^-$, F9-102.2 hybridoma antibody. The latter idiotypic interaction was used to define a new idiotype termed GA-1 idiotype. Such heterologous idiotypic interaction turns out to provide a useful strategy for identifying a common idiotype that is a minor population of serum antibodies.

Subsequent studies demonstrated that the GA-1 idiotype is an interstrain cross-reactive idiotype. All mouse strains tested with the exception of CE/J express the GA-1 idiotype.[21] The functional antigenic determinants responsible for the induction of GA-1 idiotypic antibodies were identified as GA-related determinants because GA and GA-containing polymers GAT and GLA[40] are able to induce the GA-1 idiotype (Table II). This situation is analogous to the CGAT idiotype, which is induced with GT-related determinants. Furthermore, GA and GLA[40], which lack GT-related determinants, do not induce the CGAT idiotype whereas GT and GLT[15], which lack GA-related determinants, do not induce GA-1 idiotype. These data indicate that CGAT and GA-1 are distinct idiotypes present on two different populations of anti-GAT antibodies. The fact that GAT induces both CGAT and GA-1 idiotypes indicates that these GT- and GA-related antigenic moieties are present on GAT molecules and that both act in an immunogenic fashion to induce the corresponding major and minor idiotypes.

The GA-1 idiotype is similar to the CGAT idiotype in that it is a family composed of idiotypically related but nonidentical GA-reactive antibodies; individual members of the family possess the common GA-1 idiotype and a set of private idiotypic specificities (Table IV). This conclusion is based on the fine idiotypic specificities of 10 GA-reactive hybridoma antibodies.[22] Eight hybridoma antibodies were derived from DBA/2 mice. Five of the DBA/2 hybridoma antibodies belong to GA-1 idiotypic family. This suggests that GA-1 is a major idiotype of the DBA/2 anti-GA response.

3.2. GA-2 Idiotype and Its Relationship to GA-1 Idiotype

The procedure that leads to the identification of the GA-2 idiotype is similar to that described in the previous section for the identification of the GA-1 idiotype. In this case, a GA-reactive hybridoma antibody (H51.85.2) that lacks both CGAT and GA-1 idiotypes was found to bind the guinea pig anti-idiotypic antiserum made against pooled D1.LP anti-GAT antibodies (Table IV). Therefore, in addition to anti-CGAT and anti-GA-1 idiotypic

TABLE IV
Identification of Minor Idiotypes

Test samples	Idiotype binding[a]		% inhibition of idiotype binding[b]		
	4 μl	0.4 μl	CGAT	GA-1	GA-2
D1.LP anti-GAT Ab	70	45	98	98	96
F9-102.2	95	68	4	100	100
H51.85.2	90	30	0	6	100
F27.80.11	7	1	3	6	0

[a] Idiotype binding of 10 ng ^{125}I-labeled antibodies by 4 or 0.4 μl of a guinea pig anti-idiotypic antiserum. The anti-idiotypic antiserum is made against D1.LP anti-GAT antibodies. Values in the table are percent ^{125}I-labeled ligand bound.
[b] One μg of test sample was mixed with the guinea pig anti-idiotypic antiserum. ^{125}I-labeled D1.LP antibodies (for CGAT idiotype), F9-102.2 (for GA-1 idiotype), or H51.85.2 (for GA-2 idiotype) were then added. Bound idiotypic ligands were precipitated with excess rabbit anti-guinea pig immunoglobulin antiserum. In the absence of inhibitor, 30–35% of ligand was precipitated.

activities, this antiserum contains a third population of anti-idiotypic antibodies that are responsible for the specific idiotype binding of ^{125}I-labeled H51.85.2 hybridoma antibody. This specific idiotype binding defined the GA-2 idiotype.

GA-2 idiotypic antibodies are induced by GA-related antigenic determinants, i.e., the idiotype is identified on anti-GAT, anti-GLA[40], and hybridoma anti-GA antibodies. However, the GA-2 idiotype is not a distinct idiotypic family. Rather, it is closely related to the GA-1 idiotypic family. The prototype of the GA-1 idiotype, i.e., F9-102.2 hybridoma antibody, fully expressed the GA-2 idiotype. And yet the GA-2 idiotype was not identified in a previous study. In that study, GA-1 but not GA-2 idiotypic determinants on F9-102.2 hybridoma antibody reacted with the guinea pig anti-idiotypic antiserum. The stronger GA-1 idiotypic interaction can be due to the presence of more anti-GA-1 idiotypic antibodies or high-affinity anti-GA-1 idiotypic antibodies or both. Thus, identification of the weaker GA-2 idiotype would not be possible had it not been that H51.85.2 hybridoma antibody lacks GA-1 but expresses the GA-2 idiotype.

The GA-2 idiotype is closely related to the GA-1 idiotypic family in an interesting fashion. All GA-1$^+$ idiotypic antibodies possess the GA-2 idiotype. To date, no GA-1$^+$,GA-2$^-$ hybridoma antibodies have been found. In contrast, the association of the GA-1 idiotype with GA-2$^+$ idiotypic antibodies is not stringent. Thus, the GA-2$^+$ H51.85.2 hybridoma antibody lacks the GA-1 idiotype. Another GA-2$^+$ F27-105.12 hybridoma antibody bears only 45% of GA-1 idiotypic determinants. This result suggests that diversification processes operate preferentially on V_H and V_L gene segments involved in the coding information for the GA-1 idiotype. It also indicates that GA-1 idiotypic determinants are not essential for GA binding and, for this reason, the V_H and V_L genes can tolerate these diversification processes without loss of GA reactivity. Finally, it is predicted that the H and L chains of H51.85.2 hybridoma antibody should have strong sequence homology to that of GA-1$^+$ hybridoma antibodies.[16] Further comparative sequence studies should identify the amino acid residues that are important for the construction of the GA-1 and GA-2 idiotypes.

4. Gte Idiotypic Family

The study of the CGAT idiotype strongly suggests that CGAT idiotypic antibodies are coded for by germ-line V_H and V_L genes and that regions encoding CGAT idiotypic specificities are conserved despite mouse strain diversification. It is possible that other regions not encoding CGAT idiotypic determinants have diversified during mouse strain diversification. Such events, if they occurred, might be detected as strain-specific idiotypes provided that the diversification did not alter the GT reactivity of the encoded molecules. Previous studies of anti-idiotypic antiserum made against pooled D1.LP or BALB/c anti-GAT antibodies identified only interspecies and interstrain common idiotypes. Strain-specific idiotypic determinants were not detected. It is possible that these anti-GAT antibodies do not bear sufficient and immunogenic levels of strain-specific idiotypic determinants to elicit the corresponding anti-idiotypic antibodies. In an effort to search for strain-specific idiotypes, pooled A/J anti-GAT antibodies were used to immunize a guinea pig. The anti-idiotypic antiserum contains activities specific to interspecies, interstrain, and strain-specific idiotypic determinants.[23] After adsorption with pooled DBA/2 hybridoma antibodies to remove the bulk of anti-CGAT idiotypic antibodies, it is possible to selectively detect strain-specific idiotypic determinants. These strain-specific determinants were present in both A/J and B6 anti-GAT antibodies. In order to provide a long-lasting and reliable standard for the strain-specific idiotype, a B6 hybridoma anti-GAT antibody was used as ligand in the radioimmunoassays and the idiotypic determinants detected were designated Gte idiotype.

Gte idiotypic determinants are associated with the combining sites of idiotypic antibodies that are induced by GT-related but not GA-related antigenic moieties (Table II). Genetic and strain distribution studies indicated that the expression of the Gte idiotype is controlled by $Igh-1^e$- or $Igh-1^b$-linked genes. Furthermore, $Igh-Gte$ gene has been shown to segregate together with the $Igh-NP^b$ gene that controls the production of NP^b idiotype.[24]

The interrelationship between CGAT and Gte idiotypes has been studied on hybridoma anti-GAT and anti-(T,G)-A--L antibodies of B6 origin.[19,23] The majority of CGAT$^+$ hybridoma antibodies express the Gte idiotype. However, a small fraction ($<$ 30%) of CGAT$^+$ hybridoma antibodies lacks this idiotype. Thus, the B6 V_H gene encoding CGAT idiotypic determinants also contains coding information for Gte idiotype that was established together with or after the strain diversification. The presence of CGAT$^+$,Gte$^-$ clones can be explained by the assumption that there are two separate germline structural V_H genes: one codes for CGAT idiotype and the other codes for both CGAT and Gte idiotypes. Alternatively, there may be only one germ-line V_H gene encoding both CGAT and Gte idiotypes; in this case the CGAT$^+$,Gte$^-$ clones would be products of a somatic mutation process.

5. Variation in Frequency of an Idiotypic Clone as a Basis for a Strain-Specific Idiotype

We have produced two rat monoclonal anti-idiotypic antibodies against B10 anti-(T,G)-A--L antibodies (Ju, S.-T, Pincus, S. H., and Dorf, M. E., unpublished observation). These two clones have similar or identical fine idiotopic specificity. Because the monoclonal anti-idiotopic antibodies are exquisitely specific, they can detect a minute quantity of the idiotope (designated Ig-7 idiotope) that cannot be detected with confidence by the conventional anti-idiotypic antisera prepared in guinea pigs. Strain distribution study indicates that the concentrations of Ig-7 idiotope in the anti-GAT antisera of various mouse strains differ dramatically (Table V). A/J and B10.A anti-GAT antisera have the highest levels of the idiotope, C3H/He and NZB anti-GAT antisera express moderate levels, and BALB/c, DBA/2, and SEA/GN are low Ig-7 idiotope producers. Furthermore, 100% of the GT-reactive CGAT$^+$ hybridoma antibodies of Igh^b strains and 33% (1 of 3) of GT-reactive, CGAT$^+$ C3H.SW hybridoma antibodies express Ig-7 idiotope. Ig-7 idiotope is not present in seven GT-reactive, CGAT$^+$ DBA/2 hybridoma antibodies. This difference in frequency of Ig-7 clones, although estimated on a small number of hybridomas, correlates nicely with the relative difference of Ig-7 idiotope concentrations among the corresponding strains. This correlation suggests that a strain-specific idiotype may result from variation in the frequency of idiotopic clones among different strains. The regulatory mechanisms that control the frequency of Ig-7 idiotopic clone remain unknown at present.

TABLE V
Expression of Ig-7 Idiotope on Serum and Hybridoma Anti-GAT Antibodies

Strain	*Igh* allele	Concentration of Ig-7 idiotope (μg/ml)[a]
BALB/c	a	0.4
B10.A	b	500
DBA/2	c	2.5
A/J	e	720
SEA/GN	h	2
C3H/He	j	30
NZB	n	50

No. of CGAT hybridomas	Strain	% inhibition of Ig-7 idiotope binding
18	B6 or B10	91–100
1	C3H.SW	85
2	C3H.SW	0; 15
7	DBA/2	0–5

[a]Samples were incubated with 1 μl of culture supernatant of a monoclonal anti-idiotope hybridoma for 1 hr and the mixtures were transferred into microtiter wells that were previously coated with an Ig-7 idiotope-bearing F17.174.3 hybridoma antibody. The bound anti-idiotope was measured with ^{125}I-labeled rabbit anti-rat immunoglobulin antibodies that were adsorbed with mouse immunoglobulin-conjugated immunosorbents. Concentration of Ig-7 idiotope was calculated by a standard curve generated with purified F17.174.3 antibody. The sensitivity of the assay is 0.1 μg/ml.

6. Concluding Remarks

Serological analysis of idiotypic determinants on antibody molecules is an efficient method to probe the variable-region structures of specific antibodies. These studies have provided general immunological, immunochemical, and genetic properties of the idiotypic antibodies. However, the idiotypic structures identified will remain elusive in the absence of information on the three-dimensional structure of the specific antibodies. In the BALB/c antidextran idiotypic system, amino acid sequence study has identified one or a few important residues responsible for the expression of a defined idiotypic specificity.[25] Whether such correlation between idiotypes and amino acid residues can be resolved in the more complex anti-GAT idiotypic system remains to be determined. In this regard, the many idiotypic markers that are identified in the anti-GAT idiotypic families will be extremely useful in the effort to correlate idiotypes with the amino acid sequences of anti-GAT antibodies. Finally, it is expected that the V_H and V_L DNA sequences of both germline- and somatic-derived genes will be obtained in the near future. This information will provide a better understanding of the relationship between evolutionary and somatic changes in these genes and the expression of a defined idiotype.

ACKNOWLEDGMENTS. I thank Drs. M. E. Dorf, M. Pierres, R. Germain, S. H. Pincus, and B. Benacerraf for their encouragement and invaluable suggestions.

References

1. Dorf, M. E., Plate, J. M. D., Stimpfling, J. H., and Benacerraf, B., 1975, Characterization of immune response and mixed leukocyte reactions in selected intra-H-2 recombinant strains, *J. Immunol.* **114:**602–605.

2. Gershon, R. K., Maurer, P. H., and Merryman, C. F., 1973, A cellular basis for genetically controlled immunologic-unresponsiveness in mice: Tolerance induction in T cells, *Proc. Natl. Acad. Sci. USA* **70:**250–254.

3. Kapp, J. A., Pierce, C. W., and Benacerraf, B., 1974, Genetic control of immune responses *in vitro*. III. Tolerogenic properties of the terpolymer L-glutamic acid^{60}-L-alanine^{30}-L-tyrosine^{10} (GAT) for spleen cells from nonresponder (H-2^s and H-2^q) mice, *J. Exp. Med.* **140:**172–184.

4. Kapp, J. A., Pierce, C. W., DelaCroix, F., and Benacerraf, B., 1976, Immunosuppressive factor(s) extracted from lymphoid cells of nonresponder mice primed with L-glutamic acid^{60}-L-alanine^{30}-L-tyrosine^{10} (GAT). I. Activity and antigenic specificity, *J. Immunol.* **116:**305–309.

5. Thèze, J., Kapp, J. A., and Benacerraf, B, 1977, Immunosuppressive factor(s) extracted from lymphoid cells of nonresponder mice primed with L-glutamic acid^{60}-L-alanine^{30}-L-tyrosine^{10} (GAT). III. Immunochemical properties of the GAT-specific suppressive factor, *J. Exp. Med.* **145:**839–856.

6. Germain, R. N., Ju, S.-T., Kipps, T. J., Benacerraf, B., and Dorf, M. E., 1979, Shared idiotypic determinants on antibodies and T cell derived suppressor factor specific for the random terpolymer L-glutamic acid^{60}-L-alanine^{30}-L-tyrosine^{10}, *J. Exp. Med.* **149:**613–622.

7. Kapp, J. A., Araneo, B. A., Ju, S.-T., and Dorf, M. E., 1981, Immunogenetics of monoclonal suppressor T cell products, in: *Immunoglobulin Idiotypes* (C. A. Janeway, Jr., E. E. Sercarz, and H. Wigzell, eds.), Academic Press, New York, pp. 387–396.

8. Lei, H. Y., Ju, S.-T., Dorf, M. E., and Waltenbaugh, C., 1983, Regulation of immune response by I-J gene products. III. GT-specific suppressor factor is composed of separable I-J and idiotype-bearing chains, *J. Immunol.* **130:**1274–1279.

9. Ju, S.-T., Dorf, M. E., and Benacerraf, B., 1979, Idiotypic analysis of anti-GAT antibodies. III. Determinant specificity and immunoglobulin class distribution of CGAT idiotype, *J. Immunol.* **122:**1054–1059.

10. Ju, S.-T., Kipps, T. J., Thèze, J., Benacerraf, B, and Dorf, M. E., 1978, Idiotypic analysis of anti-GAT antibodies. I. Presence of common idiotypic specificities in both responder and nonresponder mice, *J. Immunol.* **121:**1034–1039.

11. Ju, S.-T., Benacerraf, B., and Dorf, M. E., 1978, Idiotypic analysis of antibodies to poly(Glu^{60}Ala^{30}Tyr^{10}): Interstrain and interspecies idiotypic cross-reactions, *Proc. Natl. Acad. Sci. USA* **75:**6192–6196.

12. Somme, G., Leclercq, L., Petit, C., and Thèze, J., 1981, Genetic control of the immune response to the L-Glu^{60}-L-Ala^{30}-L-Tyr^{10} (GAT) terpolymer. V. Three types of idiotypic specificities on BALB/c anti-GAT antibodies, *Eur. J. Immunol.* **11:**493–498.

13. Ju, S.-T., Cramer, D. V., and Dorf, M. E., 1979, Idiotypic analysis of anti-GAT antibodies. V. Distribution of an interspecies cross-reactive idiotype, *J. Immunol.* **123:**877–883.

14. Bothwell, A. L. M., Paskind, M., Reth, M., Imanishi-Kari, T., Rajewsky, K., and Baltimore, D., 1981, NP^b family of antibodies: Somatic mutation evident in a gamma-29 variable region, *Cell* **24:**625–637.

15. Crews, S., Griffin, J., Huang, H., Calame, K., and Hood, L., 1981, A single V$_H$ gene segment encodes the immune response to phosphorylcholine: Somatic mutation is correlated with the class of the antibody, *Cell* **25:**59–66.

16. Ruf, J., Tonnelle, C., Rocca-Serra, J., Moinier, D., Pierres, M., Ju, S.-T., Dorf, M. E., Thèze, J., and Fougereau, M., 1983, Structural basis for public idiotypic specificities of monoclonal antibodies directed against poly(Glu^{60},Ala^{30},Tyr^{10})n (GAT) and poly(Glu^{60},Ala^{40})n (GA) random polymers, *Proc. Natl. Acad. Sci. USA* **80:**3040–3044.

17. Ju, S.-T., and Dorf, M. E., 1979, Idiotypic analysis of anti-GAT antibodies. IV. Induction of CGAT idiotype following immunization with various synthetic polymers containing glutamic acid and tyrosine, *Eur. J. Immunol.* **9:**553–560.

17a. Ju, S -T., Pincus, S. H., Kunar, J., and Dorf, M. E., 1984, Immunoselection of B-cell hybridomas with anti-idiotypic antisera to study the role of heavy and light chains for idiotype expression and antibody activity, *J. Immunol.* **132:**2485–2490.

18. Ju, S.-T., Pierres, M., Waltenbaugh, C., Germain, R. N., Benacerraf, B., and Dorf, M. E., 1979, Idiotypic analysis of monoclonal antibodies to poly-(Glu^{60}Ala^{30}Tyr^{10}), *Proc. Natl. Acad. Sci. USA* **76:**2942–2946.

19. Ju, S.-T., Pincus, S. H., Stocks, C. J., Jr., Pierres, M., and Dorf, M. E., 1982, Idiotypic analysis of hybridoma antibodies to branched synthetic polymer (Tyr,Glu)-Ala-Lys: Idiotypic relationship with antibodies to linear random polymer (Glu^{60},Ala^{30},Tyr^{10}), *J. Immunol.* **128:**545–550.

20. Leclercq, L., Mazie, J., Somme, G., and Thèze, J., 1982, Monoclonal anti-GAT antibodies with different fine specificities express the same public idiotype, *Mol. Immunol.* **19:**1001–1007.

21. Ju, S.-T., Pierres, M., Germain, R. N., Benacerraf, B., and Dorf, M. E., 1979, Idiotypic analysis of anti-GAT antibodies. VI. Identification and strain distribution of the GA-1 idiotype, *J. Immunol.* **123:**2505–2510.

22. Ju, S.-T., Pierres, M., Germain, R., Benacerraf, B., and Dorf, M. E., 1980, Idiotypic analysis of anti-GAT antibodies. VII. Common idiotype on hybridoma antibodies to poly(Glu^{60}Ala^{40}), *J. Immunol.* **125:**1230–1236.

23. Ju, S.-T., Pierres, M., Germain, R. N., Benacerraf, B., and Dorf, M. E., 1981, Idiotypic analysis of anti-GAT antibodies. VIII. Comparison of interstrain and allotype-associated idiotypic specificities, *J. Immunol.* **126:**177–182.

24. Ju, S.-T., and Dorf, M. E., 1981, Idiotypic analysis of anti-GAT antibodies. IX. Genetic mapping of the Gte idiotypic markers within the Igh-V locus, *J. Immunol.* **126:**183–186.

25. Schilling, J., Clevinger, B., Davie, J. M., and Hood, L., 1980, Amino acid sequence of homogenous antibodies to dextran and DNA rearrangements in heavy chain V-region gene segements, *Nature* **283:**35–37.

14

Cross-Reacting Idiotypes in the Human System

Henry G. Kunkel

1. Introduction

One of the most striking phenomena regarding anti-idiotypic antisera and monoclonal antibodies is the remarkable cross-reactions observed. This is certainly true in the human system. These cross-reactions extend well beyond simple immunoglobulin variable regions but also involve ordinary cell receptors as well as the T-cell receptors for specific antigens. In fact, the latter cross-reaction between immunoglobulins and T-cells receptors has been misleading and led to the broad impression that similar V genes are involved. Current evidence indicates that this is not the case.[1,2] Much of the work in the human system has been carried out on autoantibodies, particularly those that appear in monoclonal form. Idiotypic cross-reactions are striking in these autoantibodies, and this may be a special characteristic of these antibodies. In this discussion a number of these autoantibody systems will be reviewed with special emphasis on the chemical basis for certain of the cross-reacting idiotypes (CRI). In addition, recent work on T-cell-specific idiotypes and CRIs will be discussed.

2. Idiotypic Cross-Reactions among the Cold Agglutinins

The first description of a CRI system in any species was that for cold agglutinin antibodies in unrelated humans[3,4] and this remains one of the most striking. These autoantibodies appear in monoclonal form and lead to hemolytic anemia through destruction of the patient's red blood cells. The antigen involved in most cases is the I antigen which is a part of the blood group system. Another group of cold agglutinins involves the Pr antigen of red blood cells. Two distinct CRI systems are involved for these two different specificities.

Henry G. Kunkel (Deceased) • The Rockefeller University, New York, New York.

Most of the work on cold agglutinins has been carried out with rabbit antisera but some of this work has been confirmed recently with monoclonal antibodies. Certain highly selected antisera, after thorough absorption with pooled IgM and IgG, show high specificity for cold agglutinin proteins with I specificity. Figure 1 shows this specificity in terms of precipitin reactions. In this study no monoclonal IgM protein without this activity showed precipitin lines (more than 70 such proteins were examined). It should be emphasized that other antisera showed some specificity for these cold agglutinins, but this activity was lost following very thorough absorption with normal IgM. Such antisera detected primarily rare V-region subgroups and were very different from the selected type, as illustrated in Fig. 1, where the reactivity could not be absorbed out even when huge amounts of normal immunoglobulins were added.

An important point regarding this cold agglutinin's CRI in addition to the high specificity is that multiple antigens are involved. Figure 2 shows an agar plate with the same absorbed antiserum shown in Fig. 1, but in this case the Fab fragments of the proteins were utilized and optimal conditions arranged to show subrelationships between these proteins. The spurs observed in Fig. 2 demonstrate that at least three different antigenic groups can be distinguished. These minor but clearcut differences have not been as readily shown in the current commonly utilized radioimmune and ELISA assays. Individual monoclonal antibodies would not be expected to show these differences and this remains an important aspect in making comparisons.

The Pr cold agglutinins also showed a CRI that was entirely different than that for the I cold agglutinins.[5] the Pr type are of special interest because they illustrate the ever-present problem of distinguishing CRI reactions which involve hypervariable regions, usually in the vicinity of the combining site, from uncommon V-region subgroups. The Pr cold agglutinins all appear to have the same type of κ light chain which is clearly distinguishable from other κ types by sequence analysis.[6] This type of light chain is also found in low incidence in all normal individuals and is clearly present in proteins lacking cold agglutinin activity. Specific antibodies to these light chains are rather readily obtained and would be present in many Pr antisera either alone or together with a true CRI. Moderate absorption of the antiserum which might appear to be adequate would probably not remove these antibodies and the antiserum would be considered a CRI type when it in reality was specific for a non-hypervariable-region antigen reflecting a κ light-chain subgroup. Many presumed CRIs reported in the mouse and human system may be of this type. In addition, this type of subgroup antigen in reacting with its antibody might be blocked by antigen. Many investigators in the field consider antigen inhibition as entirely indicative of an idiotypic system. This is definitely not the case. Studies with Rh antibodies have shown that

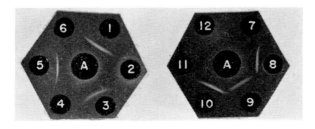

FIGURE 1. Specific reaction of an absorbed cold agglutinin antiserum with six different cold agglutinins. Macroglobulins without this activity failed to react. A, Absorbed anti-cold agglutinin; 1–12, different macroglobulins; 1, 3, 5, 8, 9, 10, cold agglutinins.[3]

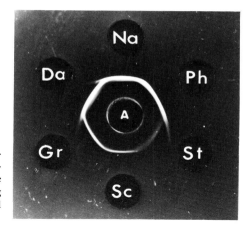

FIGURE 2. Cross-idiotypic reactions among cold agglutinins under optimal conditions for observing fine differences. Spurs indicate that multiple antigens are
involved in this CRI. The reaction with the immunizing
antigen βm is not shown. A, βm absorbed anti-cold
agglutinin.

the Rh antigen will block the reaction of Rh antibodies with antibodies to several common
light- and heavy-chain subgroups.[7]

3. Idiotypic Cross-Reactions among the Anti-γ-globulins

These are the most common of the autoantibodies both in the human and in the mouse.
They also represent the most common activity appearing in monoclonal form in disease. As
a result they represent a particularly good system for cross-idiotypic studies. Earlier work
with rabbit antisera clearly showed the occurrence of widely distributed cross-idiotypes in
this system.[8] At least three types were delineated in human sera. The Po group was a
minor type that showed a CRI that clearly distinguished this group. Sequence analyses of
the V regions of the heavy and light chains showed remarkable similarities with virtually
identical hypervariable areas, especially of the heavy chains.[9] Approximately 15% of the
anti-γ-globulins belonged to this subtype.

The Wa group represented the major type, with approximately 70% of the monoclonal
anti-γ-globulins included, and it is evident that this type is a significant component of the
anti-γ-globulins in rheumatoid arthritis sera. It has the striking characteristic that all the
proteins have very similar light chains, which are of the V_κIIIb subgroup.[10] This subgroup
of κ chains is readily recognized by specific antisera which were described and correlated
with amino acid sequences a number of years ago.[11] The rabbit antisera which defined
the Wa group of anti-γ-globulins appear to have had one type of antibody which recognized
these light chains only in association with μ heavy chains, because absorption with V_κIIIb
light chains as well as IgG and IgA proteins with light chains of this type did not remove
the Wa group specificity.[10] In addition, these antisera also contained other specificities that
more closely resembled a classical CRI but exactly which dominated is not apparent; the
use of monoclonal antibodies has clarified the issue considerably. Figure 3 shows the amino
acid sequence of light chains of two of these anti-γ-globulins as compared to the prototype
sequence of a typical V_κIIIb protein.[12] The three sequences are very similar with only two

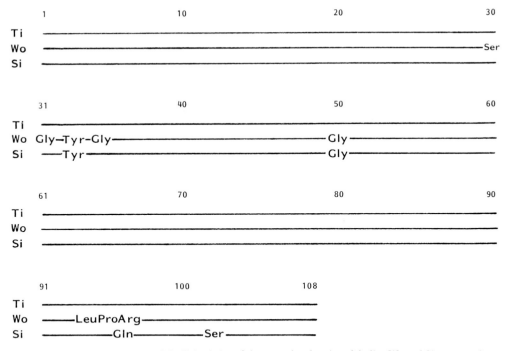

FIGURE 3. Amino acid sequence of the light chains of the monoclonal anti-γ-globulins Wo and Si, compared to a prototype V$_κ$ IIIb light chain (Ti).

positions which might be specific for the anti-γ-globulins. Sequence analyses[12] of the heavy chains of the same two proteins showed wide differences, especially in all the hypervariable areas, in striking contrast to the Po group described above. The only similarity present was in the J segment; studies are currently under way on the heavy chains of a third Wa protein to establish the significance of this finding. It appears likely that the Wa specificity defined by the rabbit antisera reflects a nonspecific V$_κ$IIIb light chain with a specific heavy-chain J segment. Also this combination may provide the combining specificity for the Fc portion of IgG. Recombination experiments with V$_κ$IIIb light chains of proteins without anti-γ-globulin activity would answer these questions, but these are particularly difficult with IgM antibodies.

Studies carried out with Dr. Pernis[13] have demonstrated that the Wa-type rabbit antisera reacted specifically with stimulated B cells from rheumatoid arthritis patients. It was clear that isolated polyclonal rheumatoid factors from patients with rheumatoid arthritis had a high content of proteins of this specificity. Thus, it was evident that a broadly reactive type of CRI was involved.

Recently, monclonal antibodies have been produced by Dr. Posnett in our laboratory to proteins of the major Wa group.[14,15] Figure 4 shows the reactivity of four of these with various proteins, including members of the specific group. Various patterns are observed with the different monoclonals in this radioimmunoassay. The first pattern shows total private idiotypy with reactions only with the immunizing protein and slight reaction with the heavy chains of this protein. The second pattern is an anti-V$_\kappa$IIIb antibody that was obtained in this fusion. The antibodies react with the light chains of the immunizing protein and four other light chains known to be of the V$_\kappa$IIIb type.[10] They also react with IgG, IgA and other IgM proteins of this light-chain type. These antibodies give the appearance of a CRI; they react with a small population of normal immunoglobulins with these light chains ($\sim$ 5–10%) but react with a much higher proportion of rheumatoid factors of both the monoclonal and the polyclonal type. However, in reality they just represent a V-region subgroup based on framework residues of the light chains. The earlier studies with rabbit antisera clearly recognized antibodies of this type which reacted with a high proportion of rheumatoid factors. These antibodies could be readily absorbed out leaving the CRI that was well recognized. A third type of pattern is also illustrated in Fig. 4. This does not relate to the V$_\kappa$IIIb system since various IgM proteins with such light chains do not show binding. It shows considerable specificity for anti-γ-globulins but does not react with all anti-γ-globulins. This appears to represent a monoclonal antibody with a true CRI specificity. A fourth type of pattern was also recognized. Here there is IgM specificity that relates closely to V$_\kappa$IIIb light chains but the antibody does not recognize IgG, IgA, or free light chains of this specificity. This type of restriction to IgM proteins was frequently observed in this study and suggests that possibly a portion of the constant area of IgM is involved in the antigenic site along with the V region. However, other possibilities are perhaps more likely. In the case illustrated, the V$_\kappa$IIIb light chain probably assumes a configuration after binding chains of IgM that is specific.

No monoclonal antibody was obtained in this sutdy that exactly duplicates the pattern of reactivity obtained with the earlier studies with rabbit antisera. It would appear that a mixture of these antibodies is involved as might be expected. V$_\kappa$IIIb reactivity solely on

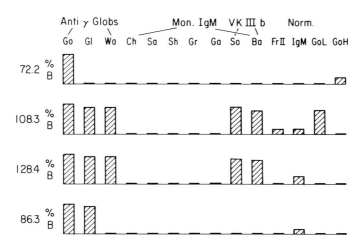

FIGURE 4. Percent binding by ELISA assay of four different monoclonal antibodies against various proteins illustrated by the bars. The proteins, listed at the top, consist of three isolated IgM anti-γ-globulins, seven IgM monoclonal proteins lacking anti-IgG activity, FrII, normal IgM, and heavy and light chains of anti-γ-globulin Go, the immunizing protein. Two nonspecific IgM proteins with V$_\kappa$IIIb light chains are also shown at the top.

TABLE I

Percent Positive Cells by Fluorescence with Two Monoclonal Antibodies (86.3
and 108.1) after Stimulation with PWM of Rheumatoid Arthritis and Normal
Lymphocytes[a]

		Hemagglutination titer	% positive cells	
			86.3	108.1
RA	1	20,000	16.4	18.3
	2	15,000	22.6	24.2
	3	12,000	14.2	16.0
	4	800	14.8	16.8
	5	20	10.2	12.0
	6	0	11.6	14.6
	7	0	9.5	12.9
Normal	1	—	0.4	0.1
	2	—	1.2	0.8
	3	—	0.6	1.1

[a] Antibody 108.1 is reactive with V_κIIIb light chains.

IgM proteins certainly represents one component of the system but others are involved
which gave the rabbit antisera their high specificity for anti-γ-globulins that was observed.

Recently, a report appeared[16] suggesting the finding of a monoclonal antibody produced against a mixed population of rheumatoid factors that shows high specificity for anti-
γ-globulins of all types with little or no reaction with normal immunoglobulins. A surprising feature of this study is that two proteins of ours were utilized which have been
completely sequenced through the V regions of the heavy and light chains. These proteins
were considered totally different in our earlier CRI studies and their sequences in both
framework and hypervariable areas are very different. The explanation for their common
reactivity with this monoclonal antibody which is so highly specific remains a mystery.
Perhaps it is necessary to involve the internal image concept[17] where the antibody sees the
internal image of the antigen, in this case the Fc fragment of IgG, and structurally dissimilar antibodies would be specifically recognized. This situation would be analogous to the
situation where anti-idiotypic antibodies made against an antibody to a specific antigen such
as insulin also react with ordinary insulin receptors.[18] The structure of the latter has not
been defined but it is unlikely that it resembles antibody to insulin. The only apparent
common property of the two molecules is that they bind insulin. In the current situation,
sequence data are available and, if the work can be confirmed, show that two very different
anti-γ-globulins can show similar reactivity with a highly specific monoclonal antibody.

Thus, a wide spectrum of monoclonal antibodies are becoming available in the anti-
γ-globulin system showing quite different CRI specificities. These range from those involving the V_κIIIb light chains, which are the least specific, to the uniquely specific type mentioned above.

One of the most interesting findings with the monoclonal antibodies against anti-γ-
globulins is their reaction selectively with proteins in rheumatoid arthritis sera that lack
anti-γ-globulin activity. High levels of V_κIIIb light-chain-containing immunoglobulins
appear to be present in such sera even in the absence of anti-γ-globulins. This is also true

of the other two antibodies illustrated in Fig. 4. Table I shows this type of reactivity utilizing the Pernis procedure of staining mitogen-stimulated B cells with the various antibodies by the fluorescent antibody technique. It is clear that the cells from certain patients with rheumatoid arthritis show a high percentage of stained cells even when no rheumatoid factor was found in the serum by hemagglutination analyses with red cells coated with IgG. This is of special interest because the occurrence of rheumatoid factor-negative cases of rheumatoid arthritis has always been thought to diminish the significance of rheumatoid factors in the disease. The occurence of the CRI detected with antibody 86.3 in these negative cases suggests that related proteins are present. It may be that these are similar to rheumatoid factors but are of such low binding affinity for IgG that they are not picked up by the serological methods utilized for rheumatoid factor analysis. The high levels of cells producing $V_\kappa IIIb$ immunoglobulins in rheumatoid arthritis are also of interest.

4. Other Systems with Broadly Cross-Reactive Idiotypes

Another remarkable CRI system has been observed for thyroglobulin antibodies.[19] Rabbit antisera have been obtained to isolated thyroglobulin antibody purified from a patient with chronic thyroiditis. These antibodies reacted with a high percentage of thyroglobulin antibodies from all of a large number of patients examined and not with other immunoglobulins. Table II shows the correlation of reactivity with the thyroglobulin antibody titer for different thyroiditis sera. If these antibodies were removed from these sera on

TABLE II

Inhibition of Binding in Thyroglobulin Antibody–Anti-idiotype System by IgG of Various Thyroiditis Sera[a]

Serum No.	Thyroid test (maximum dilution)	% inhibition IgG (µg)					
		1	5	10	50	250	500
101	> × 409,600	16	39	41	58	62	60
102	> × 409,600	6	25	30	54	49	60
103	> × 409,600	5	24	46	49	64	61
104	> × 409,600	1	8	22	37	62	67
105	> × 409,600	0	20	16	35	52	53
106	> × 409,600	0	0	0	21	41	45
107	× 6,400	0	0	8	30	57	61
108	× 6,400	0	0	0	31	41	46
109	× 400	0	0	7	12	34	43
110	× 400	0	0	0	0	16	30
111	× 20	0	0	5	15	27	41
112	< × 20	0	0	12	18	48	55
113	< × 20	0	0	4	17	31	26
114	< × 20	0	0	0	0	3	19
115	< × 20	0	0	0	0	4	0

[a]From Ref. 19.

thyroglobulin columns, the reactivity completely disappeared. Thus, these workers clearly had produced a very broadly reactive CRI which showed little or no interaction with normal immunoglobulins.

Also, in the DNA antibody system a definite CRI has been found.[20] A monoclonal antibody has been obtained which showed increased reactivity with the sera of eight of nine SLE patients with anti-native DNA antibodies and much lower reactivity for SLE sera without detectable DNA antibodies. Control sera showed very low reactivity. This study was hampered by the lack of monoclonal band sera from which to obtain pure anti-DNA antibodies for comparative studies as in the anti-γ-globulin system. The antibody reacted with a significant proportion but not all of the DNA antibody purified from SLE serum. CRI antibodies also have been obtained[21] from human monoclonal antibodies. This is a very complete story in which the monoclonal DNA antibodies have replaced the homogeneous antibodies that proved so useful in the cold agglutinin and anti-γ-globulin systems and was missing in the DNA system described above. Evidence for different CRI determinants was clear.

5. Characterization of Idiotypic Receptors on T Cells

Rapid progress has been made recently in obtaining anti-idiotypic antibodies to T-cell clones either produced with IL-2 or naturally occurring as T-cell leukemias. This work is proceeding in the human system very rapidly and basic answers regarding the T-cell receptors and their mechanism of variability should soon be available. A number of T-cell clones have been obtained from *in vitro* allostimulated T cells to which idiotype-specific monoclonal antibodies have been obtained.[22] These antibodies specifically block allostimulation and have thus far been clone specific. They have proven very useful for the characterization of the receptor on the T-cell clone. In general, molecules of approximately 90,000 daltons have been obtained under nonreducing conditions which, under reducing conditions, split into two components of approximately 43,000 to 49,000 daltons.[22] Clones with different properties have given similar molecules.

Our own studies in this area have been carried out on T–T hybrids with specific properties and also with T-cell leukemias, with and without specific activities. Antibodies made to the latter have proven of special interest. The large number of cells available from these leukemia patients makes this system especially useful for detailed chemical analyses. Anti-idiotype-like antibodies have been obtained from immunization of mice with two different leukemic cells and one T–T hybrid. These antibodies only react with the immunizing cell and not with other normal or leukemic T cells or other types of cells. All of these antibodies have given molecules that in general are similar, i.e., heterodimers are obtained by disulfide bond reduction of a parent molecule. One of these (Su) has been studied in special detail.[23] Figure 5 shows a molecule of approximately 80,000 daltons which on reduction gives two bands of unequal intensity at approximately 43,000 and the other at 38,000. In two-dimensional gels utilizing isoelectric focusing in the second dimension each band splits into closely related subunits.

A second monoclonal antibody to the above Su leukemic cells is of special interest because in addition to having high specificity for the immunizing cell it shows reactivity

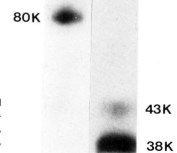

FIGURE 5. SDS gels of the molecules precipitated from the labeled membranes of the T cells of leukemia Su with the anti-idiotypic antibodies made to these cells. The band on the left, approximately 80K, is seen prior to reduction and this dissociates to two bands on the right, 43K and 38K, after reduction.

with a small population of normal T cells, approximately 2% in all normal individuals. The monoclonal antibody described above and illustrated in Fig. 5 does not show this reaction with normal cells. Gel analyses indicate, however, that the same molecules are brought down by the two antibodies. In addition, removal of the antigen with one antibody removes reactivity with the other. Both antibodies are modulated by T3 or Leu-4 T-cell antibodies. Thus, it is apparent that the two antibodies react with the same molecules but at different sites. It seems highly likely that the one sees a private idiotype and the second probably a CRI. None of the antibodies react with B cells or immunoglobulins.

Private idiotype monoclonal antibodies of this type may prove useful in the therapy of these T-cell leukemias.

6. Summary

Various human cross-reactive idiotype systems have been reviewed, some of which are remarkable in their unique specificity for and broad occurrence among proteins with a given antibody activity. Cold agglutinins, anti-γ-globulins, thyroglobulin antibodies, and DNA antibodies show these wide specificities. These are all autoantibodies, and possibly this is related to their special cross-reactions. The anti-γ-globulins have been studied in greatest detail and numerous monoclonal antibodies are available, defining specific types of cross-reactions. Many of these proteins have the V_κIIIb-type light chains as determined by both antigenic and sequence analysis; the chains occur at low incidence among normal immunoglobulins. This type of light chain together with J-segment similarities in the heavy chain appear to confer anti-γ-globulin activity despite marked differences in the heavy-chain hypervariable areas. V_κIIIb proteins as well as cross-reactive idiotypes were found at increased incidence in rheumatoid arthritis cases that were negative for anti-γ-globulin activity.

Clonotypic antibodies against T-cell clones and T-cell leukemic cells are proving particularly informative regarding private and public idiotype-like molecules on T cells. Disulfide-linked heterodimers are clearly involved.

References

1. Kraig, E., Kronenberg, M., Kapp, J. A., Pierce, C. W., Abruzzini, A. F., Sorensen, C. M., Salemson, L. E., Schwartz, R. H., and Hood, L. E., 1983, T and B cells that recognize the same antigen do not contain detectable heavy-chain variable gene transcripts, *J. Exp. Med.* **158**(1):210–227.
2. Kronenberg, M., Kraig, E., Siu, G., Kapp, J. A., Kappler, J., Marrack, P., Pierce, C. W., and Hood, L.,1983, Three T cell hybridomas do not contain detectable heavy-chain variable gene transcripts, *J. Exp. Med.* **158**(a):210–227.
3. Williams, R. C., Kunkel, H. G., and Capra, J. D., 1968, Antigenic specificities related to cold agglutinin activity of gamma M globulins, *Science* **161**:379.
4. Kabat, E. A., and Mayer, M. M., 1961, *Experimental Immunochemistry* Thomas, Springfield, Ill.
5. Feizi, T., Kunkel, H. G., and Roelcke, D., 1974, Cross idiotypic specificity among cold agglutinins in relation to combining activity for blood group-related antigens, *Clin. Exp. Immunol.* **18**:283–293.
6. Wang, A. C., Fudenberg, H. H., Wells, J. V., and Roelcke, D., 1973, A new subgroup of the kappa chain variable region associated with anti-Pr cold agglutinins, *Nature (New Biol.)* **243**:126.
7. Kunkel, H. G., Joslin, F., and Hurley, J., 1976, Blocking of certain antigenic sites in the Fab region by combination of univalent fragments of Rh antibodies with red cell antigens, *J. Immunol.* **116**:1532–1535.
8. Kunkel, H. G., Agnello, V., Joslin, F. G., Winchester, R. J., and Capra, J. D., 1973, Cross idiotypic specificity among monoclonal IgM proteins with anti-γ-globulin activity, *J. Exp. Med.* **137**:331.
9. Capra, J. D., and Kehoe, J. M., 1974, Structure of antibodies with shared idiotypy: The complete sequence of the heavy chain variable regions of two IgM antigamma globulins, *Proc. Natl. Acad. Sci. USA* **71**:4032–4036.
10. Kunkel, H. G., Winchester, R. J., Joslin, F. G., and Capra, J. D., 1974, Similarities in the light chains of anti-γ globulins showing cross-idiotypic specificities, *J. Exp. Med.* **139**:128–136.
11. McLaughlin, C. L., and Solomon, A., 1972, Bence–Jones proteins and light chains of immunoglobulins, *J. Biol. Chem.* **247**:5017.
12. Andrews, D. W., and Capra, J. D., 1981, Complete amino acid sequence of variable domains from two monoclonal human anti-gamma globulins of the Wa cross-idiotypic group: Suggestion that the J segments are involved in the structural correlate of the idiotype, *Proc. Natl. Acad. Sci. USA* **78**:3799–3803.
13. Bonagura, V. R., Kunkel, H. G., and Pernis, B., 1982, Cellular localization of rheumatoid factor idiotypes, *J. Clin. Invest.* **69**:1356–1365.
14. Kunkel, H. H., Posnett, D. N., and Pernis, B., 1983, Anti-Igs and their idiotypes: Are they part of the immune network? in: *Immune Networks* (C. A. Bona and H. Kohler, eds.), *Ann. NY Acad. Sci.* **418**:324–329.
15. Posnett, D. N., Pernis, B., and Kunkel, H. G., 1984, Dissection of the anti-γ globulin idiotype system with monoclonal antibodies, in preparation.
16. Pasquali, J. L., Urlacher, A., and Storck, D., 1983, A highly conserved determinant on human rheumatoid factor idiotypes defined by a mouse monoclonal antibody, *Eur. J. Immunol.* **13**:197–201.
17. Westen-Schnurr, I. (ed.), 1982, *Idiotypes, Antigens on the Inside,* Roche Press, Basel.
18. Sege, K., and Peterson, P. A., 1978, Use of anti-idiotypic antibodies as cell-surface receptor probes, *Proc. Natl. Acad. Sci. USA* **75**:2443–2447.
19. Matsuyama, J., Fukumori, J., and Tanaka, H., 1983, Evidence of unique idiotypic determinants and similar idiotypic determinants on human antithyroglobulin antibodies, *Clin. Exp. Immunol.* **51**:381–386.
20. Solomon, G., Schiffenbauer, J., Keiser, H. D., and Diamond, B., 1983, The use of monoclonal antibodies to identify shared idiotypes on human antibodies to native DNA from patients with systemic lupus erythematosus, *Proc. Natl. Acad. Sci. USA* **80**:850.
21. Shoenfeld, Y., Isenberg, D. A., Rauch, J., Madaio, M. P., Stollar, B. D., and Schwartz, R. S., 1983, Idiotypic cross reactions of monoclonal human lupus autoantibodies, *J. Exp. Med.* **158**(3):718–730.
22. Meuer, S.C., Fitztgerald, K. A., Hussey, R. E., Hodgdon, J. C., Schlossman, S. F., and Reinherz, E. L., 1983, Clonotypic structures involved in antigen specific human T cell function: Relationship to the T3 molecular complex *J. Exp. Med.* **157**:705.
23. Bigler, R., Fisher, D., Wang, C. Y., and Kunkel, H. G., 1983, Two types of clonotypic monoclonal antibodies to the cells of a human T cell leukemia, *J. Exp. Med.* **158**(3):1000–1003.

PART III
REGULATION OF IDIOTYPES

15

Genetic and Environmental Control of B-Cell Idiotype Expression

DORITH ZHARHARY, RICHARD L. RILEY,
BARBARA G. FROSCHER, AND NORMAN R. KLINMAN

1. Introduction

Since the earliest demonstrations that the immune system of an individual has the capacity to recognize its own antibody variable regions, the potential role of such anti-idiotypic recognition in the regulation of immune responses has gained considerable attention.[1,2] Studies which have utilized the passive transfer of anti-idiotypic antibodies have defined several levels at which anti-idiotypic recognition can affect immune responsiveness.[3-12] These include the inhibition of antigenic stimulation of idiotype-positive cells,[3-5] the direct stimulation of idiotype-positive cells,[5-8] the elimination of B cells of the appropriate idiotype from within the mature B-cell repertoire,[9,10] and the enhancement of the expression of idiotype-positive cells.[11,12] Finally, the physiological relevance of idiotypic recognition has been demonstrated by the finding that such recognition becomes a predominant feature of the immune system subsequent to immunization.[13]

Although the potential importance of idiotype recognition in immune responsiveness is now clearly recognized, many fundamental aspects of this regulatory mechanism remain unresolved. First, it is not clear whether idiotypic recognition, at a level consistent with regulatory function, normally exists before antigenic stimulation. Second, it is not clear whether idiotypic recognition, in the absence of antigenic stimulation, plays any role in shaping the primary B-cell repertoire. Obtaining answers to these questions is made far more difficult by the presence of maternal antibodies in neonates and the continuous presence of ubiquitous environmental or self antigens. This may ensure the existence of a sub-

DORITH ZHARHARY, RICHARD L. RILEY, BARBARA G. FROSCHER, AND NORMAN R. KLINMAN • Department of Immunology, Scripps Clinic and Research Foundation, La Jolla, California 92037.

stantial background of anti-idiotypic reactivity which would be superimposed on the emerging immune system, particularly with respect to certain sets of reactivities..

One experimental finding is consistent with the conclusion that "natural"or preexisting anti-idiotypic recognition plays a minimal role in the immune system of normal, young, conventionally reared mice. The experiments which have led to this tentative conclusion represent the controls carried out in a large series of experiments which originally demonstrated the onset of anti-idiotypic recognition following conventional antigenic stimulation.[13] The results of these experiments are presented in Fig. 1. These experiments utilized the fragment culture system to assess the relative capabilities for supporting hapten-specific B-cell responses of mice which had been only carrier-primed versus those which had been hapten- as well as carrier-primed. It can be seen that mice immunized with 2,4-dinitrophenyl-hemocyanin (DNP-Hy) together with Hy, developed the capacity to specifically suppress responses of primary, syngeneic DNP-specific B cells. Importantly, the suppression was long-lived, specific only for DNP-reactive B cells, and did not suppress secondary B cells. That this antigen-induced suppression is idiotype-specific is inferred from control experiments which demonstrated that primary DNP-specific B cells derived from donors (CB.20) differing only in the allotype–idiotype-linked genetic locus were not at all suppressed in hapten–carrier-primed recipients. Indeed, the frequency of response of such allotype–idiotype-mismatched donors upon transfer to hapten–carrier-primed recipients was precisely the same as the frequency of response of their B cells in allotype-syngeneic recipients which had only been carrier-primed. The fact that responses of such B cells are identical in syngeneic and allotypically mismatched carrier-primed recipients also demonstrates that idiotype-specific suppression of this type does not exist in the syngeneic host prior to priming with the relevant determinant itself. This latter finding has now been confirmed for a large number of antigenic determinants.

Although the above experiments are indicative of a minimal role for idiotypic recog-

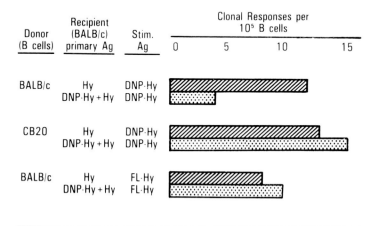

FIGURE 1. Antibody-specific immunoregulation. 4×10^6 donor cells were transferred to each recipient. All donor and recipient strains are of the $H\text{-}2^d$ haplotype. Cultures were stimulated *in vitro* with DNP-Hy at 10^{-6} M DNP or fluorescein-Hy (FL-Hy) at 10^{-6} M FL. Positive foci were detected by assaying culture fluids for DNP- or FL-specific antibody.

nition prior to antigenic stimulation, their relevance to the issue as a whole may be limited since: (1) "natural" anti-idiotypic regulatory mechanisms may be too subtle to be detected by the assay method employed, (2) the "positive" control in the above experiments has not yet formally been proven to be idiotype-specific, and (3) the "background" levels of B-cell responsiveness being assessed may already reflect the consequences of anti-idiotypic shaping of the primary B-cell repertoire. Furthermore, anti-idiotypic shaping of the repertoire and immune responsiveness may obtain mainly for clonotypes which recognize self and environmental antigenic determinants and such recognition may not be addressed by the antigens chosen for the above experiments.

In order to assess the role of anti-idiotypic recognition in B-cell responsiveness, we have utilized two experimental approaches. The first approach is a derivative of the aforementioned experiments. Since antigen-induced anti-idiotypic suppression is long-lived, it would seem likely that such suppression would accumulate in normal individuals as a result of environmental antigenic encounters. Thus, while such encounters might have a minimal effect in the 2- to 3-month-old control animals used above, much greater effects may be anticipated in aged individuals. The extent to which aged mice display accumulated immunoregulatory dampening of immune responses could thus be used as a gauge for the potential role of anti-idiotypic responsiveness generated as a result of environmental antigens during the lifetime of an individual. The second approach constitutes a direct assessment of the potential role of all environmental mechanisms, including anti-idiotypic recognition, in shaping the B-cell repertoire. In this approach, we have evaluated the repertoire as it is expressed in cells of the B-cell lineage generated in the bone marrow of adult animals at a stage in B-cell development prior to surface immunoglobulin expression. It is assumed that this cell population would represent the B-cell repertoire as it would be expressed in the absence of most environmental influences, since such influences as antigenic or anti-idiotypic interactions would be dependent on the recognition of cell surface immunoglobulin. The comparison of this repertoire with that of the mature B cells in the spleen would thus define the limits of the effects of any environmental influence of repertoire expression.

2. Anti-Idiotypic Recognition and the Immunodeficiency of Aging

The diminution in humoral responsiveness of aged individuals is well established.[14–16] A major contributor to this immunodeficiency has been shown to be the result of impaired T-cell function.[14,17–19] In order to determine whether diminished B-cell responses were also resultant from accumulated immunoregulation, we tested directly the possibility that, within the aged environment, anti-idiotypic immunoregulation would preexist, and that such immunoregulation could be transferred by cells from aged individuals.[20] Figures 2 and 3 present the results of this experimental test. These experiments were set up much as the aforementioned experiments which tested antigen-induced anti-idiotype-specific immunoregulation, except that aged carrier-primed recipients were assessed in the absence of hapten priming. Thus, the response to DNP of spleen cells from young unimmunized BALB/c or allotype-different B10.D2 mice was compared in Hy-primed aged versus young BALB/c recipients. The findings presented in Fig. 2 demonstrate that, even in the absence of hapten–carrier priming, the response of young primary BALB/c B cells is suppressed in aged BALB/c recipients, whereas the response of B cells

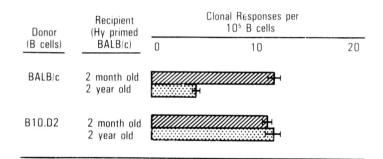

FIGURE 2. Antibody-specific immunoregulation in aged mice. 3×10^6 spleen cells were transferred to mice that were primed with Hy at either 2 months or 2 years of age. Data represent a minimum of six recipeints for each group. Data are presented as the frequency of positive fragment cultures per 10^5 B cells present in these cultures calculated on the basis that 40% of the donor spleen cells are B cells and the homing and stimulation efficiency of the splenic focus system is 4%. Error bars represent S.E.M. The frequency of DNP-specific B10.D2 B cells responsive to DNP-Hy in Hy-primed B10.D2 recipients is $12.8/10^5$ B cells.

from young (Igh) allogeneic B10.D2 donors is completely normal in aged BALB/c recipients. In Fig. 3 it is demonstrated that this apparent idiotype-specific suppression, which preexists in aged individuals, can be transferred to carrier-primed young individuals by the injection of high numbers of spleen cells from naive aged donors. It would appear from these results that the prediction that aged individuals may accumulate an anti-idiotypic immunoregulatory potential is correct. Indeed, it is likely that this immunoregulatory mechanism accounts for much of the observed immunodeficiency in the primary humoral immune responsiveness of aged individuals. This finding of a preexistent anti-idiotypic dampening of B-cell responses of aged individuals is not inconsistent with findings by others that both idiotypic and anti-idiotypic responses are suppressed in aged individuals,[22,22] although some laboratories have reported increased anti-idiotypic responses with aging.[23,24] Since the controls for the above experiments included primed syngeneic young individuals or spleen cells from naive syngeneic young individuals, it is again apparent that

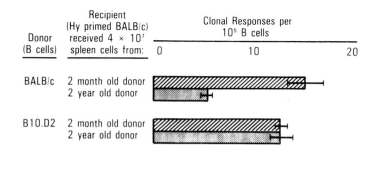

FIGURE 3. Antibody-specific immunoregulation by aged mouse spleen cells. See legend to Fig. 2.

the existence of such anti-idiotypic immunoregulatory phenomena, prior to antigenic stimulation in young individuals, is minimal. However, the demonstration that such anti-idiotypic recognition does accumulate "naturally," presumably as the result of environmental antigenic contacts in conventional individuals, also implies that such immunoregulatory phenomena, though minimal, may also exist in young individuals and may be far more pronounced for environmentally ubiquitous antigens.

Given the apparent preexistence of anti-idiotypic recognition in unprimed aged individuals, the next question which was addressed was whether or not the primary B-cell repertoire of aged animals evidences any effects of anti-idiotypic shaping of the B-cell repertoire. This question was addressed by transferring sIg⁻ bone marrow cells, which include mainly the generative pool of B cells, unfractionated bone marrow cells and spleen cells from either aged or young mice into carrier-primed young mice and determining the overall frequency of hapten-responsive B cells in each source.[25] Findings from these experiments are shown in Table I. It can be seen that, whereas the frequencies of DNP-specific B cells in the old and young sIg⁻ bone marrow subpopulation and the total bone marrow population are similar, the frequency of cells responsive to DNP is substantially lower in the spleen of aged individuals than in the spleen of young animals. Thus, it would appear that the generation of primary B cells in aged individuals is not significantly altered. However, a substantial diminution in the responsiveness of these cells is introduced as B cells emerge from the bone marrow to the periphery of an aged individual. While this finding does not prove that an enhanced anti-idiotypic immunoregulation in aged individuals is indeed shaping the primary B-cell repertoire by the elimination of emerging B cells, the finding is consistent with such an interpretation. If this interpretation is correct, then the presumptive phenotype of repertoire alteration by anti-idiotypic recognition would be normal numbers of antigen-responsive or idiotype-positive B cells in both the sIg⁻ and whole bone marrow pools, but reduced numbers of B cells of given idiotypes in the mature B-cell pool. This phenotype would not be unexpected if anti-idiotypic repertoire regulation required interaction of B cells with idiotype-specific T cells and the penetration of such T cells into the bone marrow were minimal. Given the above provocative preliminary findings, several

TABLE I

Frequency of DNP-Specific B Cells in BALB/c Mice[a,b]

	No. of clones analyzed	No. of cells injected	Average frequency per 10^6 cells injected[c]
Young			
Spleen	55	24×10^6	2.3 ± 0.28
Bone marrow	48	32×10^6	0.94 ± 0.1
sIg⁻ bone marrow	59	112×10^6	0.57 ± 0.13
Old			
Spleen	92	93×10^6	1.1 ± 0.28
Bone marrow	94	82×10^6	0.84 ± 0.19
sIg⁻ bone marrow	109	285×10^6	0.4 ± 0.06

[a]From Ref. 25.
[b]4×10^6 spleen cells, 5×10^6 bone marrow cells, or 10 ts 10^6 sIg⁻ bone marrow cells were transferred to each recipient mouse. Antibody-producing clones were detected by RIA of culture fluids collected from days 10–21 of culture.
[c]Numbers represent mean ± S.E.

experiments could be devised to test these postulates such as: (1) extension of these analyses to other antigens including environmental antigens, and (2) cell transfer studies to determine whether T cells of aged individuals can reproduce the observed phenotype in younger individuals.

3. Idiotypic Selection of Newly Emerging B Cells

Several years ago it was demonstrated that the neonatal administration of anti-idiotypic antibody could not only induce long-term suppression of responsiveness of B cells with that idiotype, but could also cause a marked, long-term depletion of B cells of that idiotype from within the mature B-cell repertoire.[9] More recently, it has been demonstrated that neonatal administration of anti-idiotypic antibodies can cause a long-term enhancement of responsiveness of B cells of that idiotype as well.[11] In order to determine the level at which passively administered anti-idiotypic antibody affects B-cell repertoire expression, we have recently carried out a series of experiments in which anti-TEPC15 (T15) antibody was administered neonatally to BALB/c mice.[26] The T15 idiotype is normally the predominant idiotype found in responses to phosphocholine (PC) of BALB/c mice.[3,9,10] The results indicate that BALB/c mice, 2–3 months after this treatment, are depleted of $T15^+$ B cells both in their mature splenic B-cell population and in the sIg^+ B-cell population of the bone marrow. Importantly, little depletion of B cells of this idiotype was observed in the sIg^- population of the bone marrow. It should be noted, however, that BALB/c mice treated with anti-idiotypic antibodies have relatively low concentrations of serum anti-PC antibody and therefore the depletion of B-cell populations could either be the direct result of anti-idiotypic treatment or of tolerance to environmental antigens which otherwise would have been blocked by serum antibodies. This latter explanation would be consistent with recent demonstrations that neonatal anti-idiotypic treatment has a prolonged effect even in nude mice.[27]

Because the administration of anti-idiotypic antibodies can have a profound effect on repertoire expression, it becomes highly important to ascertain whether similar environmentally induced alterations of repertoire expression are naturally occurring processes during repertoire development in the absence of artificially induced anti-idiotypic immunoregulatory phenomena. At the present time, little information exists concerning this question. One experimental observation relevant to this question is that two anti-DNP-specific clonotypes which are expressed as dominant clonotypes within the early neonatal B-cell repertoire of BALB/c mice are also expressed, but at a relatively lower frequency, during the adult life of BALB/c mice.[28] Thus, it does not appear that early expression of B cells of a given idiotype in the mature B-cell repertoire predisposes for either the inordinant expansion or the elimination of the expression of the same clonotype later in life.

4. Comparison of Clonotypes in Developing Bone Marrow and Mature Spleen

Perhaps the most direct test of the general postulate that anti-idiotypic recognition significantly affects repertoire expression is the comparison of the expression of identifiable clonotypes in the developing sIg⁻ bone marrow B-cell population as opposed to the mature bone marrow B-cell population or the B-cell population in the spleen. In these experiments, the developing repertoire was assessed by analyzing cells of the B-cell lineage obtained from adult bone marrow after removal of immunoglobulin-bearing cells by rosetting with red cells coated with anti-mouse immunoglobulin. The *bona fides* of these "prereceptor" sIg⁻ B cells have been demonstrated by the fact that, *in situ*, this subpopulation is totally unaffected in mice whose mature B cells of a given idiotype or antigenic specificity have been eliminated by *in vivo* anti-idiotypic suppression or tolerance.[29] Isolated prereceptor B cells are also immature in that they behave similarly to fetal and neonatal B cells by the criteria of their tolerance susceptibility *in vitro* and the fact that upon stimulation they give rise to clones producing only IgM and/or IgA antibodies, but not IgG antibodies. It is presumed that subsequent to isolation and transfer to carrier-primed recipients, such cells acquire sIg and are triggered by antigen in the milieu of maximized carrier help provided by the fragment cultures.

Extensive analysis of the antibody specificity repertoire expressed by B cells at this relatively early stage of development has now been accomplished for a variety of antigens. In previous studies, the primary splenic B-cell repertoire of BALB/c mice has been established for the hemagglutinin protein (HA) of the influenza virus strain PR8.[30,31] The anti-HA antibody repertoire of mature splenic B cells is extremely diverse and probably consists of greater than 100 distinct clonotypes. Experiments analyzing the responses of prereceptor B cells to influenza virus HA also suggest that the anti-HA prereceptor B-cell repertoire is highly diversified.[32,33] In our experiments the maturation and stimulation of HA-responsive BALB/c prereceptor B cells occur within the milieu of splenic fragments derived from recipients which are allogeneic to the BALB/c donor cells at immunoglobulin heavy-chain loci. Therefore, potential environmental effects of idiotype-specific regulatory mechanisms presumably would be minimal in these experiments. Thus, these experiments indicate that prior exposure to antigen- or idiotype-mediated regulatory mechanisms is apparently not required for diversification of the developing anti-HA repertoire per se.

Of particular relevance to questions of anti-idiotypic control of B-cell repertoire expression are the analyses of B-cell responses to several antigens characterized by predominant idiotypic or clonotypic families.[3,34–37] In responses to PC and α(1,3)-dextran (DEX) in BALB/c mice and to (4-hydroxy-3-nitrophenyl) acetyl (NP) in mice with the Igh^b heavy-chain haplotype, the T15, λ-DEX, and NP^b clonotype families, respectively, are already present in relatively high proportion in the prereceptor B-cell repertoire.[26,38–40] Similar findings have also been reported by other laboratories using polyclonal stimulation *in vitro* and analyses of the NP^b idiotype and the 460 idiotype.[41,42] Therefore, the high frequency of expression of B cells of these particular clonotype families in the mature B-cell populations need not rely upon an inordinant expansion of these clonotypes by either environmental or idiotypic selection.

In several instances, however, the comparison of the prereceptor B-cell repertoire with that of the mature B-cell population does indicate that regulatory processes, acting within the environment of developing B cells, can influence B-cell repertoire expression. As indicated above, λ-bearing B-cell clones comprising the NP^b and λ-DEX idiotype families are expressed in relatively high frequencies in both the prereceptor B-cell repertoire and mature splenic B-cell repertoires. However, B-cell precursors capable of expressing κ-bearing antibodies specific for NP in Igh^b mice and DEX in Igh^a mice are found in greater proportion in the prereceptor B-cell pools of these animals than in the mature splenic B-cell compartments. It is of interest that the mechanisms responsible for the diminished frequency of κ anti-NP antibodies in Igh^b mice appear to be different from the mechanisms responsible for the diminished frequency of κ anti-DEX antibodies in Igh^a mice. Similar frequencies of prereceptor B cells capable of expressing κ anti-NP antibodies are found in splenic fragment experiments employing recipients which are either syngeneic or allogeneic at immunoglobulin heavy-chain loci with the donor prereceptor B cells. Thus, by the criteria stated above for antigen-induced anti-idiotype reactivity, the diminution in the frequency of κ anti-NP B-cell clones within the spleens of Igh^b mice is probably not the result of idiotype-mediated regulation. Furthermore, the low proportion of NP-specific, κ-positive antibody-secreting clones is observed even at the level of sIg^+ B cells within the bone marrow. As indicated, the likely anti-idiotypic mechanisms responsible for the diminution of reactive B cells in the spleens of aged mice do not extend either to the generative prereceptor B-cell populations or to the bone marrow of aged mice.

The reduction of emerging B cells in Igh^a mice which express κ-bearing anti-DEX antibodies is, however, quite different, and may represent a paradigm for anti-idiotypic selection against the expression of certain specificities within the mature B-cell repertoire. In this case prereceptor B cells of this specificity cannot be observed if transfers are carried out to carrier-primed syngeneic recipients and can only be observed if cells are transferred to carrier-primed allotype-allogeneic recipients. Furthermore, B cells of this specificity do exist in relatively high frequency in sIg^+ cells in the bone marrow, but not in the spleen. The suppression of the stimulation of these B cells in carrier-primed syngeneic recipients demonstrates the existence, even in young Igh^a mice in the absence of overt antigenic stimulation, of an idiotype-specific immunosuppression for κ-bearing antibodies specific for DEX. This may not be unexpected since DEX is an abundant environmental antigen. Nonetheless, in every respect, the phenotype of expression of precursor cells capable of expressing κ anti-DEX antibodies in Igh^a mice is consistent with the picture observed for a vast array of specificities seen in the spleen of aged mice and is a system which should permit a more detailed investigation of the potential role of anti-idiotypic recognition in shaping the B-cell repertoire.

5. Conclusion

Overall, the findings discussed above are generally unfavorable to the view that naturally occurring anti-idiotypic recognition generally exists in the environment of the developing repertoire in the absence of overt antigenic or anti-idiotypic induction and implies that such recognition would, therefore, play little role in shaping the primary B-cell repertoire, particularly of young mice. On the other hand, it is quite clear that such recognition (1) does accumulate during the lifetime of individuals, (2) may exist for certain antigenic specificities relatively early in life, and (3) may play a determinative role in shaping the repertoire in aged individuals. At the present time, however, the effects of such recognition are measureable only as a diminution in certain antibody specificities and have yet to be demonstrated as an important "natural" mechanism for the up-regulation of any given idiotype. To the extent that predominant idiotypes have been examined, they appear to preexist in high frequency even at the prereceptor (sIg^-) B-cell level.

Although the above statements apply to studies concerning the shaping of the primary B-cell repertoire, they are not intended to be inclusive of effects which may follow antigenic stimulation. For example, it is clear that, in certain situations, idiotypes which are relatively infrequent within the primary B-cell repertoire, rapidly dominate the response subsequent to antigenic stimulation. This phenomenon was first demonstrated for antibodies bearing the T15 idiotype in certain recombinant inbred strains which expressed the Igh[a] heavy chain[43] and has subsequently been demonstrated in the response to azophenylarsonate in A/J mice.[44] Furthermore, for certain specificities, the serum response to antigen is proportionately lower than the representation of B cells of given idiotypes in the B-cell repertoire.[28,43] Since anti-idiotypic regulatory events appear to be generated very soon after antigenic stimulation,[13] it is very likely that such regulatory phenomena may play a highly important role in the ultimate representation of antibodies in the serum as well as the expression of secondary or primary B cells within the repertoire subsequent to antigenic stimulation.

ACKNOWLEDGMENT. Supported by Grants AG-01514 and AI-15797 from the National Institutes of Health. D.Z. is the recipient of a Chaim Weizmann Postdoctoral Fellowship from the Weizmann Institute of Science. R.L.R. is the recipient of an Arthritis Postdoctoral Fellowship from the Arthritis Foundation.

References

1. Rodkey, L. S., 1974, Studies of idiotypic antibodies: Production and characterization of auto-anti-idiotypic antiserum, *J. Exp. Med.* **139**:712–720.
2. Jerne, N., 1971, Toward a network theory of the immune system, *Ann. Immunol. (Paris)* **125**:373–389.
3. Köhler, H., 1975, The response to phosphorylcholine: Dissecting an immune response, *Transplant. Rev.* **27**:24–56.
4. Hart, D. A., Wang, A. L., Pawlak, L. L., and Nisonoff, A., 1972, Suppression of idiotypic specificities in adult mice by administration of antiidiotypic antibody, *J. Exp. Med.* **135**:1293–1300.
5. Eichmann, K., 1978, Expression and function of idiotypes on lymphocytes, *Adv. Immunol.* **26**:194–254.
6. Trenkner, E., and Riblet, R., 1975, Induction of antiphosphorylcholine antibody formation by anti-idiotypic antibodies, *J. Exp. Med.* **142**:1121–1132.
7. Kelsoe, G., Reth, M., and Rajewsky, K., 1980, Control of idiotype expression by monoclonal anti-idiotypic antibodies, *Immunol. Rev.* **52**:75–88.
8. Bluestone, J. A., Auchincloss, H., Jr., Cazenave, P.-A., Ozato, K., and Sachs, D. H., 1982, Anti-idiotypes to monoclonal anti-H-2 antibodies. III. Syngeneic anti-idiotypes detect idiotypes on antibodies induced by *in vivo* administration of xenogeneic anti-idiotypes, *J. Immunol.* **129**:2066–2068.
9. Accolla, R. S., Gearhart, P. J., Sigal, N. H., Cancro, M. P., and Klinman, N. R., 1977, Idiotype-specific neonatal suppression of phosphorylcholine responsive B cells, *Eur. J. Immunol.* **7**:876–881.
10. Köhler, H., Kaplan, D., Kaplan, R., Fung, J., and Quintans, J., 1979, Ontogeny of clonal dominance, in: *Cells of Immunoglobulin Synthesis* (B. Pernis and H. J. Vogel, eds.), Academic Press, New York, pp. 357–369.
11. Hiernaux, J., Bona, C., and Baker, P. J., 1981, Neonatal treatment with low doses of anti-idiotypic antibody leads to the expression of a silent clone, *J. Exp. Med.* **153**:1004–1008.
12. Rubenstein, L. J., Yeh, M., and Bona, C., 1982, Idiotype-anti-idiotype network. II. Activation of silent clones by treatment at birth with idiotypes is associated with the expansion of idiotype-specific helper T cells, *J. Exp. Med.* **156**:506–520.
13. Pierce, S. K., and Klinman, N. R., 1977, Antibody specific immunoregulation, *J. Exp. Med.* **146**:509–519.

14. Makinodan, T., 1970, Age related changes in antibody forming capacity, in: *Tolerance, Autoimmunity and Aging* (M. M. Sigel and R. A. Good, eds.), Thomas, Springfield, Ill., pp. 3–17.

15. Callard, R. E., Basten, A., and Waters, L. K., 1977, Immune function in aged mice. II. B cell function, *Cell Immunol.* **31**:26–36.

16. Zharhary, D., Segev, Y., and Gershon, H., 1977, The affinity and spectrum of cross-reactivity of antibody production in senescent mice: The IgM response, *Mech. Ageing Dev.* **6**:385–392.

17. Krosgrud, R. L., and Perkins, E. H., 1977, Age related changes in T cell function, *J. Immunol.* **118**:1607–1611.

18. Segre, D., and Segre, M., 1976, Humoral immunity in aged mice. II. Increased suppressor T cell activity in immunologically deficient old mice, *J. Immunol.* **116**:735–738.

19. Goidl, E. A., Innes, J. B., and Weksler, M. E., 1976, Immunological studies of aging. II. Loss of IgG and high avidity plaque-forming cells and increased suppressor activity in aging mice, *J. Exp. Med.* **144**:1037–1048.

20. Klinman, N. R., 1981, Antibody-specific immunoregulation and the immunodeficiency of aging, *J. Exp. Med.* **154**:547–551.

21. Kishimoto, S., Takahima, S., and Mizumachi, H., 1976, *In vitro* immune response to the 2,4,6-trinitrophenyl determinant in aged C57BL/6J mice: Changes in the humoral immune response to, avidity for the TNP determinant and responsiveness to LPS effect with aging, *J. Immunol.* **116**:294–300.

22. Flood, P. M., Urban, J. L., Kripke, M. L., and Schreiber, H., 1981, Loss of tumor-specific immunity with age, *J. Exp. Med.* **154**:275–290.

23. Szewczuk, M. R., and Campbell, J. R., 1980, Loss of immune competence with age may be due to auto-anti-idiotypic antibody regulation, *Nature* **286**:164–166.

24. Siskind, G. W., Goidl, E. A., Schrater, A. F., Thorbecke, G. J., and Weksler, M. E., 1982, The role of auto-anti-idiotype antibody in the regulation of the immune response, *Cell. Immunol.* **66**:34–42.

25. Zharhary, D., and Klinman, N., 1983, Antigen responsiveness of the mature and generative B cell populations of aged mice, *J. Exp. Med.* **157**:1300–1308.

26. Klinman, N. R., and Stone, M. R., 1983, The role of variable region gene expression and environmental selection in determining the anti-phosphorylcholine B cell repertoire. *J. Exp. Med.* **158**:1948.

27. Etlinger, H. M., 1981, The origin of immunological networks, in: *The Immune System: Festschrift in Honor of Niels Kaj Jerne on the Occasion of His 70th Birthday,* Volume I (C. M. Steinberg and I. Lefkovits, eds.), Karger, Basel, pp. 14–20.

28. Denis, K. A., and Klinman, N. R., 1983, The genetic and temporal control of neonatal antibody expression, *J. Exp. Med.* **157**:1170–1183.

29. Klinman, N. R., Schrater, A. F., and Katz, D. H., 1981, Immature B cells as the target for *in vitro* tolerance induction, *J. Immunol.* **126**:1970–1973.

30. Cancro, M. P., Gerhard, W., and Klinman, N. R., 1978, Diversity of the primary influenza specific B cell repertoire in BALB/c mice, *J. Exp. Med.* **147**:776–787.

31. Cancro, M. P., Wylie, D. E., Gerhard, W., and Klinman, N. R., 1979, Patterned acquisition of the antibody repertoire, *Proc. Natl. Acad. Sci. USA* **76**:6577–6581.

32. Wylie, D. E., and Klinman, N. R., 1981, Assessing repertoire diversity in precursors to mature B cells, in: *Proceedings of the Second International Conference on B lymphocytes in the Immune Response* (N. R. Klinman, E. Mosier, I. Scher, and E. Vitetta, eds.), Elsevier/North-Holland, Amsterdam, pp. 63–68.

33. Riley, R. L., Wylie, D. E., and Klinman, N. R., 1983, B cell repertoire diversification precedes immunoglobulin receptor expression, *J. Exp. Med.* **158**:1733.

34. Lieberman, R., Potter, M., Mushinski, W., Humphrey, W., Jr., and Rudikoff, S., 1974, Genetics of a new IgV$_H$ (T15 idiotype) marker in the mouse regulating natural antibody to phosphorylcholine, *J. Exp. Med.* **139**:983–1001.

35. Blomberg, B., Geckeler, W., and Weigert, M., 1972, Genetics of the antibody response to dextran in mice, *Science* **177**:178–180.

36. Mäkelä, O., and Karajalainen, K., 1977, Inherited immunoglobulin idiotypes of the mouse, *Immunol. Rev.* **34**:119–138.

37. Stashenko, P., and Klinman, N. R., 1980, Analysis of the primary anti-NP response, *J. Immunol.* **125**:531–537.

38. Klinman, N. R., Riley, R. L., Stone, M. R., Wylie, D. E., and Zharhary, D., 1983, The specificity rep-

ertoire of pre-receptor and mature B cells, in: *Proceedings of the International Conference on Immune Networks.* (C. A. Bona and H. Kohler, eds.) Annals of New York Academy of Sciences. **418:**130–139.

39. Riley, R. L., and Klinman, N. R. NP-specific repertoires of pre-receptor (sIg⁻) and mature B cells. Fed. Proc. **42:**941 (Abstr.)

40. Froscher, B. G., and Klinman, N. R., Immunoregulation in the development of the Dex-specific B cell repertoire in BALB/c mice, (submitted).

41. Nishikawa, S., Toshitada, T., and Rajewsky, K., 1983, The expression of a set of antibody variable regions in lipopolysaccharide-reactive B cells at various stages of ontogeny and its control by anti-idiotypic antibody, *Eur. J. Immunol.* **13:**318–325.

42. Juy, D., Primi, D., Sanchez, P., and Cazenave, P. A., 1983, The selection and maintenance of the V region determinant repertoire is germ-line encoded and T cell independent, *Eur. J. Immunol.* **13:**326–331.

43. Cancro, M. P., Sigal, N. H., and Klinman, N. R., 1978, Differential expression of an equivalent clonotype among BALB/c and C57BL/6 mice, *J. Exp. Med.* **147:**1–12.

44. Sigal, N. H., 1982, Regulation of azophenylarsonate-specific repertoire expression. I. Frequency of cross-reactive idiotype positive B cells in A/J and BALB/c mice, *J. Exp. Med.* **156:**1352–1365.

16

Quantitative Estimates of Diversity, Degeneracy, and Connectivity in an Idiotypic Network among T Cells

K. Fey, M. M. Simon, I. Melchers, and K. Eichmann

1. Introduction

We have previously described a series of limiting dilution experiments in which several T-cell types of a number of different antigenic specificties were analyzed.[1-5] In these studies, we obtained data on the precursor frequencies of antigen-recognizing T-helper cells, antigen-recognizing cytotoxic T cells, and of suppressor T cells that regulate their differentiation and expression as functional effector cells (reviewed in Ref. 5). Thus, these experiments not only provided information on T-cell precursor frequencies in normal and immunized mice but also on their regulation by suppression.[5,6] The quantitative and qualitative data obtained in these experiments strongly suggest that a suppressive network exists among normal T cells, and the data can be used to generate estimates on the diversity and degeneracy of receptors as well as on the connectivity in such a network.

Qualitatively, the idiotypic network among T cells can be described as follows. In the virgin state T cells interact with one another through mutual idiotypic recognition. If a certain minimum number of cells is present most of them will become engaged in a network of interacting cells and this situation is suppressive for all members of the network. The affinity requirements (i.e., the specificity) for suppressive interactions among virgin T cells are not very high so that the critical cell number is rather low and, therefore, all virgin T cells are suppressed as well as participate in the suppression of other T cells at all times.

When an antigen enters the system for the first time it will compete with idiotypic recognition between cells and will be bound to the receptors of those T cells which have an

K. Fey, M. M. Simon, I. Melchers, and K. Eichmann • Max Planck Institute for Immunobiology, Freiburg, Federal Republic of Germany.

affinity toward the antigen that exceeds the affinity of the network interactions these T cells happen to be exposed to at the present time. Thus, relatively high-affinity antigen-binding T cells are released from the suppressive network and become responsive to the activating signals required for differentiation into effector cells (primary response).

Subsequent to activation, such T cells or their progeny undergo further maturation which results in the requirement of higher-affinity idiotypic interactions in order for network suppression to be successful. Thus, infrequent populations become demonstrable which are not integrated into the network of the frequent virgin cells and which are selected for high affinity to previously experienced antigen (memory cells). Thus, when the T cells of a conventionally raised adult mouse are examined for reactivity with a given complex antigen such as SRBC, multiple populations of T cells will be revealed in most cases; in addition to the majority of suppressed virgin T cells, less frequent populations of greater affinity toward the antigen are demonstrable which are not susceptible to the suppressor cells that suppress the frequent virgin cells, but which may possess their own set of less frequent suppressor cells.

This hypothesis contains both network and nonnetwork elements. Particularly the assumption of a maturation step that makes T cells differentially sensitive to suppression was necessary because network arguments alone could not accommodate all experimental observations.

Most of the experimental evidence that leads to the formulation of this hypothesis has been summarized in a previous review[5] and only some essential points shall be repeated here (Section 2). The aims of the present chapter are (1) to show that the experimentally demonstrable T-cell populations of different frequencies are indeed qualitatively distinct populations, (2) to use their various frequencies for a mathematical analysis of diversity and degeneracy of antigen recognition and of idiotype recognition among T cells as well as of connectivity in a T-cell network, and (3) to analyze mathematically whether cluster formation among T cells can indeed lead to a cell concentration-dependent shift from response modes to suppressive modes as observed experimentally.

2. Previous Experimental Evidence on Frequency of Precursor and Suppressor Cells

Figure 1 shows a schematic representation of the typical result obtained when polyclonally activated T cells of an adult conventional mouse are subjected to limiting dilution in the presence of T-cell growth factors, and subsequently assayed for a typical T-cell function such as help in the antibody response to SRBC[3] or cytotoxicity for hapten-modified syngeneic cells.[6,7] We observe several response modes (negative slopes) interrupted by several zones of suppression (positive slopes). We have previously shown that the use of the negative slopes to estimate precursor frequencies for effector cells is mathematically correct.[6] The frequencies are very similar for different T-cell types and typical numbers are given in the figure. Furthermore, the cutoff points and the shapes of the positive slopes provide unequivocal information for the estimation of suppressor cell frequencies. This analysis revealed that suppressor cell frequencies are approximately 20-fold greater than effector cell frequencies in each response mode.[6] Thus, looking at the T cells recognizing

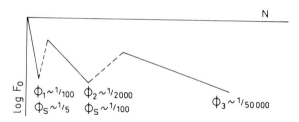

FIGURE 1. Schematic representation of the typical result of a limiting dilution experiment of polyclonally activated T cells. Lymph node T cells are diluted into microtiter wells containing irradiated syngeneic spleen cells as fillers. Concanavalin A is included for the first 2 days, then removed and T-cell growth factors are added for an additional 5–7 days. Thereafter T-cell effector functions are determined such as cytotoxicity on ^{51}Cr-labeled target cells or help for PFC formation in a subsequent culture of B cells with antigen. The results are plotted as the logarithm of the fraction of negative cultures, log F_0, versus the number of cells per culture, N. For details see Refs. 3 and 7. T-effector frequencies are determined by minimal χ^2 method for the negative slopes whereas T-suppressor frequencies are determined by a fitting procedure described in Ref. 6.

a given complex antigen, we observe effector cells of graded decreasing precursor frequencies so that usually two to three frequencies can be measured. In addition, one or two suppressor frequencies can be determined.

In addition to these observations, three previously described results are of major importance for the generation of our network model:

1. After *in vivo* and *in vitro* immunization polyclonally activated T-effector precursors appear in a single response mode corresponding to the most frequent population of normal T cells but with diminished or abrogated suppressor cell frequencies.[7] This gave rise to the proposal that antigen releases antigen-specific T-effector precursors from the suppressive network by competing with idiotypic binding among T cells.[5]

2. Specific antigen activation *in vitro* in most experiments preferentially reveals the responder cells in the infrequent precursor populations, suggesting that they represent a high-affinity selection from the virgin pool.[5]

3. Typing of the different T precursor populations for Lyt markers suggested the rare types to be more mature than the frequent pool.[1,2] The latter findings gave rise to the notion that the frequent and rare precursor populations represent virgin and memory T cells, respectively.

3. Present Results

3.1. Different Response Modes Represent Distinct T-Cell Populations

It is essential for the present model that the different response modes observed define different T precursor populations whose increasing affinity is in inverse correspondence to their decreasing frequency.* Because of the lack of an appropriate method to determine T-cell affinity to antigens, we rely on indirect experimental attempts to show that the different response modes cannot be manifestations of one and the same T-cell population.

   To this end, we performed a series of experiments in which the question was asked whether cloned (homogeneous) cytotoxic T cells, when titrated in limiting dilution with and without admixture of heterogeneous T cells, can give rise to multiple response modes. Figure 2 shows that this is not the case. A T-cell clone titrated alone gives rise to straight limiting dilution lines without any sign of suppression. In addition, when diluted together with a 10-fold excess of polyclonally activated heterogeneous T cells, the cloned T cells give rise to a single response mode followed by a single suppressive positive slope. These results, as well as others,[8] suggest that cells which appear in several distinct response modes belong to different clonal populations.

3.2. Analysis of the Repertoire

Assumption 1: A Random Repertoire

   As shown above, our experimental data suggest that the different frequencies (Fig. 1) characterize distinct populations of antigen-recognizing effector T cells. Thus, an antigen is recognized by several populations of T cells that occur at graded frequencies of, for exam-

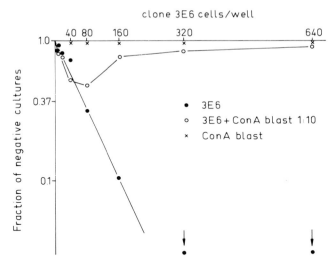

FIGURE 2. Limiting dilution analysis of cloned cytotoxic T cells (clone 3E6) from strain B6 female with specificity for B6 male (H-Y) target cells. Clone 3E6 was diluted alone or as a mixture with a 10-fold excess of Con A-activated B6 female T cells. Con A blasts alone show no deetectable H-Y-reactive CTL under the conditions used (round-bottom microtiter wells, B6 female filler cells). Whereas log $F_0(N)$ for 3E6 cells alone is a straight line (single hit), the mixture shows a single response mode followed by a single suppressive mode.

---

*This is the weakest point of our model: There is only circumstantial evidence to conclude different affinities for the various T-cell populations. On the other hand, there is nothing to argue against this assumption which, in addition, makes sense.

ple, $\phi_1 = 1/100$, $\phi_2 = 1/2000$, $\phi_3 = 1/100,000$. Each of the two frequent effector populations is sensitive to its own suppressor cell population which occurs at corresponding frequency ($\sim 20 \times \phi_E$). This observation can in principle be interpreted in two different ways. Either the T-cell repertoire is unequally distributed (selected) so that clones with receptors for different antigenic determinants, or for the same antigenic determinant but with distinct idiotypes, occur at grossly different frequencies. In this case, each suppressor population would totally discriminate the idiotypes of its effector population from that of the others. Alternatively, the T-cell receptor repertoire is random so that each receptor occurs with approximately the same frequency. In that case, the different populations would have to recognize a given antigen with different affinities such that frequency and affinity would be inversely related. Our major argument to favor the second possibility is that no indication for an unequally distributed (nonrandom) repertoire can be found when T-cell precursor frequencies for different antigens are compared.[4,5] Furthermore, we find no evidence for clonal expansion of T cells following administration of antigen, which would be a prerequisite for a selected repertoire.[7] We point out that our assumption of a random repertoire is critical and a basis for all further discussion in this chapter.

Assumption 2: A Symmetrical Network

Symmetrical networks were first formulated for the immune system by Hoffmann.[9] A brief mathematical derivation is presented in Appendix A. The time-dependent evolution of the concentration of idiotype i within the stable virgin state is determined by the negative feedback of anti-idiotypes j on idiotype i. The strength of the interaction between i and j is proportional to a coefficient k_{ij} and to the product of the concentrations of i and j. The symmetry of the model lies in the fact that no distinction is made between idiotypes i and anti-idiotypes j such that $k_{ij} = k_{ji}$.

If the total repertoire in the system consisted of n idiotypes ($i = 1 \ldots n$, $j = 1 \ldots n$), the probability for the stability of the virgin state increases with an increasing number of idiotypes j that can feed back an idiotype i or, formally, with an increasing proportion of k_{ij} coefficients that are not equal to 0. This proportion is defined as the connectance C of the system, and the mean number of idiotypes interacting with each clone is given by $C \cdot n$. C values that provide a high probability for stability would be, for example, 0.1 to 0.2 for $n = 30$ or 10^{-3} for $n = 10^6$.[10]

All further discussion and calculations are based on the assumption of symmetry. This includes the possibility that cells are divided into different classes only some of which can exert suppression whereas others participate in the network as noneffective bystanders.

3.3. Diversity, Degeneracy, and Connectivity

The affinity distribution of antibody molecules recognizing a single antigen is usually described as a continuum from many species with low- to a few with high-affinity recognition. Thus, the minimal difference in affinity to one antigen between two different antibody molecules is very small which is a reflection of a very high degree of diversity in the antibody system. In contrast, our data on T-cell frequencies indicate a discontinuous distribution of affinities even for complex antigens rather than a continuous one, suggesting pronounced minimal affinity differences between two different receptors and, perhaps, a lesser degree of diversity.

Because the least frequent T cells (most specific, highest affinity) we can detect in our assays occur at frequencies in the order of 10^{-5}, we conclude that the repertoire consists of a minimum number of 10^5 different receptor molecules. We cannot exclude the possibility that T cells of even lower frequency exist and escape our detection, so that this number is clearly a minimal estimate. Since, however, most antigens are successfully recognized by T cells of much greater frequency (10^{-2}, 10^{-3}), we can be certain that in most cases antigen recognition happens with a lower than maximal degree of discrimination (lower affinity, less precise fit).

This situation is best reflected by a T-cell receptor that consist of a limited number M of variable subsites each of which can be occupied by N different structural elements which can make contact with a corresponding number of complementary structural elements at a corresponding number of subsites on the antigen. This is illustrated in Fig. 3. The number of functionally different receptors would then be N^M. Successful antigen recognition by an effector T cell would require binding in at least K subsites, where $1 \leq K \leq M$.

We can now use our experimentally determined effector cell frequencies ϕ_{E1}, ϕ_{E2}, ϕ_{E3} to calculate M, N, and K. We construct several equations to do so. The first equation describes the minimal size of the repertoire

$$N^M = R \ (= 10^5) \tag{1}$$

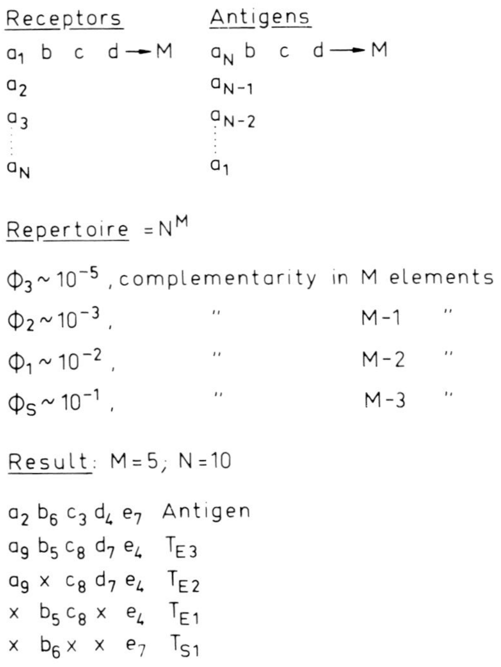

Receptors   Antigens

a_1 b c d $\rightarrow$ M a_N b c d $\rightarrow$ M

a_2 a_{N-1}

a_3 a_{N-2}

$\vdots$ $\vdots$

a_N a_1

Repertoire $= N^M$

$\phi_3 \sim 10^{-5}$, complementarity in M elements

$\phi_2 \sim 10^{-3}$,   "   M-1   "

$\phi_1 \sim 10^{-2}$,   "   M-2   "

$\phi_S \sim 10^{-1}$,   "   M-3   "

Result: M=5; N=10

a_2 b_6 c_3 d_4 e_7 Antigen

a_9 b_5 c_8 d_7 e_4 T_{E3}

a_9 x c_8 d_7 e_4 T_{E2}

x b_5 c_8 x e_4 T_{E1}

x b_6 x x e_7 T_{S1}

FIGURE 3. Essential elements used for the calculation of the T-cell repertoire and its degeneracy. Receptors and antigens are depicted as consisting of M reactive subsites each containing 1 to N different structural elements. Complementarity is generated when the coefficients of corresponding elements of the receptor and the antigen add up to $N + 1$. From this follows a repertoire size N^M. Most precise recognition requires complementarity in all M subsites, but recognition is also possible with complementarity in less than M subsites. This is somewhat simplified compared to the approach described in the text, using only two variables M and N. Using the experimentally determined frequencies, a set of equations is constructed (see text and appendices) that can be solved by $M = 5$, $N = 10$. For successful antigen recognition, at least 3 of the 5 subsites have to be complementary whereas for successful suppressive recognition, complementarities in 2 are sufficient. Examples for each type of receptor are shown such that the coefficients of complementary subsites add up to $N + 1 = 11$ and irrelevant subsites are denoted by x. It should be clear that a single receptor can appear in all four categories depending on its degree of complementarity to antigen or to another receptor.

If the most frequent population recognizes antigen with K subsites (minimal successful recognition), the size of this population is:

$$\frac{M \cdot (M - 1) \cdots (M - (K + 1))}{K!} \cdot (N - 1)^{M-K}$$

$$= \binom{M}{K} \cdot (N - 1)^{M-K} = \phi_{E1} \cdot R \quad (2)$$

The term $(N - 1)^{M-K}$ describes all possibilities to have $N - 1$ elements in each of the $(M - K)$ noncomplementary subsites. The term

$$\binom{M}{K} = \frac{M!}{K!(M - K)!}$$

describes all possible choices of K subsites out of M.

The next T-cell population shall recognize antigen with $K + 1$ subsites. It therefore has the size:

$$\binom{M}{K + 1} \cdot (N - 1)^{M-(K+1)} = \phi_{E2} \cdot R \quad (3)$$

A corresponding fourth equation can be derived for the determination of ϕ_{E3}. This frequency describes the size of the least frequent population recognizing antigen with K + 2 subsites.

Thus, we have four equations for three unknown variables M, N, and K so that each variable is unequivocally defined and can be calculated. Indeed, each variable is overdefined so that, if the model were totally senseless, the set of equations would presumably turn out to be unsolvable. This is not the case, however, and for our data ($\phi_{E1} = 100^{-1}$, $\phi_{E2} = 2000^{-1}$, $\phi_{E3} = 10^{-5}$) the set of equations can be solved by $M = 5$, $N = 10$, and $K = 3$. This would mean that T-cell receptors consist of 5 subsites, each with 10 variable elements and that minimal successful antigen recognition would require complementarity to the antigen in 3 of the 5 subsites.*

We now use these established rules to interpret the suppressive modes (Fig. 1): the cells which recognize antigen are themselves recognized by other cells which, in part, may have receptors that represent internal images of the antigen but, for the larger part, have receptors unlike the antigen that have complementarity at subsites different from those used for antigen recognition (Fig. 3). The exact calculation of the size of the suppressive population as well as a Monte Carlo simulation of a limiting dilution experiment is shown in Appendix B. This calculation shows that an effective ratio $\phi_S/\phi_E = 20$, as determined

---

*Given $R = 10^5$, our result $M = 5$, $N = 10$ may seem trivial but it is not. Given only equation (1), many different choices for M and N would satisfy $N^M = 10^5$. This unequivocal result from the four equations is an unexpected coincidence with the customary use of powers at 10 to describe large numbers.

experimentally (Ref. 6, and see above), can only be obtained if for the minimal effective suppressive recognition between T cells, complementarity in $K - 1$ ($= 2$) subsites is sufficient. Suppressive recognition is thus one step less precise (of lower affinity) than antigen recognition.

On the basis of this model it is readily possible to calculate the connectivity among T cells. If the minimal effective suppressive recognition requires complementarity in 2 subsites, one cell will not be recognized by $(N - 1)^M + 5 \cdot (N - 1)^{M-1}$ other cells. Thus,

$$C = 1 - \frac{(N - 1)^M + 5 \cdot (N - 1)^{(M-1)}}{N^M}$$

or, in our example, $C = 0.08$. In other words, each idiotype can be recognized by 8% of the other idiotypes. Figure 4 shows a histogram of connectivities for recognition in 0 to 5 subsites. It is evident that recognition in 1 subsite would involve approximately 33% of all T cells, but no experimental evidence exists to indicate that such interactions have any functional consequences. A connectivity of 0.08 would be far in excess of values estimated to confer a high degree of stability to the system.[10]

3.4. A Preliminary Approach to Describing the Suppressed State

In our experiments (see Fig. 1) it appears that when T cells are titrated, critical cell concentrations are reached above which suppression sets in rapidly whereas below which hardly any suppression is observed. This situation is reminiscent of the "phase transitions" seen among identical molecules in physics and is in contrast to a behavior expected if different functionally defined cells interacted with one another according to the mass interaction law. In the latter case, a given number of effector T cells (T_E) would coexist with a given number of suppressor T cells (T_S) and the interaction between them would result in the functional neutralization of T_E. Such a model would lead to an equilibrium between "free" and "bound" T_E and T_S and to some form of monotonous increase or, at best, a smooth decrease of functionally active T_E with increasing cell number. In our experiments,

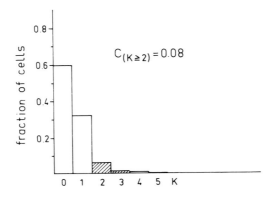

FIGURE 4. Diagram showing the proportion of cells whose receptors have complementarity to that of a single cell in 0 to 5 receptor subsites. We define the connectivity (C) of a cell to be equal to the proportion of the total cells that has complementarity to its receptor in 2 or more subsites, because this seems to be the minimum requirement for a functionally relevant (suppressive) recognition. For calculations of the proportions see appendices.

free (functionally active) T_E show a sudden decrease after a critical cell number is reached (see Fig. 1).

We have previously shown that the frequencies of T_S ($\sim 20 \times T_E$) as well as the saturating behavior of the number of T_S necessary for suppression are by themselves incompatible with functionally specialized T_S. In this chapter we make some highly simplified assumptions for the generation of a suppressed state and ask the question whether with these simple assumptions for suppressive cell interactions phase transition phenomena can occur. For our calculations we assume that every cell can participate in suppression. Each cell can interact with given numbers of others (connectivity) and the strength of interaction depends on the degree of complementarity. All cells engaged in interactions are suppressed. Thus, in contrast to suppression depending on specialized suppressor cells, the number of cells participating in suppression becomes unlimited. As will be shown below (see Fig. 5), this leads to a critical total cell number N^* above which every additional cell becomes integrated into suppressive cell clusters. When N^* is reached in a cell titration experiment, a single hit response mode will abruptly come to an end. We like to stress that the term *cluster* as used herein does not at all mean physical clumps of cells sticking together, because their interaction potentials may very well have ranges exceeding the mean diameter of a cell.

On the side, we were also interested in analyzing whether or not, by assuming that a cell can make strong interactions with a few and weak interactions with many partners, several response modes can be generated. The calculations show that this is not the case and that only a single N^* is generated. Thus, with this totally symmetrical network model we cannot satisfactorily account for our observations of several response modes. This is the reason why we have to postulate an antigen-induced maturation step that makes T cells differentially sensitive to suppression (see above).

To keep the mathematical analysis manageable, we assume receptors with two structural elements 0 and 1, where 0 shall be complementary to 1. Thus, as shown in Fig. 5, four species of receptors are generated: $a = (0.0)$; $b = (1.1)$; $c = (0.1)$; $d = (1.0)$. The total number of cells shall be large enough so that $n_a \simeq n_b \simeq n_c \simeq n_d = N/4$. In this system each member has no complementarity to 25%, a single complementarity to 50%, and a double complementarity to the remaining 25% of the other members of the system (Fig. 5).

For reasons of symmetry it is clear that the number of free cells $n_i(N)$ in each species is the same. We describe the interactions as potentials of a fixed limited range without assuming any heterogeneity in the details of the interaction potentials. For the sake of simplicity we calculate in one dimension. The symmetrical interactions between species i and j with the distance x are therefore described by the potential energy:

$$V_{ij}(x) = E_{ij} \qquad \text{when } x \leq R_{ij}$$

$$V_{ij}(x) = 0 \qquad \text{when } x > R_{ij}$$

Hence, there are two energies $Eab = Ecd = E_1$ and $Eac = Ead = Ebc = Ebd = E_2$ ($< E_1$), and two ranges R, correspondingly (Fig. 5). The system shall be at equilibrium and each interaction shall occur according to its thermodynamic probability. The various states of the system can then be calculated by minimizing its free energy $F = E - T \cdot S$

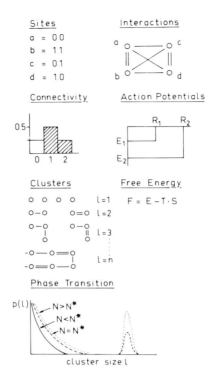

FIGURE 5. Essential elements used in the model of suppression. See text for full details.

(E = total energy, S = entropy, and T = parameter of equilibration). The system seeks a state of balance between its tendency to minimize its total energy and to maximize its entropy.

The results are obtained with the method of cluster integrals, which adds up all possible distances between several members and calculates their contribution. In this way we can estimate linear and circular clusters in one dimension (Fig. 5). The results are then extrapolated to three dimensions. For circular formations we obtain, in a fixed volume, a critical cell number N^* at which a phase transition occurs. Until N^* is reached the main part of the cells remains in clusters of the size $l = 1$ (single cells) and the probability of finding larger clusters decreases with increasing cluster size. After N^* is reached ($N = N^*$), each number of additional cells ΔN ($N = N^* + \Delta N$) will be integrated into larger clusters $l \simeq N/\ln N$. This is schematically illustrated in Fig. 5. The calculation is presented in detail in Appendix C.

We emphasize again that this is a *very* simplified version of a presumably very complicated and heterogeneous set of cell interactions. A mathematical analysis of more complex clusters with more than 2 interactions per cell is hopelessly complicated, however. In spite of this, we feel that more sophisticated symmetrical interaction models, although they may behave differently in detail, will also result in critical cell concentrations at which a phase transition from response to suppression occurs. Taken together, we think that a network model of multiple symmetrically interacting cells, with suppression being the result of cluster formation, provides an appropriate interpretation of our experimental data.

4. Appendix A

The equations for a symmetrical $(+/-)$ network model were given by Hoffman[9] as

$$\dot{x}_+ = (k_1 \cdot e_1 \cdot x_+ \cdot x_-) - (k_2 \cdot e_2 \cdot x_+ \cdot x_-) - (k_3 \cdot e_3 \cdot x_+ \cdot x_-^2)$$

$$- ((k_4 \cdot x_+) + S) \qquad (1)$$

$$\dot{x}_- = (k_1 \cdot e_1 \cdot x_+ \cdot x_-) - (k_2 \cdot e_2 \cdot x_+ \cdot x_-) - (k_3 \cdot e_3 \cdot x_- \cdot x_+^2)$$

$$- ((k_4 \cdot x_-) + S)$$

These equations describe the interaction of an idiotypic set of cells, X_+, and its anti-idiotypic partner, X_-. The dynamical system given by (1) has four stable states. The virgin state, where both concentrations are low, is governed by the balance between the so-called IgM-mediated killing term, which is negative and linear in both variables $(-k_2 \cdot e_2 \cdot x_+ \cdot x_-)$, and the source term S. The virgin state can therefore be described by the reduced equations

$$\dot{x}_+ = ((-k_2 \cdot e_2 \cdot x_+ \cdot x_-) + S) \qquad (1')$$

$$\dot{x}_- = ((-k_2 \cdot e_2 \cdot x_+ \cdot x_-) + S)$$

This has been extended to more than two partners to see how the stability of the virgin state is influenced by extended interactions

$$\dot{x}_i = -x_i \cdot \sum_{j=1}^{n} k_{ij} \cdot x_j + S \qquad (2)$$

One may generate the coefficients k_{ij} of the interaction matrix randomly with the conditions $0 \le k_{ij} \le 1$ and $k_{ij} = k_{ji}$. One gets stable equilibria almost certainly if the system has a sufficient connectance C. That means that a fraction C of all n^2 coefficients k_{ij} remains greater than 0.

5. Appendix B

We consider the effective ratio R_{eff} of the frequencies of suppressive cells and effector cells in our model. The effectors shall recognize the antigen in K of M structural elements on the receptor. Each element is taken from a set of N different units. This set contains for each unit also its complementary counterpart. The suppressive recognition shall be due to the same mechanism.

To produce $R_{\text{eff}} \gg 1$ the suppressor cells have to be more degenerate with respect to their targets than the effector cells. One may look at the following example:

$$Ag = (a, b)$$

$$T_E = (\bar{a}, x) \; (I); \quad (x, \bar{b}) \; (II)$$

One has $M = 2$, $K = 1$ and therefore

$$\phi_E = \frac{2(N - 1)}{N^2}$$

Further $a \in \{a, \bar{a}, b, \bar{b}, \ldots\}$.

If the suppressors recognize the targets in one element one gets four sets of T_S:

$$(a, y) \; (III); \quad (y, \bar{x}) \; (IV); \quad (y, b) \; (V); \quad (\bar{x}, y) \; (VI)$$

In this case (III) and (IV) are directed against (I), and (V) and (VI) against (II). (III) contains $(N - 1)$ members all directed against each member of (I). The chance that an effector is from (I) is ½. The same arguments hold for (V) so R_{eff} (III, V) = ½. The set (IV) contains $(N - 1)$ cells directed against a special element of (I). The chance to find an effector to be just this cell is $1/(2 \cdot (N - 1))$. The same applies to (VI). It follows that R_{eff} (total) is of the order of 1.

In Fig. 6 a Monte Carlo simulation for the case of $M = 3$ and $N = 10$ is plotted. One has two effector sets with $K = 2$ and $K = 3$. The frequent set is recognized by the suppressors in one element. Arguments like those above lead to $R_{\text{eff}} = 10$. The number of T_S required to suppress a culture was set equal to $A = 24$. The fraction of negative wells $F_0(N)$ was simulated with the help of a random number generator generating to 60 times N receptors, (60 wells). Figure 7 is made by a multiple Poisson analysis[6] with homoge-

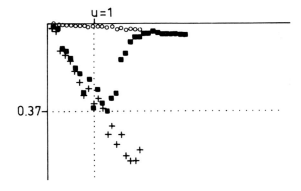

FIGURE 6. Computer printout of a Monte Carlo simulation for a hypothetical case $M = 3$, $N = 10$ (see Fig. 3). Sixty wells were simulated for each cell concentration. Horizontal axis, cells per well; vertical axis, log F_0; vertical dotted line, u = multiplicity of $T_E = 1$; horizontal dotted line, log F_0 = log 0.37; +, effector cells complementary to the antigen in 2 subsites; (○), effector cells complementary to the antigen in 3 subsites; (■), experimental curve if suppression required recognition between frequent cells in 1 receptor subsite. These conditions lead to $R_{\text{eff}} = 10$. A (= number of cells needed for suppression) assumed as 24.

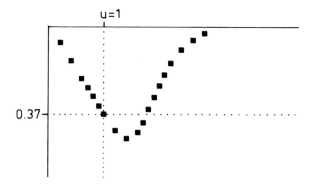

FIGURE 7. Computer printout of an analytical reproduction by multiple Poisson analysis of a homogeneous T_E/T_S population with $R = 10$, $A = 20$. Symbols and axes as in Fig. 6.

neous T_E, T_S and exact $R = 10$, $A = 20$. The estimation of R_{eff} is fairly good although in its derivation it was assumed that every cell occurs according to its mean value $\phi \cdot N$, neglecting all fluctuations.

6. Appendix C

We calculate the thermodynamical states of a one-dimension system of N interacting cells represented by their equally distributed receptors $a = (0, 0)$, $b = (1, 1)$, $c = (0, 1)$, and $d = (1, 0)$. N shall be large enough so that $n_a = n_b = n_c = n_d = N/4$ holds. 0 and 1 are complementary structural units. The position of cell i is denoted by x_i with $-L \leq x_i \leq L$. For the potential energy the step function

$$V_{ij}(x_i, x_j) = -\epsilon_{ij} \cdot \theta(-|x_i - x_j| + r_{ij})$$

$$\theta(y) = 1 \quad \text{if } y \geq 0; \quad \theta(y) = 0 \quad \text{if } y < 0$$

is taken. Strong interaction is given by $\epsilon_{ij} = \epsilon_1$ and $r_{ij} = r_1$ for $i, j = a, b$ or c, d. A weak interaction occurs if $i, j = a, c$ or a, d or b, c or b, d; then $\epsilon_{ij} = \epsilon_2$ and $r_{ij} = r_2$.

One assumes thermal equilibrium and therefore the existence of an equilibrium constant β whose value is not known. One can then calculate the canonical partition function $Z(\beta, L, N)$. The free energy is given by $F = -\beta \ln Z$. Because we are only interested in some qualitative properties of the model simple factorizing functions of β are omitted.

One gets

$$Z(\beta, L, N) = (n_a! \cdot n_b! \cdot n_c! \cdot n_d!)^{-1} \cdot \int_{-L}^{L} dx_1 \int_{-L}^{L} dx_2 \cdots \int_{-L}^{L} dx_N e^{-\beta \cdot \Sigma_{i<j} V_{ij}(x_i, x_j)}$$

$$(1)$$

where the integrations over the momenta p_i have already been carried out, giving a factorizing function of β. With the help of $Z(\beta, L, N)$ one can calculate the grand canonical partition function Ψ by

$$e^{\Psi(\beta,L,\alpha)} = \sum_{N=0}^{\infty} Z(\beta, L, N)e^{-\alpha \cdot N} \tag{2}$$

In a more explicit version one had to use $\alpha_1, \ldots, \alpha_4; n_a \ldots n_d$ instead of $\alpha; N$; we omit that and use the symmetry explicitly.

(1) and (2) can be calculated by a modified version of the cluster integral method.[11,12] One defines

$$F_{ij}(x_i, x_j) = e^{-\beta \cdot V_{ij}(x_i, x_j)} - 1$$

and

$$b_l(l_i) = \int_{-L}^{L} dx_1 \cdots \int_{-L}^{L} dx_l \left(\sum_{\text{c.g.}} \prod_{i<k} F_{ik}(x_i, x_k) \right) \tag{3}$$

where the sum in (3) is taken over all connected graphs with l-cells with fixed numbers l_i of cells of sort a, b, c, d.

Then one gets

$$Z(\beta, L, N) = \sum_{\text{config.}} \prod_{l(l_i)} \frac{b_l(l_i)^{m_l(l_i)}}{m_l(l_i)! \, S_l^{m_l(l_i)}} \qquad \text{with} \sum lm_l(l_i) = N \tag{4}$$

The sum is taken over all configurations. S means the symmetry of the graph $l(l_i)$ (example: with interacting identical cells $S(l) = l!$). With the help of (4) one can write

$$\Psi(\beta, L, \alpha) = \sum_{l=1}^{\infty} \sum_{(l_i)} \frac{b_l(l_i)}{S_l(l_i)} \cdot e^{(-\alpha \cdot l)} \tag{5}$$

Because of $N = -\partial\Psi/\partial\alpha$ it follows

$$N = \sum_{l=1}^{\infty} l \cdot C_l \qquad \text{with } C_l = \sum_{(l_i)} \frac{b_l(l_i)}{S_l(l_i)} \cdot x^l$$

and $\tag{6}$

$$x = e^{-\alpha}$$

C_l is the contribution of all clusters of size l with different combinations of l_i. The contribution of a single chain $(a\text{-}b\text{-}c\text{-}b\text{-} \cdots)$ of length l with ν strong and μ weak interactions is

$$V \cdot (r_1 E_1)^\nu \cdot (r_2 E_2)^\mu$$

where $E_i = e^{\beta \epsilon_i} - 1$, V is the volume $= 2L$, and $\nu + \mu = l - 1$.

If one connects the first and last member of a chain to a circle one gets one additional E_i and a certain restriction in the phase space of all member positions x_i. We use the following trick to estimate this. The *mean* distance of the outer members of the chain is 0 and one has a superposition of equal distributions each with $\sigma = r/3^{1/2}$ (if two partners are in interaction the special form of the potential leads to an equal distribution of the distance with the mean 0 and $\Delta x\epsilon(-r/2, r/2)$). According to the central limit theorem the distance of the extreme partners approaches a Gaussian with $\sigma = [r \cdot (l - 1)^{1/2}]/3^{1/2}$. One has to ask for a large probability for this distance to be in a domain with length r around 0 and gets therefore a factor proportional to $l^{-1/2}$ caused by the phase space restriction. A plausible extension to three dimensions yields $l^{-3/2}$.

One can therefore estimate an upper bound for the contribution of a single circle in three dimensions to be

$$V \cdot (r_1 E_1)^\nu \cdot (r_2 \cdot E_2)^\mu \cdot E_i \cdot l^{-3/2} \cdot \kappa \tag{7}$$

where κ is a constant factor. For an alternating circle (a-c-a-c $\cdots$) one gets $(l/2)!^2/2l$ different graphs and $S = (l/2)!^2$. This gives

$$\frac{b_l}{S_l} = V \cdot (r_2 E_2)^{l-1} \cdot E_2 \cdot \frac{x^l}{l^{3/2} \cdot l} \cdot \kappa \tag{8}$$

and for a chain

$$\frac{b_l}{S_l} = (E_2 \cdot r_2)^{(l-1)} \cdot V \cdot \frac{x^l}{l^{3/2}} \tag{9}$$

because the number of graphs is l times larger. If we restrict ourselves to "weak" circles one can replace any a by b and c by d giving an additional factor 2^l and the total contribution

$$C_l = \frac{V}{r} \cdot \text{const.} \frac{\overline{x}^l}{l^{5/2}} \quad \text{with } \overline{x} = 2 \cdot r_2 \cdot E_2 \cdot e^{-\alpha}$$

One can now see the onset of a phase transition by the following argument[13]:

$$N = \frac{V}{r} \cdot \sum_{l=0}^{l_{max}} \frac{\overline{x}^l}{l^{3/2}} \cdot \text{const.} \tag{10}$$

where the upper summation limit is replaced by some large finite l_{max}. The sum converges up to $x = 1$ where one gets

$$N^* = \text{const.} \frac{V}{r} \cdot 2.61 \tag{11}$$

the cluster size distribution is decreasing $P_l = \overline{x}^l/l^{5/2}$. Only an infinitesimal increase in x, $x \rightarrow l + \epsilon$, generates a large cluster $l/\ln l \gtrsim \epsilon^{-1}$ while the decreasing part is not affected.

All additional ΔN cells, $N = N^* + \Delta N$, can be placed in the sum (10) by such an ϵ. So one comes to an equilibrium between an undisturbed "gas" of small clusters with the main contribution on $l = 1$ and a well-separated large cluster. An inspection of the chain contributions shows roughly a pole $N \cong \dfrac{1}{1-x}$ in the neighborhood of $\bar{x} = 1$ so that one can achieve any N by a broadening distribution in l without a phase transition.

Finally we show that the main contributions in our model come from those clusters, where weak as well as strong connections are present in the same cluster. By this reason one gets only one critical value N^*.

Consider the total contribution of all circles of size l with pure weak interactions

$$\frac{\displaystyle\prod_{k=0}^{l/2-1} (2n - k)^2}{l} \cdot (E_2 \cdot r_2)^{(l-1)} \cdot E_2 \cdot \frac{V}{l^{3/2}} \cdot \kappa$$

where n $= N/4$, and compare it with clusters of size l built up like $a\text{-}b\text{-}c\text{-}a\text{-}b\text{-}c \cdots$ with all possible insertions (for example a replacement of c by d).

$$\frac{\displaystyle\prod_{k=0}^{l/3-1} (n - k)^3}{l \cdot \frac{2}{3}} \cdot (E_2 \cdot r_2)^{(2l/3)} \cdot (E_1 \cdot r_1)^{l/3} \cdot \frac{V \cdot 2^{(2l/3+1)}}{l^{3/2}} \cdot \kappa' \cdot r_i^{-1}$$

where κ' is a constant factor. One gets a major contribution of the latter clusters if $2E_2r_2 < E_1r_1$. The maximal contribution will depend on the ratio E_1r_1/E_2r_2.

References

1. Eichmann, K., Falk, I., Melchers, I., and Simon, M. M., 1980, Quantitative studies on T cell diversity. I. Determination of the precursor frequencies of two types of streptococcus A-specific helper cells in non-immune, polyclonally activated splenic T cells, *J. Exp. Med.* **152**:477.
2. Goronzy, J., Schäfer, U., Eichmann, K., and Simon, M. M., 1981, Quantitative studies on T cell diversity. II. Determination of the frequencies and Lyt phenotypes of two types of precursor cells for alloreactive cytotoxic T cells in polyclonally and specifically activated splenic T cells, *J. Exp. Med.* **153**:857.
3. Melchers, I., Fey, K., and Eichmann, K., 1982, Quantitative studies on T cell diversity. III. Limiting dilution analysis of precursor cells for T helper cells reactive to xenogeneic red blood cells, *J. Exp. Med.* **156**:1587.
4. Eichmann, K., Goronzy, J., Hamann, U., Krammer, P. H., Kuppers, R., Melchers, I., Simon, M. M., and Zahn, G., 1982, Clonal analysis of helper and cytolytic T cells: Multiple independently regulated precursor sets at frequencies suggesting a limited repertoire, in: *Isolation, Characterization and Utilization of T Lymphocyte Clones* (C. G. Fathman and F. W. Fitch, eds.), Academic Press, New York, p. 233.
5. Eichmann, K., Fey, K., Kuppers, R., Melchers, I., Simon, M. M., and Weltzien, H. U., 1983, Network regulation among T cells: Conclusions from limiting dilution experiments, *Springer Semin. Immunopathol.* **6**:7-32.
6. Fey, K., Melchers, I., and Eichmann, K., 1983, Quantitative studies on T cell diversity. IV. Mathematical analysis of multiple limiting populations of effector and suppressor T cells, *J. Exp. Med.* **158**:40-52.
7. Hamann, U., Eichmann, K., and Krammer, P. H., 1983, Frequencies and regulation of trinitrophenyl-specific cytotoxic T precursor cells: Immunization results in release from suppression, *J. Immunol.* **130**:7.

8. Weyand, C., Goronzy, J., and Hämmerling, G., 1981, Recognition of polymorphic H-2 domains by T lymphocytes. I. Functional role of different H-2 domains for the generation of alloreactive cytotoxic T lymphocytes and determination of precursor frequencies, *J. Exp. Med.* **154**:1717.

9. Hoffmann, G. W., 1975, A theory of regulation and self–non-self discrimination in an immune network, *Eur. J. Immunol.* **5**:638.

10. Hoffmann, G., 1982, The application of stability criteria in evaluating network regulation models, in: *Oscillatory Dynamics in the Immune Response* (C. DeLisi and J. Hiernaux, eds.), CRC Press, Boca Raton, Fla., pp. 137–162.

11. Landau, L. D., and Lifschitz, E. M., 1966, *Theoretische Pysik V*, Akademie Verlag, Berlin.

12. Huang, K., 1966, *Statistical Mechanics,* Wiley, New York.

13. Becker, R., 1966, *Theorie der Wärme,* Springer-Verlag, Berlin.

17

Expression of Anti-MHC Idiotypes in Immune Responses

SUZANNE L. EPSTEIN, JEFFREY A. BLUESTONE, AND
DAVID H. SACHS

1. Introduction

Major histocompatibility complex (MHC) antigens are the targets of immune attack recognized during graft rejection and graft-versus-host (GVH) reactions. Therefore, a knowledge of the nature of anti-MHC receptors may allow specific intervention to alter the course of these clinically important reactions. The MHC antigens also function as stimulators and targets of allogeneic reactions such as mixed lymphocyte reactions and cell-mediated lympholysis, and as restriction elements for immune responses to foreign antigens. Thus, the generation and regulation of a wide variety of immune responses is governed by the recognition of this set of antigens. Both of these considerations have given impetus to the study of lymphocyte receptors for histocompatibility antigens.

The unique functional properties of MHC antigens have led to suggestions on theoretical grounds that the anti-MHC repertoire may have a privileged status in the immune system, perhaps with more fundamental significance than the response repertoire to an arbitrary foreign antigen. This concept was proposed originally for development of both T- and B-cell repertoires.[1] It has recently been supported for the T-cell repertoire by models involving thymic influence,[2] while the significance of the MHC in B-cell repertoire development remains uncertain at present.[3–5] Overall, the central role of self tolerance to MHC and the strikingly high reactivity to allogeneic MHC determinants suggest the possibility of special regulation of the anti-MHC repertoire.

For these reasons, studies of anti-MHC idiotypes are of particular interest. Such studies have been in progress for a number of years in a variety of laboratories. The initial results of these studies suggested extensive sharing of anti-MHC idiotypes by T and B

SUZANNE L. EPSTEIN, JEFFREY A. BLUESTONE, AND DAVID H. SACHS • Transplantation Biology Section, Immunology Branch, National Cancer Institute, Bethesda, Maryland 20205.

cells[6-8] and led to great excitement. However, such studies proved difficult to reproduce[9] (and N. Shinohara and D. H. Sachs, unpublished data) and have not yet been confirmed by studies with currently available reagents or with monoclonal idiotypes.

Two major possibilities are apparent to explain these difficulties. First, MHC antigens bear complex sets of specificities, and responses to them may involve receptors of great heterogeneity. In addition, it is difficult to purify an antibody fraction with a particular specificity from alloantiserum. With such heterogeneous antibody populations from conventional alloantisera as sources of idiotype, production of anti-idiotypic reagents is very difficult, and may be quite variable. Second, conventional alloantibody populations may be contaminated with soluble T-cell products. Thus, anti-idiotypes raised against heterogeneous antibody might also include antibodies directed against T-cell receptors that are not necessarily similar to antibody idiotypes.

The availability of monoclonal antibodies has allowed a new approach to the study of anti-MHC idiotypes, and avoids the problems of lack of reproducibility and unknown idiotypic complexity of the reagents used. An unlimited supply of homogeneous idiotype is available for detailed characterization, including protein sequencing and molecular biological studies and for the production of anti-idiotype. In addition, if monoclonal antibody used for the production of anti-idiotype is prepared from tissue culture supernatants, it is not likely to be contaminated with T-cell products or factors. Using monoclonal antibodies, the reexamination of the questions outlined above has in fact led to a great deal of information about the complexity and nature of the expressed anti-MHC repertoire.

This chapter will cover studies of anti-MHC idiotypes performed by this laboratory and its collaborators, with the emphasis on anti-Ia (class II) systems but also with some discussion of anti-H-2 (class I) systems. Other aspects of the class I idiotypic systems have been reviewed more extensively elsewhere.[10] The discussion will focus on idiotype expression in B-cell responses, with brief mention of the available information on T-cell responses. The serology of idiotypes as expressed in both conventional alloantibody populations and on monoclonal antibodies will be discussed. *In vivo* manipulation with anti-idiotypes will also be considered as an avenue for investigation of the control and manipulation of idiotype expression and possible network effects. The responder capability of various genetic strains will be reviewed with regard to responses to antigen and responses to anti-idiotype priming.

2. Production and Characterization of Anti-Idiotypes

Anti-idiotypes have been prepared against a variety of anti-Ia and anti-H-2 monoclonal antibodies. Indicated in Table I are the monoclonal antibodies used, the alloimmunizations used to produce them, and their specificities.

The immunization protocols for production of anti-idiotypic sera, purification of the anti-idiotypic antibodies, and testing for specificity of their reactivities have been described in detail elsewhere.[11-13] For most of the work to be discussed in this chapter, xenogeneic anti-idiotypes were used. In brief, monoclonal antibodies were purified from culture supernatant, emulsified in complete Freund's adjuvant, and used to immunize miniature swine and rabbits. The resulting activity was monitored by hemagglutination assays on antibody-coated sheep erythrocytes. After repeated boosts and bleeds, pools of serum were used for purification of anti-idiotype. First, activity against constant-region determinants (and pos-

TABLE I

Summary of Monoclonal Anti-MHC Antibodies Used to Generate Anti-Idiotypes

Hybridoma lines	Responding strain	Immunizing strain	Specificity	Cross-reactions	Ig class	Reference
Anti-class I						
3-83	BALB/c	C3H/HeJ	K^k, D^k	K^b, s, p, q, r	IgG2a,κ	16
11-4.1	BALB/c	CKB	K^k	K^q, p, r	IgG2a,κ	18
16-3-22	C3H.SW	C3H/HeJ	K^k	None	IgG2a,κ	16
12-2-2	C3H.SW	C3H/HeJ	K^k, D^k	K^q, p, r	IgM,κ	16
36-7-5	A.TL	A.AL	K^k	None	IgG2a,κ	16
H142-23	BALB/c	CBA	K^k, D^k	K^b, s, q, r (p)	IGg2b,κ	45
H100-30	BALB/c	CBA	K^k, D^k	b, s, q, r	IgG2b,κ	45
28-13-3	C3H/HeJ	C3H.SW	K^b	f	IgM,κ	46
28-14-8	C3H/HeJ	C3H.SW	D^b	L^d, D^q, L^q	IgG2a,κ	46
30-5-7	BALB/c.H-2^{dm2}	BALB/c	L^d	L^q, D^q	IgG2a,κ	46
23-10-1	BALB/c.H-2^{dm2}	BALB/c	L^d	L^q, D^q	IgM,κ	46
Anti-class II						
17-3-3	C3H.SW	C3H/HeJ	I-E^k	r	IgG2a,κ	47
14-4-4	C3H.SW	C3H/HeJ	I-E/C^k	d, p, r	IgG2a,κ	46
10-2.16	CWB	C3H	I-A^k	f, r, s	IgG2b,κ	18
25-9-17	C3H	C3H.SW	I-A^b	b, d, p, q	IgG2a,κ	48
28-16-8	C3H	C3H.SW	I-A^b	b, d	μ,κ	48

sibly common V-region determinants) was removed by affinity chromatography on columns of Sepharose conjugated with myeloma proteins and with normal mouse serum immunoglobulin. Then specific anti-idiotypic antibody was positively selected by absorption to and elution from columns of idiotype-Sepharose. Syngeneic and allogeneic anti-idiotypes were produced by immunization with conjugates of idiotype coupled to KLH with glutaraldehyde.[14] It should be noted that these methodologies could result in preparations containing both combining site-related and non-combining site-related anti-idiotopes.

The specificity of purified anti-idiotypes was tested by hemagglutination assays and by enzyme-linked immunosorbent assays (ELISA). In all cases, it was possible to generate reagents with activity specific for the immunizing idiotype and not for other monoclonal antibodies of the same isotype and allotype. Yields ranged from 50 to 500 μg/ml of serum. Although background reactivity of anti-idiotypes with other monoclonal antibodies or myelomas was quite low, residual reactivity with normal mouse serum (NMS) was difficult to eliminate by absorption, so ELISA tests were performed in the presence of NMS. This could reflect either a nonspecific serum effect or the expression in sera of low amounts of immunoglobulins expressing cross-reactive idiotopes on antibodies of unrelated specificity, as has been described in other systems.[15]

3. Prevalence of Monoclonal Antibody Idiotypes in Alloantisera

Immune responses to MHC antigens are quite complex, which may explain the failure to produce detectable anti-idiotypic activity upon immunization with heterogeneous alloantibody populations in most cases. Such complexity reflects both the existence of multiple alloantigens differing between immunization partners, and the presence of multiple immunogenic determinants on individual alloantigens. In addition, there is possible idiotypic complexity of receptors expressed in response to a single allogeneic determinant. The actual extent of heterogeneity in alloimmune responses and the contribution of each of these factors to idiotypic complexity have been difficult to assess with heterogeneous reagents.

A major concern in the use of monoclonal antibodies for studies of idiotype is that an arbitrarily selected clone may not reflect a significant portion of the overall response; it might represent a rare clonotype, perhaps a somatic mutant. Thus, one of the first questions addressed using monoclonal idiotypes has been that of prevalence of particular idiotypes in alloantisera. The hope was that patterns might emerge, and certain idiotypes might prove common enough to serve as markers for studies of V-region expression, like the classical cross-reactive idiotypes (CRIs) seen in response to hapten and protein antigens (reviewed elsewhere in this volume).

Our studies of monoclonal idiotypes have demonstrated examples of idiotypes both widely expressed ("public") in alloantiserum responses and rarely expressed or undetectable ("private"). The best-characterized example of a public anti-MHC idiotype is that of anti-Ia.7 antibodies as represented by monoclonal antibody 14-4-4[16] (Table I). This idiotype was found to be readily detected in responses of C3H.SW mice to Ia.7, and to be specifically absorbed from appropriate sera by Ia.7-bearing cells.[12] Idiotype expression was readily detected in almost all individual mice tested (Fig. 1). The proportion of anti-Ia.7 antibody that in fact bore idiotype in pooled alloantibody populations was estimated by two methods. First, anti-idiotype was able to inhibit approximately 40% of the Ia.7-specific binding to cells as detected on the fluorescence-activated cell sorter.[12] Second, passage of anti-Ia.7 antibody through a column of Sepharose conjugated with anti-idiotype removed approximately 30% of the activity.[17] Thus, both combining-site-related and non-site-related techniques demonstrated that a sizable fraction of the antibody produced expressed at least some idiotopes cross-reactive with 14-4-4. Of course these measurements do not indicate how many molecules bear the entire 14-4-4 idiotype.

This system thus represents an anti-Ia system with a CRI similar to those studied in responses to certain other classical antigens, and demonstrates that not all responses to MHC determinants are hopelessly complex, nor are they subject to inordinate individual variation. With CRIs like 14-4-4 as markers, studies of the regulation and genetics of expression of anti-MHC receptors could be undertaken.

Several other anti-Ia monoclonal idiotypes have been studied in this laboratory. In the case of 17-3-3, another anti-I-E,[16] no significant idiotype was detected in appropriate alloantisera above the background levels seen in normal mouse sera (S. L. Epstein and D. H. Sachs, unpublished data). With 10-2.16,[18] an example of an anti-I-A antibody, idiotype could be detected only at marginal levels in a minority of immunized animals (S.T. Ildstad, S. L. Epstein, and D. L. Sachs, unpublished data). Thus, each of these monoclonal antibodies appears to represent idiotypes expressed only rarely in the response to antigen. Two anti-I-A^b antibodies will be discussed below (Section 4).

A number of monoclonal antibodies directed against class I MHC antigens have also been used for studies of alloimmune responses. Most of the anti-idiotypes prepared against anti-H-2 monoclonal antibodies detected relatively private idiotypes as determined by either the site-specific antigen-binding inhibition assay or the non-site-specific idiotype-binding inhibition assay. One exception was found using xenogeneic anti-idiotype prepared against

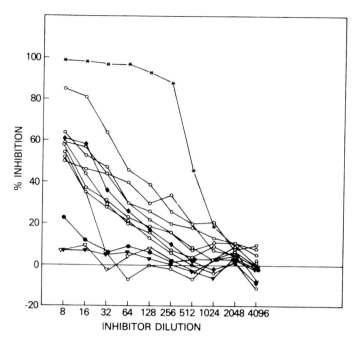

FIGURE 1. Penetrance of 14-4-4 idiotype expression in individual C3H.SW anti-C3H immune mice. C3H.SW mice were grafted with C3H tail skin and multiply boosted with C3H splenic lymphocytes. Inhibition ELISA employs 14-4-4 monoclonal antibody-coated plates and pig anti-idiotype as described previously.[12] Inhibitors are as follows: (∗), purified 14-4-4; (▼), purified 17-3-3; (●), C3H.SW normal serum; (◆), C3H.SW anti-C3H pool; (O), C3H.SW anti-C3H individual sera. In other experiments (see Fig. 5), one individual C3H.SW anti-C3H response has been found that was negative for the 14-4-4 idiotype, of a total of 10 tested.

an anti-H-2K^b monoclonal antibody (28-13-3). The 28-13-3 idiotype was expressed in all C3H and CBA/J mice immunized with H-2K^b tissue which were tested (J. A. Bluestone, unpublished data). The idiotype expression was allotype-linked, and idiotype was expressed on both IgG and IgM antibodies. In addition, the anti-H-2L idiotype, 23-10-1, has also proven to be detectable in alloantisera.[19] In this case, the idiotype sharing was detectable by inhibition of binding to antigen, but not by inhibition ELISA assays for idiotopes.

Several explanations can be given for the contrasting instances of public and private idiotypes observed. First, alloantisera to MHC antigens contain antibody of multiple fine specificities, in varying proportions. Antibodies of identical or very closely related fine specificity would be most likely to share idiotype, though antibodies of differing specificity are also observed to share idiotype in the course of an immune response.[15] Thus, an apparently rare idiotype may actually represent an antibody specific for a determinant of low immunogenicity. (Of course, even in the case of common idiotypes, the determinant recognized is only one of many recognized during the immune response, which can even be directed against a whole haplotype difference.) If this explanation is correct, such an idiotype should be more readily detectable in antibody populations enriched for the particular specificity, and this has in fact been shown for one case.[20]

Another explanation, which may apply in other cases, is a difference in the degree of somatic diversification required to arrive at a particular V-region sequence. Public idiotypes, such as 14-4-4, 23-10-1, and 28-13-3, may have V-region sequences identical to or very similar to germ-line V regions. Private idiotypes, on the other hand, for example 17-3-3 or 3-83, may be products of somatic mutation, making it less likely that the same events will arise in most individual animals responding to the antigen. The fact that two of the public idiotypes are IgM monoclonal antibodies, which are thought to display less somatic mutation than IgGs,[21] is also suggestive. In the case of the family of anti-Ia.7 monoclonal antibodies, the predominance of the 14-4-4 idiotype on antibodies of this fine specificity makes it seem unlikely that much somatic mutation is required to give products with these idiotopes. While some evidence makes this model likely, sequence data and molecular biologic studies are needed to evaluate it definitively.

4. Idiotype Sharing among Monoclonal Antibodies

In addition to studies of heterogeneous serum responses, idiotope sharing has been analyzed by testing of panels of monoclonal antibodies specific for the same antigen. This approach has the advantage that topographic regions of the antigen molecule can be defined by competitive binding analysis, which permits more precise comparisons of fine specificity than are possible for mixed sera.

An example is the analysis of a panel of anti-I-E monoclonal antibodies[22] for shared idiotype. Some of the antibodies recognized determinants corresponding to Ia.7 by strain distribution, while some recognized other determinants on the I-E antigen. Three epitope clusters (I, II, and III) could be distinguished by competitive binding.[23] In fact, even anti-Ia.7 antibodies fell into all three clusters, indicating that the antibodies see distinct determinants on the antigen, even though they cannot be distinguished by strain typing.

As shown in Fig. 2, xenogeneic anti-idiotype to 14-4-4 recognized four of the monoclonal antibodies specific for epitope cluster I and none of those specific for cluster III. In a more sensitive combining-site-related assay using excess anti-idiotype as inhibitor, all five of the anti-cluster I antibodies showed idiotypic cross-reactions with 14-4-4, but the anti-cluster III antibodies were still negative. Presumably the fifth antibody (40H) shares idiotopes detected only by a lower titered component of the heterogeneous anti-idiotype.

Studies of this type have also revealed idiotype sharing in several other cases. In the same study cited above,[22] anti-Ia.1 monoclonal antibodies were shown to express shared idiotopes in addition to private ones. Also, 25-9-17 which recognizes the I-A^b antigen of B6 but not bm12 has been shown to share idiotopes with 34-5-3.[24] With anti-H-2K^k monoclonals, the 3-83 idiotype was not shared by any of a panel tested in an initial study,[11] but a subsequent test of a panel including monoclonal antibodies of the same epitope specificity did detect sharing.[20]

The conclusion of such studies is that idiotope sharing between monoclonal antibodies generally correlates with fine specificity, although exceptions to this generalization have been seen.[22] The receptor repertoire for recognition of at least some MHC epitopes appears to involve highly penetrant expression of certain idiotypes, just as had been seen for responses to certain haptens. Such behavior may reflect the frequent expression of one or a few germline *V* genes and their close somatic relatives. This information supports the

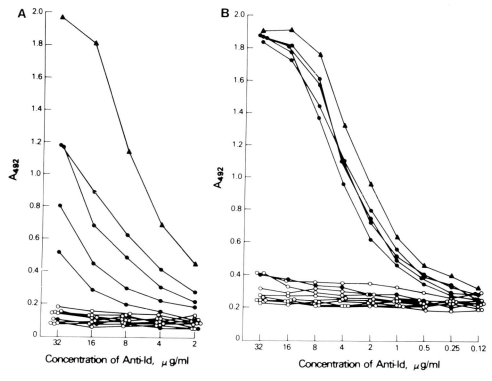

FIGURE 2. Binding of I-E^k-specific monoclonal antibodies with pig or rabbit anti-idiotypic antibodies to anti-Ia.7 monoclonal antibody 14-4-4. I-E^k-specific monoclonal antibody-coated plastic plates were incubated with various dilutions of rabbit (A) or pig (B) anti-idiotypic antibodies to 14-4-4. Bound antibodies were revealed by ELISA using either horseradish peroxidase-coupled goat anti-rabbit immunoglobulin (A) or rabbit anti-pig immunoglobulin (B). Specificities are indicated as epitope cluster I and epitope cluster III, as defined previously (see Ref. 23). Plates were coated with 14-4-4 (▲), anti-cluster I (●), or anti-cluster III (○). (Adapted from Ref. 22.)

idea that at least part of the complexity in anti-MHC responses results from the large number of immunogenic epitopes recognized in a response.

5. Alteration of Idiotype Expression by *in Vivo* Treatment with Anti-Idiotype

One of the major hopes of studies of idiotype regulation is that it will prove possible to alter the course of immune responses, either suppressing deleterious responses or inducing desirable ones, by clonally specific means. This approach has been applied to a number of systems, and the findings have been reviewed elsewhere.[25] The discussion here relates to observations in selected anti-MHC systems.

When animals were treated *in vivo* with small quantities of xenogeneic anti-idiotype without adjuvant, striking effects were noted. In all systems we have examined, material was induced which reacted with anti-idiotype prepared in a variety of xenogeneic hosts. Such material (termed Ab3 after Urbain *et al.*,[26] although generated here across a species barrier) could include antibodies structurally related to the original idiotype (idiotope-positive), which might or might not bind the relevant antigen, and also anti-anti-idiotype formed as a consequence of a conventional immune response to the foreign material injected (the anti-idiotype). The latter antibodies would not be expected to resemble idiotype in structure.

At least a portion of the response appeared to consist of idiotope-positive antibodies rather than anti-anti-idiotype, since (1) xenogeneic anti-idiotype from a variety of animal species was reactive, but would not be expected to share V regions, and (2) quantitative levels of the response were influenced by allotype-linked genes, an unlikely result for an overall response to anti-idiotype V regions.

The nature of the Ab3 molecules induced by anti-idiotype treatment has been evaluated using monoclonal Ab3 antibodies generated from mice treated with xenogeneic anti-11-4.1 idiotype.[27] Four monoclonal antibodies were generated and analyzed for idiotype, H-2K^k antigen-binding activity, and amino acid sequence homology to 11-4.1, the Ab1 monoclonal antibody. All four of the monoclonal antibodies shared at least some idiotopes with 11-4.1, since rabbit, pig, goat, and in one case (J1-8-1) mouse anti-11-4.1 idiotype bound to these antibodies. When examined structurally, three of the four monoclonal Ab3's differed extensively from the original idiotype in both their heavy- and light-chain N-terminal amino acid sequences. In addition, none of these three Ab3's bound H-2K^k antigen. Although we expect there will be sequence homologies responsible for the shared idiotypes, such structural correlations may not be apparent until much more of the Ab3 amino acid sequences have been determined. The remaining Ab3 monoclonal antibody (J1-8-1) exhibited extensive homology to the original idiotype. The H-chain N-terminal amino acid sequence was identical through the 39th residue although the light-chain sequence was quite different. Neither the native immunoglobulin nor the isolated H chains bound detectably to H-2K^k antigen. However, the reassociation of J1-8-1 heavy chains with 11-4.1 light chains resulted in the recovery of significant H-2K^k antigen-binding activity. These results suggest that a significant portion of antigen-nonbinding Ab3 molecules induced by anti-idiotype may resemble, idiotypically and structurally, the original idiotype and therefore may participate in an antigen-independent regulation of the immune response.

In some systems examined, a readily detected component of the response was specific for the original antigen, even though the mice had never been exposed to the antigen. When C3H.SW mice were primed with affinity-purified pig anti-14-4-4 idiotype and their sera tested by flow microfluorometry, the sera were found to contain specific anti-I-E activity (Fig. 3). The penetrance of such induced anti-Ia activity was 100% in anti-idiotype-primed mice, but no such activity was seen in mice primed with control xenogeneic immunoglobulins. This response persisted for up to 9 months after priming without subsequent boosting (Fig. 4). No activity could be detected in cytotoxic assays of such sera, and subsequent analysis showed that IgG1 dominated over IgG2 in the response. While all animals produced detectable antigen-specific activity, the majority of the Ab3 did not bind antigen, as shown by absorption experiments.[17] Rabbit anti-14-4-4 could also prime for specific anti-I-E activity, but appeared to be somewhat less efficient.

When animals treated with anti-idiotype were subsequently immunized by skin graft-

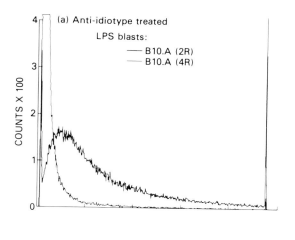

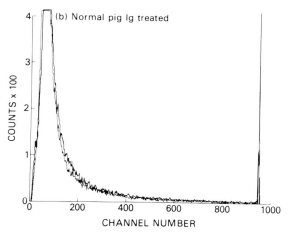

Figure 3. Detection by FMF of specific serum anti-I-E activity after *in vivo* treatment with anti-idiotype. Histograms of number of cells detected vs. fluorescence intensity are shown. Target cells are LPS blasts from B10.A(2R) or B10.A(4R). (Top) Serum from C3H.SW mouse treated with pig anti-14-4-4 idiotype. (Bottom) Serum from C3H.SW mouse treated with normal pig immunoglobulin. (Reproduced from Ref. 17.)

ing, an alteration in their idiotype expression was seen in the antigen-specific response. This has been demonstrated for the anti-H-2K^k system with the 3-83 idiotype.[28] An idiotype like 3-83 that is rare in the usual response to antigen showed a marked enhancement of expression in previously primed animals, even though they had not expressed significant antigen-binding activity before skin grafting. In the case of a public idiotype like 14-4-4, priming increased the fraction of the response to subsequent grafting that was idiotype-positive. Thus, the expressed anti-MHC repertoire can be intentionally altered by idiotypic manipulation.

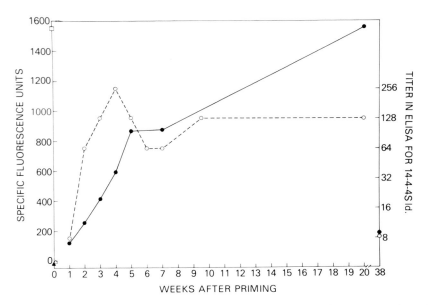

FIGURE 4. Time course of response after *in vivo* treatment with anti-idiotype. Responses are shown for an individual C3H.SW mouse treated with pig anti-14-4-4. (●—●), anti-I-E in fluorescence units above background in FMF assay (shown on left ordinate); (▲), staining with preimmune serum; (□), with 14-4-4; (△), staining reagent alone. (○---○), titer in inhibition ELISA for the 14-4-4 idiotype (shown on right ordinate), defined as last dilution giving greater than 40% inhibition. Detection reagent was rabbit anti-14-4-4. (Reproduced from Ref. 17.)

The mechanism of *in vivo* effects of anti-idiotype is not well understood, but some information has been obtained in the anti-H-2K system. One approach to analyzing the mechanism of Ab3 induction was to alter the anti-idiotype molecules. Since the Fc moiety of immunoglobulin is thought to play an important role in some immune responses, F(ab′)₂ fragments of rabbit anti-11-4.1 were generated and examined in the *in vivo* induction of Ab3. Although the F(ab′)₂ fragments were found to bind the original idiotype equally well as did the whole rabbit anti-idiotype, administration of these fragments did not lead to Ab3 induction.[10] Although these results suggested that the Fc portion of the xenogeneic anti-idiotype might be involved in Ab3 induction, these same fragments when coupled to keyhole limpet hemocyanin (KLH), induced levels of Ab3 equivalent to those induced by the whole anti-idiotype molecule. Therefore, xenogeneic Fc determinants may act as carrier determinants recognized by T-helper cells required in the induction of Ab3 molecules. Finally, attempts have been made in several of the H-2K systems to induce Ab3 by treating *in vivo* with syngeneic or allogeneic anti-idiotype. To date, we have been unable to reproduce the profound *in vivo* effects of anti-idiotype using the mouse reagents, even when these reagents were coupled to KLH to provide additional carrier determinants.

The prolonged time course of the response to anti-idiotype, without adjuvants or boosting, suggests that it is not just a conventional immune response to the xenogeneic anti-idiotype, but more likely a receptor-specific alteration in the balance of precursors for the response.

6. Genetic Control of Idiotype Expression

Studies of classical idiotypic systems have demonstrated the usefulness of V-region genetic markers for analysis of receptor repertoires. Recently, indirect evidence has accumulated for both regulatory[29] and structural gene[30,31] differences between strains that differ in their phenotype of idiotype expression. It would be of particular interest to have genetic markers for anti-MHC receptors, to allow analysis of the control of these responses, and of the V gene families involved.

The genetic loci associated with control of idiotype expression in many systems have been shown to be linked to the heavy-chain allotype and κ light-chain loci.[32,33] In addition, loci elsewhere in the genome may regulate idiotype expression, as has been demonstrated in the levan system.[34] The heavy- and light-chain-linked effects are most easily explained by structural V genes, but could also include instances of nearby regulatory DNA sequences or immunoregulatory effects of gene products such as anti-idiotypes.

Thus, genetic control of idiotype expression in anti-MHC systems was first examined by tests for allotype-linked effects. Examination of idiotype expression in responses to antigen requires a predominant idiotype like 14-4-4 that can be detected in the responses of unmanipulated animals. Preliminary analyses of appropriate immune sera had indicated that while C3H.SW $(Igh\text{-}C^j)$ mice expressed substantial levels of idiotype, none was detected in sera of B10 mice $(Igh\text{-}C^b)$. It should be noted that B10 mice respond well to Ia.7 and in fact to epitope cluster I, so this failure to express idiotype does not appear to be due to poor responder capability or to an Ir gene effect. When responses of C3H.SW mice were compared to those of the allotype-congenic strain CWB,[35] a clear difference was seen (mean for C3H.SW 44 ± 18%, mean for CWB 17% ± 10%). The mean for CWB sera was not different statistically from the mean for preimmune sera.[12] Thus, the level of expression of 14-4-4-related idiotopes is influenced by allotype-linked genes. Of course, additional control by light-chain-associated or background genes is possible, and has not been assessed to date.

Certain individual CWB sera gave values suggestive of low-level idiotope expression, but near the detection limit of the ELISA. To confirm that such sera in fact expressed idiotopes, isoelectric focusing (IEF) was performed, followed by overlay with radioiodinated anti-idiotype. As shown in Fig. 5, a discrete set of bands could be seen for the 14-4-4 monoclonal antibody itself (lane 1), corresponding to the equally spaced set of bands usually seen for monoclonal antibody, due to posttranslational charge modifications. C3H.SW anti-C3H antibodies (lanes 4, 17) showed a very limited pattern, implying that only a small number of clones are involved in the idiotope-positive response. Lane 18 shows a C3H.SW anti-C3H sample that was idiotype-negative both by ELISA and by IEF, the only such C3H.SW response seen. CWB antibody from an individual (lane 15) giving the highest value in the ELISA also showed a definite banding pattern, while no distinct bands were seen for an individual (lane 16) that appeared negative for idiotype. The isoelectric points of the CWB antibodies were different from those expressed in C3H.SW; this may be due to charge differences contributed by the allotypically different constant regions, to V-region differences, or to both. Thus, CWB mice are capable of expressing some determinants reactive with anti-idiotype to 14-4-4, but they do not ordinarily express significant amounts of these idiotopes in the response to Ia.7. The expression of these V regions is presumably under some kind of regulatory control.

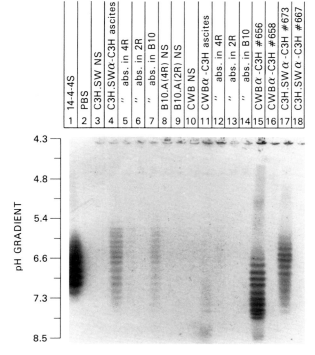

FIGURE 5. Idiotype detection following isoelectric focusing. Antibodies were focused on slab gels as described previously.[28] Gels were subjected to sodium sulfate precipitation, glutaraldehyde cross-linking, and were then overlayed with iodinated pig anti-14-4-4 idiotype. After washing, gels were dried and bands revealed by autoradiography.

In vivo priming with anti-idiotype (see Section 5) was next used as another measure of genetic differences between V-region repertoires of different strains. All strains expressed Ab3 in response to anti-idiotype treatment, with some quantitative differences.[17] The Ab3 molecules expressed in different strains may have different sequences, however, and this possibility is supported by results of tests for induced activity specific for I-E. By this measure, the differences among strains were striking. Presumably, the requirement for antigen binding imposes more stringent restrictions on the V regions that can be used. The strain must put together multiple idiotopes into a suitable combining site, or perhaps must express a particular critical idiotope.

As shown in Fig. 6, B10 mice failed to express I-E-specific activity among their Ab3, while CWB mice expressed just as much activity as C3H.SW mice. Thus, CWB mice respond to anti-idiotype priming by producing antigen-binding idiotype, but express little idiotype in response to antigen. At least two interpretations are possible: first, the response to anti-idiotype priming may not be under allotype-linked control at all; this model is rendered unlikely by results presented below. Second, a recombination in allotype-linked genes could have occurred during the derivation of the CWB strain, such that either structural or regulatory genes were picked up that encourage high levels of expression of the 14-4-4 idiotype when the stimulus is idiotype specific, but expression of this idiotype is not favored

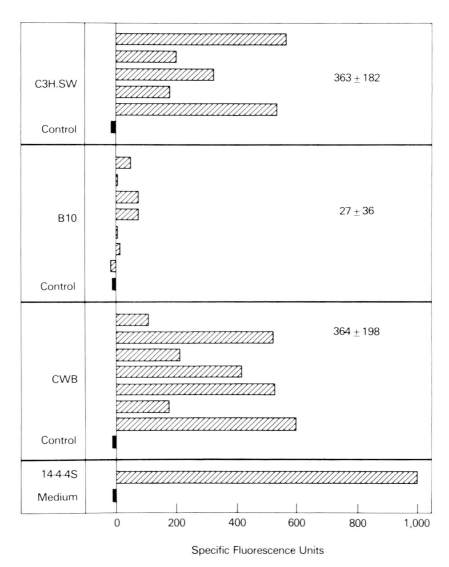

FIGURE 6. Induction of anti-I-E by anti-idiotype in different strains of mice. Bleedings were taken 4 weeks after treatment. Specific fluorescence units calculated as units on 2R-4R cells. Test sera: shaded bars, individual sera from mice treated with pig anti-idiotype; solid bars, mean values for three sera from mice treated with normal pig immunoglobulin. Controls: shaded bar = 14-4-4S culture supernatant; solid bar = medium. Mean ± S.D. for each group of anti-idiotype-treated mice shown to the right of bars. (Reproduced from Ref. 17.)

when antigen is the only stimulus. Additional control by light-chain genes or other background genes is also possible.

In *vivo* priming can also be compared for an allotype-congenic pair on a different genetic background. The A.SW-b strain was derived by backcrossing B10.MBR to A.SW, with selection for the Igh-C^b allotype (D. H. Sachs, unpublished data). Responses of A.SW and A.SW-b to anti-idiotype priming and also to alloimmunization are being analyzed, with the hope of clarifying the role of allotype-linked genes in control of these responses. Examination of other strain combinations is in progress, to determine the possible effects of background genes, and possibly light chain genes, on the response to priming.

Control of idiotype expression in each of these situations, the response to antigen and the response to anti-idiotype priming, could be mediated by structural V genes, or by regulatory elements mapping near the *Igh* loci. Distinguishing between these possibilities will require structural analysis to determine whether the same sequences are expressed in the different strains or whether idiotype expression is due to serologically cross-reactive structures. In addition, molecular biological analyses which are in progress should allow comparison of the V-region genes available to each strain in the germ line.

7. Comparison of Xenogeneic and Syngeneic Anti-Idiotypes

The role, if any, of idiotype–anti-idiotype interactions or network effects in regulating naturally occurring immune responses would necessarily be mediated by autologous anti-idiotype. Some evidence has been reported for the possibility that such anti-idiotype production does occur.[36] However, production of syngeneic anti-idiotype for use in studies of immune modulation has usually involved hyperimmunization to idiotype, rather than purification of spontaneous anti-idiotype from animals responding to antigen. We have compared the specificity of syngeneic anti-idiotype prepared in this way to xenogeneic anti-idiotype.

In general, the syngeneic reagents did not detect all the idiotopes detected by the xenogeneic anti-idiotype. The syngeneic reagents were able to detect Ab3 molecules induced by the xenogeneic reagents.[37] However, in all of the anti-H-2 systems examined, the mouse reagents did not detect the cross-reactive idiotopes in alloantisera and on other monoclonal antibodies which were detected by the xenogeneic anti-idiotypes.

Syngeneic anti-14-4-4 failed to detect cross-reactive idiotypes on other anti-Ia.7, cluster I monoclonal antibodies readily detected by xenogeneic reagents.[38] Thus, the syngeneic response was essentially private in nature, and did not include activity against the widely shared idiotopes. Similar results have also been obtained for 25-9-17.[24]

These results agree with those in some other anti-MHC systems, such as anti-Ia.2,[39] but contrast with reactivities of syngeneic anti-idiotypes in other non-MHC systems, such as anti-nitrophenylacetyl, which do detect the cross-reactive public idiotopes.[40] One exception among anti-MHC systems has been described, a public anti-Ia.1 idiotype detected by syngeneic anti-idiotype (M. Pierres *et al.*, unpublished data). These results may indicate that in MHC systems, certain receptors are common enough that the syngeneic animal is tolerant to those idiotopes, whereas receptors for other foreign antigens might not be common enough to result in such tolerance.

It is possible that neither xenogeneic anti-idiotype nor syngeneic anti-idiotype raised by hyperimmunization reflects the precise spectrum of fine specificities that would be recognized by spontaneously occurring autologous anti-idiotype. Nonetheless, the different types of reagents are useful for different purposes. For example, xenogeneic anti-idiotypes have been crucial in revealing the degree of sharing among anti-MHC receptors even in the presence of private idiotypic determinants (Sections 3 and 4). They are also more suitable in some cases for *in vivo* manipulation of immune responses, as described in Section 5. Studies of internal immune networks, however, are probably best approached by the use of syngeneic systems.

8. T Cells and Idiotype Expression

Among biologically and clinically important alloreactions, many are mediated by T lymphocytes, and as mentioned in the Introduction, early evidence suggested idiotype sharing by T and B cells. For these reasons, the anti-MHC idiotypic systems described above have been used to search for T cells, the receptor idiotypes of which might cross-react with antibody idiotypes, and to study T-cell participation in control of anti-MHC responses.

Approaches used to search for an idiotype-positive T cell have included testing the effects of anti-idiotype on bulk mixed lymphocyte reactions (MLR) or cell-mediated lympholysis (CML) reactions, of anti-idiotype plus complement killing of cells responding in MLR or CML, and of pretreatment of animal with anti-idiotype on their subsequent MLR, CML, or skin graft rejection reactions (J. A. Bluestone, unpublished data; S. L. Epstein, unpublished data). Screening of a number of alloreactive T-cell clones of appropriate specificities has also been performed (J. A. Bluestone, unpublished data). In no case was a consistent effect of anti-idiotype observed that could be attributed to the presence of idiotype-positive T cells in the responding population. Thus, idiotype sharing by alloreactive T and B cells, if it exists, is at best rather rare.

A role of T cells had been shown for the antibody response to *in vivo* treatment with anti-idiotype in the nuclease system.[41] This was confirmed in an anti-H-2K^k idiotypic system by the deficient response observed in nude mice.[42] In addition, a T-cell role may explain the response to KLH-conjugates of syngeneic anti-idiotype but not to unconjugated anti-idiotype (see Section 3), and also the adoptive transfer of idiotypic dominance by T cells.[43] In each of these cases, the participating T cells need not express idiotype; they could instead be carrier specific or anti-idiotypic in nature, and provide help for the response.

In summary, we have no evidence to date for idiotype sharing by T and B cells of the same specificity, but there is evidence in several responses for an idiotype-specific T-cell role in the control of idiotype expression in anti-MHC systems.

9. Conclusion

The development of monoclonal antibodies has greatly facilitated the analysis of responses to complex antigens such as transplantation antigens. New reagents have allowed more precise definition of antigenic specificities than was possible with conventional antisera, and thus have allowed comparison of receptors having the same specificity. In at least some cases, the receptors expressed in response to a particular determinant appear to belong to families, not to complex sets that differ in each individual. From the point of view of using anti-idiotype to manipulate immune responses, this situation is more encouraging than had been suggested by the great difficulty in reproducing reagents prepared with heterogeneous idiotypes. The overall results, however, do not imply that the anti-MHC receptor repertoire is simple. Not all systems show idiotypic sharing, and even in families that do, there are private idiotopes distinguishing the various clones, perhaps as a result of somatic mutation.

Anti-idiotypes prepared against monoclonal idiotypes have proved useful for studies of the regulation of anti-MHC immunity. The results of *in vivo* treatment are suggestive of perturbation of a preexisting network of idiotypes, the expression of which can be influenced by exogenous treatment. In any case, such treatment allows manipulation of the immune response by altering expression of part of the repertoire. Similar manipulation to aid in revealing T cells with a particular idiotype has not been successful in this laboratory to date, but is worthy of further study.

Future directions include studies of the mechanism regulating idiotype expression of anti-MHC responses. Conditions may be identified which lead to suppression of idiotype in addition to induction. Cellular requirements for development of responses to antigen or to anti-idiotype will be examined, and adoptive transfer experiments used to analyze genetic restrictions among the responding subpopulations, with the previously established genetics as a basis.

Further genetic studies will include both fine-specificity analysis of responses to MHC antigens in different strains, and also studies of which individual idiotopes are expressed by the different strains. The idiotypic markers will also allow direct analysis of the location and complexity of V-region gene families coding for anti-MHC receptors. We are currently pursuing these questions by analysis of DNA from mouse strains exhibiting different patterns of expression of the anti-Ia.7 public idiotype (Section 6), to detect possible V-region gene polymorphisms. With the use of V-region probes developed from the hybridoma cell lines, the V-region genes used in these anti-Ia receptors will be identified and characterized.

The existence of V-region genetic markers for alloreceptors will allow both serological and molecular biological approaches to the question of whether anti-MHC receptors on B cells have an exceptional status, or possess unusual characteristics. Is allogeneic MHC just a special case of foreign antigen, or is there something unique about this repertoire, even at the B-cell level? Are anti-MHC germ-line V genes clustered, or scattered among other V genes?

Further attempts to define idiotypes on alloreactive T cells, either cross-reactive with B-cell idiotypes or distinct, will employ T-cell clones selected both by idiotype-specific means and by fine specificity. In addition, studies will continue on the possible relationship between receptors for allogeneic MHC and for self MHC determinants. Self MHC determinants function both as restriction elements in responses to viruses and haptens and as the targets of autoimmune responses. The relationship between the receptors for MHC antigens in the various types of responses is unclear at this point. Some studies have reported that receptors for self and allogeneic MHC share idiotype,[44] but this remains to be examined for a system defined by a monoclonal idiotype to eliminate the ambiguities of reagent complexity.

The fundamental role of MHC antigens in the immune system has led to great interest in the nature of anti-MHC receptors. While it remains unclear what contribution idiotypic manipulation will make to solving the problem of organ transplantation, such studies should provide a fuller understanding of histocompatibility systems and their recognition in general, an understanding which is crucial to our overall view of immune regulation.

References

1. Jerne, N. K., 1971, The somatic generation of immune recognition, *Eur. J. Immunol.* **1**:1–9.
2. Bevan, M. J., and Fink, P. J., 1978, The influence of thymus H-2 antigens on the specificity of maturing killer and helper cells, *Immunol. Rev.* **43**:3–41.
3. Wylie, D. E., Sherman, L. A., and Klinman, N. R., 1982, Participation of the major histocompatibility complex in antibody recognition of viral antigens expressed on infected cells, *J. Exp. Med.* **155**:403–414.
4. Katz, D. H., 1980, Adaptive differentiation of lymphocytes: Theoretical implications for mechanisms of cell–cell recognition and regulation of immune responses, *Adv. Immunol.* **29**:138–207.
5. Singer, A., and Hodes, R. J., 1982, Major histocompatibility complex-restricted self-recognition in responses to trinitrophenyl-Ficoll: Adaptive differentiation and self-recognition by B cells, *J. Exp. Med.* **156**:1415–1434.
6. McKearn, T. J., 1974, Anti-receptor antiserum causes specific inhibition of reactivity to rat histocompatibility antigens, *Science* **183**:94–96.
7. Binz, H., and Wigzell, H., 1975, Shared idiotypic determinants on B and T lymphocytes reactive against the same antigenic determinants. I. Demonstration of similar or identical idiotypes on IgG molecules and T-cell receptors with specificity for the same alloantigens, *J. Exp. Med.* **142**:197–211.
8. Ramseier, H., Aguet, M., and Lindemann, J., 1977, Similarity of idiotypic determinants of T- and B-lymphocytes receptors for alloantigens, *Immunol. Rev.* **34**:50–88.
9. Krammer, P., 1981, The T cell receptor problem, *Curr. Top. Microbiol. Immunol.* **91**:179–215.
10. Bluestone, J. A., Auchincloss, H., Jr., Epstein, S. L., and Sachs, D. H., 1984, Idiotypes of anti-MHC monoclonal antibodies, in: *Idiotypy* (H. Köhler, P.-A. Cazenave, and J. Urbain, eds.), Academic Press, New York, pp. 243–269.
11. Sachs, D. H., Bluestone, J. A., Epstein, S. L., and Ozato, K., 1981, Anti-idiotypes to monoclonal anti-H-2 and anti-Ia hybridoma antibodies, *Transplant. Proc.* **13**:953–957.
12. Epstein, S. L., Ozato, K., Bluestone, J. A., and Sachs, D. H., 1981, Idiotypes of anti-Ia antibodies. I. Expression of the 14-4-4S idiotype in humoral immune responses, *J. Exp. Med.* **154**:397–410.
13. Sachs, D. H., Bluestone, J. A., Epstein, S. L., Kiszkiss, P., Knode, M., and Ozato, K., 1981, Idiotypes of anti-MHC monoclonal antibodies, in: *Immunoglobulin Idiotypes and Their Expression: ICN–UCLA Symposia on Molecular and Cellular Biology*, Volume XX (C. A. Janeway, Jr., E. E. Sercarz, and H. Wigzell, eds.), Academic Press, New York, pp. 751–757.
14. Buttin, G., Le Guern, G., Phalente, L., Lin, E. C. C., Medrano, L., and Cazenave, P.-A., 1978, Production of hybrid lines secreting monoclonal anti-idiotypic antibodies by cell fusion on membrane filters, *Curr. Top. Microbiol. Immunol.* **81**:27–36.
15. Oudin, J., and Cazenave, P.-A., 1971, Similar idiotypic specificities in immunoglobulin fractions with different antibody functions or even without detectable antibody function, *Proc. Natl. Acad. Sci. USA* **68**:2616–2620.
16. Ozato, K., Mayer, N., and Sachs, D. H., 1980, Hybridoma cell lines secreting monoclonal antibodies to mouse H-2 and Ia antigens, *J. Immunol.* **124**:533–540.
17. Epstein, S. L., Masakowski, V. R., Bluestone, J. A., Ozato, K., and Sachs, D. H., 1982, Idiotypes of anti-Ia antibodies. II. Effects of in vivo treatment with xenogeneic anti-idiotypes, *J. Immunol.* **129**:1545–1552.
18. Oi, V. T., Jones, P. P., Goding, L. A., Herzenberg, L. A., and Herzenberg, L. A., 1978, Properties of monoclonal antibodies to mouse allotypes, H-2 and Ia antigens, *Curr. Top. Microbiol. Immunol.* **81**:115–129.
19. Ozato, K., Epstein, S. L., Bluestone, J. A., Sharrow, S. O., Hansen, T., and Sachs, D. H., 1983, The

presence of a common idiotype in anti-H-2 immune sera as detected by anti-idiotype to a monoclonal anti-H-2 antibody, *Eur. J. Immunol.* **13**:13–18.

20. Bluestone, J. A., Auchincloss, H., Jr., Sachs, D. H., Fibi, M., and Hämmerling, G. J., 1983, Anti-idiotypes against monoclonal anti-H-2 antibodies. VI. Detection of shared idiotypes among monoclonal anti-H-2 antibodies, *Eur. J. Immunol.* **13**:489–495.

21. Gearheart, P. J., Johnson, N. D., Douglas, R., and Hood, L., 1981, IgG antibodies to phosphorylcholine exhibit more diversity than their IgM counterparts, *Nature* **291**:29–34.

22. Devaux, C., Epstein, S. L., Sachs, D. H., and Pierres, M., 1982, Cross-reactive idiotypes of monoclonal anti-Ia antibodies: Characterization with xenogeneic anti-idiotypic reagents and expression in anti-H-2 humoral responses, *J. Immunol.* **129**:2074–2081.

23. Pierres, M., Devaux, C., Dosseto, M., and Marchetto, S., 1981, Clonal analysis of B and T cell responses to Ia antigens. 1. Topography of epitope regions of I-A^k and I-E^k molecules analysed with 35 monoclonal alloantibodies, *Immunogenetics* **14**:481–495.

24. Melino, M. R., Epstein, S. L., Sachs, D. H., and Hansen, T. H., 1983, Idiotypic and fluorometric analysis of the antibodies which distinguish the lesion of the I-A mutant B6.C-H-2^{bm12}, *J. Immunol.* **131**:359–364.

25. Sacks, D. L., Kelsoe, G. H., and Sachs, D. H., 1983, Induction of immune responses with anti-idiotypic antibodies: Implications for the induction of protective immunity, *Springer Semin. Immunopathol.* **6**:79–97.

26. Urbain, J., Wikler, M., Franssen, J. D., and Collignon, C., 1977, Idiotypic regulation of the immune system by the induction of antibodies against anti-idiotypic antibodies, *Proc. Natl. Acad. Sci. USA* **74**:5126–5130.

27. Bluestone, J. A., Krutzsch, H. C., Auchincloss, H., Jr., Cazenave, P.-A., and Sachs, D. H., 1982, Comparative analysis of monoclonal anti-H-2K^k idiotype and idiotype-positive molecules induced by in vivo anti-idiotype treatment, *Proc. Natl. Acad. Sci. USA* **79**:7847–7851.

28. Bluestone, J. A., Epstein, S. L., Ozato, K., Sharrow, S. O., and Sachs, D. H., 1981, Anti-idiotypes to monoclonal anti-H-2 antibodies. II. Expression of anti-H-2K^k idiotypes on antibodies induced by anti-idiotype or H-2K^k antigen, *J. Exp. Med.* **145**:1305–1318.

29. Primi, D., Juy, D., and Cazenave, P.-A., 1981, Induction and regulation of silent idiotype clones, *Eur. J. Immunol.* **11**:393–398.

30. Siekevitz, M., Gefter, M. L., Brodeur, P., Riblet, R., and Marshak-Rothstein, A., 1982, The genetic basis of antibody production: The dominant anti-arsonate idiotype response of the strain A mouse, *Eur. J. Immunol.* **12**:1023–1032.

31. Takemori, T., Tesch, H., Reth, M., and Rajewsky, K., 1982, The immune response against anti-idiotope antibodies. I. Induction of idiotype-bearing antibodies and analysis of the idiotope repertoire, *Eur. J. Immunol.* **12**:1040–1046.

32. Pawlak, L. L., Mushinski, E. B., Nisonoff, A., and Potter, M., 1973, Evidence for the linkage of the IgC$_H$ locus to a gene controlling the idiotypic specificity of anti-p-azophenylarsonate antibodies in strain A mice, *J. Exp. Med.* **137**:22–31.

33. Laskin, J. A., Gray, A., Nisonoff, A., Klinman, N. R., and Gottlieb, P. D., 1977, Segregation at a locus determining an immunoglobulin genetic marker for the light chain variable region affects inheritance of expression of an idiotype, *Proc. Natl. Acad. Sci. USA* **74**:4600–4604.

34. Stein, K. E., Bona, C., Lieberman, R., Chien, C. C., and Paul, W. E., 1980, Regulation of the anti-inulin antibody response by a non-allotype linked gene, *J. Exp. Med.* **151**:1088–1102.

35. Klein, J., and Herzenberg, L. A., 1967, Congenic mouse strains with different immunoglobulin allotypes. I. Breeding scheme, histocompatibility tests, and kinetics of γG2a-globulin production by transferred cells for C3H.SW and its congenic partner CWB/5, *Transplantation* **5**:1484–1495.

36. Kelsoe, G., and Cerny, J., 1979, Reciprocal expansions of idiotypic and anti-idiotypic clones following antigenic stimulation, *Nature* **279**:333–334.

37. Bluestone, J. A., Auchincloss, H., Jr., Cazenave, P.-A., Ozato, K., and Sachs, D. H., 1982, Anti-idiotypes to monoclonal anti-H-2 antibodies. III. Syngeneic anti-idiotypes detect idiotopes on antibodies induced by in vivo administration of xenogeneic anti-idiotypes, *J. Immunol.* **129**:2066–2068.

38. Epstein, S. L., and Sachs, D. H., 1983, Use of monoclonal antibodies for studies of anti-Ia receptor idiotypes, in: *Ir Genes, Past, Present, and Future* (C. W. Pierce, S. E. Cullen, J. A. Kapp, B. D. Schwartz, and D. C. Shreffler, eds.), Humana Press, Clifton, N.J., pp. 81–90.

39. Grützmann, R., and Hämmerling, G. J., 1982, Idiotypic relationship of anti-Ia.2 antibodies, *Eur. J. Immunol.* **12**:307–312.
40. Kelsoe, G., Reth, M., and Rajewsky, K., 1980, Control of idiotype expression by monoclonal anti-idiotypic antibodies, *Immunol. Rev.* **52**:75–88.
41. Miller, G. M., Nadler, P. I., Asano, Y., Hodes, R. J., and Sachs, D. H., 1981, Induction of idiotype-bearing, nuclease-specific helper T cells by in vivo treatment with anti-idiotype, *J. Exp. Med.* **154**:24–34.
42. Auchincloss, H., Jr., Bluestone, J. A., and Sachs, D. H., 1983, Anti-idiotypes against anti-H-2 monoclonal antibodies. V. *In vivo* anti-idiotype treatment induces idiotype-specific helper T cells, *J. Exp. Med.* **157**:1273–1286.
43. Sachs, D. H., Bluestone, J. A., Epstein, S. L., and Rabinowitz, R., 1983, Idiotypes of anti-MHC antibodies, in: *Immune Networks* (C. A. Bona and H. Köhler, eds.), *Ann. NY Acad. Sci.* **418**:265–271.
44. Nagy, Z. A., Elliott, B. E., Carlow, D. A., and Rubin, B., 1982, T cell idiotypes recognizing self-major histocompatibility complex molecules: H-2 specificity, allotype linkage, and expression on functional T cell populations, *Eur. J. Immunol.* **12**:393–400.
45. Lemke, H., and Hämmerling, G. J., 1981, Topographic arrangement of H-2 determinants defined by monoclonal hybridoma antibodies, in: *Monoclonal Antibodies and T Cell Hybridomas* (G. J. Hämmerling, U. Hämmerling, and J. F. Kearney, eds.), Elsevier/North-Holland, Amsterdam, pp 102–109.
46. Sachs, D. H., Mayer, N., and Ozato, K., 1981, Hybridoma antibodies directed toward murine H-2 and Ia antigens, in: *Monoclonal Antibodies and T Cell Hybridomas* (G. J. Hämmerling, U. Hämmerling, and J. F. Kearney, eds.), Elsevier/North-Holland, Amsterdam, pp. 95–101.
47. Sachs, D. H., El-Gamil, M., Arn, J. S., and Ozato, K., 1981, Complementation between I region genes is revealed by a hybridoma anti-Ia antibody, *Transplantation* **31**:308–311.
48. Ozato, K., and Sachs, D. H., 1981, Monoclonal antibodies to mouse MHC antigens. III. Hybridoma antibodies reacting to antigens of the H-2^b haplotype reveal genetic control of isotype expression, *J. Immunol.* **126**:317–321.

18

Murine Plasmacytoma MOPC315 as a Tool for the Analysis of Network Regulation

M315 Idiotopes Are Inducers and Targets of Immunoregulatory Signals

RICHARD G. LYNCH AND GARY L. MILBURN

1. Introduction

A great deal of what is presently known about antibody molecules, their idiotypes, and their genes has come from studies of neoplastic antibody-producing cells. Typically, such studies have used an approach in which a myeloma cell provided the investigator with large quantities of a single, specific, readily purified macromolecule, e.g., an antibody, an RNA, or an immunoglobulin gene. This strategy has been successfully used to establish the primary, secondary, and tertiary structures of antibody molecules,[1-3] to develop the molecular probes that specifically detect immunoglobulin genes and RNAs,[4] and to identify the chromosomal location,[5] and the molecular organization and nucleotide sequences of immunoglobulin genes.[6,7]

The development of drug-sensitive myeloma cell lines and hybridization of these cells with normal antibody-producing cells[8] have provided investigators access to large quantities of monoclonal antibodies from virtually anywhere in the B-cell repertoire.[9] This development has now made it possible to begin to identify the precise structural basis of idiotypy.[10-12] In addition, the application of recombinant DNA technology to the study of neoplastic B cells has provided important, new information about the alterations in immu-

RICHARD G. LYNCH AND GARY L. MILBURN • Department of Pathology, University of Iowa College of Medicine, Iowa City, Iowa 52242.

noglobulin gene structure that accompany B-cell development.[6,7] Thus, neoplastic B cells have been widely and productively employed during the past 15 years to establish the structures of immunoglobulin proteins and the organization of immunoglobulin genes as they exist in a more or less fixed state in each clone. More recently, neoplastic B cells have been successfully used to study dynamic aspects of immunoglobulin expression such as immunoglobulin gene activation[13] and T-cell-mediated regulation of B-cell proliferation, differentiation, and imunoglobulin expression.[14-18]

While large gaps exist in our understanding of the processes by which B cells attain immunocompetency, it is generally assumed that the developmental steps that occur prior to the expression of surface membrane heavy and light chains occur independently of antigen and network regulation. Once a B cell becomes immunocompetent its further growth and differentiation are highly regulated processes. Helper and suppressor T cells, macrophages, lymphokines, anti-idiotypic antibodies, specific antigens, hormones, and a large number of other factors have been shown to contribute to the regulation of B-cell proliferation and differentiation. Thus, B cells are responsive to a vast array of external influences. While a great deal is already known about the conditions that alter the intensity of these influences, little is known about the events that occur within the target B cell following the arrival of the regulatory signals at the cell surface.

Visualization of the biochemical events that occur in a B cell following receipt of an immunoregulatory signal has been hampered by the lack of large numbers of purified, antigen-specific B cells for study. In conventional immune cell samples, e.g., spleen cells, the B cells of particular interest comprise a minor fraction of the entire sample. Efforts to establish *in vitro* cell lines of antigen-specific, normal B cells have been generally unsuccessful, although some progress has recently been reported.[19]

In contrast, many murine myeloma cells have defined antigen-binding properties[20] and are readily propagated *in vivo* and *in vitro*. This laboratory has established the feasibility of using murine myeloma cells to analyze immunoreguatory mechanisms.[14,17,21-23] These studies have shown that murine myeloma cells can function as inducers and targets of immunoregulatory signals and can be productively used to study the mechanisms involved in antigen-specific, isotype-specific, and idiotype-specific regulation.

Our studies of idiotypic regulation have, for the most part, used the 2,4,6-trinitrophenyl (TNP)-specific, BALB/c plasmacytoma MOPC315. The IgAλ_2 anti-TNP antibody (M315) produced by MOPC315 has been extensively characterized in terms of its structure[24,25] and its hapten-binding properties.[26,27] The studies discussed in this chapter review: (1) the characteristics of the immune responses of BALB/c mice to M315, and (2) the influence that the anti-M315 immune responses exert on the proliferation, differentiation, and immunoglobulin expression of MOPC315 cells. While MOPC315 has been most extensively studied, it is clear from the literature that other neoplastic antibody-producing cells are responsive to a variety of immunoregulatory signals.[28-38]

2. Immunoregulatory Responses Induced in BALB/c Mice Immunized with M315

A multiplicity of immunoregulatory responses have been identified in BALB/c mice immunized with M315. The availability of large quantities of specifically purified M315, its constitutive polypeptide chains, and proteolytic fragments have allowed considerable progress to be made in the analysis of these responses. The following subsections will review our present understanding of these responses.

2.1. Protection against Challenge with Myeloma Cells

In 1972 it was reported that BALB/c mice immunized with purified M315 were rendered resistant to challenge with otherwise lethal numbers of MOPC315 cells.[39] The transplantation resistance to subcutaneous challenge was specific for M315. Mice challenged with MOPC460, another IgA anti-TNP myeloma, developed progressively lethal tumors. In contrast, mice immunized with M460 were resistant to challenge with MOPC460 cells but were not resistant to MOPC315 cells. However, this idiotype-specific tumor immunity could be overcome by challenge with large numbers of myeloma cells. Subsequent development of a sensitive and quantitative MOPC315 spleen colony assay[40] demonstrated that the systemic resistance to challenge was considerably greater than the subcutaneous resistance. In the original studies mice were immunized with M315[39] but it was later demonstrated that mice immunized with either L^{315} or V_L^{315} also exhibited an Id^{315}-specific resistance to myeloma cell challenge.[41]

The mechanism of Id^{315}-specific tumor immunity is still incompletely understood but some elements of the mechanism have been identified. Resistance to challenge with MOPC315 cells appears to involve a short-lived, thymus-dependent T cell.[42] Surgical resection of the thymus gland after immunization abrogates the protective immunity but does not influence the expression of anti-idiotypic antibodies.[42] Evidence has been presented for participation of an L^{315}-specific T cell in the protective immunity.[11] Preliminary evidence suggests a cytostatic rather than a cytotoxic effector mechanism (G. L. Milburn and R. G. Lynch, unpublished observations). While anti-idiotypic antibodies may play a role in protective immunity when they are present, they are not required[41] nor have they been sufficient in themselves in the studies reported thus far.[43]

While further studies are required before the precise mechanism of protective immunity is clearly defined the studies thus far indicate that a complex, T-cell-dependent mechanism inhibits the clonal expansion of MOPC315 cells. This suppressor circuit is different both in effect and in specifity from the suppressor T-cell circuit discussed below (Section 2.4) that mediates the inhibition of M315 synthesis and secretion by MOPC315 cells.

2.2. Induction of Anti-Idiotypic Antibodies

In 1971 Sirisinha and Eisen[44] reported that BALB/c mice immunized with purified M315 developed antibodies specific for the DNP-binding site of M315. It was subsequently shown that antibodies specific for M315 were also induced in mice immunized with Fab^{315},[45] DNP-affinity-labeled M315,[46] or L^{315}.[46] Three major classes of specificities have been identified in the anti-M315 antibodies present in these mice.

One population of antibodies is specific for a combinatorial ($V_L^{315} + V_H^{315}$) determinant(s) of the M315 paratope. Antibodies with this specificity have been detected in mice immunized with M315[44,47] or Fab 315.[45]

A second population of antibodies, specific for a combinatorial ($V_L^{315} + V_H^{315}$) determinant(s) that appears to be located outside of the M315 paratope, has been identified in mice immunized with M315,[47] Fab 315,[45] or DNP-affinity-labeled M315.[46]

Antibodies that are L^{315}-specific develop in mice immunized with free L^{315}.[46] These antibodies bind to free L^{315} but bind poorly, or not at all, to L^{315} when it is associated with H^{315}.[46] The L^{315}-specific antibodies do not bind to the M315 molecules expressed on the surface of MOPC315 cells. Since mice immunized with L^{315} do not develop antibodies that bind combinatorial determinants on M315, and L^{315}-specific antibodies do not react with MOPC315 cells, the tumor immunity that is induced by immunization with L^{315} is effected in the absence of M315-reactive antibodies. This finding is one of several observations that tends to minimize the potential for any direct role of antibody in Id^{315}-specific tumor immunity. Although the studies to date have failed to identify a direct role for anti-idiotypic antibodies in protective immunity, further studies are clearly warranted since there are numerous examples in the literature in which administration of anti-idiotypic antibodies leads to the expression of idiotype-specific suppressor T-cell effects.

One effector function of anti-Id^{315} antibodies has been identified. Polyclonal and monoclonal anti-Id^{315} (combinatorial, $V_L^{315} + V_H^{315}$) antibodies have been shown to modulate the surface membrane expression of M315 on MOPC315 cells.[48] These studies showed that anti-Id^{315}–M315 immune complexes formed on the surface of MOPC315 cells and were rapidly shed. When an *in vitro*-adapted line of MOPC315 cells was cultured in the continuous presence of anti-Id^{315} antibodies for up to several weeks no effect could be detected on the growth properties of the cells nor on the secretion of M315. The ultrastructural properties of the MOPC315 cells were not altered and the only effect observed was the continued clearance of surface membrane M315 in a treadmill fashion. Reutilization of cleared anti-Id^{315} antibodies did not occur. When anti-idiotypic antibodies were consumed, or removed from the culture, surface membrane expression of M315 recovered within 2 hr. In preliminary studies the addition of normal lymphoid cells and accessory cells to cultures of MOPC315 that contained anti-Id^{315} antibodies neither influenced the modulation of surface M315 nor resulted in additional effects. While it is possible, and perhaps likely, that the *in vivo* presence of anti-Id^{315} antibodies may influence the expression of other Id^{315}-specific regulatory circuits, the only direct effector function established for anti-Id^{315} antibodies thus far is their ability to modulate the surface membrane expression of M315 on MOPC315 cells.

2.3. Induction of Anti-IgA Antibodies

In 1978 Odermatt *et al.*[47] observed that about 30% of BALB/c mice immunized with M315 developed antibodies that appeared to be specific for a determinant(s) located in the second and/or third homology regions of the constant region of the α heavy chain. An effector function for the anti-IgA antibodies has not been established but it is of considerable interest that under these circumstances of hyperimmunization some BALB/c mice develop antibodies specific for one of their own heavy chains.

2.4. Inhibition of Synthesis and Secretion of M315 by MOPC315 Cells

In the original demonstration of protective immunity against challenge with MOPC315 cells[39] it was observed that some of the immunized mice developed tumors which were progressive but which were not accompanied by the appearance of M315 in the serum. However, when such tumors were transplanted to nonimmunized mice many of the tumors that developed were accompanied by the expected high levels of circulating M315. In subsequent studies[49] it was demonstrated that M315-immunized mice developed idiotype-specific suppressor T cells that inhibited secretion of M315 but did not influence MOPC315 proliferation. Secretory inhibition could be adoptively transferred to normal mice with M315-immune T cells. There were several interesting aspects of these studies. (1) Unlike the Id^{315}-specific suppressor T cell that inhibited the clonal proliferation of MOPC315 cells,[39,42] the T cell that inhibited secretion did not influence MOPC315 proliferation. (2) The T cell that suppressed M315 secretion did not influence the cytological differentiation of MOPC315 from lymphocytoid to plasmacytoid cells. In an earlier study[53] it had been shown that MOPC315 cells differentiated during *in vivo* growth in normal BALB/c mice. The finding that the T cell that suppressed M315 secretion did not influence the cytological differentiation of MOPC315 cells suggested that inhibition of M315 secretion was effected at a late stage in differentiation. Other experiments demonstrated that the inhibition of M315 secretion was reversible, suggesting that inhibition was mediated at the level of the actual secretory cell. (3) Since the inhibition of M315 secretion occurred across the 0.2-μm pores of the diffusion chamber membrane, and occurred even after removal of contaminating accessory cells from the MOPC315 ascites cells in the chambers, it was proposed that a soluble suppressive factor acted directly on the MOPC315 secretory cell.[52]

Recently, significant progress has been made in further characterization of the suppressor T cells that inhibit M315 secretion and in identification of some of the cellular and molecular events that mediate the effect. An *in vitro* system was established in which T cells from M315-immunized mice were examined for their ability to influence a tissue culture-adapted line of MOPC315 cells.[15] As shown in Table I the immune T cells did not influence the viability or surface membrane expression of M315 compared to normal T cells, but did effect a striking inhibition of M315 secretion. The suppression of M315

TABLE I
Effect of Id^{315}-Specific T Cells on MOPC315 Cells in Vitro

Effector : MOPC315 cell ratio[a]	Effector cells	Viability	Percentage of MOPC315 with surface M315	Percentage of MOPC315 cells that secrete M315
MOPC315 cells alone	None	93 ± 2[b]	89 ± 2	44 ± 3
50 : 1	Normal spleen T cells	86 ± 3	89 ± 2	41 ± 5
100 : 1	Normal spleen T cells	85 ± 5	84 ± 3	40 ± 4
200 : 1	Normal spleen T cells	83 ± 5	82 ± 3	38 ± 3
50 : 1	RA315-immune spleen T cells	78 ± 3	82 ± 4	36 ± 4
100 : 1	RA315-immune spleen T cells	78 ± 5	79 ± 5	8 ± 2
200 : 1	RA315-immune spleen T cells	76 ± 2	77 ± 5	3 ± 2

[a] MOPC315 cell number was typically 10^5 viable cells/ml, and the effector cell number was adjusted according to the ratio indicated.
[b] Mean $\pm$ 1 S.E.M. for three experiments.

secretion was dependent on the dose of immune T cells and virtually total inhibition could be achieved. The effector cells were shown to be Lyt-1$^-$2$^+$ and were enriched by adsorption to Id^{315}-Sepharose columns. Immune T cells cocultured with MOPC315 cells inhibited secretion as early as 6 hr after mixing. Since the myeloma cells were secreting M315 at the time that the suppressor cells were added to the culture, the suppressor T cells acted directly on the actual antibody-secreting cell rather than on a secretory precursor.

Incorporation of [^{3}H] leucine into secreted and intracellular M315 was inhibited more than 90% in the presence of suppressor T cells. The suppression of M315 synthesis was shown to be selective. Studies performed in a diffusion apparatus in which the T cells were separated from the MOPC315 cells by a Millipore membrane provided a means to study incorporation into total protein and M315 protein by MOPC315 cells. When the cells were incubated in separate compartments of the chambers for 48 hr and then pulsed with [^{3}H] leucine for 24 hr, a decrease of approximately 50% in total protein synthesis was observed and the entire decrement could be accounted for by the decrease in M315 synthesis (Table II). When suppressed MOPC315 cells were removed from the diffusion chambers and cultured in the absence of T cells, secretion of M315 was reestablished. In all of the studies discussed above the T cells were isolated from BALB/c mice that had been immunized with affinity-purified M315.

In a recent study[51] we have established that the suppressor T cell is specific for a V_H^{315} idiotope(s).[51] In competitive inhibition studies the suppressor T cells were prevented from inhibiting M315 synthesis and secretion when M315 or V_H^{315}-containing fragments

TABLE II
Depletion and Enrichment of Id^{315}-Specific T Cells

Effector : MOPC315 cell ratio	Treatment of added RA315-immune T cells	Percentage of MOPC315 cells that secrete M315
MOPC315 cells alone	No treatment	43 ± 3[a]
50 : 1	No treatment	12 ± 3
100 : 1	No treatment	8 ± 3
200 : 1	No treatment	3 ± 1
50 : 1	Id^{460} absorption[b]	16 ± 4
100 : 1	Id^{460} absorption	10 ± 5
200 : 1	Id^{460} absorption	7 ± 2
50 : 1	Id^{315} absorption[c]	35 ± 3
100 : 1	Id^{315} absorption	36 + 5
200 : 1	Id^{315} absorption	34 ± 6
12 : 1	Eluted from Id^{315} absorbant[d]	11 ± 5
25 : 1	Eluted from Id^{315} absorbant	4 ± 4
50 : 1	Eluted from Id^{315} absorbant	1 ± 1

[a]Mean ± 1 S.E.M. for three experiments.
[b]RA315-immune spleen T cells were passed over an Id^{460}-Sepharose 6MB column, and the nonadherent cells were used as effectors.
[c]RA315-immune spleen T cells were passed over an Id315-Sepharose 6MB column, and the nonadherent cells were used as effectors.
[d]Cells that adhered to the Id^{315}-Sepharose 6MB column were eluted with soluble RA315 in PBS at a concentration of 2 mg/ml.

of M315 were added to the cultures. In addition, the induction of the V_H^{315}-specific suppressor T cell can be achieved by immunization with purified V_H^{315}.[51] Thus, in this suppressor circuit, a V_H^{315}-recognition event occurs at both inductive and effector stages.

The selective nature and the kinetics of inhibition of M315 synthesis suggested a transcriptional or translational mechanism of control. To address this issue polyadenylated RNA was isolated from control and suppressed MOPC315 cells. The RNA was electrophoresed in a 1.2% agarose gel under denaturing conditions, transferred to nitrocellulose membranes, and probed for RNA sequences complementary to cloned DNA fragments specific for α heavy- or λ_2 light-chain gene segments.[17] When polyadenylated RNA isolated from nonsuppressed and suppressed MOPC315 cells was hybridized to a ^{32}P-labeled probe specific for α constant-region sequences, autoradiography revealed three major transcipts of 1.7, 2.1, and 3.0 kb in length (Fig. 1, lane 1). We observed that the pattern of α-transcript banding was comparable in suppressed (Fig. 1, lanes 2 and 4) and nonsuppressed (Fig. 1, lanes 1 and 3) MOPC315 cells. Qualitative differences were not detected whether MOPC315 cells were cocultured directly with (Fig. 1, lanes 1 and 2) or membrane-segregated from (Fig. 1, lanes 3 and 4) these suppressor T cells.

Analysis of the same RNA preparations with a hybridization probe specific for the λ_2 light-chain constant region revealed a single complementary transcript of 1.2 kb in length. This corresponds to the mature-sized λ_2 mRNA transcript previously reported[52] and appears in lanes using RNA isolated from direct coculture (Fig. 2, lane 1) or membrane-segregated cocultures (Fig. 2, lane 3) with normal T lymphocytes. Polyadenylated RNA recovered from suppressed MOPC315 cells had a marked reduction in the amount of λ_2 transcript (Fig. 2, lanes 2 and 4). When the autoradiograms were analyzed by densitometric techniques, the quantity of λ_2 transcripts from suppressed cells was less than 10% of the control lane although precise measurement could not be made from the low image density. These findings demonstrated that suppressor T cells and a diffusible product of the suppressor cells produced a marked reduction in the expression of λ_2 mRNA in MOPC315 cells.[17]

When examined in a cell-free translation system the α-chain mRNA from suppressed MOPC315 cells was shown to be initiated and served as a template for a mature-sized α

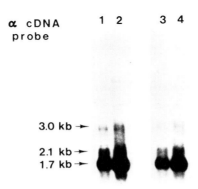

FIGURE 1. The effect of culturing MOPC315 cells with normal T cells (lanes 1 and 3) or Id^{315}-specific T-suppressor cells (lanes 2 and 4) in direct cocultures (lanes 1 and 2) or membrane-segregated cocultures (lanes 3 and 4) on the α heavy-chain mRNA.

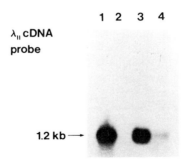

λ_{II} cDNA
probe

1.2 kb ⟶

FIGURE 2. The effect of culturing MOPC315 cells with normal T cells (lanes 1 and 3) or Id[315]-specific T-suppressor cells (lanes 2 and 4) in direct cocultures (lanes 1 and 2) or membrane-segregated cocultures (lanes 3 and 4) on the λ_2 light-chain mRNA.

polypeptide.[17] The presence of a functional α heavy-chain mRNA and the apparent absence of heavy-chain polypeptide synthesis in the suppressed myeloma cells presented a paradox. Furthermore, it was surprising that while the suppressor T cells were specific for a V_H^{315} idiotope,[51] the conspicuous alteration of mRNA expression was at the level of the light chain. In an effort to account for these findings we have proposed a model in which the light-chain polypeptide functions as a regulatory subunit of the immunoglobulin molecule (Fig. 3).[17] In normal immunoglobulin-secreting cells the expression of the light and heavy polypeptide chains occur as independent events, but the precise steps in the assembly of the secretory IgA molecule from the synthesized chains have not been completely defined. In the suppressed myeloma cell, the absence of the light-chain polypeptide appears to prevent full expression of the heavy-chain gene by a mechanism that operates distal to the occurrence of a functionally intact heavy-chain mRNA.[17] These findings are consistent with a model in which light-chain polypeptides, once synthesized and released from their polysomes, either: (1) facilitate the release of the heavy-chain polypeptides from their polysomes, or (2) protect heavy chains from degradation. This mechanism could also account for many of the patterns of heavy- and light-chain expression that have been observed in neoplastic B cells (discussed in Ref. 17). Moreover, a regulatory role of light chain in the full expression of immunoglobulin is consistent with the changes that occur in the transition of a pre-B cell to an immunocompetent B cell (discussed in Ref. 17). The proposed model describes a mechanism in which regulation of expression of one chain of a two-chain protein, in effect, regulates expression of the other chain and, therefore, the whole molecule.

An interesting aspect of light-chain mRNA regulation in MOPC315 cells is the finding of coordinate regulation of the normal λ_2 mRNA and the truncated λ_1 mRNA.[16] In MOPC315 cells an aberrantly rearranged λ_1 gene produces a truncated mRNA that is translated into a rapidly degraded short λ_1 light-chain polypeptide.[55] Analysis of a poly-adenylated RNA preparation with a hybridization probe specific for the λ_1 constant region revealed a single complementary species in nonsuppressed MOPC315 cells (Fig. 4). Because a large portion of the coding sequence for the variable region is absent from this anomalous λ_1 transcript[54] it is easily distinguished from λ_2 mRNA by its smaller size (1.0 kb). When suppressed MOPC315 cells were examined we observed that changes in the

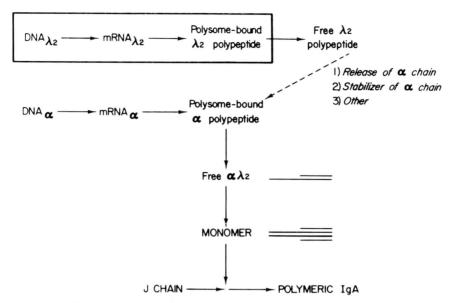

FIGURE 3. This model, consistent with the data presented here, outlines the independent biosynthesis of immunoglobulin light and heavy chains. It also depicts the role of the light chain as a stabilizer of the heavy chain or as a facilitator of its release. The box outlines the level at which a regulatory event may occur after the myeloma cell receives the suppressive signal from the Id^{315}-specific T cell. The absence of the light chain prevents the *full* expression of the heavy chain.

concentration of the λ_1 transcript precisely paralleled those observed for λ_2 mRNA.[16] Since the concentration of α heavy-chain mRNA in suppressed MOPC315 cells is not significantly different from nonsuppressed MOPC315 cells the inhibition of light-chain mRNA expression is relatively selective and is not merely a result of nonspecific RNA degradation. These findings suggest that the suppressor T cells selectively inhibit the expression of λ_2 and λ_1 light-chain mRNAs in MOPC315 cells. To produce such an effect, the suppressive factors must either decrease the rate of synthesis of light-chain-specific transcripts or enhance the rate of degradation of these transcripts in the nucleus or cytoplasm of the target cell. Since the aberrantly rearranged λ_1 gene in MOPC315 cells is located on the chromosome homologous to that of the productively rearranged λ_2 gene[54] the coordinate regulation of λ_2 and λ_1 mRNAs appears to be mediated by a *trans* mechanism.

The considerable nucleotide sequence homology between λ_1 and λ_2 constant-region genes[55,56] as well as between coding and upstream elements of λ_1 and λ_2 variable regions provides a structural basis for coordinate regulation of the λ family of light chains. Coordinate *trans* regulation of λ_2 and λ_1 gene expression implies the existence of a λ-specific regulatory molecule. It is of interest that Abbas *et al.*[57] observed independent regulation of M11 ($\gamma_{2b}\kappa$) and M315 ($\alpha\lambda_2$) expression in a myeloma–myeloma hybrid line (MPC11 × MOPC315) exposed to suppressor T cells specific for the corresponding idiotype. While the molecular details of suppression in those studies were not investigated, the findings are of particular interest since one of the immunoglobulin molecules expressed a κ light chain, while the other expressed a λ_2 light chain. One possible way to account for independent

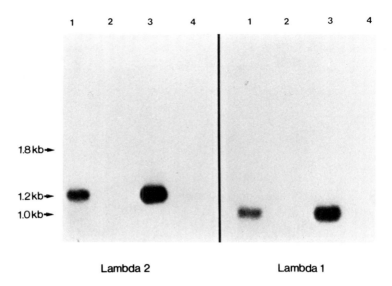

FIGURE 4. The effect of culturing MOPC315 cells with normal T cells (lanes 1 and 3) or ID[315]-specific T-suppressor cells (lanes 2 and 4) in direct cocultures (lanes 1 and 2) or membrane-segregated cocultures (lanes 3 and 4) on the λ_2 and λ_1 mRNA.

regulation in a cell producing two immunoglobulins is by a light-chain class-specific mechanism. Further studies are needed to examine this possibility.

A predicted consequence of light-chain class-specific suppression by idiotype-specific T cells would be suppression of Id$^+$ cells regardless of the changing heavy-chain class commitment of the clone. If a similar mechanism operated for the regulation of κ light-chain expression, then it might be possible to regulate immunoglobulin expression of the entire B-cell repertoire by a mechanism in which an idiotype-specific encounter activated the expression of either a κ or a λ regulatory molecule.

2.5. Induction of Idiotype-Specific Helper Cells

In an interesting series of studies Jorgensen and Hannestad[46,58,59,60] have identified a $V_L{}^{315}$-specific, Mitchisonian-type helper T cell in BALB/c mice immunized with M315, DNP-affinity-labeled M315, L[315], $F_V{}^{315}$ or $V_L{}^{315}$. These $T_H{}^1$ cells mediate a carrier helper effect when transferred with NIP-primed B cells into irradiated recipients that are challenged with NIP$_5$-M315.[46] The $V_L{}^{315}$-specific helper T-cell response is controlled by genes linked to the *H-2* complex.[59] Since the target B cells of the $V_L{}^{315}$-specific helper T cell in the studies of Jorgensen and Hannestad are conventional, nonneoplastic B cells, their findings provide evidence that the immunoregulatory cells induced in mice immunized with M315 also function in conventional immune responses and are not simply artifacts of immunization with myeloma proteins. Recognition of the antigenic site by the $V_L{}^{315}$-specific T cells is not dependent on L[315] conformation,[60] but L[315] conformation is required for recognition by anti-L^{315} antibodies. Furthermore, induction of V_L^{315}-specific T_H^1 cells follows immunization with V_L^{315} or $F_V^{315(46)}$ whereas these proteins fail to induce anti-V_L^{315} antibodies.[61] Rohrer et al.[18] have identified Ly-1^+2^-, Qa-1^+ L^{315}-specific helper T cells in BALB/c mice immunized with M315. These have been shown to be T_H^2 cells that enhance secretory differentiation of MOPC315 cells without affecting their proliferation. This cell is a helper cell counterpart to the Ly-1^-2^+, V_H^{315}-specific suppressor cell that inhibits M315 secretion without affecting MOPC315 proliferation.

As proposed by Jorgensen and Hannestad[46] the preferential activation of T cells by immunoglobulin variable-region domains could be of fundamental importance in network regulation.[62] This issue warrants further study in light of: (1) the small quantity of soluble V_L^{315} that is required to induce suppression of M315-specific DTH responses (Section 2.6 and Ref. 11) and (2) the finding that V_L and V_H fragments of immunoglobulins can be generated spontaneously in vivo.[63]

2.6. Induction and Regulation of M315-Specific Delayed-Type Hypersensitivity (DTH)

Sakato et al.[11] have shown that BALB/c mice immunized with 60 μg of M315 in complete Freund's adjuvant exhibit a DTH response when challenged 10 days later with 10 μg of M315. The response was shown to be M315-specific and had typical features of a murine DTH response. Interestingly, a single intravenous injection of 100 μg of soluble M315 or F_V^{315} was found to stimulate the development of suppressor T cells that blocked induction of the M315-specific DTH response.

In an elegent study Sakato et al.[11] used a battery of monoclonal immunoglobulin light chains to investigate the specificity of the DTH suppressor cells. They found that the suppressor cells could also be induced by soluble L^{315} or V_L^{315} but not by the monoclonal λ_1 light chains isolated from the TNP-specific myeloma T952 or the TNP-specific hybridoma MA-13. The major structural difference between L^{315}, L^{952}, and L^{8-13} is the amino acid triplet located at positions 94, 95, and 96 in the third hypervariable loop.[11] Thus, the T cells (or their precursors) that suppress M315-specific DTH appear to recognize only a site that includes the third hypervariable loop of L^{315}. Since the fully reduced and S-alkylated L^{315} failed to induce the suppressor T cell, it was proposed that the suppressor cells (or their precursors) recognized the tertiary structure of V_L^{315}, not simply the key amino acid triplet in the third hypervariable region. This detail contrasts with the V_L^{315}-specific helper T cells described by Jorgensen and Hannestad (discussed in Section 2.5 and Ref. 50) that appear to recognize unfolded L^{315}.

Another interesting aspect of the studies of Sakato et al.[11] was the finding that immunoglobulin molecules reconstituted by pairing L^{315} with heterologous H chains were effective inducers of the suppressor cell. As discussed by Sakato et al.[11] such heterologous recombinant molecules could be considered, in network terms, as nonspecific, parallel sets of idiotypes. Conceivably, if a B cell produced such molecules it might come under the regulatory control of the V_L^{315}-specific suppressor T cell because it expressed the regulatory idiotope located in the third hypervariable loop of L^{315}. Such a B cell would not be DNP-specific and, since it shared only the light-chain idiotopes with M315, it would have a different idiotype from M315. As proposed by Sakato et al.[11] regulatory interactions of this type could account for the frequent finding, originally described by Oudin and Cazenave,[64] that some antibodies elicited by an antigen fail to bind that antigen but express an idiotope in common with the antigen-binding antibodies.

3. Summary and Concluding Remarks

This chapter has reviewed the immunoregulatory responses that develop in BALB/c mice immunized with the BALB/c myeloma protein M315. A multiplicity of highly specific T-cell and B-cell responses have been identified. While it is clear that a great deal is yet to be learned about the mechanisms that underlie many of these responses much progress has already been made. It is also clear that the study of neoplastic B cells provides a powerful experimental system in which to analyze the precise molecular events that mediate immunoregulatory processes. These studies have begun to visualize the participation of different variable-region domains of M315 in different immunoregulatory circuits. The diversity of effects that have been observed to follow engagement of surface membrane M315 on MOPC315 cells by various immunoregulatory effectors is strong evidence that the surface membrane immunoglobulin molecules function as focusing devices for regulatory signals rather than as simple transducers.

While the use of myeloma cells to study immunoregulatory mechanisms is sometimes viewed with skepticism, the anomalous features of these cells often permit observations to be made that probably would never be possible with normal cells. The most recent example is the coordinate regulation of λ_2 and λ_1 gene expression in MOPC315 cells discussed in Section 2.4. Rather than being limitations, the aberrant features of neoplastic B cells often provide the most interesting information.

There are a number of important, unanswered questions raised by some of the studies reviewed above. What is the relationship between the various L^{315}-specific regulatory T cells? What is the important molecule in the suppression of λ-mRNA expression? Where is it made, how does it act, and what is its chemical structure? What is the mechanism of Id^{315}-specific tumor immunity? Studies addressing these questions should continue to develop new and useful information about the nature of immunoregulatory mechanisms. A more general question is the relevance of the MOPC315 system to idiotypic network regulation. In this regard the recent studies of Amor et al.[65] are of interest. They found that BALB/c mice immunized with a monoclonal anti-Id^{315} (combinatorial, $V_L^{315} + V_H^{315}$) antibody (Ab2) developed anti-anti-Id^{315} antibodies (Ab3) that bound DNP when the Ab3 contained λ light chains but did not bind DNP when Ab3 contained κ light chains. These findings suggest that the idiotypic network is not close-ended for a given idiotypic system but must be connected with other systems. While network regulation is obviously complex, the MOPC315 system appears to be a useful model with which to identify and analyze the elements that underlie the complexity.

ACKNOWLEDGMENTS. The studies from this laboratory that were reviewed above were supported by USPHS Research Grants CA-32275 and CA-17114. Various aspects of these studies have been carried out in this laboratory over the past 10 years by James W. Rohrer, Bernhard Odermatt, Michael J. Daley, Maureen Frikke, Howard B. Urnovitz, Katie R.

Williams, Sandra Bridges, Howard M. Gebel, Allan Mueller, and Ruth Mordhorst. The authors are grateful to Dr. Michael Potter, National Cancer Institute, who provided us with the plasmacytomas used in these studies, to Dr. Joseph M. Davie, Washington University, who provided many useful reagents, to Dr. Herman N. Eisen, Massachusetts Institute of Technology, and Professor Ernest Simms, Washington University, who provided cell lines, encouragement, and useful discussion in the early phase of these studies, and to Vicki Brown and Betty Perry for secretarial help in the preparation of the manuscript.

References

1. Kabat, E. A., Wu, T. T., and Bilofsky, H., 1979, *Sequences of Immunoglobulin Chains,* National Institute of Health Publication 80-2008.
2. Edelman, G. M., Cunningham, B. A., Gall, W. E., Gottlieb, P. D., Rutishauser, U., and Waxdal, M. J., 1969, The covalent structure of an entire γG immunoglobulin molecule, *Proc. Natl. Acad. Sci. USA* **63:**78–85.
3. Amzel, L. M., and Poljak, R. J., 1979, Three-dimensional structure of immunoglobulins, *Annu. Rev. Biochem.* **48:**961–967.
4. Hozumi, N., and Tonegawa, S., 1976, Evidence for somatic rearrangement of immunoglobulin genes coding for variable and constant regions, *Proc. Natl. Acad. Sci. USA* **73:**3628–3632.
5. Erikson, J., Finan, J., Nowell, P. C., and Croce, C. M., 1982, Translocation of immunoglobulin V_H genes in Burkitt lymphoma, *Proc. Natl. Acad. Sci. USA* **79:**5611–5615.
6. Tonegawa, S., Brock, C., Hozumi, N., Matthyssens, G., and Schuller, R., 1979, Dynamics of immunoglobulin genes, *Immunol. Rev.* **36:**73–94.
7. Leder, P., and Seidman, J. G., 1978, The arrangement and rearrangement of antibody genes, *Nature* **276:**790–795.
8. Köhler, G., and Milstein, C., 1975, Continuous cultures of fused cells secreting antibodies of predefined specifications, *Nature* **256:**495–497.
9. Kenneth, R. H., McKearn, T. J., and Bechtol, K. B. (eds.), 1980, *Monoclonal Antibodies,* Plenum Press, New York.
10. Potter, M., Pawlita, M., Mushinski, E., and Feldmann, R.J., 1981, Structure of idiotypes and idiotopes, in: *Immunoglobulin Idiotypes* (C. A. Janeway, Jr., E. E. Sercarz, and H. Wigzell, eds.), Academic Press, New York, pp. 1–20.
11. Sakato, N., Semma, M., Eisen, H. N., and Azuma, T., 1982, A small hypervariable segment in the variable domain of an immunoglobulin light chain stimulates formation of anti-idiotypic suppressor T cells, *Proc. Natl. Acad. Sci. USA* **79:**5396–5400.
12. Schilling, J., Clevinger, B., Davie, J. M., and Hood, L., 1980, Amino acid sequence of homogeneous antibodies to dextran and DNA rearrangements in heavy chain V-region gene segments, *Nature* **285:**35–40.
13. Parslow, T. G., and Granner, D. K., 1982, Chromatin changes accompany immunoglobulin K gene activation: A potential control region within the gene, *Nature* **299:**449–451.
14. Lynch, R. G., Rohrer, J. W., Odermatt, B. O., Gebel, H. M., Autry, J. R., and Hoover, R. G., 1979, Immunoregulation of murine myeloma cell growth and differentiation: A monoclonal model of B cell differentiation, *Immunol. Rev.* **48:**45–80.
15. Milburn, G. L., and Lynch, R. G., 1982, Immunoregulation of murine myeloma in vitro, *J. Exp. Med.* **155:**852–861.
16. Parslow, T. G., Milburn, G. L., Lynch, R. G., and Granner, D. K., 1983, Suppressor T cell action inhibits the expression of an excluded immunoglobulin gene, *Science* **220:**1389–1391.
17. Milburn, G. L., Parslow, T. G., Goldenberg, C., Granner, D. K., and Lynch, R. G., 1984, Idiotype-specific T cell suppression of light chain mRNA expression in MOPC-315 cells is accompanied by a post-transcriptional inhibition of heavy chain expression, *J. Cell. Mol. Immunol.* **1:**115–123.
18. Rohrer, J. W., Gershon, R. K., Lynch, R. G., and Kemp, J. D., 1984, The enhancement of B lymphocyte secretory differentiation by an Ly 1^+, 2^-; Q_a-1^+ helper T cell subset that sees both antigen and determinants on immunoglobulin, *J. Cell. Mol. Immunol.* **1:**50–62.

19. Aldo-Benson, M., and Scheiderer, L., 1983, Long-term growth of lines of murine dinitrophenyl-specific B lymphocytes in vitro, *J. Exp. Med.* **157**:342–347.
20. Potter, M., 1977, Antigen-binding myeloma proteins of mice, *Adv. Immunol.* **25**:141–211.
21. Rohrer, J. W., and Lynch, R. G., 1978, Antigen-specific regulation of myeloma cell differentiation in vivo by carrier-specific T cell factors and macrophages, *J. Immunol.* **121**:1066–1074.
22. Hoover, R. G., Gebel, H. M., Dieckgraefe, B. K., Hickman, S., Rebbe, N., Hirayama, N., Ovary, Z., and Lynch, R. G., 1981, Occurrence and potential significnce of increased numbers of T cells with Fc receptors in myeloma, *Immunol. Rev.* **56**:115–139.
23. Hoover, R. G., and Lynch, R. G., 1983, Isotype-specific suppression of IgA: Suppression of IgA responses in BALB/c mice by Tα cells, *J. Immunol.* **130**:521–523.
24. Dugan, E. S., Bradshaw, R. A., Simms, E. S., and Eisen, H. N., 1973, Amino acid sequence of the light chain of a mouse myeloma protein (MOPC-315), *Biochemistry* **12**:5400–5416.
25. Francis, S. H., Leslie, R. G. Q., Hood, L., and Eisen, H. N., 1974, Amino acid sequence of the variable region of the heavy (alpha) chain of a mouse myeloma protein with anti-hapten activity, *Proc. Natl. Acad. Sci. USA* **71**:1123–1127.
26. Eisen, H. N., Simms, E. S., and Potter, M., 1968, Mouse myeloma proteins with anti-hapten antibody activity: The protein produced by plasma cell tumor MOPC-315, *Biochemistry* **7**:4126–4134.
27. Inbar, D., Hochman, J., and Givol, D., 1972, Localization of antibody-combining sites within the variable portions of heavy and light chains, *Proc. Natl. Acad. Sci. USA* **69**:2659–2662.
28. Meinke, G. C., McConakey, P. J., and Spiegelberg, H. L., 1974, Suppression of plasmacytoma growth in mice by immunization with myeloma protein, *Fed. Proc.* **33**:792.
29. Sugai, S., Palmer, D. W., Talal, N., and Witz, I. P., 1974, Protective and cellular immune responses to idiotypic determinants on cells from a spontaneous lymphoma of NZB/NZW$_{F1}$ mice, *J. Exp. Med.* **140**:1547–1558.
30. Eisen, H. N., Sakato, N., and Hall, S. J., 1975, Myeloma proteins as tumor-specific antigens, *Transplant. Proc.* **7**:209–214.
31. Beatty, P. G., Kim, B. S., Rowley, D. A., and Coppleson, L. W., 1976, Antibody against the antigen receptor of a plasmacytoma prolongs survival of mice bearing the tumor, *J. Immunol.* **116**:1391–1396.
32. Bosma, M. J., and Bosma, G. C., 1977, Prevention of IgG$_{2A}$ production as a result of allotype-specific interaction between T and B cells, *J. Exp. Med.* **145**:743–748.
33. Bankert, R. B., Mayers, G. L., and Pressman, D., 1978, Clearance and re-expression of a myeloma cell's antigen-binding receptors induced by ligands known to be immunogenic or tolerogenic for normal B lymphocytes: A model to study membrane events associated with B cell tolerance, *Eur. J. Immunol.* **8**:512–519.
34. Kans, J., D'Ottavio, R., and Köhler, H., 1981, Mechanism of neonatal idiotype suppression. III. Delayed maturation of plasmacytoma stem cells in neonatally suppressed hosts, *J. Immunol.* **127**:509.
35. Fu, S. M., Chiorazzie, N., Kunkel, H. J., Halper, J. P., and Harris, S. R., 1978, Induction of in vitro differentiation and immunoglobulin synthesis of human B leukemic lymphocytes, *J. Exp. Med.* **148**:1570–1578.
36. Miller, R. A., Maloney, D. G., Warnke, R., and Levy, R., 1982, Treatment of λ B cell lymphoma with monoclonal antiidiotype antibody, *N. Engl. J. Med.* **306**:517–522.
37. Suemura, M., Ishizaka, A., Kobatake, S., Sugimura, K., Maeda, K., Nakanishi, K., Kishimoto, S., Yanamura, Y., and Kishimoto, T., 1983, Inhibition of IgE production in B hybridomas by IgE class-specific suppressor factor from T hybridomas, *J. Immunol.* **130**:1056–1060.
38. Kresina, T. F., Baine, Y., and Nisonoff, A., 1983, Adoptive transfer of resistance to growth of an idiotype-secreting hybridoma by T cells from idiotypically suppressed mice, *J. Immunol.* **130**:1478–1482.
39. Lynch, R. G., Graff, R., Sirisinha, S., Simms, E. S., and Eisen, H. N., 1972, Myeloma proteins as tumor specific transplantation antigens, *Proc. Natl. Acad. Sci. USA* **69**:1540–1544.
40. Daley, M. J., Bridges, S., and Lynch, R. G., 1978, MOPC-315 spleen colonization: A sensitive quantitative in vivo assay for idiotype-specific immune suppression of MOPC-315, *J. Immunol. Methods* **24**:47–56.
41. Jorgensen, T., Gaudernack, G., and Hannestad, K., 1980, Immunization with the light chain and the V$_L$ domain of the isologous myeloma protein 315 inhibits growth of mouse plasmacytoma MOPC-315, *Scand. J. Immunol.* **11**:29–35.
42. Daley, M. J., Gebel, H. M., and Lynch, R. G., 1978, Idiotype-specific transplantation resistance to MOPC-315: Abrogation by post-immunization thymectomy, *J. Immunol.* **120**:1620–1624.

43. Frikke, M. J., Bridges, S. H., and Lynch, R. G., 1977, Myeloma-specific antibodies: Studies of their properties and relationship to tumor immunity, *J. Immunol.* **118**:2206–2212.
44. Sirisinha, S., and Eisen, H. N., 1971, Autoimmune antibodies to the ligand binding sites of myeloma proteins, *Proc. Natl. Acad. Sci. USA* **68**:3130–3135.
45. Tungkanak, R., and Sirisinha, S., 1976, Immunogenicity of Fab fragment of protein-315 for BALB/c mice, *J. Immunol.* **117**:1664–1667.
46. Jorgensen, T., and Hannestad, K., 1977, Specificity of T and B lymphocytes for myeloma protein 315, *Eur. J. Immunol.* **7**:426–431.
47. Odermatt, B. O., Perlmutter, R., and Lynch, R. G., 1978, Molecular heterogeneity and fine specificity of BALB/c antibodies elicited by isologous myeloma protein, *Eur. J. Immunol.* **8**:858–865.
48. Milburn, G. L. and Lynch, R. G., 1983, Anti-idiotypic regulation of IgA expression in myeloma cells, *Molec. Immunol.,* **20**:931–940.
49. Rohrer, J. W., Odermatt, B. O., and Lynch, R. G., 1979, Immunoregulation of murine myeloma: Isologous immunization with M315 induces idiotype-specific T cells that suppress IgA secretion by MOPC-315 cells in vivo, *J. Immunol.* **122**:2011–2019.
50. Rohrer, J. W., Vasa, K., and Lynch, R. G., 1977, Myeloma cell immunoglobulin expression during in vivo growth in diffusion chambers: Evidence for repetitive cycles of differentiation, *J. Immunol.* **119**:861–866.
51. Lynch, R. G. and Milburn, G. L., 1983, Id^{315}-specific T cells that suppress MOPC-315 IgA synthesis recognize a $V_H{}^{315}$ idiotope, *Fed. Proc.* **42**:688.
52. Bothwell, A., Paskind, M., Schwartz, R., Sonenshein, G., Gefter, M., and Baltimore, D., 1981, Dual expression of λ genes in the MOPC-315 plasmacytoma, *Nature* **290**:65.
53. Schwartz, R., Sonenshein, G., Bothwell, A. and Gefter, M., 1981, Multiple expression of Ig λ-chain encoding RNA species in murine plasmacytoma cells, *J. Immunol.* **126**:2104.
54. Hozumi, N., Wu, G., Murialdo, H., Baumal, R., Mosmann, T., Winberry, L., and Marks, A., 1982, Arrangement of λ light chain genes in mutant clones of the MOPC-315 mouse myeloma cells, *J. Immunol.* **129**:260–266.
55. Max, E., Maizel, J. and Leder, P., 1981, The nucleotide sequence of a 5.5-kilobase DNA segment containing K immunoglobulin J and C region genes, *J. Biol. Chem.* **256**:5116–5120.
56. Selsing, E., Miller, J., Wilson, R., and Storb, U., 1982, Evaluation of mouse immunoglobulin λ genes, *Proc. Natl. Acad. Sci. USA* **79**:4681–4685.
57. Abbas, A., Burakoff, S., Gefter, M., and Green, M., 1980, T lymphocyte mediated suppression of myeloma function *in vitro*. III. Regulation of antibody production in hybrid myeloma cells by T lymphocytes, *J. Exp. Med.* **152**:969–978.
58. Jorgensen, T., and Hannestad, K., 1979, T helper lymphocytes recognize the V_L domain of the isologous mouse myeloma protein 315, *Scand. J. Immunol.* **10**:317–323.
59. Jorgensen, T., and Hannestad, K., 1981, H-2 linked genes control immune response to V-domains of myeloma protein 315, *Nature* **228**:396–397.
60. Jorgensen, T., and Hannestad, K., 1982, Helper T cell recognition of the variable domains of a mouse myeloma protein (315), *J. Exp. Med.* **155**:1587–1596.
61. Helman, M., Shreier, I., and Givol, D., 1976, Preparation and subfractionation of isologous and heterologous anti-idiotypes, using F_V fragments, *J. Immunol.* **117**:1933–1937.
62. Jerne, N. K., 1974, Towards a network theory of the immune system, *Ann. Immunol. (Paris)* **125C**:373–389.
63. Solomon, A., and McLaughlin, C. L., 1969, Bence-Jones proteins and light chains of immunoglobulins, *J. Biol. Chem.* **244**:3399–3404.
64. Oudin, J., and Cazenave, P.-A., 1971, Similar idiotype specificities in immunoglobulin fractions with different antibody functions or even without detectable antibody function, *Proc. Natl. Acad. Sci. USA* **68**:2616–2620.
65. Amor, M., Mariamé, B., Voegtlé, D., and Cazenave, P.-A., 1982, The idiotypic network: The murine MOPC-315 anti-DNP system, *Ann. Immunol. (Paris)* **133**:255–262.

19

Idiotypic Suppression of B-Cell-Derived Tumors

Models for Lymphocyte Regulation

ABUL K. ABBAS AND GINA MOSER

1. Introduction

The expression of idiotypic determinants on immunoglobulin-producing monoclonal neoplasms has been recognized for over a decade. Tumor idiotypes have two major applications: they are surface determinants against which highly specific immunity can be induced and used for therapy, and they are targets for immunoregulatory cells and antibodies, so that the tumors can serve as models for the regulation of nonneoplastic lymphocytes. Since the first demonstration of idiotype-specific tumor immunity against murine myelomas,[1] the general validity of this approach has been convincingly established by numerous investigators. It is now clear that anti-idiotypic antibodies and/or T lymphocytes can suppress the growth or mediate the rejection of murine and human B-cell lymphomas and leukemias,[2,3] a variety of antibody-secreting myelomas,[4,5] and "hybridomas" produced by fusion of immune B lymphocytes and drug-marked myelomas.[6] The clinical applicability of such approaches is limited by the problem of producing specific anti-idiotypic antibodies and effector T lymphocytes against individual neoplasms. However, modern advances in techniques for long-term cell culture and somatic cell hybridization may well make it feasible to direct immunotherapeutic regimens against the idiotypic determinants present on B-cell-derived neoplasms.

The concept that tumors of immunocompetent cells are valid models for normal lymphocytes has been rigorously tested only during the last 5 years or so. It is, in fact, remarkable that neoplasms frequently remain susceptible to physiologic regulatory stimuli, and

ABUL K. ABBAS AND GINA MOSER • Departments of Pathology, Harvard Medical School and Brigham and Women's Hospital, Boston, Massachusetts 02115.

are not "frozen" in terms of differentiative stage or function.[7] Tumors possess a number of properties which can be exploited to analyze mechanisms that cannot be reliably studied with normal cells. Specifically, they are autonomous, relatively homogeneous, and can be readily manipulated. Physiologic immunocompetent cells, in contrast, are highly heterogeneous, constantly differentiating, and are interacting with one another, so that molecular mechanisms of immune regulation are difficult to define in normal immune responses. The value of tumors as models for normal cells extends beyond analyses of lymphocyte function, since monoclonal neoplasms can be used to explore cell–cell or ligand–receptor interactions, recognition patterns, and signal transduction in many biologic systems, such as the effects of hormones on target cells.[8] Clearly, the physiologic relevance of such studies is limited to the extent that any tumor resembles its nonneoplastic cellular counterpart. Although this caveat is of obvious importance, the similarities between tumors and normal cells have been proved by direct experimentation in numerous instances.[7]

Our laboratory's interest in the use of murine myelomas as models for studying idiotypic regulation was stimulated by two unrelated sets of observations. First, we and others showed that myelomas (and, more recently, hybridomas) that produced antibodies of defined hapten specificities could be functionally suppressed by tolerogenic hapten–carrier conjugates and immune complexes.[9–11] Moreover, the inhibition of myeloma cells was similar to the inactivation of normal hapten-specific B lymphocytes and antibody-secreting cells in terms of kinetics, reversibility, and the requisite properties of tolerogenic hapten-carriers.[12] Second, there was increasing evidence that idiotype-specific resistance to transplantable myelomas may be mediated by T lymphocytes rather than anti-idiotypic antibodies, suggesting that idiotype-reactive immunoregulatory cells can have profound effects on the relevant tumor targets.[13] Based on such studies, we initiated attempts to selectively generate idiotype-reactive T lymphocytes with different functional properties and to analyze their effects on idiotype-expressing myelomas in vitro. This review is aimed at highlighting the many similarities between immune responses to myeloma idiotypes and "physiologic" idiotypes, and the potential value as well as the limitations of myelomas as models for normal immunoglobulin-producing cells.

2. The Induction and Specificity of Idiotype-Reactive T Lymphocytes

The prototype immunoglobulin-producing tumor we have used for the majority of our studies is a culture-adapted cloned line of the mineral oil-induced BALB/c myeloma, MOPC315, which secretes an IgA,λ_2 antibody specific for 2,4-dinitrophenol and 2,4,6-trinitrophenol (TNP). At any time, 30–60% of the cells secrete sufficient antibody to be detectable in reverse hemolytic plaque assays and 50–75% of the tumor cells express membrane receptors, as measured by rosette formation with haptenated erythrocytes that is specifically inhibitable by anti-idiotypic antibody. The basis for the observed microheterogeneity in this MOPC315 line is unresolved; it cannot be attributed to cell cycle-related variations or the presence of functionally different clones within the parent tumor. It is known that repeated immunization of isologous mice with affinity-purified M315 IgA induces anti-idiotypic antibody as well as a variety of idiotype-reactive T lymphocytes (suppressor, helper, and possibly cytolytic or cytostatic T cells).[13] The goal of our experiments was to selectively generate distinct functional subsets of idiotype-specific T cells. We, therefore, immunized BALB/c mice subcutaneously or intravenously with syngeneic splenocytes to which the myeloma protein was covalently coupled, employing an approach first used to induce hapten-reactive effector or suppressor T lymphocytes.[14] These experiments[15] showed that subcutaneous immunization with idiotype-coupled cells primed animals for delayed hypersensitivity (DH) responses, which could subsequently be elicited by a challenge with either aqueous myeloma protein or idiotype-coupled cells (Fig. 1). As expected, this form of immunity could be transferred to naive animals with T lymphocytes. In contrast, intravenous immunization with idiotype-coupled cells induced T lymphocytes which: (1) suppressed priming for DH, and (2) inhibited antibody secretion by the myeloma targets following coculture (Fig. 2). Thus, the consequences of immunizing mice with myeloma idiotype-coupled cells are essentially identical to what has been described in a variety of hapten systems, i.e., the idiotype functions like a foreign antigen under these conditions. Studies from other laboratories suggest that the idiotype-specific T cells mediating DH and suppressor T lymphocytes (Ts) may recognize distinct determinants on the immunoglobulin molecule, but the biologic significance of this finding remains unclear. Moreover, we have been unable to generate idiotype-specific proliferating or cytolytic T lymphocytes in isologous mice, although it is likely that both functional T-cell types specific for immunoglobulin idiotypes can be induced by appropriate immunization.

Our subsequent experiments have focused on the regulation of myeloma function by idiotype-specific Ts. Suppressor cells induced by a single intravenous immunization with M315-coupled splenocytes inhibit immunoglobulin synthesis and secretion by MOPC315 targets by 40–60% following 3–4 days of coculture.[15] Based on concepts of Ts pathways

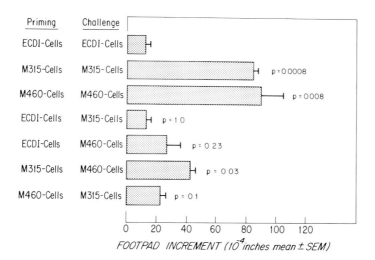

FIGURE 1. Idiotype-specific delayed hypersensitivity. Groups of three to five BALB/c mice were immunized subcutaneously with 3×10^7 syngeneic splenocytes to which M315 or M460 protein was covalently coupled using the carbodiimide, ECDI. Control mice received ECDI-treated cells. Seven days later animals were challenged in one footpad with 2×10^7 cells, as shown; footpads were measured 24 hr later and the difference between challenged and unchallenged is shown. Note that optimal DH is elicited by priming and challenge with the same protein; the marginal reaction of M315-primed mice to M460 may reflect partial idiotype cross-reactivity between these myeloma immunoglobulins. Data from Ref. 15.

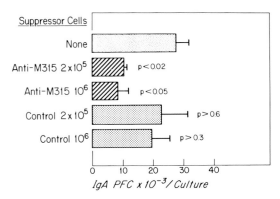

FIGURE 2. Suppression of MOPC315 cells by idiotype-specific Ts. MOPC315 cells (10^5) were cocultured for 4 days with nylon wool-nonadherent splenic T lymphocytes from BALB/c mice injected 7 days previously with M315-coupled splenocytes ("anti-M315") or with ECDI-treated splenocytes ("control"). IgA PFC were measured by a reverse hemolytic plaque assay. Anti-M315 Ts significantly inhibit IgA secretion; in the same cultures, viable myeloma cell recoveries and percent of MOPC315 cells forming rosettes with TNP-coated erythrocytes are the same as normal (not shown). Data from Ref. 15.

developed largely by analyses of suppression of azobenzenearsonate and later in nitrophenyl-specific contact sensitivity or DH (reviewed in Ref. 16), we reasoned that such an immunization protocol might lead to the generation of first-order "Ts_1" which differentiate into effector Ts during the coculture with myeloma targets. We, therefore, attempted to induce effector Ts by immunizing mice subcutaneously with M315-coupled cells and administering soluble extracts of Ts_1 cells intravenously; an identical protocol has previously been used to induce hapten-specific effector Ts.[17] The T cells induced by such an approach inhibited antibody secretion by myeloma targets more rapidly and to a greater extent than Ts_1 cells (Table I), and have been operationally defined as effector Ts.[18] Both Ts_1 and effector Ts are specific for the myeloma idiotype, as shown by reciprocal suppression of idiotypically dissimilar myelomas and binding to idiotype-coated immunosorbents (Table II). Moreover, effector Ts have the expected Lyt-1^-2^+ phenotype, whereas Ts_1 function can be abrogated by treatment with either anti-Lyt-1 or anti-Lyt-2 antibody + complement, implying that these cells express both surface markers or that T lymphocytes bearing the two markers participate in the differentiation of Ts_1 to effector Ts *in vitro*.

The ability to generate idiotype-specific Ts apparently representing different stages of

TABLE I

Kinetics of Suppression of MOPC315 Cells by Idiotype-Specific Ts_1, Effector $Ts^{a,b}$

	IgA PFC/10^3 viable MOPC315 cells (mean ± S.E.)		
T lymphocytes (2 × 10^6)	Day 1	Day 2	Day 4
None	432 ± 29	461 ± 23	490 ± 25
Normal	453 ± 53	485 ± 45	455 ± 40
Ts_1	434 ± 26	284 ± 37	<u>137 ± 45</u>
Effector Ts	<u>181 ± 24</u>	<u>115 ± 30</u>	<u>83 ± 27</u>

^aData from Ref. 18.
^bMOPC315 cells (10^5) were cultured alone or with 2 × 10^6 normal BALB/c splenic T lymphocytes, or T cells ("Ts_1") from mice injected 7 days previously with 5 × 10^7 M315-coupled syngeneic splenocytes intravenously, or T cells ("effector Ts") from mice given 3 × 10^7 M315-coupled cells subcutaneously on day 7 and soluble extracts of Ts_1 cells intravenously daily from day 7 for 5 days. IgA PFC were assayed after 1, 2, and 4 days of coculture. Groups showing significant inhibition ($P <$ 0.001 compared to myeloma cells alone) are underlined; data are pooled from four experiments. Effector Ts induce significant suppression within 1 day whereas Ts_1 after 4 days of coculture.

TABLE II
Specificity of M315-Reactive Ts[a]

T lymphocytes (2 × 10^6)	% suppression of IgA PFC induced by	
	Ts[1]	Effector Ts
Ts, untreated	58.2	70.8
Ts, depleted on M315-coated dish	5.9	5.6
Ts, depleted on M460- or MPC11-coated dish	45.9	69.7

[a] 10^5 MOPC315 cells were cocultured with Ts[1] for 4 days or effector Ts for 2 days, and IgA PFC/10^3 viable myeloma cells assayed. (See legend to Table I.) In some groups prior to coculture the T cells were adhered to plastic dishes coated with M315, M460, or MPC11 myeloma proteins, as described in Refs. 15 and 18.

a suppressor pathway (Table III) is similar to results with hapten-reactive Ts, and emphasizes the resemblance between isologous myeloma idiotypes and foreign antigens. In addition, previous studies of the suppression of physiologic antibody responses have focused on "afferent" and "efferent" Ts. The experiments with myeloma cells, which are autonomous and, therefore, insusceptible to any form of "afferent" suppression, indicate that the kinetics of suppression mediated by Ts[1] and effector Ts are different. Such a result suggests that in situations where immune suppression is only observed if Ts are added early in the response, the delay may be due to the need for Ts[1]-like cells to differentiate into effector Ts rather than the effects of Ts on immune induction ("afferent" suppression). Thus, differences in kinetics of inhibition do not necessarily imply differences in the cellular targets of suppression, and it is conceivable that most or all forms of T-lymphocyte-mediated suppression are due to effector Ts which can be generated by various experimental protocols. It should, however, be pointed out that in the myeloma idiotype system, there is no formal proof to date for differentiation of Ts[1] to effector Ts *in vitro,* or for the existence of intermediate cell types in this suppressor pathway.

TABLE III
Properties of M315-Reactive Ts[1], Effector Ts[a]

	Ts[1]	Effector Ts
Induced by	M315-coupled spleen cells i.v.	M315-coupled spleen cells s.c. + extract of Ts[1] cells i.v.
Kinetics of suppression	40–60% inhibition of IgA PFC after 3–4 days of coculture	40–70% inhibition in 1–2 days, 90% by 4 days
Surface phenotype	Thy-1+, Lyt-1+2+ (or Lyt-1+ and Lyt-2+ cells required to generate effector Ts *in vitro*)	Thy-1+, Lyt-1−2+
Specificity	Bind to M315- but not M460- or MPC11-coated dishes	Bind to M315- but not M460- or MPC11-coated dishes
Suppression by secreted factors	None demonstrated	Demonstrated in Marbrook cultures and with cell-free culture supernatants

[a] Based on data in Refs. 15, 18, 21.

3. Mechanisms of Action of Idiotype-Specific Ts

The greatest value of using monoclonal neoplasms as targets for immune regulation is that such systems allow one to analyze subcellular mechanisms of suppression in far more detail than is feasible with physiologic immune responses. Experiments employing Ts_1 and effector Ts with MOPC315 targets have revealed the following significant features.

1. The Ts are neither cytostatic nor cytolytic for myeloma cells. Lynch and co-workers have shown that T lymphocytes induced by multiple immunizations with myeloma protein in adjuvant also inhibit antibody production without affecting viable tumor cell recovery,[19] although other investigators have observed clonal inhibition using similar protocols.[5]

2. The Ts block antibody secretion without altering the expression of membrane receptors[15] or the synthesis of nonantibody proteins; whether this reflects a true selectivity in Ts-mediated effects, differences in the sensitivities of the various assays, or longer half-lives of receptor immunoglobulin and nonantibody proteins compared to secretory immunoglobulin is presently unknown.

3. Suppressibility of myeloma targets is not related to their position in the cell cycle. Thus, in the MOPC315 tissue culture line routinely passaged *in vitro,* 70–75% of the cells are in G_1, as measured by propidium iodide staining of nuclear DNA and quantitative analysis by flow cytometry. Cells blocked in G_2 with colcemid (such that $> 75\%$ are in G_2) are as suppressible by effector Ts as the original cell line following brief coculture with Ts (Michael Kauffman and Abul Abbas, unpublished observations). These experiments have also revealed that antibody secretion and receptor expression by the cells of this particular tumor line are not influenced by the cell cycle.

In order to further analyze the mechanism of action of idiotype-specific Ts, we have used a somatic cell hybrid line prepared by fusing two BALB/c myelomas, MOPC315 (IgA,λ_2) and MPC11 (IgG2b,κ). The majority of the cells ($> 95\%$) express both antibodies on their surfaces by double immunofluorescence, 40–50% form hemolytic plaques using protein A-coated erythrocytes as indicators and either anti-IgA, anti-IgG, or a mixture of both as developing sera, and $> 90\%$ of the two immunoglobulins synthesized show homologous heavy-chain–light-chain combinations.[20] The goal of our experiments was to use this cloned line producing two idiotypically unrelated immunoglobulins as the target for Ts_1 specific for either idiotype. Such studies revealed that each Ts inhibited secretion of only the idiotype that was recognized on the cell surface (Table IV). Although the suppression observed was only partial, the properties of the hybrid cell line support the view that Ts selectively inhibit production of one of two antibodies made by the cell. Moreover, in parallel experiments we showed that TNP-specific, syngeneic cytolytic T lymphocytes recognize TNP-proteins bound to myeloma cells bearing receptors for the hapten. Such cytolytic T cells do not inhibit IgG secretion by parent MPC11 cells even in the presence of TNP-proteins, but induce a comparable reduction in IgA and IgG secretion by the double-secreting hybrid cells.[20] This result indicates that, within the limits of the assay, the hybrid cells that express TNP-specific (IgA) receptors must also be secreting IgG, strengthening the view that the selective effects of anti-idiotypic Ts truly represent selective inhibition of the secretion of one or the other idiotype. Although the mechanism underlying this phenomenon is unclear, a possible clue comes from the recent work of Milburn, Lynch, and

TABLE IV
Idiotype-Specific Suppression of MOPC315, MPC11, and Double-Secreting MOPC315–MPC11
Hybrid Tumor Cells[a,b]

Myeloma cells (10^5)	T lymphocytes (10^6)	PFC/10^3 myeloma cells (mean ± S.E.)	
		IgA	IgG
MOPC315	None	656 ± 41	0
MOPC315	Anti-M315 Ts	363 ± 22	
MOPC315	Anti-MPC11 Ts	567 ± 142	
MPC11	None	0	691 ± 45
MPC11	Anti-M315 Ts		692 ± 47
MPC11	Anti-MPC11 Ts		371 ± 45
MOPC315–MPC11 hybrid	None	498 ± 37	547 ± 25
MOPC315–MPC11 hybrid	Anti-M315 Ts	248 ± 47	607 ± 77
MOPC315–MPC11 hybrid	Anti-MPC11 Ts	445 ± 50	357 ± 36

[a]Data from Ref. 20.
[b]Myeloma cells, as shown, were cultured for 4 days with 10^6 thymic T lymphocytes from normal BALB/c mice or mice injected 7 days previously with 5×10^7 M315- or MPC11-coupled syngeneic splenocytes intravenously. Aliquots of cultures were assayed for IgA or IgG PFC; groups showing significant suppression compared to myeloma cells alone are underlined. Similar results have been obtained with splenic Ts$_1$.

their colleagues, who have shown that Ts block the transcription of light-chain but not heavy-chain DNA (see Chapter 18). Thus, one can predict that idiotype-specific Ts would induce selective inhibition in hybrid cells where the two immunoglobulins have different light chains (e.g., MOPC315 and MPC11) but would have a nonselective effect if the two parent lines produced the same immunoglobulin light chain. Attempts to formally test this hypothesis by constructing appropriate somatic cell hybrids are currently in progress.

4. Suppressor Factors and the Role of Accessory Cells in Suppression of Idiotype of Secretion

A major problem in analyzing the interaction between Ts and their specific targets has been the heterogeneity of suppressible immunocompetent cells. Myelomas obviously offer one approach toward such a goal, and we reasoned that any studies of Ts–myeloma interactions would be greatly simplified if suppression was mediated by cell-free molecules, as has been shown for a variety of suppressor cells. In order to test this possibility, attempts were made to suppress myeloma function across cell-impermeable membranes. These experiments revealed the surprising result that myeloma cells were only suppressed by idiotype-specific effector Ts if nonimmune accessory cells were present together with the tumor targets.[21] In addition, only the Ia-positive subset of accessory cells was functional, even though there was no requirement for histocompatibility matching between the myeloma and accessory cells (Fig. 3). As expected, depletion of Ia-bearing or plastic-adherent cells from the Ts population abrogated suppression in cocultures (i.e., when Ts and myeloma targets were in direct contact), and the suppression was completely restored by the

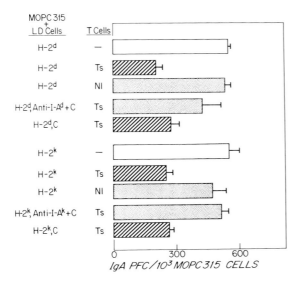

FIGURE 3. Role of I-A-positive accessory cells in Ts-mediated suppression of MOPC315 cells across cell-impermeable membranes. MOPC315 cells (2×10^5) were cultured with 4×10^5 low-density splenoctyes (LD cells, specific gravity $<$ 1.082 on discontinuous albumin gradients) purified from normal H-z^d (BALB/c) or H-2^k (CBA or B10.BR) mice in the inner chambers of double-chamber Marbrook vessels. In the outer chamber (separated by 0.2-μm Nucleopore membranes) were 2×10^7 normal BALB/c spleen cells (NI) or spleen cells from mice immunized to generate M315-specific effector Ts. In some groups, LD cells were treated with a monoclonal anti-I-A^d (MKD6) or anti-I-A^k (10.2.16) + complement, or complement alone. IgA secretion by myeloma cells was measured after 2 days. Note that significant suppression of PFC ($P < 0.001$, hatched bars) is only seen in the presence of Ia-positive LD cells of either H-2 haplotype. Data pooled from three experiments, and taken from Ref. 21.

addition of nonimmune accessory cells (Fig. 4). The properties of the accessory cells involved in the effector phase of Ts-mediated inhibition are listed in Table V. It is noteworthy that this phenomenon is exquisitely idiotype-specific, and does not represent yet another example of nonspecific immunosuppression induced by macrophages that are themselves activated by Ts. More recent experiments have shown that Ts factors generated in one culture specifically inhibit MOPC315 cells in a second culture only in the presence of nonimmune accessory cells. Such results suggest that a possible role of nonimmune cells is to "present" suppressor factors to the targets. This also implies that targets of T-cell-mediated suppression are not passive recipients of immunoregulatory signals, but may participate by actively recognizing Ts-derived factors on appropriate presenting cells.

5. Future Prospects of Myeloma Idiotype Regulation

The analysis of idiotypic regulation of B-cell-derived tumors, which was largely stimulated by its potential value for immunotherapy, has provided significant insights into the mechanisms of functional regulation of B lymphocytes. The requirements for generation of idiotype-specific T cells and the operation of Ts pathways in this system of immunoregulation are strikingly similar to what has been previously demonstrated in physiologic immune responses. The homogeneity of tumors has allowed us to answer questions that cannot be addressed with nonneoplastic immunocompetent cells. Moreover, the combination of immunologic and molecular biologic techniques is already providing clues to the mode of action of Ts. Finally, the autonomous nature of neoplastic targets has revealed a hitherto unsuspected role for accessory cells in T-lymphocyte-mediated suppression of mye-

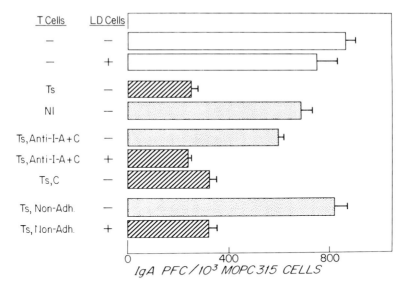

FIGURE 4. Role of nonimmune accessory cells in suppression of MOPC315 cells: Ts–myeloma cocultures. MOPC315 cells (10^5) were cocultured with 2×10^6 splenic T lymphocytes from normal BALB/c mice (Nl) or mice immunized to generate M315-specific effector Ts. In some groups the Ts were treated with anti-I-A^d (MKD6) antibody + complement or complement alone, or depleted of plastic-adherent cells (45 min adherence at 37°C). "LD cells" refer to 10^5 nonimmune syngeneic low-density splenocytes purified on albumin gradients. Note that significant suppression ($P < 0.001$, hatched bars) is induced by Ts; this is abrogated by depletion of either I-A-bearing or adherent cells from the Ts population, and is restored by the addition of nonimmune low-density splenocytes. Data from Ref. 21.

loma secretion. As these experimental systems are developed, it is likely that neoplasms will provide increasingly definitive answers to issues of Ts–target interactions, recognition of Ts-derived factors, and the biochemical basis of functional regulation. Perhaps the greatest value of tumors will be demonstrated if they suggest phenomena that are only later shown to be operative in physiologic immune responses, just as myeloma genes and antibodies have been invaluable for our understanding of normal immunoglobulins and the genes encoding them.

TABLE V

Properties of Accessory Cells Involved in Idiotype-Specific Ts-Mediated Suppression[a]

Present in thioglycollate-induced peritoneal exudates, nonimmune low-density splenocytes; absent in high-density splenocytes

Radioresistant (1500 R)

Plastic adherent

Ia-positive, not MHC restricted; activity correlates with stimulating ability of cell populations in fully allogeneic mixed lymphocyte reactions

Present in Fc receptor-positive and negative subsets of low-density splenocytes

Effect not abrogated by indomethacin

[a]Modified from Ref. 21.

ACKNOWLEDGMENTS. We thank Dr. Mark Greene for his substantive contributions to this work, Ms. Sheldon Smith for technical assistance, and Ms. Valerie Sherman for invaluable help in the preparation of the manuscript. The authors' research is supported by NIH Grant AI-16349. G.M. is the recipient of an NIH postdoctoral fellowship.

References

1. Lynch, R. G., Graff, R. J., Sirisinha, S., Simms, E. S., and Eisen, H. N., 1972, Myeloma proteins as tumor-specific transplantation antigens, *Proc. Natl. Acad. Sci. USA* **69:**1540–1545.
2. Vitetta, E. S., Krolick, K. A., and Uhr, J. W., 1982, Neoplastic B cells as targets for antibody-ricin A chain immunotoxins, *Immunol. Rev.* **62:**159–183.
3. Miller, R. A., Maloney, D. G., Warnke, R., and Levy, R., 1982, Treatment of B-cell lymphoma with monoclonal anti-idiotypic antibody, *N. Engl. J. Med.* **306:**517–522.
4. Beatty, P. G., Kim, B. S., Rowley, D. A., and Coppelson, L. W., 1976, Antibody against the antigen receptor of a plasmacytoma prolongs survival of mice bearing the tumor, *J. Immunol.* **116:**1391–1396.
5. Flood, P. M., Phillipps, C., Taupier, M. A., and Schreiber, H., 1980, Regulation of myeloma growth *in vitro* by idiotype-specific T lymphocytes, *J. Immunol.* **124:**424–430.
6. Kresina, T. F., Baine, Y., and Nisonoff, A., 1983, Adoptive transfer of resistance to growth of an idiotype-secreting hybridoma by T cells from idiotypically suppressed mice, *J. Immunol.* **130:**1478–1482.
7. Abbas, A. K., 1982, Immunologic regulation of lymphoid tumor cells: Model systems for lymphocyte function, *Adv. Immunol.* **32:**301–368.
8. Sato, G. H., and Ross, R. (eds.), 1979, *Hormones and Cell Culture,* Cold Spring Harbor Laboratory, Cold Spring Harbor, N.Y.
9. Abbas, A. K., and Klaus, G. G. B., 1977, Inhibition of antibody production in plasmacytoma cells by antigen, *Eur. J. Immunol.* **7:**667–674.
10. Abbas, A. K., and Klaus, G. G. B., 1978, Antigen–antibody complexes suppress antibody production by mouse plasmacytoma cells *in vitro, Eur. J. Immunol.* **8:**217–220.
11. Boyd, A. W., and Schrader, J. W., 1980, Mechanisms of effector-cell blockade. I. Antigen-induced suppression of Ig synthesis in a hybridoma cell line, and correlation with cell-associated antigen, *J. Exp. Med.* **151:**1436–1451.
12. Abbas, A. K., 1979, Antigen and T lymphocyte mediated suppression of myeloma cells: Model systems for regulation of lymphocyte function, *Immunol. Rev.* **48:**245–264.
13. Lynch, R. G., Rohrer, J. W., Odermatt, B., Gebel, H. M., Autry, J. M., and Hoover, R. G., 1979, Immunoregulation of murine myeloma cell growth and differentiation: A monoclonal model of B cell differentiation, *Immunol. Rev.* **48:**45–80.
14. Battisto, J. R., and Bloom, B. R., 1966, Dual immunological unresponsiveness induced by cell membrane-coupled hapten or antigen, *Nature* **212:**156–158.
15. Abbas, A. K., Perry, L. L., Bach, B. A., and Greene, M. I., 1980, Idiotype-specific T cell immunity. I. Generation of effector and suppressor T lymphocytes reactive with myeloma idiotypic determinants, *J. Immunol.* **124:**1160–1166.
16. Germain, R. N., and Benacerraf, B., 1981, A single major pathway of T-lymphocyte interactions in antigen-specific immune suppression, *Scand. J. Immunol.* **13:**1–10.
17. Sy, M.-S., Nisonoff, A., Germain, R. N., Benacerraf, B., and Greene, M. I., 1981, Antigen- and receptor-driven regulatory mechanisms. VIII. Suppression of idiotype-negative *p*-azobenzenearsonate-specific T cells results from the intereaction of an anti-idiotypic second-order T suppressor cell with a cross-reactive idiotype-positive *p*-azobenzenearsonate primed T cell target, *J. Exp. Med.* **153:**1415–1425.
18. Abbas, A. K., Takaoki, M., and Greene, M. I., 1982, T lymphocyte-mediated suppression of myeloma function in vitro. IV. Generation of effector suppressor cells specific for myeloma idiotypes, *J. Exp. Med.* **155:**1216–1221.
19. Milburn, G. L., and Lynch, R. G., 1982, Immunoregulation of murine myeloma in vitro. II. Suppression of MOPC-315 immunoglobulin secretion and synthesis by idiotype-specific suppressor T cells, *J. Exp. Med.* **155:**852–862.

20. Abbas, A. K., Burakoff, S. J., Gefter, M. L., and Greene, M. I., 1980, T lymphocyte-mediated suppression of myeloma function in vitro. III. Regulation of antibody production in hybrid myeloma cells by T lymphocytes, *J. Exp. Med.* **152**:969–978.
21. Moser, G., Tominaga, A., Greene, M. I., and Abbas, A. K., 1983, Accessory cells in immune suppression. I. Role of I-A-positive accessory cells in effector phase idiotype-specific suppression of myeloma function, *J. Immunol.* **131**:1728–1733.

20

Idiotype and Anti-Idiotype Regulation of Antipolyfructosan Response

Role of Regulatory Idiotopes

CONSTANTIN A. BONA

1. Network Theory

The key element of the network theory of the immune system proposed by Jerne[1] is the potential importance of receptor-specific regulation of the immune response.

The first postulate of this theory is that the immune system represents a collection of clones, each capable of binding an antigenic determinant through its combining site, designated as paratope, and each capable of being recognized by some other element of the system because it displays one or more idiotopes. Accordingly, the clones can speak one to another using an idiotypic dictionary.

The second postulate of the network concept is that for each antibody expressing a given paratope and idiotope ($Ab_1 = p_1i_1$) there exists a complementary clone producing antibody able to bind to i_1 ($Ab_2 = p_2i_2$). In the steady state, the i_1 molecules stimulate the clones bearing p_2 receptors to secrete Ab_2 antibodies which through their paratope (p_2) suppress the expansion of Ab_1 clones. This type of $Ab_1 \rightleftarrows Ab_2$ interaction with the resultant suppression of Ab_1, represents the characteristic pattern of the steady-state immune network. Antigen upsets this equilibrium by inducing the proliferation of Ab_1. Ab_1 can now initiate the synthesis of a "cascade" of complementary anti-Id antibodies: Ab_2–anti-Id, Ab_3–anti(anti-Id), Ab_4–anti[anti(anti-Id)] antibodies, etc.[2,3]

The third postulate of the network theory is that among the multitude of steric struc-

CONSTANTIN A. BONA • Department of Microbiology, Mount Sinai School of Medicine, New York, New York 10029.

tures exhibited by the variable regions of antibody molecules conventionally designated as idiotopes, one could find shapes which are similar if not identical to epitopes of foreign antigens. These particular idiotopes represent the internal images of the antigen. The notion of internal image was introduced as a statistical necessity to explain the stimulation of Ab_1-producing clones (antiepitopes) by immunoglobulin in nonimmunized animals, i.e., the production of "natural" antibodies. An immunoglobulin molecule bears several idiotopes which are recognized by xenogeneic, allogeneic, syngeneic, and auto-anti-Id antibodies. Syngeneic and auto-anti-Id antibodies are restricted in their recognition to a few idiotopes,[4] suggesting that not all antigenic determinants of the V region are immunogenic in an autologous system. We have previously proposed that only the idiotopes which function as autoimmunogens play a role in idiotypic regulation of the immune response.

2. Regulatory Idiotopes

We designated these idiotopes "regulatory idiotopes."[3,5] The concept of regulatory idiotopes emerged from a study of the antigen-binding properties of various members of an idiotypic network pathway in which the initiator was ABPC48 (A48), a $\beta2 \rightarrow 6$ fructosan-binding monoclonal protein. This protein shares idiotopes with UPC10, another $\beta2 \rightarrow 6$ fructosan-binding monoclonal protein.[6] The V_H gene of UPC10 probably derives from a recently cloned pV_H 441-4 germline gene.[7] This germline gene encodes a hydrophobic leader peptide and the first 98 amino acids are identical to the leader peptide sequence of UPC10 and the V region of the mature heavy chains of the UPC10 and MOPC173 proteins. The V_H A48 gene probably derives from this germline gene as well because the V_H A48 sequence is very similar to UPC10. the D genes of A48, UPC10, and MOPC173 are quite different from one another and the COOH-terminal protein of each variable region is encoded by distinct J genes.[7] These results would suggest that the idiotypic sharing of A48 and UPC10 depends, at least in part, on V-gene similarities, although the contribution of L chains remains to be evaluated.

A study of the immunochemical properties of the various members of the idiotypic pathway of the A48 Id system showed that Ab_1 and Ab_3 shared idiotopes and that both were bound by Ab_2 and Ab_4. Although the binding affinity of Ab_4 for Ab_1 was lower than that of Ab_4 for Ab_3, our results[3] as well as those obtained in the rabbit by Wickler and colleagues[2] indicate that Ab_4 resembles Ab_2 (Table I).

To explain these results, we postulated that Ab_1 molecules (p_1i_1) express a special set of idiotopes, regulatory idiotopes (ri), as well as conventional idiotopes.

The Ab_2 antibodies (p_2i_2) produced in an autologous system subsequent to immunization with Ab_1 will be mainly directed against ri because only ri are immunogenic in an autologous system. Ab_2 lacks ri but the antibodies Ab_3 (p_3i_3) produced in response to immunization with Ab_2 will express regulatory idiotopes (actually, they are p_3 ri). Indeed, we have found that polyclonal Ab_3 as well as several monoclonal Ab_3 expressed A48 idiotopes.[8] Because the majority of Ab_3 are actually p ri antibodies, the Ab_4 produced subsequent to immunization with Ab_3 is principally made up of anti-ri antibodies (like Ab_2), rather than anti-i_3 antibodies. Our experimental results showed that 60% of Ab_4 bind to Ab_1.

Recently, Sachs et al.[9] suggested an alternative explanation for preferential induction

TABLE I

Binding of Radioactive Ab_1 and Ab_3 to Plates Coated

With Ab_2 and Ab_4

Microtiter plates coated with	Bound ligand	
	$[^3H]$-Ab_1	$[^{125}I]$-Ab_3
BALB/c Ig (10 μg)	105	1,130 ± 110
Ab_3 (10 μg)	110 ± 8	ND
Ab_2 (10 μg)	1386 ± 142	22,944 ± 1374
Ab_4 (150 μg Ig fraction)	524 ± 19	8,713 ± 271

of Id-bearing molecules in animals immunized with polyclonal Ab_2. Their explanation is based on two assumptions:

1. Difference between paratopic homogeneity and idiotypic heterogeneity of polyclonal Ab_2 will lead to a substantial activation of Ab_i after administration of Ab_2 into a naive animal. In contradistinction, the immunization with a monoclonal Ab_2 in which the concentration of paratope and idiotope is equal can lead to the synthesis of anti-Ab_2 (true $Ab_3 = p_3i_3$) as well as Ab_1.

2. The antigen specificity of idiotopes induced by the administration of Ab_2 depends on the nature of idiotopes with which Ab_2 molecules interact. The Ab_2s which interact with i_1 associated with paratope induce mainly antibodies of similar specificity to Ab_1 whereas Ab_2s which interact with framework-associated Ab_1 idiotopes might induce Id-bearing molecules with diverse specificity.

The studies of Goldberg et al.[8] have suggested that A48 idiotopes shared with UPC10 (a BL-binding protein), $\beta 2 \rightarrow 6$, and $\beta 2 \rightarrow 1$ fructosan-binding monoclonal proteins are not paratope associated. In fact, it is very difficult to conceive that anti-Id antibodies can selectively discriminate during the clonal activation, clones which express paratope or framework-associated idiotopes on their immunoglobulin receptor. More likely, the binding of Ab_2 to Id-bearing immunoglobulin receptor will randomly activate the clones independent of their antigen specificity.

Furthermore, Legrain and Buttin[10] have shown that in Northern blot analysis carried out under low- and high-stringency conditions, the poly(A) mRNA from five monoclonal Ab_3 antibodies hybridized with the pV_H 441-4 germ-line gene probe. Two hybridoma poly(A) mRNA which did not hybridize produced antibodies specific for only the individual idiotopes of Ab_2 which can be considered true Ab_3 (p_3i_3). The Legrain–Buttin experiment constitutes an important test of the regulatory idiotope concept since they used monoclonal anti-A48 Id antibodies for immunization. Their results indicate that A48 Id$^+$ B cells are activated in preference to anti-A48 Id-specific B cells.

Therefore, the regulatory idiotopes represent a special set of idiotopes which are characterized by several criteria:

1. They function as autoimmunogens and are able to induce the synthesis of auto-anti-Id antibodies.

2. They are shared by several members of an idiotypic pathway and could be shared
   by antibodies with different specificities.
3. Clones expressing these idiotopes possess the potential of becoming dominant possibly because regulatory T cells specific for them are present prior to immunization
   or may be elicited in the course of an immune response.[11]

An extensive analysis of immunochemical and functional properties of regulatory idiotopes was carried out in the A48 Id anti-$\beta2\rightarrow6$ fructosan system.

3. Polymorphism of the A48 Id System

We have previously shown that UPC10, the other $\beta2\rightarrow6$ fructosan-binding monoclonal protein, shares the A48 Id.[6] Recently, the V_H germ-line gene encoding the UPC10–
MOPC173 gene family was cloned and sequenced.[7] The hydrophobic leader peptide and
the first 98 amino acid residues of the mature UPC10 V_H segment are identical to the
amino acid sequence predicted by the pV_H 441 germ-line gene clone. These structural data
can provide invaluable information for the eventual localization of the A48–UPC10
idiotopes.

Therefore, we studied the expression of A48–UPC10 idiotopes on monoclonal antibodies (MAbs) obtained from BALB/c mice in which A48 Id$^+$ clones were activated: (1)
subsequent to the pretreatment at birth with A48 Id$^+$ monoclonal protein (series 1); (2)
subsequent to the administration at birth of minute amounts of anti-A48 Id antibodies
(series 2); and (3) in adult BALB/ mice producing Ab^3 antibodies in response to the immunization with anti-A48 Id–KLH conjugate (series 3).

Interestingly, among 19 MAbs which expressed the A48 Id six bound to BL but not
to inulin, whereas eight bound to both BL and inulin. Since inulin contains only $\beta2\rightarrow1$
fructosan linkages while BL contains both $\beta2\rightarrow6$ and $\beta2\rightarrow1$ fructosan linkages, those
MAbs which bind BL but not inulin should be considered specific for $\beta2\rightarrow6$ linkages. The
inulin-binding myeloma proteins display antigenic cross-reactivity by binding both types of
linkages (8); thus, MAbs binding to both BL and inulin can be considered similar to inulin-
binding myeloma proteins. Therefore, we observed that some MAbs obtained subsequent
to altering the steady-state configuration of the A48 Id network differ from A48 since they
bind to both $\beta2\rightarrow6$ and $\beta2\rightarrow1$ linkages. However, it should be mentioned that they also
differ from inulin-binding myeloma proteins because they exhibit a high binding activity
to BL and low binding to inulin. Among the antibodies of series 3, only two of five bound
to BL (8) (Table II).

Two approaches were utilized in characterizing the A48 Id expressed on these MAbs.
In the first approach, we prepared syngeneic anti-Id antibodies against A48, UPC10, and
a MAb from each series: 1-5-1, 2-11-3, and 3-76-42. The antibodies were ^{3}H-labeled and
their binding to purified anti-Id antibodies studied.

The study of the binding of ^{3}H-labeled antibodies to anti-Id antibodies indicated that
A48 bears at least two sites shared with UPC10 (designated A48$_1$ and A48$_2$). By contrast,
1-5-1 and 2-11-3 MAbs express the A48$_1$ site; the 3-76-42 expresses only the A48$_2$ site.
The second approach was to study the inhibition of binding of Id to anti-Id by BL. In this
study, we found that A48, UPC10, and 1-5-1 bear antigen-inhibitable and antigen-non-

TABLE II

Binding Activity of A48 Id$^+$ Monoclonal Antibodies

Origin of monoclonal antibodies		BL	Inulin
Spontaneous myelomas	A48	+ +	−
	UPC10	+ + +	−
	W3082	+ +	+ + +
BALB/c mice	1-5-1	+ +	−
injected at birth with 10 μg A48	1-3-1	+ + +	−
BALB/c mice	2-1-1	+ +	±
injected at birth with 0.01 μg anti-A48	2-1-3	+ + +	+
	2-7-3	+ +	+
	2-11-3	+ + +	+
	2-28-3	+	+
	2-32-3	+ +	−
BALB/c mice	3-76-1	±	−
hyperimmunized with anti-A48-KLH conjugate	3-76-12	−	−
	3-76-24	−	−
	3-76-38	±	±
	3-76-42	−	−

inhibitable sites; 2-11-3 and 3-76-42 expressed only an antigen-noninhibitable idiotope[8] (Table III). Since 3-76-42 MAb which is an Ab$_3$ without BL-binding activity and expresses only A48$_2$ and the antigen-noninhibitable site, we concluded that the A48 regulatory idiotope(s) is not associated with the combining site. One may ask where the regulatory idiotopes are located on the V$_H$ segment. Auffrey *et al.*[12] recently reported the amino acid sequence of the V$_H$ segments of A48 and UPC10. A comparison of these sequences indicated a strong homology for the H$_V$I segment, one amino acid substitution in H$_V$II (position 63), and three amino acid substitutions in the D segment. In addition, while A48 uses the J$_H$3 segment, UPC10 uses the J$_H$2 segment. Therefore, the specificity for the $\beta2 \rightarrow 6$ linkages of these two monoclonal proteins can be related to H$_V$I and/or H$_V$II or to a particular three-dimensional structure resulting from joining of different D and J seg-

TABLE III

Summary of Studies Regarding the Expression of Various Idiotopes on MAbs

Monoclonal antibodies	Idiotopes identified with syngeneic anti-Id antibodies		Idiotopes identified by ability of BL to inhibit Id–anti-Id interaction		
A48	A48$_1$	A48$_2$	A48 I^a	A48 NI	U10 I
UPC10	A48$_1$	A48$_2$	A48 NI	U10 I	U10 NI
1-5-1	A48$_1$		A48 I	A48 NI	U10 I
2-11-3	A48$_1$		A48 NI	U10 NI	
3-76-42	A48$_2$		A48 NI	U10 NI	

^{a}I, idiotope antigen-inhibitable; NI, idiotope antigen-noninhibitable.

ments. Since 2-11-3 and 3-76-42 MAbs do not express A48 and UPC10 antigen-inhibitable idiotopes, and because of differences in D and J segments of A48 and UPC10, the regulatory idiotopes which are antigen noninhibitable probably are located in FrI or FrII segments of the V_H region. Further studies should be carried out to substantiate this hypothesis.

4. Expression of A48 Idiotopes on Parallel Sets

One prediction of the regulatory idiotope model was the expression of such determinants on antibodies lacking BL-binding activity. So far, A48 idiotopes expressed on antibodies without BL-binding activity have been observed only on polyclonal or MAbs obtained from animals producing Ab_3. In order to test if these regulatory idiotopes are expressed on antibodies with other specificities, we studied the expression of A48 idiotopes on 198 murine and 80 human myeloma proteins. In this study, we found that only MOPC167, and IgA,κ phosphocholine (PC)-binding monoclonal protein, was able to:

1. Inhibit the binding of labeled A48 to anti-A48 Id antibodies in RIA and ELISA assays
2. Bind to anti-A48 Id antibodies using alkaline phosphatase-labeled MOPC167 and plastic plates coated with anti-A48 Id antibodies in an ELISA assay or by using ^{3}H-labeled goat anti-mouse IgA in RIA
3. Absorb out anti-A48 antibodies subsequent to passage over an MOPC167-Sepharose 4B column (Table (IV)

These results clearly indicated that some determinants expressed on MOPC167 were recognized by anti-A48 Id antibodies.

It should be mentioned that MOPC511, another PC-binding myeloma protein, did not cause the inhibition of A48 to anti-A48. Like MOPC167, MOPC511 expresses the same V_H region and the light chain derived from MOPC167 germ-line genes. Only six amino acid differences were reported between mature MOPC167 and MOPC511 V_L chains and the $V\kappa167$ germline gene.[13] This suggests that the light-chain V region can contribute to the antigenic determinants of MOPC167 recognized by anti-A48 Id antibodies. A comparison of previously reported amino acid sequences of MOPC 167, A48, and UPC10 shows a certain degree of homology only in the FrI segment. The availability of only a partial sequence of the UPC10 V_L segment (i.e., only the sequence of the first 30 amino acids was reported[14]) and the complete lack of information on the sequence of the A48 V_L chain do not allow any speculation on the localization of regulatory idiotopes on MOPC167. However, the study of the inhibition of binding of labeled MOPC167 to anti-A48 Id antibodies by BL, PC, A48, UPC10, and 3-76-42 MAb had suggested that the $A48_2$ site and/or antigen-noninhibitable A48 idiotope was shared with MOPC167. Indeed, whereas BL and PC did not inhibit the binding of MOPC167 to anti-A48 Id antibodies, A48 and 3-76-42 strongly inhibited this binding at 0.1–10 $\mu g/ml$[8] (Table IV).

Ids shared among antibodies specific for different epitopes borne by the same antigen molecule, antibodies with different antigen specificities, or even with immunoglobulins with unknown antigen-binding activity, were reported in several systems (see data reviewed in Ref. 15). These results as well as our data on the expression of regulatory idiotopes on

TABLE IV
Expression of A48 Id on MOPC167, a Phosphocholine-Binding Myeloma Protein

A. Direct binding (measured by binding of ^{3}H goat anti-IgA)

Microtiter plates coated with	Ligand	Binding of [^{3}H]anti-IgA (cpm)
—	—	123 ± 50
Anti-A48 Id antibodies	A48	2856 ± 142
	MOPC167	2783 ± 47
	MOPC460	398 ± 18

B. Inhibition of binding of [^{3}H]-A48 to anti-A48 Id antibodies

Inhibitor	Amount required for 50% inhibition (µg)
A48	5
W3082	>5000
MOPC167	50

C. Inhibition of binding of alkaline phosphatase MOPC167 to anti-A48 Id antibodies

Inhibitor	Amount required for 50% inhibition (µg)
BL	>10
PC-chloride	>10
UPC10	10
A48	1
3-76-42	0.1

antibodies with different specificities, strongly substantiate the concept that some segments of DNA can be shared by *V* genes encoding different antigen specificities.

The shared idiotopes among antibodies with different specificities could explain the increased level of so-called nonspecific immunoglobulins in various infectious diseases. The bulk of immunoglobulins responsible for hypergammaglobulinemia actually are composed of specific antibodies against the causative infectious agents and probably of parallel sets sharing idiotopes.

5. Activation of A48 Id$^+$ Clones Subsequent to Administration at Birth of Minute Amounts of Anti-A48 Id Antibodies

Immunization of BALB/c mice with BL elicits a vigorous T-independent antibody response.[16] Subsequent to immunization with BL, two families of antibodies are produced. One family resembles A48 or UPC10 and binds only to $\beta2\rightarrow6$ fructosan. However, A48 and UPC10 idiotopes are not expressed in a significant amount on anti-$\beta2\rightarrow6$ fructosan antibodies synthesized during a conventional immune response, suggesting that A48 and UPC10 Id$^+$ clones represent a silent or minor fraction of the anti-$\beta2\rightarrow6$ fructosan repertoire. The production of these antibodies is not related to a particular allotype. In addition, the anti-$\beta2\rightarrow6$ fructosan antibody response occurs very early in ontogeny because 1-week-old animals immunized with BL mount a meager but significant response.

The second family of antibodies binds to $\beta2\rightarrow1$ fructosan and displays a cross-reactivity for $\beta2\rightarrow6$ linkages. They share the IdXs (i.e., G, B, and A) of inulin-binding myeloma proteins. The expression of these IdXs is associated with the Igl^a allotype. The clones producing anti-$\beta2\rightarrow1$ antibodies probably belong to the Lyb-5$^+$ subset since mice bearing the *xid* defect cannot synthesize anti-$\beta2\rightarrow1$ antibodies. In addition, a substantial ontogenic delay of this response was observed.

In previous studies, we have shown that an A48 Id$^+$ response can be observed in BALB/c mice treated at birth with minute amounts of anti-A48 Id antibodies and immunized 1 month later with BL [17] (Table V). Recently, Rubinstein and Bona [18] have shown that activation of A48 Id$^+$ in animals treated at birth with anti-A48 Id antibodies is independent of *MHC* gene complex control because an A48 Id response was observed in BALB.B and BALB.K. As expected, this response is not associated with a particular allotype as was assessed by studying the occurrence of A48 Id$^+$ molecules in CAL.20 and BAB.14. The CBB R4 mice bearing $V_H{}^b$ and $C_H{}^a$ also developed an A48 Id$^+$ response.

The A48 Id$^+$ component of the anti-BL response varies between 30 and 70% in animals treated at birth with anti-A48 Id antibodies. This treatment causes a long-lasting activation of A48 Id precursors since an A48 Id$^+$ response was still detected in 12-week-old BALB/c mice which were treated at birth with anti-A48 Id antibodies. This activation is related to the direct interaction of anti-A48 Id antibodies with the A48 Id$^+$ immunoglobulin receptor of the precursor cells. Indeed, an A48 Id$^+$ response can be obtained in lethally irradiated BALB/c mice infused with highly purified B cells from mice treated at birth with anti-A48 Id antibodies. The infusion of T cells together with B cells does not alter the A48 Id$^+$ response.

It might be envisioned that the interaction of anti-A48 Id antibodies with the immunoglobulin receptor of B cells bearing A48 Id mimics the binding of a T-independent antigen to the cellular receptors. Therefore, an antibody molecule with a combining site specific for antigenic determinants of the immunoglobulin receptor (i.e., isotype, allotype, and idiotype) can function as a T-independent antigen and stimulate the proliferation of B cells in the absence of T-cell help. However, this proliferation does not suffice for the maturation of precursors into immunoglobulin-producing cells.

6. Requirement of Challenge with Antigen or Anti-Id Antibodies for the Activation of A48 Id$^+$ Anti-BL Antibody-Secreting Cells

Mice treated at birth with minute amounts of anti-A48 Id antibodies cannot mount an anti-BL immune response without an antigenic challenge.[16] This observation suggests that the parenteral administration of anti-A48 Id antibodies at birth causes an alteration of balance of $\beta2\rightarrow6$ fructosan-reactive clones with a preferential expression of A48 Id$^+$ clones. However, only the binding of the antigen to the cellular receptor of clones primed by anti-Id antibodies induced the maturation of the A48 Id$^+$ precursors into anti-$\beta2\rightarrow6$ fructosan antibody-producing cells. Thus, the antigenic challenge seemed to be critical for the occurrence of A48 Id$^+$ molecules in the sera of the animals treated at birth with anti-A48 Id antibodies.

One may ask if the BL immunization can be replaced by an anti-Id challenge which mimics the antigen. Rubinstein *et al.*[19] investigated this hypothesis by studying the effect of injection of several monoclonal anti-A48 Id antibodies in animals treated at birth with

TABLE V
Specificity of Activation of A48 Id⁺ Anti-BL Clones by Anti-A48 Id Antibodies

Mice pretreated at birth	Immunization	A48 Id$^+$ molecules (μg/ml)
—	BL[a]	0.004 ± 0.002
0.01 μg anti-A48	BL	0.430 ± 0.162
0.01 μg anti-A48	TNP-Ficoll	0.002 ± 0.001
0.01 μg anti-384[b]	BL	0.048 ± 0.014

[a]Mice were 4 weeks of age at the time of immunization with 20 μg BL or 10 μg TNP-Ficoll.
[b]MOPC384 is an IgA,κ, methyl β-galactoside-binding myeloma protein which does not share A48 idiotypes.

polyclonal anti-Id antibodies. One anti-Id antibody (i.e., 17-38) was found to be able to induce an anti-BL response when 1–100 μg was injected intravenously into the mice. The antigenlike challenge properties of this MAb do not seem to be related to a particular isotype because other IgM anti-A48 Id MAbs lacked this property.

As expected, when this MAb was injected into 1-month-old mice, an anti-$\beta2\rightarrow6$ fructosan PFC response was observed, whereas when it was injected into 3-month-old animals, both anti-inulin and anti-BL responses were increased. The idiotypic analysis of these antibodies showed that in both groups of animals, the A48 Id$^+$ component was suppressed. Actually, in 1-month-old mice, only A48 and UPC10 Id$^-$anti-BL PFC were observed, whereas in 3-month-old mice, only W3082 IdX anti-$\beta2\rightarrow1$ and $\beta2\rightarrow6$ fructosan PFC were observed (Table VI).

The most likely explanation of the ability of 17-38 monoclonal anti-A48 Id antibody to elicit an anti-BL or anti-inulin response in mice treated at birth with anti-A48 Id antibodies is that it carries the internal image of the antigen.

There are several examples which suggest that anti-Id antibodies represent the inter-

TABLE VI
Summary of PFC and IEF Results in Mice Treated at Birth with Anti-A48 Id and Challenged with BL or 17-38

Treatment at birth	Challenged with	Age of mice	PFC response					IEF pattern	
			BL	A48 Id$^+$	U10 Id$^+$	Inulin	W3082 Id$^+$	BL	Inulin
—	BL	1	+	−	−	−	−	BALB/c spectrotype	—
Anti-A48 Id	BL	1	+	+	+	−	−	"UPC10-like" spectrotype	—
Anti-A48 Id	17-38	1	+	−	−	−	−	BALB/c spectrotype	—
—	BL	3	+	−	±	+	+	BALB/c spectrotype	BALB/c J606 spectrotype
Anti-A48 Id	BL	3	+	+	+	ND	ND	BALB/c and CXBJ spectrotype	CXBJ spectrotype
Anti-A48 Id	17-38	3	+	−	±	+	+	BALB/c spectrotype	BALB/c J606 spectrotype

nal images of the antigen and that they can bind to the cellular receptor for the antigen and even mimic the functions of the antigen (see data reviewed in Ref. 20).

However, our results showed that only the clones specific for BL or inulin can be stimulated, whereas A48 Id clones which generally are expressed subsequent to BL stimulation were supressed subsequent to challenge with 17-38. At first glance, these results are paradoxical. However, the most intriguing property of all immunoglobulin molecules is their dual function: to recognize an antigen by virtue of their paratopes and to be immunogenic by virtue of their idiotopes in autologous system. Keeping in mind the dualism of immunoglobulin molecules, the effect of the challenge with 17-38 MAb can be easily explained. Indeed, through its paratope, this anti-Id antibody suppressed the A48 Id^+ precursors activated at birth and through its idiotope(s) stimulated the A48 Id^- anti-$\beta2{\rightarrow}6$ and anti-$\beta2{\rightarrow}1$ fructosan-reactive clones.

Therefore, the anti-Id antibodies carrying the internal image of the antigen not only can stimulate some clones and function as vaccines but also can suppress other clones which belong to a family of antibodies exhibiting a polymorphic Id system.

7. Id-Induced Id Response Subsequent to the Administration at Birth of A48 Id^+ MAbs

As long as the immune system is at steady state, a delicate balance exists between the clones which is established through fragile idiotypic links. This balance can be upset by antigen, Id, and anti-Id.

In further experiments, Rubinstein et al.[6] studied the effect of administration at birth of A48 Id^+ antibodies on the expression of the A48 Id. The injection of 10 ng A48 monoclonal protein followed 1 month later by immunization with BL led to activation of A48 Id^+ anti-BL clones. These clones became dominant, since certain individuals expressed this Id on $> 90\%$ of the anti-BL PFC assays. These results suggest that the A48 regulatory idiotopes shared by Ab_1 (i.e., A48 and UPC10) and by Ab_3 (i.e., 3-76-42) play an important role in this Id-induced Id response (Table VII).

TABLE VII

Idiotype-Induced Idiotype Response by Pretreatment of Newborn BALB/c Mice with Monoclonal Antibodies Bearing A48 Idiotypes

Treatment at birth with	Anti-BL response		A48 Id
$-^a$	5.0	$\pm$ 8.6[b]	$< 1^b$
A48	37.1	$\pm$ 21.7	173.3 ± 63.3
UPC10	1.1	$\pm$ 0.4	12.0 ± 6.4
3-76-42	3.6	$\pm$ 0.8	27.7 ± 5.0

^{a}Mice were immunized at 1 month with 20 μg BL.
$^b\mu$g/ml expressed as mean $\pm$ SEM.

It should be pointed out that this response was (1) Id specific since the administration at birth of MOPC460, a TNP-binding monoclonal protein, led to an increased 460 Id anti-TNP response but not to an increased A48 Id anti-BL response; and (2) the activation of A48 Id required antigenic stimulation. This latter observation, which is in agreement with data reported by various investigators,[21,22] clearly demonstrated that the Id-induced Id response is not related to a mitogenic effect.

Rubinstein et al.[6] have shown that the dominance of A48 Id$^+$ anti-BL clones in mice injected at birth with 10 μg of A48 monoclonal protein is related to the expansion of A48 Id-specific helper T cells. Indeed, when Lyt-1.2 helper T cells from animals injected at birth with A48 were infused together with B cells into lethally irradiated BALB/c mice, an A48 Id anti-BL PFC response was observed subsequent to immunization with BL. The A48 Id specificity of these Lyt-1.2 T cells was proved in experiments performed in nude mice. The infusion of these cells into nude mice helped the B cells to develop an IgM anti-TNP PFC response subsequent to immunization with A48-TNP conjugate. By contrast, MOPC384-TNP conjugate did not elicit an anti-TNP PFC response. MOPC384 is an IgA,κ protein bearing an unrelated Id.

Therefore, these results demonstrated that the administration after birth of A48 Id$^+$ monoclonal proteins as well as of minute amounts of anti-A48 Id antibodies had a similar effect leading to the activation of A48 Id$^+$ clones. However, the mechanisms responsible for the activation of A48 Id$^+$ clones subsequent to these distinct manipulations were essentially different. Whereas the anti-Id antibodies exert their effect directly on A48 Id$^+$ precursors of B cells, the administration of A48 monoclonal proteins induced the expansion of A48 Id-specific helper T cells. These helper T cells probably selectively expand the A48 Id B cells subsequent to antigen stimulation. The input of the antigen into the host might generally result in a diverse antibody response. These antibodies can react with different affinity with all the epitopes that the host encounters. Our results demonstrating the dominance of A48 Id$^+$ clones in the animals treated at birth with A48 Id$^+$ MAbs strongly indicate that the idiotypic interactions may severely limit the clones which potentially can be stimulated by antigens. Several factors determine which particular clone will be chosen for the response to an antigen such as the genetic background, previous contact with the antigen, and amount of antigen exposure. Our data clearly showed that the T cells also play an important role in determining which set of clones are expanded, suggesting that the principal function of Id-specific regulatory T cells is the fine tuning of the immune response.

8. Idiotypic Influence on the Development of the Immune System

The experimental data on the Id-determined expansion of A48 Id helper T cells and the dominance of A48 Id clones subsequent to the parenteral injection after birth of A48 Id$^+$ MAbs suggested that, in general terms, the passive influx of maternal Id in the immune system of the fetus can influence clonal expansion, favoring those clones which produce Ids similar to the dominating maternal ones. In order to verify this hypothesis, we tested the effects of in utero exposure of Id on the anti-BL clones. For this study, we chose UPC10 instead of A48 because (1) it is an IgG2a and therefore can traverse placenta, (2) it shares A48 idiotopes, and (3) UPC10, like A48 Id, are not expressed on anti-BL antibodies. In

TABLE VIII

Activation of U10 Id Clones by in Utero Exposure to UPC10 Monoclonal Protein

Treatment	Anti-BL PFC/ spleen	UPC10 Id⁺ (%)
Females injected with UPC10	13,170 ± 4,658[a]	30 ± 15
Progeny from females injected with UPC1O	5,500 ± 1,622	93 ± 3
Progeny from females	40,000 ± 15,558	9 ± 9

[a]Mean ± S.E.M.

these experiments, female mice were intravenously injected with 100 μg UPC10 during mating and throughout pregnancy. The progeny were immunized 1 month after birth with 20 μg of BL and the anti-BL response was measured. Whereas mice originating from females not injected with UPC10 as well as mothers injected with UPC10 did not develop a significant UPC10 Id⁺ response, the progeny originating from mothers injected with UPC10 developed a significant Id response (Table VIII). This response was not associated with a particular *MHC* or *IghC* gene complex because it was observed in BALB/c as well as BAB.14 and BALB.B.

These observations clearly indicate that the passive influx of maternal Id into the fetus via placenta or colostrum has a profound influence on the development of UPC10 Id⁺ anti-BL response. In physiological terms, it is clearly an advantage to have the immunological experience of the mother-to-be transmitted to the newborn resulting in the expansion of the precursors and therefore in a more vigorous response against the pathogens prevailing in the species. This also indicates that the inheritance of acquired immunity is not related solely to passive acquisition of maternal antibodies but also to priming the immune system of progeny to a more vigorous response against the antigens which have been encountered by the mother.

References

1. Jerne, N. K., 1974, Towards a network theory of the immune response, *Ann. Immunol. (Inst. Pasteur)* **125C**:373–389.
2. Winkler, M., Franssen, J. D., Collignon, C., Leo, O., Mariaimé, B., van de Walle, P., de Groote, D., and Urbain, J., 1979, Idiotypic regulation of the immune system: Common idiotypic specificities between idiotopes and antibodies raised against anti-idiotypic antibodies in rabbits, *J. Exp. Med.* **150**:184–195.
3. Bona, C. A., Heber-Katz, E., and Paul, W. E., 1981, Idiotype anti-idiotype regulation. I. Immunization with a levan binding myeloma protein leads to the appearance of auto-anti(anti-idiotypes) antibodies and to the activation of silent clones, *J. Exp. Med.* **153**:951–967.
4. Rodkey, L. S., 1980, Autoregulation of immune response via idiotypic network interactions, *Microbiol. Res.* **49**:631–659.
5. Paul, W. E., and Bona, C., 1982, Regulatory idiotopes and immune networks: A hypothesis, *Immunol. Today* **3**:230–234.
6. Rubinstein, L. J., Yeh, M., and Bona, C. A., 1982, Idiotype–anti-idiotype network. II. Activation of silent

clones by treatment at birth with idiotypes is associated with the expansion of idiotype-specific helper T cells, *J. Exp. Med.* **156**:506–521.

7. Ollo, R., Auffrey, C., Sikorov, J. L., and Rougeon, F., 1981, Mouse heavy chain variable region: Nucleotide sequences of a germ line V_H gene segment, *Nucleic Acids Res.* **9**:4098–4109.

8. Goldberg, B., Paul, W. E., and Bona, C., 1983, Idiotype–antiidiotype regulation. IV. Characterization of regulatory idiotopes on β2-6 fructosan binding monoclonal antibodies and monoclonal proteins with different antigen specificities, *J. Exp. Med.* **158**:515–528.

9. Sachs, D. L., Kelsoe, G. H., and Sachs, D. H., 1983, Induction of immune response with anti-idiotypic antibodies: Implications for the induction of protective immunity, *Springer Semin. Immunopathol.* **6**:79–97.

10. Legrain, P., and Buttin, G., 1983, The level of expression and the molecular distribution of ABPC48 idiotopes in levan or anti-idiotope primed BALB/c mice, in: *Immune Networks* (C. Bona and H. Kohler, eds.), *Ann. NY Acad. Sci.* **418**:290–296

11. Bona, C., 1984, Regulatory idiotopes, in: *Idiotype Manipulation in Biological Systems* (H. Kohler, P. A. Cazenave, and J. Urbain, eds.), Academic Press, New York, pp. 29–41.

12. Auffrey, C., Sikorov, J. L., Ollo, R., and Rougeon, F., 1981, Correlation between D region structure and antigen-binding specificity: Evidence from the comparison of closely related immunolobulin V_H sequence, *Ann. Immunol. (Inst. Pasteur).* **132D**:77–88.

13. Selsing, E., and Storb, W., 1981, Somatic mutation of immunoglobulin light-chain variable region genes, *Cell* **25**:45–58.

14. Kabat, E. A., Wu, T. T., and Bilofsky, H., 1979, *Sequence of Immunoglobulin Chains,* U.S. Department of Health, Education and Welfare.

15. Bona, C., 1981, *Idiotype and Lymphocytes,* Academic Press, New York.

16. Bona, C., Lieberman, R., Chien, C. C., Mond, J., House, S., Green, I., and Paul, W. E. 1978, Immune response to levan. I. Kinetics and ontogeny of anti-levan and anti-inulin antibody response and of expression of cross-reactive idiotype, *J. Immunol.* **120**:1436–1442.

17. Hiernaux, J., Bona, C., and Baker, T. J., 1981, Neonatal treatment with low doses of anti-idiotypic antibodies leads to the expression of a silent clone, *J. Exp. Med.* **153**:1006–1008.

18. Rubinstein, L. J., and Bona, C., 1983, Idiotype–anti-idiotype network. III. Genetic control of activation of A48Id silent clones subsequent to manipulation of the immune network, in: *Immune Networks* (C. Bona and H. Kohler, eds.), *Ann. N Y Acad. Sci.* **418**:97–109.

19. Rubinstein, L. J., Goldberg, B., Hierneux, J., Stein, K. G., and Bona, C., 1983, Idiotype–anti-idiotype regulation. V. The requirement for immunization with antigen or monoclonal anti-idiotypic antibodies for the activation of β2→6 and β2→1 polyfructosan reactive clones in BALB/c mice treated at birth with minute amounts of anti-A48 idiotype antibodies, *J. Exp. Med.* **158**:1129–1144.

20. Bona, C., and Pernis, B., 1983, Immune networks, in: *Fundamental Immunology* (W. E. Paul, ed.), Raven Press, New York, pp. 577–592.

21. Kelsoe, G., Reth, M., and Rajewsky, K., 1981, Control of idiotype expression by monoclonal anti-idiotype and idiotype-bearing antibody, *Eur. J. Immunol.* **11**:418–423.

22. Heyman, B., Andrighetto, G., and Wigzell, H., 1982, Antigen-dependent IgM mediated enhancement of the sheep erythrocytes response in mice, *J. Exp. Med.* **155**:994–1009.

21

Idiotype-Specific T Cells

Role in Regulation

Mary McNamara, Heinz Kohler, and Susan Smyk

1. The Necessity for Idiotope-Specific T Helpers

The nature of T-cell receptors is among the most controversial questions in contemporary immunology. The key problem lies in the hypothesis that T-cell receptors are encoded by genes which are homologous to immunoglobulin gene segments.[1-3] Data that are pertinent for this issue come from four different approaches: (1) serological identification of T-cell surface proteins or T-cell-derived factors, (2) functional impairment or stimulation of T-cell activities induced by idiotype-specific antibodies, (3) demonstration of immunoglobulin linkage for T-cell-specific functions, and (4) analysis of the immunoglobulin gene segment arrangement in specific T-cell clones. Among the strongest supportive evidence for the immunoglobulinlike structures of T-cell receptors is the sharing of idiotopes among B and T cells. For example, some anti-idiotypic[4-8] and anti-V_H framework sera[9] effect T-cell functions and bind to antigen-specific factors made by T cells.[10,11] In a set of recent experiments we have obtained evidence that T-helper cells (Th) can recognize idiotypes as carrier-determinants for a hapten-specific B cell.[12,13] These Th can be induced by idiotype- and antigen-specific priming procedures. The specificity of idiotype recognition is somewhat unique and clearly different from that of B cells responding to immunization with idiotype.[14,15] It appears that the idiotype-recognizing Th recognize idiotopes primarily on the heavy chain and that these idiotopes are involved in the binding site of the target idiotype immunoglobulin.

The structural and genetic basis of B–T-cell idiotype sharing might not consist of structural and genetic identities for B- and T-cell receptors. The serological idiotype sharing, observed in many instances, and the functional use of idiotype as targets for T–B-cell interactions might be simply due to idiotypic cross-reactivity. In other words, T-cell recep-

Mary McNamara, Heinz Kohler, and Susan Smyk • Department of Molecular Immunology, Roswell Park Memorial Institute, Buffalo, New York 14263.

tors look like B-cell idiotypes because they mimic the three-dimensional shapes of idiotopes. The potential of idiotopes to mimic or to be mimicked by other structures seems to be a very general feature of idiotopes since antigens are mimicked by idiotopes creating the universe of internal images.[16]

The physiological necessity of idiotype-recognizing Th is not immediately apparent. Some suggestions have been made; Bottomly and co-workers[17,18] have hypothesized that a special type of Th is needed to maintain the dominant expression of a B-cell idiotype; the induction of auto-anti-idiotypic antibody[19] is likely to require idiotope–carrier recognition. We would like to suggest here that the role of idiotype-recognizing Th should be understood as part of the recognition and representation of internal antigen images. Since the encounter of external antigens is infrequent, the evolutionary maintenance of immunity depends on the constant interactions of idiotopes and idiotope internal images. In the case of Th which recognize an idiotope on the heavy chain of T15 and M167[13,14] the internal image of an antigen might be the physiological target. If this reasoning is correct, the dominant expression of certain B-cell idiotypes is necessary for the evolutionary maintenance of certain important internal images. In this context the pair of idiotype–anti-idiotype B–T interactions becomes the maintenance procedure for antigen images.

In some recent experiments, we probed the maintenance requirements by T-helper cells for the dominant T15 idiotype. We are basing our experiments and the interpretation of data on the assumption that the T15/M167-specific T-helper cells play the role of the internal T-cell anti-image of T15.

We have found that there is a direct correlation between the level of T15 B-cell expression and the frequency of T cells which recognize the T15/M167 idiotope. Furthermore, primary B cells appear to be relatively independent of T-helper cells in their T15 dominance expression while secondary B cells do exhibit a relative need for T15-recognizing T cells.

2. Results

2.1. Induction and Specificity of Idiotype-Recognizing T-Helper Cells

In order to study the function of idiotype-recognizing Th, we first investigated the induction pathway of these cells and their fine specificity. The ways in which these cells can be stimulated is important in discerning the role of idiotype-recognizing T cells in immunoregulation.

We used priming with phosphocholine (PC) in order to induce the Th. Antigen stimulation is a natural occurrence in an immune response; thus, this method of induction mimics a physiological event. We found that PC-Hy priming of NBF_1 males stimulated a population of Th which can recognize the similar but idiotypically distinct myelomas, T15 and M167 (Table I). PC-Hy priming does not induce T-cell help nonspecifically, however. PC-primed T cells do not provide help for the anti-PC hybridoma 104, which, unlike M167, has a very different heavy and light chain from T15. This finding indicates that while the T15/M167-recognizing Th are not idiotype-specific in the conventional sense, they do seem to be heavy-chain idiotope-specific.

We next investigated the fine specificity of these T15/M167-recognizing T cells. We

TABLE I
Specificity of PC-Hy-Induced T-Helper Cells

NBF$_1$ male donor treatment[a]	In vitro antigen[b]	In vitro inhibitor[c]	Anti-TNP-positive wells[d]	Percent inhibition[e]
PC-Hy	—	—	3	—
	TNP-T15	—	30	—
	TNP-M167	—	33	—
	TNP-104	—	6	—
	TNP-T15	PC	2	93
		T15	4	87
		M167	2	93
	TNP-M167	PC	4	88
		T15	12	64
		M167	2	90

[a]Donor NBF$_1$ males were primed with 100 μg Hy in CFA i.p. 8 weeks before use and 100 μg PC-Hy in IFA i.p. 4 weeks before use. T cells were prepared by nylon wool purification followed by treatment with anti-Ly-2 + complement. 1.2×10^6 Ly-2$^-$ T cells were injected into athymic, *nu/nu* recipients.
[b]The splenic fragment cultures were immunized *in vitro* with TNP$_7$-T15, TNP$_{12}$-M167, or TNP$_{19}$-104 at 10^{-8} M TNP.
[c]PC was used as an *in vitro* inhibitor at a concentration of 10^{-7} M. Affinity-purified proteins T15 and M167 were used as *in vitro* inhibitors at 10^{-9} M protein.
[d]48–96 fragment cultures were assayed for anti-TNP activity on days 9 and 12 by ELISA.
[e]Percent inhibition was calculated by the formula: [1 − (percent positive cultures with inhibitor/percent positive cultures without inhibitor)] $\times$ 100.

were interested in the target of recognition of the Th. Knowing the specificity of Th is important for understanding how T cells recognize and regulate B cells. We performed a series of inhibition experiments, using as *in vitro* inhibitors PC and unconjugated T15 and M167 to block the help for the T15 and M167 carriers attached to the TNP hapten. As can be seen in Table I, PC hapten could inhibit the response to both idiotypes. Furthermore, both T15 and M167 could inhibit the response to either idiotype equally well, indicating that the idiotype-recognizing Th recognize a target determinant in the PC-binding site and that a single Th population recognizes an idiotope shared by the T15 and M167 molecules. Other data from our laboratory[13] showed that the major part of the shared determinant is located on the T15 and M167 heavy chains. Collectively, these data demonstrate that the conventional idiotype specificity of B cells and their products is not found with T cells. T cells appear to be idiotype-nonspecific, recognizing instead a cross-reactive idiotope shared by groups of idiotypes. T cells, by recognizing key idiotypes in a constantly mutating B-cell repertoire, would be able to control the B-cell idiotype repertoire. By doing this, T cells would concentrate on so-called "regulatory idiotopes."[13,14,20]

2.2. Frequency of Idiotype-Recognizing Th in T15$^+$ and T15$^-$ Mice

Previously we have shown[13,14] that T15/M167-recognizing T cells can be induced in both idiotype-positive and idiotype-negative mice. To quantitatively establish the difference in the frequency of T15/M167-recognizing Th in these two groups of mice, we performed limiting dilution analysis on PC-primed T cells from NBF$_1$ male and BALB/c mice. We transferred graded doses of Ly-2$^-$ T cells from the two groups of mice to

BALB/c *nu/nu* recipients. Splenic fragment cultures were prepared and the supernatants analyzed for anti-TNP activity. The Poisson distribution was used to determine the frequency of T15- and M167-recognizing Th. Using the splenic homing efficiency of 30%,[13] the frequencies of T15- and M167-recognizing T cells in NBF_1 males were estimated at 1/35,000 and 1/85,000, respectively; in BALB/c mice, the frequencies of T15- and M167-recognizing cells were estimated at 1/9570 and 1/16,800. The NBF_1 male and BALB/c frequencies differ significantly from each other, taking into account experimental variation. The reduced frequency of T15/M167-recognizing T cells in immune-defective NBF_1 mice may be caused by a lack of T-cell priming by αPC B cells.

2.3. Time-Dependent Establishment of T15 Dominance

The collaboration of anti-PC B cells with idiotype-recognizing T cells in the establishment of T15 dominance was further investigated. Secondary B cells and Th from an immunodefective NBF_1 male mouse were used. Previously we had shown[21] that primary B cells together with carrier-primed T cells from either $T15^+$ or $T15^-$ donors respond with a T15-dominant response. When, however, secondary PC-primed B cells are used, the appearance of T15 dominance is delayed. KLH-primed NBF_1 male T cells fail to provide help for a T15-dominant anti-PC response with secondary PC-primed B cells. But if the recipient mice, reconstituted with male NBF_1 T cells and PC-primed B cells, are rested for 3 weeks after cell transfer before being challenged with the PC antigen, the anti-PC response on day 27 has recovered the T15 dominance (Table II). These data, demon-

TABLE II
T15 Dominance Recovers with Time after Cotransfer of Secondary B Cells and Primed T Cells from Male MBF₁ Mice

KLH-primed T-cell donor[a]	BALB/c B-cell donor[b]	Day of assay[c]	Anti-PC PFC/ spleen[d]	Percent T15 clonotype[e]
2×10^6 NBF₁ female	Unprimed	8	1,500 ± 2,000	97
		27	4,800 ± 6,100	88
	PC-primed	8	10,800 ± 7,800	90
		27	15,000 ± 9,500	85
2×10^7		27	5,900 ± 3,400	96
2×10^6 NBF₁ male	Unprimed	8	5,283 ± 1,115	98
		27	11,400 ± 4,700	90
	PC-primed	8	37,550 ± 19,777	48
		27	19,733 ± 2,386	90
2×10^7		27	4,900 ± 900	97

[a]NBF₁ mice were primed with 100 μg KLH in CFA 4 weeks before use.
[b]Eight-week-old BALB/c mice were injected i.p. with 100 μg PC₄₅-BSA in CFA 6 weeks before use as B-cell donors. Purified B cells were prepared by elimination of T cells from spleen cell suspensions by anti-Thy-1.2 and complement treatment. 650-R 8-week-old NBF₁ male mice served as recipients. Recipients received 2×10^6 T cells, 5×10^6 B cells, and 50 μg PC₃₀-KLH i.v.
[c]Adoptively transferred NBF₁ males were either immunized on the day of cell transfer or 21 days later and assayed on day 8 or 27, respectively.
[d]Five days after cell transfer and immunization, recipient spleens were assayed for anti-PC PFC by hemolytic plaque analysis.
[e]Percent T15 was determined by inhibition of plaque formation by the addition of purified T15-specific hybridoma product, F63, to the plaquing mixture.

strating slower establishment of T15 dominance with NBF$_1$ male T cells, correlate well with the data above on the lower frequency of T15/M167-recognizing Th in the NBF$_1$ male. A reduced number of these idiotype-specific T cells would necessarily indicate a delayed appearance of T15 dominance.

3. Discussion

According to Jerne's network hypothesis,[16] the immune response is regulated by specific T–B-cell collaboration. These interactions occur via complementary idiotypic–anti-idiotypic receptor recognition. Specific B-cell responses are regulated by T cells which recognize B-cell idiotypes. These T cells play an immunoregulatory role by either suppressing or enhancing the immune response. T-suppressor cells have been widely studied[22–25] and their role in suppression of specific antibody responses has been well documented. Conversely, the role of idiotype-recognizing Th in immune regulation is uncertain. One proposed function of these Th which has received experimental support is the maintenance of idiotype clonal dominance.[17,18] Bottomly et al. found that PC-primed B cells require a special auxiliary T cell in order to maintain T15 idiotype dominance. Likewise, Woodland and Cantor[26] found that idiotype-specific T cells are needed for the induction of idiotype-positive B memory cells. In our laboratory, we have demonstrated the existence of these idiotype-recognizing Th[12–14] and shown that they can be induced by antigen, idiotype, or anti-idiotype priming. The latter finding provides further evidence that idiotype-specific Th play a significant role in the regulation of the B-cell response.

In the study discussed here, we pursue the question of the regulation of clonal dominance by studying both the dominant idiotype-producing B cell as well as the idiotype-recognizing Th involved in its regulation. With this experimental approach, we analyze the Th directly by using a hapten–carrier idiotype as antigen. Limiting dilution analysis demonstrates the existence of a single Th population which recognizes both T15 and M167 idiotypes. Inhibition experiments indicate that the target of recognition for this Th population is a determinant on the T15 and M167 H chains which is involved in the PC-binding site. Interestingly, this finding is different from that of Jorgensen and Hannestad,[27] who found that Th recognize the variable region of the light chain of the myeloma protein 315. For these T cells which recognize 315, the V$_L$ region is the most antigenic. These findings indicate that in the 315 system, immunoregulation by T cells might work at the level of the light chain, whereas in our system, the heavy chain constitutes the major part of the target recognized by the T cells. Both findings, however, demonstrate that B and T cells seem to "see" idiotypes differently. B cells (antibodies) recognize "complete" idiotypic determinants, formed by heavy- and light-chain association, while T cells prefer to recognize isolated heavy- or light-chain determinants.

The requirement for these idiotype-recognizing T-helper cells for the dominant expression of the T15 idiotype was next addressed. Contrary to other reports[17,18] which found that T cells from T15$^-$ mice (NBF$_1$ males) cannot support an anti-PC response which is T15 dominant, we found that carrier-primed donor T cells from these mice can, in time, provide help for a T15-dominant anti-PC response by adoptively transferred secondary B cells. The appearance of T15 dominance is seen if the reconstituted recipients are challenged 3 weeks after reconstitution.

TABLE III
Frequencies of Idiotype-Recognizing T-Helper Cells

PC-primed Th cell donor[a]	In vitro antigen[b]	Precursor frequency of carrier-specific T cells[c]
NBF$_1$ male	TNP-T15	1:35,000
	TNP-M167	1:85,000
BALB/c	TNP-T15	1: 9570
	TNP-M167	1:16,800

[a]T-helper cell donors were primed as in Table I. Ly-2$^-$ T-helper cells were prepared as in Table I and injected into BALB/c, *nu/nu* recipients.
[b]TNP$_7$-T15 or TNP$_{12}$-M167 were used as *in vitro* antigens at 10^{-8} M TNP.
[c]The precursor frequency of T15- and M167-recognizing T-helper cells was calculated using the Poisson distribution and linear regression analysis.

The delay in the establishment of T15-idiotype dominance can be explained by our finding on the significant difference in frequency of T15/M167-recognizing Th in NBF$_1$ male (T15$^-$) mice versus BALB/c (T15$^+$) mice. NBF$_1$ males have a substantially lower number of these Th than do BALB/c mice. The inefficiency of NBF$_1$ males to establish T15 dominance could be attributed to the reduced number of Th capable of recognizing the T15 idiotype (Table III).

The lower frequency of T15/M167-recognizing T cells in NBF$_1$ males could be due to the lack of circulating anti-PC antibodies in the defective NBF$_1$ males; there are no anti-PC antibodies available to "educate" the Th to recognize T15 or M167. Priming with PC antigen or idiotype does induce the generation of idiotype-specific help[12]; however, since the priming is a transient phenomenon rather than a continuing influence (as circulating antibody would be) the level of idiotype-recognizing T-cells in the T15$^-$ mice will remain substantially lower than in the T15$^+$ mice. In this hypothesis, the T-cell repertoire would be secondarily formed and be dependent on the expression of B-cell idiotypes.

These experimental findings and the resulting hypothesis raise the question of why the T15/M167-recognizing Th induce T15 dominance over M167 dominance or T15/M167 codominance. This selective promotion of the T15 idiotype must be dependent on the developmental state of the T15 and M167 B cells. The T15 B cells are more numerous than the latter because of selective maturation in ontogeny and may be in an advanced developmental state. Thus, the T15/M167-recognizing Th effectively induce only T15 dominance.

References

1. Jensenius, J. C., and Williams, A. F., 1982, the T lymphocyte antigen receptor-paradigm lost, *Nature* **300**:583.
2. Kronenberg, M., Davis, M. M., Early, P. W., Hood, L. E., and Watson, J. D., 1980, Helper and killer T cells do not express B cell immunoglobulin joining and constant region gene segments, *J. Exp. Med.* **152**:1745.
3. Cayre, Y., Pallidino, M., Marcu, K., and Stavnezer, J., 1981, Expression of an antigen receptor on T cells does not require recombination at the immunoglobulin J$_H$-Cμ locus, *Proc. Natl. Acad. Sci. USA* **78**:3814.
4. Binz, H., and Wigzell, H., 1977, Antigen-binding, idiotypic T lymphocyte receptors, *Contemp. Top. Immunobiol.* **7**:113.

5. Julius, M. H., Cosenz, H., and Augustin, A. A., 1978, Evidence for endogenous production of T cell receptor bearing idiotypic determinants, *Eur. J. Immunol.* **8**:484.
6. Kim, B. S., 1979, Mechanisms of idiotype suprression. I. *In vitro* generation of idiotype-specific suppressor T cells by anti-idiotype antibodies and specific antigen, *J. Exp. Med.* **149**:1371.
7. Miller, G. G., Nadler, P. I., Asano, Y., Hodes, R. J., and Sachs, D. H., 1981, Induction of idiotype-bearing nuclease-specific helper T cells by *in vivo* treatment with anti-idiotype, *J. Exp. Med.* **154**:24.
8. Eichmann, K., and Rajewsky, K., 1975, Induction of T and B cell immunity by anti-idiotypic antibodies, *Eur. J. Immunol.* **5**:661.
9. Rajewsky, K., and Eichmann, K., 1977, Antigen receptors of T helper cells, *Contemp. Top. Immunobiol.* **7**:69.
10. Bach, B. A., Greene, M. I., Benacerraf, B., and Nisonoff, A., 1979, Mechanisms of regulation of cell-mediated immunity. IV. Azobenzenearsonate-specific suppressor factor(s) bear cross-reactive idiotypic determinants the expression of which is linked to the heavy-chain allotype linkage group of genes, *J. Exp. Med.* **149**:1084.
11. Tada, T., and Okumura, K., 1979, The role of antigen-specific T cell factors in the immune response, *Adv. Immunol.* **28**:1.
12. Gleason, K., Pierce, S. K., and Kohler, H., 1981, Generation of idiotype specific T cell help through network perturbation, *J. Exp. Med.* **153**:926.
13. Gleason, K., and Kohler, H., 1982, Regulatory idiotypes: T helper cells recognize a shared V_H idiotype on phosphorylcholine-specific antibodies, *J. Exp. Med.* **156**:539.
14. McNamara, M., and Kohler, H., 1983, Idiotype recognizing T helper cells which are not idiotype-specific, *J. Exp. Med.* **158**:811–821.
15. McNamara, M., Gleason, K., and Kohler, H., 1983, Idiotype-specific T helper cells, *Ann. N.Y. Acad. Sci.* **418**:65–73.
16. Jerne, N. K., 1974, Towards a network theory of the immune response, *Ann. Immunol. (Paris)* **125C**:373.
17. Bottomly, K., and Mosier, D. E., 1979, Mice whose B cells cannot produce the T15 idiotype also lack an antigen-specific helper T cell required for T15 expression, *J. Exp. Med.* **150**:1399.
18. Bottomly, K., and Jones, F., III, 1981, Idiotypic dominance manifested during a T-dependent anti-phosphorylcholine response requires a distinct helper T cell, in: *B Lymphocytes in the Immune Response: Functional Development and Interactive Properties* (N. Klinman and D. Mosier, eds.), Elsevier/North-Holland, Amsterdam.
19. Kluskens, L., and Kohler, H., 1974, Regulation of the immune response by autogenous antibody against receptor, *Proc. Natl. Acad. Sci. USA* **71**:508.
20. Bona, C. A., Heber-Katz, E., and Paul, W., 1981, Idiotype–anti-idiotype regulation. I. Immunization with a levan-binding myeloma protein leads to the appearance of auto-anti(anti-idiotype) antibodies and to the activation of silent clones, *J. Exp. Med.* **158**:951.
21. Smyk, S., McNamara, M., Gleason, K., and Kohler, H., 1983, Time dependent establishment of T15 dominance with secondary B cell and T helper cells from T15-negative NBF_1 male mice, submitted for publication.
22. Dohi, Y., and Nisonoff, A., 1979, Suppression of idiotype and generation of suppressor T cells with idiotype-conjugated thymocytes, *J. Exp. Med.* **150**:909.
23. Bona, C., and Paul, W. F., 1979, Cellular basis of regulation of expression of idiotype. I. T-suppressor cells specific for MOPC 460 Id regulate the expression of cells secreting anti-TNP antibodies bearing 460 Id, *J. Exp. Med.* **149**:592.
24. DuClos, T. W., and Kim, B. S., 1977, Suppressor T cells: Presence in mice rendered tolerant by neonatal treatment with anti-receptor antibody or antigen, *J. Immunol.* **119**:1769.
25. Sy, M-S., Bach, B. A., Dohi, Y., Nisonoff, A., Benacerraf, B., and Greene, M. I., 1979, Antigen- and receptor-driven regulatory mechanisms. II. Induction of suppressor T cells with idiotype-coupled syngeneic spleen cells, *J. Exp. Med.* **150**:1229.
26. Woodland, R., and Cantor, H., 1978, Idiotype-specific T helper cells are required to induce idiotype-positive B memory cells to secrete antibody, *Eur. J. Immunol.* **8**:600.
27. Jorgensen, T., and Hannestad, K., 1978, T helper lymphocytes recognize the V_L domain of the isologous mouse myeloma protein 315, *Scand. J. Immunol.* **10**:317.

22

The Role of Idiotype and of Immunoglobulin in T-Cell Differentiation and Function

CHARLES A. JANEWAY, JR.

1. Introduction

A great deal of attention has appropriately been directed to the role of genes encoded in the major histocompatibility complex (MHC) in T-cell development, antigen recognition by T cells, and cell interactions involving T cells. However, it seems likely that not all T cells are under the influence of MHC-linked genes. Some T cells appear to be involved in recognition and regulation of immunoglobulin (Ig) gene products, or products of loci linked to the *Igh* genes. I have previously reviewed the characteristics of some of these cells in several different articles,[1-3] and I will not repeat those descriptions here. Rather, I would like to focus on the role of Ig and of idiotypic Ig in particular (Id) in T-cell maturation and function.

In this chapter, I propose to cover four points. First, I will describe T-cell activities that appear to depend on Ig for their expression. Second, I will compare a class of helper T (Th) cell that appears to be specific both for antigen and for self Id with the very similar or identical T cell that activates feedback suppression. Third, I will compare two distinct classes of Id-specific Th cells as an aid to their distinction, listing what I believe are most of the literature references to the two types. Finally, I will present evidence that dominant Id expression in most systems is based on antibacterial antibodies, either through cross-reactivity with the test antigen or through idiotypic relationships between the antibody produced in response to the test antigen and antibody produced to the bacterial antigen, or by both mechanisms. From this analysis, I will argue that idiotypic regulation critically involves antibacterial antibody as a primary stimulus to regulatory elements, including helper and suppressor T cells specific for Id, and that the observed patterns of idiotypic dominance are conditioned by the induced idiotypic environment in which these regulatory

CHARLES A. JANEWAY, JR. • Department of Pathology, Immunology Division, and The Howard Hughes Medical Institute, Yale University School of Medicine, New Haven, Connecticut 06510.

cells mature. A complete picture of the regulation of Id expression must include not only the regulatory cells but the inducing Ids.

2. T-Cell Function in B-Cell-Deprived Mice

Our principal tool in these studies has been the B-cell-deprived mouse. These mice are prepared by means of chronic administration of heterologous anti-mouse μ-chain antibody. These mice will be termed anti-μ-suppressed mice for convenience. It is important to emphasize that all of the studies I will review with such mice use chronic suppression, in which case essentially no B-cell function and little if any Ig are present.[4-7] In such mice, T cells recognizing antigen in the context of self MHC-encoded gene products are essentially normal in activity and specificity.[4,5,7-11] Any T-cell function detected as abnormal in such mice might reflect a pathway of development which contains at least one step dependent upon Ig, and thus may be independent of MHC gene products. I realize that this approach is open to question; even more open to question is the further supposition that T-cell activities missing in such mice are in fact functions of T cells that actually recognize or require Ig for their physiological function. However, in some cases it has been possible to show directly that this is so, and thus this assumption, initially based on indirect evidence, has now been made more credible by its direct confirmation in some of these systems. Its actual demonstration in the rest of the systems I will describe awaits further analysis.

Before turning to a description of the T-cell subsets whose activity is altered in anti-μ-treated mice, I would like to list those clearly MHC-recognizing T cells whose function has been tested and found to be within normal limits. T cells responsive to a variety of T-cell mitogens, nonself MHC gene products, and minor H antigens are all normal in activity. Likewise, MHC-restricted, antigen-specific helper activity is normal in these mice in a number of independent studies.[7-11] The only MHC-restricted T-cell function that is consistently absent in these mice is the ability to mount an antigen-specific lymph node T-cell proliferative response.[12] This appears to be due to the role of B cells in lymph node as the major antigen-presenting cell,[13,14] unlike the spleen, where antigen presentation in anti-μ-treated mice is normal.[12] All the studies detailed here deal with splenic T cells, and no example of an abnormal, MHC-restricted T cell derived from spleen has yet been observed in anti-μ-treated mice.

While conventional, MHC-restricted Th cells are normal in anti-μ-treated mice, we have shown in four different systems that a second Th cell is not present in these mice.[4,7,10,15] In two of the systems, the response to 2,4-dinitrophenyl (DNP) *in vivo* and the response to sheep red blood cells (SRBC) *in vitro*, the major change observed in the response is a delay in antibody production, which, in both cases, can be attributed to a distinct Th-cell subset. In the case of the response to DNP, this cell was shown to be antigen-specific but did not require a hapten–carrier bridge.[16] This second Th cell (ThIg) is dependent upon a conventional, MHC-restricted Th cell (ThMHC) for its effect, and this latter Th required that the hapten be physically linked to the carrier molecule. While it is our working hypothesis that ThIg in both of these systems recognize idiotypic determinants on B-cell Ig, this has not been demonstrated in either system.

In subsequent studies, anti-μ-treated mice were shown to have normal ThMHC activity for the response to T-dependent forms of the hapten PC (see Bottomly and Dunn,

Chapter 23 this volume), but lacked a Th (ThId) similar in its properties to ThIg, required for the dominant expression of the T15 Id in this response.[10] Bottomly and colleagues have now confirmed that this cell actually binds specifically to T15, thus directly demonstrating the Id specificity of this ThId cell.[17]

Finally, recent studies carried out in collaboration with Rohrer[15] have shown that anti-μ-treated mice have Th cells that promote the antigen-dependent growth of the MOPC315 tumor in diffusion chambers *in vivo* but lack a second, antigen-specific, MOPC315-binding Th cell that promotes secretory differentiation of the MOPC315 tumor cells to anti-DNP plaque-forming cells.[18]

These studies, in conjunction with other studies of McDougal *et al.*,[19] Jayaraman *et al.*,[20] Woodland and Cantor,[21] Herzenberg *et al.*,[22] and Adorini *et al.*,[23] suggest that *optimal* T-dependent B-cell activation requires two distinct Ly-1 Th cells. One, the ThMHC, recognizes antigen bound to specific B cells via a hapten–carrier bridge; this cell is present at normal levels in antigen-primed, anti-μ-treated mice. The other, ThIg, requires both the ThMHC and the antigen to which the ThIg donor was primed to observe its effects on specific B cells, although studies of Rosenberg and Asofsky[24] suggest that this cell may induce a polyclonal antibody response as well, again not requiring a hapten–carrier bridge for its effects on B cells. Nor need ThIg come from a donor primed with an antigen the B cell is capable of binding. ThIg, in several studies, is readily killed by anti-Qa-1 and complement, while ThMHC are relatively resistant to this treatment.[18,19,25] Finally, in studies by Bottomly and co-workers, this cell has been shown to be able to help B cells of a different MHC gentotype[26], to be independent of known Ir gene control[11], and to be absent from MHC-recognizing sets of Th cells.[27] Thus, it apparently carries specificity for self Id and for antigen, but not for polymorphic self MHC gene products.

Because of the similarity of ThIg to Ly-1 T cells required for the induction of feedback suppression, which are also Qa-1-positive,[25] induced by antigen,[25] and recognize their targets by means of Igh-V-linked gene products,[28] we have examined the activity of inducers of suppression in anti-μ-treated mice. Preliminary studies showed that such cells were absent or markedly reduced in such mice.[4] Likewise, previous studies by L'Age-Stehr and co-workers[29] supported the notion that induction of suppression involved T-cell recognition of Ig in a different system, as did older studies of Gershon *et al.*[30] In recent experiments, we have shown that inducers of feedback suppression, and their molecular product, Ly-1 TsiF, are essentially absent in anti-μ-treated mice.[31] Furthermore, we have shown that only one of the two chains comprising Ly-1 TsiF is missing in supernatants of Ly-1 cells from these mice. This chain is I-J$^+$ and confers Igh-V-linked restriction on the interaction of Ly-1 TsiF with its target, an Ly-12 T cell.[32] Ly-1 cells from anti-μ-treated mice produce normal levels of the antigen-binding component of Ly-1 TsiF. While it is not clear from this experiment whether antigen is required for the induction of secretion of the I-J$^+$, Igh-V-restricted chain, this seems likely since supernatants of normal Ly-1 T cells do not contain this material. Thus, these experiments suggest that an Ly-1, Qa-1-positive T cell critical in the induction of suppression is absent in anti-μ-treated mice. This cell, like the ThId, is restricted in its interaction with its target cell by products of *Igh*-linked genes.

Recently, Sacks and co-workers[33] have shown that, unlike normal mice, anti-μ-treated mice are resistant to *Leishmania*. This resistance is due to the absence of T-cell-mediated suppression, which, in transfer experiments to normal mice, can be demonstrated to be mediated by Ly-1 T cells.[34] Interestingly, these cells do not transfer suppression to

Igh-congenic recipients (D. L. Sacks, personal communication). These data, in a disease susceptiblity model, are entirely consistent with our finding that anti-μ treatment leads to the absence of Ly-1, Igh-restricted inducers of T-cell suppression.

A finding almost certainly related to the loss of inducers of suppression is that anti-μ-treated mice also fail to produce Ly-2 TsF,[31] the molecular product of Ly-2 T-suppressor-effector cells.[35] While we have no evidence to prove it, the nature of the feedback suppression pathway suggests that this result is secondary to the absence of inducers of T-cell suppression.[36]

Finally, we have examined the presence or absence of contrasuppressor T cells in anti-μ-treated mice. Remarkably, spleen cells from mice treated with anti-μ for less than 10 days after birth and placed in culture, fail to generate contrasuppressor T cells (D. R. Green, R. K. Gershon, and C. A. Janeway, unpublished data). Likewise, T cells from adult, anti-μ-treated mice, after treatment with a low dose of a monoclonal anti-Thy-1 antibody, also do not generate contrasuppressor T cells on incubation *in vitro*. These observations have led to the hypothesis that contrasuppressor T cells recognize antigen–antibody complexes, and are activated by them. This hypothesis makes a certain amount of sense. If it is true, it would suggest that the role of the contrasuppressor T cell is to permit antibody production in the face of high levels of antibody, as long as antigen is present in the system. In practice, this means that the immune response may be initiated prior to the clearance of antibody, undoubtedly of survival value in cases in which the antigen is a multiplying pathogen. We have begun to test this hypothesis. Prior data from this author[37] and others have shown that antibody can augment the response of immune cells, while it is generally suppressive of naive cells.[38] We have recently repeated this finding and shown that while neither immune cells nor antibody effectively transfer an immune response to intact recipients, a mixture of immune cells and immune serum will do so (C. A. Janeway and T. N. Marion, unpublished observations). We are currently attempting to characterize the molecules in serum and the cells involved in this transfer system.

Thus, anti-μ-treated mice lack both ThIg and a number of immunoregulatory T-cell sets. The mechanism by which anti-μ treatment achieves these effects is currently being studied, with an emphasis on attempting to demonstrate a decisive role for Ig in T-cell maturation or activation, as well as determining whether specific or nonspecific Ig is required for maturation or expression of each T-cell type. We have no evidence for two trivial explanations of our findings, direct interaction of anti-μ with T cells or dominant suppression; indeed, in all cases studied, suppression has been deficient rather than dominant in anti-μ-treated mice.

3. Are ThId and Inducers of Feedback Suppression Distinct T-Cell Sets?

As noted briefly above, two functional activities are associated with Ly-1, Qa-1$^+$ T cells that are dependent on B cells or Ig for their activation: help for dominant Id production and the induction of feedback suppression. The B-cell dependence of both cell types has been shown in a number of ways by several different investigators in several independent experimental systems. The question now to be posed is whether these two activities derive from a single population of T cells, or whether each functional activity is associated with an independent T-cell subset. It should be stated at the outset that the answer to this question is not known. These cells share most characteristics in common; the one clear difference may be more apparent than real. Data on these points are summarized in Table I.

The common characteristics are cell surface antigen phenotype, Lyt-1$^+$2$^-$, Thy-1$^+$, Qa1$^+$, susceptibility to anti-μ treatment of donors or activation by Ig or activated B cells, apparent lack of MHC restriction in interaction with target, and activation by a T-cell-derived antigen-binding factor.

The common factors probably are I-J, clearly found on inducers of suppression and reported on ThId by Jayaraman et al.[20] and by K. Bottomly (personal communication); independence from known MHC-linked Ir genes in ThId[10] and in an apparent inducer of suppression,[39,40] and antigen specificity, which has been shown clearly for ThId and is implicit in the activity of the Ly-1 cell that is I-J$^+$ and Igh-V-restricted, in that its factor is only produced by Ly-1 cells from mice twice stimulated with antigen.[41] However, precise specificity of such cells has yet to be documented in a particular experiment. Again, if the cell characterized by Herzenberg et al. in the epitope suppression system is in fact an inducer of suppression, then it is clearly antigen specific.[42]

Finally, there appears to be one clear difference between inducers of suppression and ThId. This is the specificity of each of the activities for its target. The ThId is clearly specific for classical B-cell Ig, since many investigators have removed such cells on petri dishes coated with Ig,[17,18,20,21,23] and Bottomly and Dunn[17] have inhibited such binding with free Id. The target of the ThId is clearly the B cell bearing this idiotypic Ig. Finally, while controversial, it would appear that expression of the Id is required for the activation of ThId.[43,44] On the other hand, the inducer of feedback suppression, while manifesting an Igh-V-linked restriction in its interaction with its target Ly-12 T cell[28,32,41] and being sensitive to anti-μ treatment of the donor,[31] does not apparently recognize classical idi-

TABLE I

Characteristics of ThIg and of Inducers of Feedback Suppression[a]

Characteristic	ThIg	Reference	Inducers	Reference
Ig	−	18	−	25
Thy-1	+	18	+	25
Lyt-1	+	18	+	25
Lyt-2	−	18	−	25
Qa-1	+	18	+	25
I-J	+	20	+	41
Anti-μ mice	−	7, 10	−	4, 31
Antigen specific	+	10, 11	?	39, 41
Binds idiotype	+	17, 18, 20, 21, 23	?	
Igh-V-linked restriction	?	+, 26, 60	+	28
MHC restriction	−	26, 27	−(?)	40
Ir gene control	−	11	−	40
Present in nu/nu mice	−	27	?	
Responsive to inducer factor	+	79	+	79

[a]References are not exhaustive. I have chosen certain references that directly examine these questions.

otypic determinants found on Ig.[45] Rather, it appears to recognize a cell surface molecule expressed by T cells, at least of the Ly-12 class, and also some similarly polymorphic structure on thymic epithelial cells. This Igh-V-linked restriction is apparently not influenced by the genetic origin of the Ig. Such T cells are exposed to during ontogeny, although the activity of inducers of suppression is dependent on B cells or Ig for its development.

Can these seemingly disparate observations be used to discriminate between two distinct cells types, or are these simply two manifestations of the action of a single cell type? It seems simpler to propose that these are actions of a single cell type. This cell would appear as two activities because it is assayed on two different targets. That is, using a similar receptor molecule, this cell recognizes distinct structures on distinct target cells, and thus performs distinct functions. The situation would be clarified if antigens other than SRBC were tested, since all strains of mice appear to make antibody with a shared Id in response to SRBC (G. M. Iverson, personal communication). This may account for the apparent lack of influence of Ig genotype in the ontogeny of inducers of feedback suppression in the response to SRBC.

In any case, it is important to resolve this question, since our understanding of the activation of idiotypic B cells and of suppressor pathways depends on accurately defining the nature of each cell type. Experiments using idiotypically restricted systems and cloning of the cells appear to hold the greatest promise in this direction.

4. Evidence for Two Distinct Types of Idiotype-Specific Th Cells

I have argued in the past that there are two distinct classes of Id-specific Th cells.[1–4,46] This argument is now strengthened by many experiments that clearly distinguish the two types of cells.

One of the two types of helper cell has been termed ThId, an Ly-1, Qa-1$^+$ cell that is sensitive to anti-μ treatment of the donor, and which in the MOPC315 tumor system is involved in secretory differentiation of MOPC315.[15,18] This cell shows no apparent recognition of MHC gene products. The second cell type I propose to call anti-idiotypic Th (anti-Id Th). These cells can be induced in most cases by immunization of mice with syngeneic Id-bearing Ig.[47–54] Such cells, in the MOPC315 system, are resistant to treatment of the donor with anti-μ, are Ly-1, Qa-1$^-$ cells, and promote growth of MOPC315 cells rather than secretory differentiation.[15,18] Anti-Id Th have been described by numerous authors, sometimes in systems in which the idiotypic Ig is used as a conventional carrier molecule for antihapten antibody responses,[47–49,51,53,54] and sometimes in systems in which the anti-Id Th are added directly to idiotypic B cells in the absence of antigen,[15,18,50,52,55] as in the MOPC315 system. In both types of assay, evidence has been presented that anti-Id Th are also MHC-recognizing[52,55] and under control of MHC-linked Ir genes.[51] These characteristics are summarized in Table II. In Table III, references to descriptions of each cell type are given; the author has made decisions (where possible) as to which type of cell is being described as anti-idiotypic based on the criteria for distinguishing these cells given in Table II.

As a final complication, it should be noted that yet another variant on this theme exists. In the MOPC315 system, mice immunized with MOPC315 protein actually generate both

Table II

Characteristics of Two Distinct Classes of Idiotype-Specific Helper T Cells[a]

Characteristic	ThId	Anti-Id Th
Thy-1	+	+
Lyt-1	+	+
Lyt-2	−	−
Qa-1	+	−
MHC-restricted	−	+
Foreign antigen specific	+	−
Binds idiotype	+	−
Present in anti-μ-treated mice	−	+
Activates Id$^+$ B cells without antigen	−	+

[a]For references, see text.

Table III

Published Reports of ThId and of Anti-Id Th

ThId

Woodland and Cantor, 1978[21]
Hetzelberger and Eichmann, 1978[56]
Bottomly and Mosier, 1979[43]
Adorini et al., 1979[23]
Bottomly et al., 1980[10]
Jayaraman et al., 1982[20]
Rohrer et al., 1983[18]

Other ThIg Resembling ThId

Herzenberg, et al., 1976[22]
Janeway et al., 1977[7]
Seman and Morisset, 1981[57]

Anti-Id Th

Janeway et al., 1975[47]
Sakato et al., 1977[48]
Cosenza et al., 1977[49]
Eichmann et al., 1978[50]
Jorgenson and Hannestad, 1982[51]
Gleason et al., 1981[53]
Pierce et al., 1981[54]
Kawahara et al., 1982[52]
Augustin, 1983[55]
Rohrer et al., 1983[18]

Ig- or Id-Specific Th of Uncertain Type

Kelsoe et al., 1980[58]
Cerny and Caulfield, 1981[59]
L'Age-Stehr, 1981[60]
Nutt et al., 1981[61]

a growth-promoting anti-μ-resistant Th cell and an anti-μ-sensitive Ly-1, Qa-1$^+$ Th cell required for secretory differentiation of the tumor cells. This cell appears to recognize two distinct epitopes on the MOPC315 molecule, one as self Id and one as nominal antigen, presumably the highly immunogenic private idiotope on the MOPC315 protein. By its physiological characteristics, this cell would be classified as a ThId, even though it was induced by immunization with the idiotypic Ig.

While anti-Id Th might seem to be an artifact of experimental manipulation unlikely to play a physiological role in regulating immune responses, recent data suggest that such cells may play a role in regulation of Id expression. Thus, while two different groups have observed that one cannot immunize a normal BALB/c mouse to express anti-Id Th specific for the myeloma protein TEPC15,[48,49] whose Id is present in normal BALB/c serum at significant levels ($>$ 10 μg/ml), recent studies by Kohler, Pierce, and co-workers[53,54] have suggested that such cells can be activated by immunization with the hapten phosphocholine (PC), for which TEPC15 is specific. Even more interesting, Cerny and co-workers[58,59] have shown that TEPC15-specific Th cells exist in normal BALB/c T-cell populations, and will activate B cells which have been activated by T-independent forms of PC in the absence of added antigen. It appears to be such cells that are responsible for the cyclical nature of the anti-PC response in normal mice after immunization with T-independent forms of the antigen. Why such cells are not perpetually activating Id-bearing B cells is something of a mystery. Whether these cells defined by Cerny and colleagues are ThId or anti-Id Th is not clear. Their ability to activate B cells directly suggests they may be of the anti-Id Th class. On the other hand, their ability to bind unmodified TEPC15 directly is more consistent with their being ThId. A third possibility is that both classes are involved in Cerny's system, accounting for these apparently contradictory results. Further analysis of this interesting observation is clearly important to our understanding of idiotypic regulation.

The observation that anti-Id Th specific for TEPC15 cannot be activated directly by immunization with the myeloma protein is perhaps consistent with the notion that the activity of anti-Id Th specific for dominant Ids is itself tightly regulated. Interestingly, if BALB/c mice are neonatally suppressed with anti-Id, or are raised germfree so that their serum does not contain detectable TEPC15, anti-Id Th can be activated by direct immunization with TEPC15.[48,49] Thus, balance in this system appears to be dynamic,[53,54,58,59] and to be regulated by Id expression itself.

If the physiological role of anti-Id Th is to sustain T-independent antibody responses, a role one can well imagine to be of some value in responses to bacterial antigens that do not activate conventional MHC-restricted Th cells, what is the physiological role of ThId? This is not clear at the present time. However, in two systems, it has been shown that responses develop much more rapidly in the presence than in the absence of ThId.[4,7] Given that bacteria can multiply as frequently as 3 times in an hour, the speed at which an antibody is produced may be critical in determining the outcome of an infection. While this is a plausible explanation for the existence of such cells, it may not be the true physiological explanation. This will have to await the construction of mice that have a normal immune system but lack this particular cell type. Analysis of bacterial resistance in such mice should tell us whether ThId are critical to such resistance or not, and may tell us the mechanism by which they promote such resitance.

5. Naturally Occurring Idiotype as a Primary Influence on Idiotypic Networks

As outlined above, optimal production of Id in several different systems appears to depend on a cell we have termed ThId. This cell, in turn, appears to require Id in the form of Ig for its maturation or activation. ThId will bind to Id-coated petri dishes,[17,18,20,21,23] and cannot be demonstrated in mice lacking Id expression.[10,15,43] If this is true of all idiotypic systems, then one should expect to find Ig carrying the appropriate Id in normal serum. We have analyzed one such system, which I will summarize briefly below. Several other experimental idiotypic systems now also appear to have a normal serum analog, and indeed this may be a general rule. I will describe these systems briefly at the end of this section.

As we had initially described two synergistic Th in the *in vivo* adoptive secondary anti-DNP antibody response, we sought to develop an idiotypic system in the response to this antigen. We chose BALB/c mice to study because of the availability of a variety of Ig-congenic strains. Our studies have shown the following. Using an anti-Id reagent prepared by immunization of rabbits with the BALB/c, DNP-binding myeloma MOPC460 followed by absorption and hapten-specific elution, we found that the Id defined by this reagent (Id-460) is the dominant Id in this response.[62,63] This is seen clearly by measuring Id in serum or by inhibition of plaque-forming cells. The production of Id-460 in response to DNP-OVA immunization is inherited in linkage to Igh-V and V_κ,[62] as shown by analysis of Ig-congenic and recombinant mice (Lee, Dzierzak, Riblet, and Janeway, unpublished results). Thus, expression of Id-460 is similar to expression of the CRI associated with antiarsonate responses in A/J mice.[64,65]

We reasoned that it did not make evolutionary sense for a mouse to inherit genes with which to make antibody to nonpathogenic materials, and therefore sought a different explanation for the dominance of Id-460 in the anti-DNP antibody response. Since anti-DNP antibody responses apparently require a ThId-like cell,[7,66] we thought that perhaps Id-460 would be present in normal mouse serum and would be specific, not for DNP, but for some environmental pathogen. We do indeed find significant levels of Id-460 in normal mouse serum in most strains of mice.[67] This material is Ig by several criteria. It is found at much lower levels in germfree mouse serum, suggesting that its presence may be due to exposure to environmental bacterial antigens. This material can be obtained in large amounts for analysis by producing monoclonal antibodies from LPS-activated spleen cells or from mice immunized with anti-Id-460. We used such monoclonal antibodies to screen bacteria for reactivity with Id-460 bearing Ig. We have found that the common environmental pathogen *Pasteurella pneumotropica* reacts with these monoclonal proteins as well as with normal serum Id-460. Whether this identification is unqiue to *P. pneumotropica* is not known at this time. However, this organism can induce the production of Id-460$^+$ Ig that binds almost entirely to the inducing bacterium, as well as monoclonal antibodies with the same specificity.[68] Like the normal serum Id-460, this material does not bind to DNP. Whether anti-DNP-bearing Id-460 can bind to *P. pneumotropica* still remains to be defined precisely. We are presently trying to identify the structure on this bacterium that binds to Id-460$^+$, DNP-non-binding Ig, so that we can use it as a hapten in further studies. It is interesting to note that *P. pneumotropica* can be isolated from most mice, where it is not normally pathogenic. However, it is a major cause of death in recently described severe combined immune deficient (SCID) mice (M. Bosma, personal communication) which cannot make protective antibody. Whether our Id-460$^+$ monoclonal antibodies can protect such mice remains to be seen.

We believe that this form of Id-460 is the most biologically relevant form of the Id. We would now like to determine whether this idiotypic material "sets" the idiotypic network, leading to the production of Id-460 as the dominant form of anti-DNP antibody. If so, we would like to determine the mechanism by which this occurs.

Finally, in examining other idiotypic systems described in the literature, it appears that most or all of them may be similarly based on naturally occurring antibacterial antibodies. If this is true, it would readily explain the inheritance of these particular structures. For instance, both PC[69] and dextran[70] induce the production of a dominant Id in BALB/c mice; both are bacterial antigens. In the case of PC, essentially only a single Id is produced in normal mice hyperimmunized with antigen. On the other hand, the Id associated with the response to azophenylarsonate (Ars-CRI) is present at high levels early in the response, and then declines to about 20–50% of the response.[64,65] Material carrying an idiotypic determinant shared with almost all Ars-CRI$^+$ molecules is found at the 10–20 μg/ml level in normal mouse serum, and this material again does not bind to the arsonate hapten.[71,72] It has been reported (Sato, personal communication) that this material is in fact specific for *Brucella abortus*. Finally, the response to the hapten (4-hydroxy-3-nitrophenyl) acetyl (NP) is even more peculiar. This response is initially dominated by production of a highly restricted set of antibodies that bind the immunogen NP poorly, but bind chemically related haptens much more strongly.[73] This antibody is easy to follow, as it is all λ light chain bearing.[74] On hyperimmunization with NP, the response shifts entirely to κ light chain bearing and binds NP better than related haptens.[75] Finally, the initial response is mainly IgG, and is very intense.[76] It is dominated by a closely related family of molecules that share several Ids.[77] Interestingly, immunization with anti-Id leads to the production of much Id that does not bind NP.[78] All of this suggests that the NP-specific B cells found in normal mice are in fact immunized or primed by some environmental antigen. In this case, in addition to possible activation of Id-specific regulatory cells, it seems likely that the intensity and restricted nature of the primary anti-NP antibody response reflects priming of B cells by the postulated bacterial antigen itself. This would explain not only the intensity and specificity of the response, but also its relatively poor binding affinity for NP as compared to other available anti-NP B-cell clones. Experiments with B cells from germfree mice may help to clarify this issue. In this case, the actual environmental antigen has not been identified.

From such an analysis, it seem likely that most dominant Ids are based on protective antibacterial antibodies, although exceptions to this "rule" no doubt exist. Some react directly with the bacterial antigens, some cross-react weakly, and some, like Id-460 in the anti-DNP antibody response or the Ars-CRI, appear to be antigenically unrelated. Obviously, a great deal of testing of such a generalization will be required before it can be accepted. However, it seems from the evidence cited that normal serum should be examined carefully for expression of Id, and that such naturally occurring idiotypic material should be used to examine normal flora and common pathogens to determine the environmental trigger for its production. How the two different forms of Id are related obviously also needs a great deal of clarification.

6. Summary and Conclusions

From the data summarized above, it seems safe to conclude that B cells and/or Ig produced by B cells play an important role in T-cell development and activation. These T cells belong to subpopulations that appear not to recognize antigen in the context of self MHC, or, indeed, to recognize polymorphic portions of MHC molecules at all. Rather, such cells appear to be specific for Ig and for T-cell structures encoded in *Igh-V* and V_L genes, or in related genes. Their physiological role appears to be more in fine tuning of the response than in its basic on–off strategy. For instance, ThId are not required for antibody production, but may promote early production of antibacterial antibodies. Such cells appear also to be important in suppression and in contrasuppression of antibody responses. In probing the role of B cells or Ig in T-cell development and function, we have found anti-μ-treated mice to be a most useful tool. However, such mice have limitations, and more refined strategies need to be developed to determine the mechanisms by which depletion of B cells influences T-cell development and function.

Our analysis of these mice, and of idiotypic systems, suggest the following model. T cells are activated or expanded by, and regulate, Id-bearing B cells specific for common bacterial antigens. These cells may play a critical role in inducing a prompt and appropriately regulated antibacterial antibody response. Finally, it appears likely that most dominant Ids are actually based on antibacterial antibody responses. In some cases, the system studied involves a bacterial antigen, in some cases there is cross-reactivity between the bacterial and the test antigen, and in some cases, as for Id-460 expression in anti-DNP antibody responses, we believe that the connection is via Id–anti-Id interactions.

ACKNOWLEDGMENT. Supported in part by NIH Grant AI-13766. The author is an Investigator of the Howard Hughes Medical Institute.

References

1. Janeway, C. A., Jr., 1980, Idiotypic control: The expression of idiotypes and its regulation, in: *Strategies of Immune Regulation* (E. Sercarz and A. Cunningham, eds.), Academic Press, New York, pp. 179–198.
2. Janeway, C. A., Jr., 1980, Manipulation of the immune response by anti-idiotype, *Prog. Immunol.* **4**:1149–1159.
3. Janeway, C. A., Jr., 1983, The selection of self-MHC recognizing T lymphocytes: A role for idiotypes?, *Immunol. Today* **3**:261–265.
4. Janeway, C. A., Jr., Broughton, B., Dzierzak, E., Jones, B., Eardley, D., Durum, S. D., Yamauchi, K., Green, D. R., and Gershon, R. K., 1981, Studies on T lymphocyte function in B cell deprived mice, in: *Immunoglobulin Idiotypes* (C. A. Janeway, Jr., E. Sercarz, and H. Wigzell, eds.), Academic Press, New York, pp. 661–671.
5. Lawton, A. R., Asofsky, R., Hylton, M. B., and Cooper, M. D., 1972, Suppression of immunoglobulin class synthesis in mice. I. Effects of treatment with antibody to μ-chain, *J. Exp. Med.* **135**:277–297.
6. Manning, D. D., 1975, Heavy chain isotype suppresion: A review of the immunosuppressive effects of heterologous anti-Ig heavy chain antisera, *J. Reticuloendothel. Soc.* **18**:63–97.
7. Janeway, C. A., Jr., Murgita, R. A., Weinbaum, F. I., Asofsky, R., and Wigzell, H., 1977, Evidence for an immunoglobulin-dependent antigen-specific helper T cell, *Proc. Natl. Acad. Sci. USA* **74**:4582–4586.
8. Aden, D. P., Manning, D. D., and Reed, N. D., 1974, Exclusion of cooperating T cells as targets for heterologous anti-μ antiserum, *Cell. Immunol.* **14**:307–312.

9. Gordon, J., Murgita, R. A., and Tomasi, T. B., Jr., 1975, The immune response of mice treated with anti-μ antibodies: The effect on antibody-forming cells, their precursors, and helper cells assayed *in vitro, J. Immunol.* **114**:1808–1812.

10. Bottomly, K., Janeway, C. A., Jr., Mathieson, B. J., and Mosier, D. E., 1980, Absence of an antigen-specific helper T cell required for the expression of the T15 idiotype in mice treated with anti-μ antibody, *Eur. J. Immunol.* **10**:159–163.

11. Bottomly, K., and Maurer, P. H., 1980, Antigen-specific helper T cells required for dominant production of an idiotype (ThId) are not under immune response (Ir) gene control, *J. Exp. Med.* **152**:1571–1582.

12. Ron, Y., DeBaetselier, P., Gordon, J., Feldman, M., and Segal, S., 1981, Defective induction of antigen-reactive proliferating T cells in B cell-deprived mice, *Eur. J. Immunol.* **11**:964–968.

13. Tzehoval, E., DeBaetselier, P., Ron, Y., Tartakovsky, B., Feldman, M., and Segal, S., 1983, Splenic B cells function as immunogenic antigen-presenting cells for the induction of effector T cells, *Eur. J. Immunol.* **13**:89–94.

14. Katz, M., Ron, Y., Broughton, B., and Janeway, C. A., Jr., 1984, B cells are the major antigen presenting cell in peripheral lymph node: Role in spontaneous lymphoproliferation of mice with the *lpr* gene, submitted for publication.

15. Rohrer, J. W., and Janeway, C. A., Jr., 1984, Absence of a helper cell subset in B cell deficient mice, submitted for publication.

16. Janeway, C. A., Jr., Bert, D. L., and Shen, F. W., 1980, Cell cooperation during *in vivo* anti-hapten antibody responses. V. Two synergistic Lyt-1$^+$23$^-$ helper T cells with distinctive specificities, *Eur. J. Immunol.* **10**:231–236.

17. Bottomly, K., and Dunn, E., 1983, The role of B cell Ia antigens in T cell dependent B cell activation: Ia antigen density correlates with idiotype expression, *Ann. N.Y. Acad. Sci.* **418**:230–239.

18. Rohrer, J. W., Gershon, R. K., Lynch, R. G., and Kemp, J. D., 1983, The enhancement of B lymphocyte secretory differentiation by an Ly1$^+$,2$^-$; Qa-1$^+$ helper T cell subset, that sees both antigen and determinants on immunoglobulin, *J. Mol. Cell. Immunol.* **1**: 50–62.

19. McDougal, J. S., Shen, F.-W., Cort, S. P., and Bard, J., 1982, Two Ly1 T helper cell subsets distinguished by Qa1 phenotype: The priming environment determines whether one or both subsets will be generated, *J. Exp. Med.* **155**:831–838.

20. Jayaraman, S., Swierkosz, J. E., and Bellone, C. J., 1982, T cell replacing factor substitutes for an I-J$^+$ idiotype-specific T helper cell, *J. Exp. Med.* **155**:641–646.

21. Woodland, R., and Cantor, H., 1978, Idiotype-specific T cells are required to induce idiotype-positive B memory cells to secrete antibody, *Eur. J. Immunol.* **8**:600–605.

22. Herzenberg, L. A., Okumura, K., Cantor, H., Sato, V. L., Shen, F.-W., Boyse, E. A., and Herzenberg, L. A., 1976, T cell regulation of antibody responses: Demonstration of allotype-specific helper T cells and their specific removal by suppressor T cells, *J. Exp. Med.* **144**:330–344.

23. Adornini, L. M., Harvey, M., and Sercarz, E. E., 1979, The fine specificity of regulatory T cells. IV. Idiotypic complementarity and antigen bridging interactions in the anti-lysozyme response, *Eur. J. Immunol.* **9**:906–911.

24. Rosenberg, Y. J., and Asofsky, R., 1981, T cell regulation of isotype expression: The requirement for a second Ig-specific helper T cell population for the induction of IgG responses, *Eur. J. Immunol.* **11**:705–710.

25. Cantor, H., Hugenberger, J., McVay-Boudreau, L., Eardley, D. D., Kemp, J., Shen, F.-W., and Gershon, R. K., 1978, Immunoregulatory circuits among T cell sets: Identification of a subpopulation of T-helper cells that induces feedback inhibition, *J. Exp. Med.* **148**:871–877.

26. Bottomly, K., and Mosier, D. E., 1981, Antigen-specific helper T cells required for dominant idiotype expression are not H-2 restricted, *J. Exp. Med.* **154**:411–421.

27. Bottomly, K., and Janeway, C. A., Jr., 1981, Selected populations of alloreactive T cells contain helper T cells but lack ThId, an antigen-specific helper T cell required for dominant production of the T15 idiotype, *Eur. J. Immunol.* **11**:270–274.

28. Eardley, D. D., Shen, F.-W., Cantor, H., and Gershon, R. K., 1979, Genetic control of immunoregulatory circuits: Genes linked to the Ig locus govern communication between regulatory T-cell sets, *J. Exp. Med.* **150**:44–50.

29. L'Age-Stehr, J., Tuchmann, H., Gershon, R. K., and Cantor, H., 1980, Stimulation of regulatory T cell circuits by Ig-associated structures on activated B cells, *Eur. J. Immunol.* **10**:21–26.

30. Gershon, R. K., Orbach-Arbouys, S., and Calkins, C., 1974, B cell signals which activate suppressor T cells, *Prog. Immunol.* **2:**123–134.

31. Flood, P. M., Janeway, C. A., Jr., and Gershon, R. K., 1984, B cell deprived mice are deficient in an I-J$^+$ subset of T cells required for suppression, *J. Mol. Cell. Immunol.* (in press).

32. Yamauchi, K., Chao, N., Murphy, D. B., and Gershon, R. K., 1982, Molecular composition of an antigen-specific Ly1 T suppressor inducer factor: One molecule binds antigen and is I-J$^-$; another is I-J$^+$, does not bind antigen, and imparts an Igh-variable region-linked restriction, *J. Exp. Med.* **155:**655–664.

33. Sacks, D. L., 1984, The effect of anti-μ chain antibody suppression on immunity and specific suppressor cells in *Leishmania tropica* infection, *J. Exp. Med.* (in press).

34. Howard, J. G., Hale, C., and Liew, F. Y., 1981, Immunological regulation of experimental cutaneous leishmaniasis. IV. Prophylactic effect of sublethal irradiation as a result of abrogation of suppressor T cell generation in mice genetically susceptible to *Leishmania tropica*, *J. Exp. Med.* **153:**557–568.

35. Yamauchi, K., Murphy, D. B., Cantor, H., and Gershon, R. K., 1981, Analysis of an antigen-specific H-2 restricted cell free products(s) made by "I-J$^-$" Ly-2 cells (Ly2 TsF) that suppresses Ly2 cell-depleted spleen cell activity, *Eur. J. Immunol.* **11:**913–918.

36. Green, D. R., Flood, P. M., and Gershon, R. K., 1983, Immunoregulatory T cell pathways, *Annu. Rev. Immunol.* **1:**439–463.

37. Janeway, C. A., Jr., Koren, H., and Paul, W. E., 1975, The role of thymus-derived lymphocytes in an antibody mediated hapten-specific helper effect, *Eur. J. Immunol.* **5:**17–22.

38. Uhr, W. J., and Moller, G., 1968, Regulatory effect of antibody on the immune response, *Adv. Immunol.* **8:**81–127.

39. Herzenberg, L. A., Tokuhisa, T., and Herzenberg, L. A., 1980, Carrier priming leads to hapten-specific suppression, *Nature* **285:**664–666.

40. Herzenberg, L. A., Tokuhisa, T., and Hayakawa, K., 1981, Lack of immune response (Ir) gene control for the induction of epitope-specific suppression by the TGAL antigen, *Nature* **295:**329–331.

41. Yamauchi, K., Murphy, D. B., Cantor, H., and Gershon, R. K., 1981, Analysis of antigen-specific Ig-restricted cell free material made by I-J$^+$ Ly1 cells (Ly1 TsiF) that induces Ly2$^+$ cells to express suppressive activity, *Eur. J. Immunol.* **1:**905–912.

42. Herzenberg, L. A., 1983, Allotype suppression and epitope-specific regulation, *Immunol. Today* **4:**113–117.

43. Bottomly, K., and Mosier, D. E., 1979, Mice whose B cells can not produce the T15 idiotype also lack an antigen-specific helper T cell required for T15 expression, *J. Exp. Med.* **150:**1399–1409.

44. Janeway, C. A., Jr., Bert, D. L., and Mosier, D. E., 1980, Cellular cooperation during *in vivo* anti-hapten antibody responses. VI. Evidence for an allogeneic effect replacing one of two helper T cells, *Eur. J. Immunol.* **10:**236–241.

45. Flood, P. M., Yamauchi, K., Singer, A., and Gershon, R. K., 1982, Homologies between cell interaction molecules controlled by major histocompatibility complex and Igh-V-linked genes that T cells use for communication: Tandem "adaptive" differentiation of producer and acceptor cells, *J. Exp. Med.* **156:**1390–1397.

46. Janeway, C. A., Jr., Bottomly, K., Bert, D. L., Dzierzak, E. A., and Mosier, D. E., 1980, Synergizing helper T cell sets and the regulation of antibody quality, in: *Regulatory T Lymphocytes* (B. Pernis and H. Vogel, eds.), Academic Press, New York, pp. 159–170.

47. Janeway, C. A., Jr., Sakato, N., and Eisen, H. N., 1975, Recognition of immunoglobulin idiotypes by thymus-derived lymphocytes, *Proc. Natl. Acad. Sci. USA* **72:**2357–2360.

48. Sakato, N., Janeway, C. A., Jr., and Eisen, H. N., 1977, Immune response of BALB/c mice to the idiotype of T15 and other myeloma proteins of BALB/c origin: Implications for an immune network and antibody multispecificity, *Cold Spring Harbor Symp. Quant. Biol.* **41:**719–724.

49. Cosenza, H., Julius, M. H., and Augustin, A. A., 1977, Idiotypes as variable region markers: Analogies between receptors on phosphorylcholine-specific T and B lymphocytes, *Immunol. Rev.* **34:**3–33.

50. Eichmann, K., Falk, I., and Rajewsky, K., 1978, Recognition of idiotypes in lymphocyte interactions. II. Antigen-independent cooperation between T and B lymphocytes that possess similar and complementary idiotypes, *Eur. J. Immunol.* **8:**853–857.

51. Jørgensen, T., and Hannestad, K., 1982, Helper T cell recognition of the variable domains of a mouse myeloma protein (315): Effect of the major histocompatibility complex and domain conformation, *J. Exp. Med.* **155:**1587–1596.

52. Kawahara, D. J., Marrack, P., and Kappler, J., 1982, Helper T cells specific for a VH determinant(s) are under H-2 linked Ir gene control, *Fed. Proc.* **41**:366.

53. Gleason, K., Pierce, S. K., and Kohler, H., 1981, Generation of idiotype-specific T cell help through network perturbation, *J. Exp. Med.* **153**:924–935.

54. Pierce, S. K., Speck, N. A., Gleason, K., Gearhart, P. J., and Kohler, H., 1981, BALB/c T cells have the potential to recognize the TEPC 15 prototype antibody and its somatic variants, *J. Exp. Med.* **154**:1178–1187.

55. Sim, G. K., and Augustin, A. A., 1983, Internal images of major histocompability complex antigens on T-cell receptors and their role in the generation of the T-helper cell repertoire, *Ann. NY Acad. Sci.* **418**:272–281.

56. Hetzelberger, D., and Eichmann, K., 1978, Recognition of idiotypes in lymphocyte interactions. I. Idiotypic selectivity in the cooperation between T and B lymphocytes, *Eur. J. Immunol.* **8**:846–852.

57. Seman, M., and Morisset, J., 1981, Analysis of T clones provides evidence for two distinct populations of helper T cells (Th1 and Th2) one of them participating to the isotypic regulation of the antibody response, *J. Supramol. Struct. Cell Biochem. Suppl.* **5**:86.

58. Kelsoe, G., Isaak, D., and Cerny, J., 1980, Thymic requirement for cylical idiotypic and reciprocal anti-idiotypic immune responses to a T-independent antigen, *J. Exp. Med.* **151**:289–300.

59. Cerny, J., and Caulfield, M. J., 1981, Stimulation of specific antibody-forming cells in antigen-primed nude mice by the adoptive transfer of syngeneic anti-idiotypic T cells, *J. Immunol.* **126**:2262–2266.

60. L'Age-Stehr, J., 1981, Priming of T helper cells by antigen-activated B cells: B cell-primed Lyt-1[+] helper cells are restricted to cooperate with B cells expressing the IgV$_H$ phenotype of the priming B cells, *J. Exp. Med.* **153**:1236–1245.

61. Nutt, N., Haber, J., and Wortis, H. H., 1981, Influence of Igh-linked gene products on the generation of T helper cells in the response to sheep erythrocytes, *J. Exp. Med.* **153**:1225–1235.

62. Dzierzak, E. A., Janeway, C. A., Jr., Rosenstein, R. W., and Gottlieb, P. D., 1980, Expression of an idiotype (Id-460) during *in vivo* anti-dinitrophenyl antibody responses. I. Mapping of genes for Id-460 expression to the variable region of immunoglobulin heavy-chain locus and to the variable region of immunoglobulin κ-light-chain locus, *J. Exp. Med.* **152**:720–729.

63. Dzierzak, E. A., Rosenstein, R. W., and Janeway, C. A., Jr., 1981, Expression of an idiotype (Id-460) during *in vivo* anti-dinitrophenyl antibody responses. II. Transient idiotypic dominance, *J. Exp. Med.* **154**:1432–1441.

64. Nisonoff, A., Ju, S.-T., and Owen, F. L., 1977, Studies of structure and immunosuppression of a cross-reactive idiotype in strain A mice, *Immunol. Rev.* **34**:89–118.

65. Conger, J. D., Lewis, G. K., and Goodman, J. W., 1981, Idiotype profile of an immune response. I. Contrasts in idiotype dominance between primary and secondary responses and between IgM and IgG plaque-forming cells, *J. Exp. Med.* **153**:1173–1186.

66. Janeway, C. A., Jr., 1975, Cellular cooperation during *in vivo* anti-hapten antibody responses. I. The effect of cell number on the response, *J. Immunol.* **114**:1394–1401.

67. Dzierzak, E. A., and Janeway, C. A., Jr., 1981, Expression of an idiotype (Id-460) during *in vivo* anti-dinitrophenyl antibody responses. III. Detection of Id-460 in normal serum that does not bind dinitrophenyl, *J. Exp. Med.* **154**:1442–1454.

68. Marion, T. M., Dzierzak, E. A., Lee, H.-S., Adams, R. L., and Janeway, C. A., Jr., 1983, Id-460 that does not bind 2,4-dinitrophenyl is specific for *Pasteurella pneumotropica*, *J. Exp. Med.* **159**:221–233.

69. Cozenza, H., and Kohler, H., 1972, Specific inhibition of plaque formation to phosphorylcholine by antibody against antibody, *Science* **176**:1027–1029.

70. Weigert, M., and Riblet, R., 1978, The genetic control of antibody variable regions in the mouse, *Springer Semin. Immunopathol.* **1**:133–157.

71. Wysocki, L. J., and Sato, V. L., 1981, The strain A anti-*p*-azobenzenearsonate major cross-reactive idiotypic family includes members with no reactivity toward *p*-azophenylarsonate, *Eur. J. Immunol.* **11**:823–839.

72. Hornbeck, P. V., and Lewis, G. K., 1983, Idiotype connectance in the immune system. I. Expression of a cross-reactive idiotype on induced anti-*p*-azophenylarsonate antibodies and on endogenous antibodies not specific for arsonate, *J. Exp. Med.* **157**:1116–1135.

73. Imanishi, T., and Mäkelä, O., 1974, Inheritance of antibody specificity. I. Anti-(4-hydroxy-3-nitrophenyl) acetyl of the mouse primary response, *J. Exp. Med.* **140**:1498–1510.

74. Jack, R. S., Imanishi-Kari, T., and Rajewsky, K., 1977, Idiotypic analysis of the response of C57BL/6 mice to the (4-hydroxy-3-nitrophenyl) acetyl group, *Eur. J. Immunol.* **7:**559–565.
75. Mäkelä, O., and Karjalainen, K., 1977, Inheritance of antibody specificity. IV. Control of related molecular species by one VH gene, *Cold Spring Harbor Symp. Quant. Biol.* **41:**735–741.
76. Imanishi-Kari, T., Rajnavolgyi, E., Takemori, T., Jack, R. S., and Rajewsky, K., 1979, The effect of light chain gene expression on the inheritance of an idiotype associated with primary anti-NP antibody, *Eur. J. Immunol.* **9:**324–331.
77. Karjalainen, K., 1980, Two major idiotypes in mouse anti-(4-hydroxyl-3-nitrophenyl) acetyl (NP) antibodies are controlled by "allelic" genes, *Eur. J. Immunol.* **10:**132–139.
78. Takemori, T., Tesch, H., Reth, M., and Rajewsky, K., 1982, The immune response against anti-idiotope antibodies. I. Induction of idiotope-bearing antibodies and analysis of the idiotype repertoire, *Eur. J. Immunol.* **12:**1040–1046.
79. Mattingly, J. A., Kaplan, J., and Janeway, C. A., Jr., 1980, Two distinct antigen-specific suppressor factors induced by the oral administration of antigen, *J. Exp. Med.* **152:**545–554.

23

Helper T-Lymphocyte Influences on Idiotype-Bearing B Cells

KIM BOTTOMLY AND EILEEN DUNN

1. Introduction

Lyt-1$^+$ T–B-cell interactions can be delineated best by understanding the characteristics of the individual T and B lymphocytes, including their specificity, cell surface markers, function, and requirements for activation. Previous studies have placed T cells in subsets based on functional differences and perhaps more convincingly on the expression of unique surface markers correlating with the specialized function of the subset. More recently, Lyt-1$^+$ T cells have been further delineated by their dependence on the presence of either major histocompatibility complex (MHC)-encoded determinants[1-11] or immunoglobulin (Ig)-encoded determinants.[12-34] This recognition requirement has been demonstrated both for the activation of the T-cell subset and for its subsequent interaction with the target B cell.

This chapter will review the characteristics of two such subsets of helper T (Th) cells which differ in their specificity for B-cell surface molecules: one subset of Th cells recognizing MHC-encoded determinants (Ia antigens) and referred to here for convenience as ThMHC and one subset recognizing Ig-encoded determinants (in this case idiotypic determinants) (ThId). These subsets have been shown to differ phenotypically and in their functional activity, yet the two distinct sets of Th cells act synergistically during many antibody responses, generating a response of greater magnitude and of more limited repertoire.

In describing the Th cells participating in the regulation of a T-dependent antibody response, there are several issues which, at this time, need to be addressed:

1. Are the two Th-cell subsets distinct or are the two separate activities the function of the same cell?
2. Are two Th cells necessary to activate a B cell to secrete antibody?

KIM BOTTOMLY AND EILEEN DUNN • Department of Pathology, Yale University Medical School, New Haven, Connecticut 06510.

3. What is the biological role of each Th-cell subset?
4. Does the state of maturation of the B cell limit the functional options of the Th-cell subset?

2. Review of the Subsets of Th Cells

The activation of most B cells to secrete antibody depends on the presence of Lyt-1^+2^- T cells. Previous studies looking at the specificity of the interaction have demonstrated that hapten-specific B cells could be induced to secrete antibody by carrier-specific Th cells if the hapten was physically linked to the carrier protein—the T- and B-cell specificities being on the same molecule.[35] In subsequent experiments, it was shown that T cells primed to the carrier recognized the carrier antigen in the context of syngeneic MHC-encoded determinants or Ia molecules, and therefore had specificity for both antigen and Ia.[4-11] While the activation of this Th-cell subset required recognition of antigen in the context of syngeneic Ia on the antigen-presenting cell (APC) surface, the communication between this subset and B cells based on these same recognition specificities is controversial. In most studies, T–B collaboration required T-cell recognition of antigen in the context of B-cell Ia glycoproteins.[8-11] Yet when considering the activation potential of subpopulations of B cells defined by their expression of the Lyb-5 alloantigen, it has been suggested that, whereas interactions between "classical" Th cells and Lyb-5$^-$ B cells depend on recognition of B-cell Ia, the activation of Lyb-5$^+$ B cells does not.[36,37] This may, in fact, reflect differences in B-cell receptivity to Th-cell signals based on the B cell's state of maturation or prior antigenic exposure which may influence the B cell's requirements for differentiation to secretion.[38-40] In any event, the delineation of ThMHC–B-cell interactions must take into account both the specificity and the function of the Th-cell subset as well as heterogeneity of the B cells being activated.

Finally, currently available evidence suggests the "classical" Th-cell subset does not express Qa-1 or I-J determinants, and plays a role primarily in B-cell clonal expansion.[32] The characteristics of ThMHC cells are reviewed in Table I.

Ig-recognizing Th cells have been shown to regulate antibody class,[25,26,41] allotype,[12] and idiotype[14-17,19,28,32] expression. Evidence for an Ig-recognizing cell has been well defined by measuring Id-bearing antibody response to azophenylarsonate,[14] streptococcal A carbohydrate,[15] trimethylammonium,[28] lysozyme,[17] phosphocholine (PC),[16,19] and trinitrophenyl (TNP) using MOPC315 myeloma in place of heterogeneous B-cell populations.[32]

In characterizing this subset of ThId in terms of specificity and function, it became clear that two classes of Id-recognizing cells could be generated and could be discriminated by their mode of generation and by their specificity, especially self specificities recognized. One class of Id-recognizing Th cells can be generated by direct immunization with Id in adjuvant.[42-48] These Th cells activate B cells in the presence of a hapten–carrier-linked antigen in which the Id-bearing molecules provide the carrier determinant. Furthermore, as might be expected, these cells can directly stimulate and Id-bearing B cell in the absence of antigen, since the B-cell surface Ig Id would serve to bring the two cells together.[45] Moreover, the activity of the directly immunized Id-specific cells appears to be under *H-2* gene control.[47,48] These characteristics suggest that this class of Ig-recognizing Th cells is

TABLE I
Characteristics of Two Helper T-Cell Subsets

T cells	Phenotype	Immunization protocol	T-cell activation requirements		B-cell activation requirements		Specificity of secreting cell
			Antigen	Ia	Antigen	Self specificity	
ThMHC	Ly-1$^+$, Qa-1$^-$	Carrier	Carrier	Syngeneic	Hapten–carrier	Ia	α hapten
		Idiotype	Idiotype	Syngeneic	Hapten–idiotype	Ia	α hapten
		Idiotype	Idiotype	Syngeneic	Idiotype alone	Ia	Id-bearing B cell
ThId	Ly-1$^+$, Qa-1$^+$	Carrier	Carrier	—	Carrier	Id	Id-bearing B cell
		Idiotype	Idiotype	—	—	Id	Id-bearing B cell

actually a member of the "classical" ThMHC-cell subset, with Id being recognized as antigen in the context of MHC-encoded determinants.

The second class of Id-recognizing Th cells does not require direct immunization with Id. This class of T cells can be found either in unimmunized mice expressing high levels of Id-bearing antibody[21,27] or found amplified in mice immunized with carriers unrelated to the Id molecule.[14,16,19,28,32] That the ThId-cell subset is specific for idiotypic determinants has been supported by three types of experiments. (1) The presence of these cells is detected only in mice expressing the corresponding Id. For example, anti-μ-suppressed mice, which lack B cells and their products, also are lacking ThId cells.[19,34] This suggests that the level of naturally occurring circulating Id may play a role in development (expansion and or activation) of ThId cells. (2) The ThId cells augment the antibody responses of only Id-bearing B cells. There is no selective activation of B cells bearing alternate Ids of the same specificity.[14–17,19,28] (3) The ThId cells bind to and can be removed from Id-coated plates in an Id-specific manner.[14,17,27,28,32,49]

It is important to propose, however, that not all B-cell Ig Ids need be recognized and promoted by the existence of ThId cells, but that determinants on certain Ig molecules may be important as cellular interaction molecules. This is particularly important since postulating the presence of ThId cells for each Id-bearing receptor would require large numbers of T cells, each presumably at low frequency, and the probability of a measurable interaction between such a T cell and an equally infrequent Id-bearing B cell seems negligible. It makes more sense to assume that only a limited number of "special" Ids are actually recognized by ThId cells. Furthermore, for many of the idiotypic systems where ThId cells have been defined, Id-bearing antibody is highly represented in sera or on B cells possibly due to environmental or genetic pressures. This suggests the activation and expansion of the ThId cells is a direct consequence of stimulation by frequently expressed idiotypic determinants. Thus, Id produced in sufficient concentrations leads to the activation of T and B cells specific for the idiotope. The consequence of this as put forward by Paul and Bona[50] is the further activation of the highly represented, idiotope-bearing B cells.

In addition to specificity for Ig Ids, the ThId-cell set, as described in several systems,[16,19,28,32] appears to be carrier specific. This has been shown by studies demonstrating that the functional activity of the ThId cells depends on antigen priming of the T-cell donor *in vivo* and reexposure of the T-cell population to the priming antigen in order to activate the Id-bearing B cells. Recent studies have added strength to the argument that one T cell recognizes antigen as well as Id[16,19,51,52] by demonstrating that ThId cells isolated from Id-coated plates are also carrier antigen specific.[32] Thus, both subsets of Th cells (ThMHC and ThId) appear to require recognition of two specificities to become functionally active, and they are most easily delineated by whether or not they recognize MHC- or Ig-encoded determinants.[51]

If the ThId cells recognize both carrier antigen and idiotypic determinants, does this imply that the functional activity of the cells requires simultaneous recognition of these specificities as has been suggested for the ThMHC-cell subset? It is difficult to envision this type of recognition mechanism for the ThId-cell set since the immunizing carrier is unrelated to the specificity of the Id-bearing B cell. It seems most likely that the ThId cells bind the determinants sequentially. This is further confirmed by the fact that the carrier antigen does not need to bear haptenic determinants for effective ThId–B-cell interaction.[16,19,32]

Finally, ThId cells bear Ly-1 and Qa-1[32] antigens. The presence of I-J-encoded determinants has been reported in some systems,[28] but not all.

It is well to note that the generation and expansion of the ThId cells may occur naturally,[21,27] by carrier immunization,[14,16,19,28,32] or by direct immunization with Id-bearing Igs.[42–48] For all these regimens, both classes of ThId cells may appear, yet they clearly may be distinguished by phenotype, by specificity, and, as will be discussed later in Section 6, by functional capabilities.

To further analyze the interactions of ThMHC and ThId and B cells, *in vitro* T-dependent responses were analyzed using monoclonal or enriched populations of each subset of Th cells to precisely delineate their specificity, function, and activation requirements.

3. ThMHC–B-Cell Interaction

The study of "classical" Th-cell influences on the growth, expansion, and differentiation of B cells has been approached using cloned T-cell lines. These monoclonal T cells are phenotypically Thy-1$^+$, Lyt-1$^+$2$^-$ and have been shown to be antigen [in this case ovalbumin (OVA)]-specific and to proliferate upon stimulation with OVA in the context of self I-A or I-E-encoded molecules. The characteristics of some of these cloned lines are outlined in Table II.

The clones were tested for their ability to induce antibody secretion in an *in vitro* T-dependent response using primed or unprimed B cells, cloned T cells, and evaluating an anti-PC response in the presence of PC-OVA. All the cloned T cells listed in Table II induced PC-specific B cells to secrete antibody and the requirements for helper cell activity are listed in Table III. Basically the cloned T cells are antigen-specific and I-A- or I-E-restricted in their helper cell activity[53,54] and require hapten–carrier linkage for effective T–B collaboration.[52,55] In all senses, the cloned T cells analyzed were identical in phenotype, specificity, and activation requirements to the "classical" Th cell reported previously.

Table II
Characteristics of Cloned Helper T-Cell Lines

| T-cell clone | Strain of origin | Specificities | | | Helper function |
		Antigen	Self MHC	Foreign MHC	
B6d.D2/B4	BALB/c	OVA	I-A^d	(I-A$^{k,r?}$)	+
A3a10.4	BALB/c	OVA	I-A^d		+
4.19	BALB/c	OVA	I-A^d		+
D10/G4	AKR	OVA	I-A^k	I-A^b	+
D8	AKR	OVA	I-A^k		+
D4b	BALB.B	OVA	I-A^b		+
B6B5/B2	C57BL/6	OVA	I-A^b		+
5.2	BALB/c	OVA	I-E^d		+

Taking advantage of this highly defined *in vitro* system, it was possible to look closely at the following questions:

1. Is there a preferential activation of T15-bearing B cells in the presence of cloned Th cells?
2. Are B-cell-surface Ia glycoproteins essential for T–B communication and is the level of Ia controlling this interaction?
3. Does prior antigenic history of the B-cell donor influence the mature *in vitro* response induced by cloned Th cells?

3.1. T15 Id Expression in the Presence of Cloned Th Cells

In *vivo* responses to T-dependent and T-independent forms of the hapten PC in BALB/c mice are characterized by the production of antibody bearing the T15 Id.[56,57] Eighty-five to one hundred percent of the anti-PC plaque-forming cells are T15 bearing. The Lyt-1$^+$ T-cell population required for an optimal T-dependent T15-dominated anti-PC response seen in an adoptive secondary response can be divided, on the basis of function, into two participating T-cell subsets. The "classical" ThMHC cell is required for induction of PC-specific B cells to produce antibody, and the expression of antibody bearing predominantly the T15 Id is dependent on the presence of a second Th cell (ThId). Inducing an anti-PC response *in vitro* using cloned Th cells allowed analysis of T15 expression in the absence of the ThId subset of cells. It can be seen in Table IV that the clones activated PC-specific B cells that were idiotypically heterogeneous.[49,52,54,55] This supports the *in vivo*

Table III
Requirements for Optimal OVA-Specific Helper T-Cell Function

Recognition of foreign antigen (OVA)
Recognition of syngeneic B-cell Ia glycoproteins
Hapten–carrier linkage
Threshold level of Ia molecules

TABLE IV
*Frequency of T15-Bearing B Cells Activated by Monoclonal
Helper T Cells*

B-cell source	Range of frequency of T15 Id expressed in response to PC-OVA
Normal BALB/c	20–55%
PC-primed BALB/c	7–34%
Germfree BALB/c	50–70%

data where the PC response was idiotypically heterogeneous in the absence of ThId cells.[16,19]

3.2. T–B Interaction Requires Recognition of B-Cell Ia Glycoproteins

It had been shown previously that the cloned Th cells required identity at I-A to become activated to proliferate in response to antigen.[53,58] It was important to determine whether or not the T-cell clones providing Th activity recognized antigen in the context of APC Ia and/or B-cell Ia glycoproteins. It has been reported previously that subsets of B cells, distinguished by their expression of the Lyb-5 determinant, differ in their activation by Th cells. The interaction between Th cells and Lyb-5⁻ B cells is MHC-restricted requiring Th-cell recognition of B-cell Ia, whereas the Lyb-5 cell is activated indirectly, with the MHC restriction occurring at the level of the APC.[36,37] It is significant when considering anti-PC responses that T15-bearing B cells are missing in the CBA/N mouse and appear to reside exclusively in the Lyb-5⁺ pool of B cells.[59,60] If this were the case, one might predict that the T15-bearing anti-PC response generated in the presence of Ia-recognizing Th cells would not depend on the recognition of B-cell Ia. To determine if the T-cell clones recognized B-cell Ia rather than APC Ia antigens, purified B cells from BALB/c (d) and BALB.B (b) were cultured with either Ia^d-recognizing or Ia^b-recognizing T-cell clones. APCs of both haplotypes were present in all wells. As seen in Table V, the cloned Th cells recognize syngeneic Ia glycoproteins on both T15-bearing and non-T15-bearing precursor B cells. There was a requirement for identity at all antigen concentrations tested.[54] These data demonstrate that there is a direct interaction between the cloned Th cells and PC-specific B cells and that this interaction depends on T-cell recognition of antigen and B-cell Ia glycoproteins.

3.3. T–B Collaboration is Controlled by Ia Density

While cloned Th cells clearly require B-cell Ia recognition, it is important to take into account that the density of Ia antigens on B cells is heterogeneous.[61,62] Several studies have suggested that quantitative expression of surface Ia may be critical in T-cell[67] and B-cell activation.[63–66] It seemed possible that subsets of B cells defined by means of B-cell-surface Ia expression may have different activation requirements in the presence of an Ia-recog-

TABLE V
Interaction between Cloned T Cells and B Cells is MHC-Restricted

			% of PC PFC eliminated by Y-3 + C treatment using:[a]			
		Dose of	B6 Th-cell clones		BALB/c Th-cell clones	
B cells tested	B-cell haplotype	PC-OVA ($\mu g/ml$)	Total PFC	T15$^+$ PFC	Total PFC	T15$^+$ PFC
C6BF1	$d \times b$	0.1	100	100	100	100
		20.0	100	100	100	100
BALB.B	b	0.1	100	100	NR^b	NR
		20.0	100	100	NR	NR
BALB/c	d	0.1	NR	NR	0	0
		20.0	NR	NR	0	0
BALB/c +	$d + b$	0.1	100	100	0	0
BALB.B		20.0	100	100	0	0

[a]The PFCs bearing H-2^b determinants (CB6F1 or BALB.B) were determined by treating the PFC either with complement alone or with monoclonal anti-H-2.5 antibody (Y-3) plus complement.
[b]NR, no response.

nizing cloned Th cell. In testing this possibility, our studies have shown that the optimal interaction between cloned Th cells and B cells depends on a threshold level of B-cell-surface Ia. Those B cells easily activated by cloned Th cells to secrete antibody at low antigen concentrations express relatively high-density cell surface Ia antigens as shown by their sensitivity to monoclonal anti-Ia antibody plus complement treatment (Table VI). Pretreatment of B cells with a monoclonal anti-Ia antibody and complement, selected to kill 40–60% of B cells at plateau levels, reduced the number of cells bearing high-density Ia, seen using FACS analysis, and showed a concomitant reduction in the total number of PC PFC generated in the presence of Ia-recognizing cloned Th cells.[(54)] This reduction in the total response was due to a drastic reduction in the number of non-T15-bearing B cells secreting antibody suggesting that the non-T15-bearing B cells were enriched in the B-cell pool expressing high levels of Ia glycoproteins. Thus, the non-T15-bearing subset of B cells is the most easily activated by the Ia-recognizing cloned Th cells.

When considering the question of why cloned Th cells fail to generate T15-dominated

TABLE VI
T–B Collaboration Influenced by Ia Glycoprotein Density

B cell activated in the presence of Ia^d-recognizing cloned Th cells	Pretreatment of B-cell donor (anti-Ia + complement)	Antigen	% of PC PFC response eliminated by anti-Ia plus complement pretreatment		
			Total PFC	T15$^+$ PFC	T15$^-$ PFC
CB6F1	Y17 (anti-E$_\alpha$:E$_\beta$)	PC-OVA	63	0	99
CB6F1	Y17 (anti-E$_\alpha$:E$_\beta$)	PC-BA	42	40	47
BALB/c	MKD6 (anti-Ia^d)	PC-OVA	68	8	91
BALB/c	MKD6 (anti-Ia^d)	PC-BA	38	36	38
BALB/c germfree	MKD6 (anti-Ia^d)	PC-OVA	59	52	56
BALB/c germfree	MKD6 (anti-Ia^d)	PC-BA	83	80	86

anti-PC responses *in vitro* as is seen using whole populations of Lyt-1$^+$ T cells (85–100% T15-bearing), there are two identifiable possibilities, supported by the data. (1) It may be suggested that the failure to generate a T15-dominated response is due to the fact that a minority of PC-specific precursors are T15-bearing, and the cloned Th cells activate all T15-bearing precursors capable of binding PC. The secretion of predominantly T15-bearing antibody requires a second ThId-type Th cell available *in vivo* or in whole populations of Ly-1$^+$ T cells. (2) Alternatively, the cloned Th cells distinguish between subsets of B cells and activate only those B cells with which their interaction is most efficient—in this case while the majority of the B cells activated are non-T15-bearing the majority of PC-specific precursors may be T15-bearing. Thus, T15 dominance is not observed. It seems clear that both of these explanations may be correct. This issue will be discussed further when considering the importance of ThId–B-cell interactions in Section 4.

3.4. Environmental Antigens Influence T–B Interactions

It has been suggested that environmental priming by many PC-containing bacterial antigens may (1) activate B cells in a T-independent fashion and may (2) activate almost exclusively B cells bearing the T15 Id. When considering what factors may directly influence a developing B cell *in vivo* both the form of the PC antigen and the activation requirements of the responding B cell are of consequence. As such, the continued presence of PC during B-cell development may result in the selection and expansion of responding B cells in a nonrandom fashion. Thus, the observation that non-T15-bearing B cells express primarily high quantities of Ia glycoproteins and are easily activated by Ia-recognizing cloned Th cells may reflect direct interaction between T cells, antigen, and B cells leading to the activation of certain B cells during *in vivo* maturation. The presence of these types of influences throughout *in vivo* B-cell development might produce in a population of mature cells, T15-bearing B cells whose priming with T-independent forms of PC is apparently unrelated or not associated with Ia expression and non-T15-bearing B cells which may be highly T cell dependent with the density of Ia glycoproteins playing an important role in T–B communication. The data in Table VI suggest that environmental antigens may play a role in B-cell maturation. Whereas pretreatment of normal B cells with anti-Ia and complement reduces the response to PC-OVA and drastically affects non-T15-bearing B cells, T15-bearing and non-T15-bearing cells from germfree mice are equally effected. These data suggest that the B-cell maturational environment may be important both in considering the form of the environmental antigen selectively activating different subsets of B cells and in considering the importance of T cells during continued B-cell priming.

4. ThId–B-Cell Interaction

Induction of an anti-PC response with a whole population of Lyt-1$^+$ Th cells *in vivo*[56,57] or *in vitro*[68,69] activates predominantly T15-bearing B cells (90–100%). As shown in numerous *in vivo* studies,[16,19] there are within the population of Lyt-1$^+$ T cells both ThMHC and ThId subsets. To test the relative contributions of the ThId subset, Lyt-1$^+$ T cells were added to the *in vitro* cultures containing cloned "classical" Th cells and B cells responding to PC-OVA. Since cloned Th cells induced anti-PC responses in which the majority of PFC were non-T15-bearing and since Lyt-1$^+$ cells by themselves were unable to induce anti-PC responses, it was possible to add Lyt-1$^+$ T cells and look for augmentation of the activation of T15-bearing B cells.

The addition of nylon wool-passed, thoroughly suppressor cell-depleted, Lyt-1$^+$ T cells to cultures of cloned "classical" Th cells and B cells results in an increase in the total PC-specific PFC response, and this increase is entirely due to an increase in the number of B cells secreting T15-bearing antibody (Table VII). This type of data suggested that ThId cells interacted directly with B cells by recognition of B-cell-surface T15-bearing receptors. Since it has been demonstrated *in vivo* that the ThId cells do not recognize polymorphic MHC-encoded determinants for their activation and function[70] and are not under the control of known Ir genes,[71] it appeared that MHC-encoded products were not important in the activity of this Th-cell subset. Furthermore, it might be suggested that the inability to recognize MHC-encoded determinants as a self marker might be replaced by the subset's ability to recognize Ig instead. To support this idea, it was necessary to demonstrate that ThId cells were specific for T15-bearing antibody by binding and competitive inhibition studies.

Having shown that the addition of Lyt-1$^+$ T cells to cultures containing cloned "classical" Th cells and B cells will specifically augment T15 expression, we tested whether the ThId cell actually recognized T15 idiotypic determinants. To best approach this question, a plate-binding assay was established using available hybridoma and myeloma proteins. In an initial analysis, we compared the ability of plate-adherent and plate-nonadherent Lyt-1$^+$ T-cell populations to augment the *in vitro* T15-bearing PFC response. As seen summarized in Table VII, in contrast to BSA adherent T cells, T cells obtained from T15 myeloma protein-coated plates would specifically augment the secretion of T15-bearing B cells. To better define the specificity of the ThId-cell subset, we inhibited the binding of the ThId cells to T15-coated plates using various concentrations of hybridoma or myeloma proteins. It can be concluded from these studies that the binding is specific for the T15 Id

TABLE VII
ThId Cells Are T15-Idiotype Specific

Source of ThId cells added to cloned Th cells and B cells responding to PC-OVA	Inhibitor[a]	PC PFC response		
		Total PFC	T15$^+$ PFC	T15$^-$ PFC
None	—	+ +	+	+
Ly-1 T	—	+ + + +	+ + +	+
Ly-1 T–T15 plate adherent	—	+ + + +	+ + +	+
Ly-1 T–BSA plate adherent	—	+ +	+	+
Ly-1 T–T15 plate adherent	T15	+ +	+	+
Ly-1 T–T15 plate adherent	P26	+ + + +	+ + +	+
Ly-1 T–T15 plate adherent	P24	+ +	+	+
Ly-1 T–T15 plate adherent	M460	+ + + +	+ + +	+

[a]Various concentrations of myeloma or hybridoma proteins were used to inhibit the binding of Ly-1 T cells to T15-coated plates. The adherent cells recovered from the plates were added to the *in vitro* cultures containing syngeneic B cells, cloned Th cells, and PC-OVA. P26 is a hybridoma secreting IgM anti-PC (T15$^-$) antibody; P24 is a hybridoma secreting IgM anti-PC (T15$^+$) antibody; M460 is an IgA DNP-binding myeloma protein.

in that only T15-bearing IgA and T15-bearing IgM antibodies can inhibit the binding of ThId cells to T15 IgA-coated plates.

It remains to be determined if the ThId-cell subset recognizes B-cell-surface Ig or how such an Id-specific Lyt-1$^+$ Th cell locates the appropriate B cell in the face of 10–80 μg/ml of naturally circulating T15-bearing antibody. However, it should be possible using this methodology to propagate and ultimately clone ThId cells to further explore these questions.

5. Th–Cell Influences on T-Independent Responses

B cells responding to T-independent (TI) and T-dependent (TD) forms of the hapten PC have been shown to be distinct.[72] Many studies have shown that TI responses, while relatively T-independent, are influenced by the presence or absence of T cells.[73] It was of interest to determine if the cloned ThMHC cells influence the activation of B cells responding to TI form of PC. Studies evaluating the response to PC–*Brucella abortus* (BA), a TI antigen, have shown that there is a significant augmentation of the anti-PC PFC response in the presence of cloned Th cells. When comparing the response to PC-OVA and PC-BA *in vitro*, several differences in activation requirements were noted, and these are summarized in Table VIII. Clone D8 cells both induced a response to PC-OVA and greatly augmented the response to PC-BA, TNP-BA, and TNP-Ficoll. While supernatants from clones would replace D8's amplifying effects on TI responses, they would *not* replace Th cells in a TD response to PC-OVA. Further studies with TI antigens indicated that under suboptimal antigen conditions, the responses were augmented 20- to 50-fold in the presence of D8 supernatant. It is important to note that without antigen there was no response. Moreover, in contrast to the response to PC-OVA, the cloned Th cells did not require recognition of B-cell Ia glycoproteins or OVA during the culture to mediate the augmentation of the response to PC-BA. These data suggested that two subsets of B cells differ in their requirements for activation and that a single T cell can satisfy both requirements.

TABLE VIII
Summary of Activation Requirements of TI and TD Responses in the Presence of Cloned Th Cells

	Response to PC-OVA	Response to PC-BA
Absence of cloned Th cells	No	Yes
Presence of cloned Th cells	Yes	2- to 50-fold augmentation
Requirement for Th-cell recognition of OVA during *in vitro* culture	Yes	No
Requirement for Th-cell recognition of syngeneic B-cell Ia glycoproteins	Yes	No
Requirement for presence of PC antigen during *in vitro* culture	Yes	Yes
Replacement of Th-cell requirement with supernatant from Th-cell clone	No	Yes

6. Regulation of the Antibody Response by Subsets of Th Cells

The TD anti-PC response is clearly influenced by two Th-cell subsets. These two subsets have been shown to be distinct based on the following parameters: (1) *Specificity*. The activation and function of the ThMHC cells depend on recognition of carrier antigen in the context of MHC-encoded determinants. That ThMHC cells fail to activate predominantly T15-bearing B cells attests to their lack of specificity for idiotypic determinants and suggests that other factors account for predominant T15 production. ThId cells, while apparently antigen-specific, recognize and bind T15-bearing Ig. It may be suggested that recognition of Id replaces the need to recognize self MHC-encoded determinants with B-cell-surface Id serving as a "self" marker. This concept is supported by the findings that the activity of the subset of ThId cells is not MHC-restricted and not under the control of known Ir genes.[70,71] Both activation and function of ThId cells require recognition of T15 in that ThId-cell activity can only be measured in systems expressing high levels of circulating Id. (2) *Cell surface markers*. To date, the most distinguishing difference between the two subsets of T cells is in their expression of the Qa-1 alloantigen. The ability to eliminate ThId functional activity by treatment with anti-Qa-1 antisera and complement distinguishes between ThMHC cells, ThId cells recognizing Id as a foreign antigen, and ThId cells recognizing Id as a self specificity. Only the function of the latter is eliminated.[32] (3) *Function*. There are two notable distinctions in the function of the two subsets of Th cells. The ThId-cell set, in contrast to the ThMHC-cell set, acts only on a limited number of B cells bearing the appropriate idiotypic determinant. Furthermore, while cloned ThMHC cells can activate B cells to proliferate and secrete antibody, the augmentation of the response of Id-bearing B cells by ThId cells can only occur in the presence of ThMHC cells. This suggests that the ThId subset of cells cannot by itself activate B cells to secrete antibody. This necessity for a ThMHC-cell signal seems reasonable since it might be expected in the absence of such a requirement that Id-bearing B cells would be activated by a large variety of incoming antigens unrelated to the specificity of the B cell. It might make more sense to postulate that a signal from a "classical" Th cell is required to ensure that the appropriate B cells are activated to expand and secrete antibody.

Moreover, it is apparent that the function of an Id-recognizing Th cell generated by direct immunization with Id is similar to classical ThMHC cells in that the Id-recognizing Th cells alone will activate B cells to secrete antibody.

These functional distinctions bring forth an important question. Are two Th cells necessary to activate a B cell to secrete antibody? Clearly the cloned Th MHC cells appear to provide all the necessary signals. The need for a ThId cell is still an unresolved issue but several possibilities exist as to the role of the ThId cell. The recent studies of Rohrer and co-workers[32] have demonstrated that optimal B-cell secretion is controlled by the presence of ThId cells. In their system using MOPC315 tumor cells as a B-cell source, the Qa-1⁻ "classical" Th-cell population controls clonal expansion of the tumor cells and the Qa-1⁺ ThId-cell population influences secretory differentiation. It might be argued that the presence of ThId cells either increases the number of B cells secreting Id-bearing antibody and/or increases the rate at which they secrete antibody.

Alternatively, we have shown *in vitro* that cloned ThMHC cells preferentially activate high-Ia-bearing B cells—in this system the high-Ia-density cells are mainly non-T15-bearing. This brings forth the possibility that T15-bearing B cells are present but do not express the activating quantities of Ia antigens. That the addition of ThId cells to this culture leads to an augmentation in the activation of T15-bearing B cells lends support to this possibility. Since one might consider a ThId cell as "anti-Ig" in its specificity, and since previous studies have shown that anti-Ig reagents can stimulate B cells to proliferate and to increase cell surface Ia density,[74,75] it seems possible that the ThId subset of cells may also stimulate low-Ia-density, T15-bearing B cells to proliferate and increase in Ia density. The T15-bearing B cells would now be more easily activated by cloned Ia-recognizing ThMHC cells which are absolutely required to get antibody secretion.

While both of these possibilities may be correct, it suggests that increased secretion of Id-bearing antibody either due to an increase in the number of B cells secreting or an increase in the rate of secretion has some biological importance. It might be argued that antibody bearing "regulatory idiotopes" may be important in an immune response against certain antigens or environmental pathogens. As has been shown in the PC system, the T15-bearing antibody seems to be the best in binding PC-bearing bacteria. In many systems, antibodies bearing regulatory idiotopes are found in normal serum at high levels,[76-80] and this serum antibody has been shown to be critical in protection against certain pathogens.[81,82] Therefore, both augmentation of the secretion of Id-bearing antibody early during an immune response and the maintenance of secretion late in a response in the face of decreasing antigen concentration with responses moving toward higher affinity and greater diversity may be of benefit.

Finally, the function of ThMHC and ThId subsets may be dictated by the state of maturation of a B cell. Several studies have suggested that size, age, or prior antigenic history may determine a B cell's receptivity to Th-cell signals. Our own data demonstrate that T15-bearing B cells responding to PC-BA are relatively insensitive to signals from ThId cells which will increase responsiveness to T15-bearing B cells responding to PC-OVA. Moreover, PC-BA-responding B cells are acutely sensitive to signals from ThMHC cells, yet the requirements for B cell activated by PC-BA are vastly different from those for B cells activated by PC-OVA in the presence of the same cloned Th cells. Clearly the two populations of PC-specific B cells responding to different forms of the antigen have distinct activation requirements. The relationship between Th-cell function and B-cell activation at this level is ambiguous. Further clarification in defining the parameters governing these interactions will depend on development of markers needed for identification of the individual B-cell subsets.

References

1. Jerne, H. K., 1971, The somatic generation of immune recognition, *Eur. J. Immunol.* **1**:1–9.
2. Bevan, M. J., 1978, In a radiation chimera, host H-2 antigens determine immune responsiveness of donor cytotocis cells, *Nature,* **269**:417–418.
3. Zinkernagel, R. M., Callahan, G. N., Althage, A., Cooper, S., Klein, P., and Klein, J., 1978, On the thymus in the differentiation of "H-2 self recognition" by T cells: Evidence for dual recognition?, *J. Exp. Med.* **147**:882–896.
4. Rosenthal, A. S., and Shevach, E. M., 1973, Function of macrophages in antigen recognition by guinea pig T lymphocytes. I. Requirement for histocompatible macrophages and lymphocytes, *J. Exp. Med.* **138**:1194–1212.
5. Erb, P., and Feldman, M., 1975, The role of macrophages in the generation of T-helper cells. II. The

genetic control of the macrophage–T-cell interaction for helper cell induction with soluble antigens, *J. Exp. Med.* **142**:460–472.

6. Schwartz, R. H., Yano, A., and Paul, W. E., 1978, Interaction between antigen-presenting cells and primed T lymphocytes, *Immunol. Rev.* **40**:153–180.

7. Benacerraf, B., and Germain, R. H., 1978, The immune response genes of the major histocompatibility complex, *Immunol. Rev.* **38**:70–119.

8. Katz, D. H., Graves, M., Dorf, M. E., DiMuzio, H., and Benacerraf, B., 1975, Cell interactions between histoincompatible T and B lymphocytes. VII. Cooperative responses between lymphocytes are controlled by genes in the I region of the H-2 complex, *J. Exp. Med.* **141**:263–268.

9. Sprent, J., 1978. Restricted helper function of F_1 T cells positively selected to heterologous erythrocytes in irradiated parental strain mice. II. Evidence for restrictions affecting helper cell induction and T–B collaboration, both mapping to K-end of the H-2 complex, *J. Exp. Med.* **147**:1159–1174.

10. Sprent, J., 1978, Restricted helper function of F_1 parent bone marrow chimeras controlled by K-end of H-2 complex, *J. Exp. Med.* **147**:1838–1842.

11. Marrack, P. C., Harwell, L., Kappler, J. W., Kawahara, D., Keller, D., and Swierkosz, J. E., 1979, Helper T cell interactions with Be cells and macrophages, in: *Immunologic Tolerance and Macrophage Function* (P. Barnum, J. R. Battisto, and C. W. Pierce, eds.), Elsevier/North-Holland, Amsterdam, pp. 31–44.

12. Herzenberg, L. A., Okumura, K., Cantor, H., Sato, V. L., Shen, F.-W., Boyse, E. Q., and Herzenberg, L. A., 1976. T cell regulation of antibody responses: Demonstration of allotype-specific helper T cells and their specific removal by suppressor T cells, *J. Exp. Med.* **144**:330–344.

13. Janeway, C. A., Jr., Murgita, R. A., Weinbaum, F. I., Asofsky, R., and Wigzell, H., 1977, Evidence for an immunoglobulin-dependent antigen-specific helper T cell, *Prod. Natl. Acad. Sci. USA* **74**:4582–4586.

14. Woodland, R., and Cantor, H., 1978, Idiotype-specific T cells are required to induce idiotype-positive B memory cells to secrete antibody, *Eur. J. Immunol.* **8**:600–605.

15. Hetzelberger, D., and Eichmann, K., 1978, Recognition of idiotypes in lymphocyte interactions. I. Idiotypic selectivity in the cooperation between T and B lymphocytes, *Eur. J. Immunol.* **8**:846–852.

16. Bottomly, K., and Mosier, D. E., 1979, Mice whose B cells can not produce the T15 idiotype also lack an antigen-specific helper T cell required for T15 expression, *J. Exp. Med.* **150**:1399–1409.

17. Adorini, L. M., Harvey, M., and Sercarz, E. E., 1979, The fine specificity of regulatory T cells. IV. Idiotypic complementarity and antigen bridging interactions, *Eur. J. Immunol.* **9**:906–911.

18. Eardley, D. D., Shen, F.-W., Cantor, H., and Gershon, R. K., 1979, Genetic control of immunoregulatory circuits: Genes linked to the Ig locus govern communication between regulatory T-cell sets, *J. Exp. Med.* **150**:44–50.

19. Bottomly, K., Janeway, C. A., Jr., Mathieson, B. J., and Mosier, D. E., 1980, Absence of an antigen-specific helper T cell required for the expression of the T15 idiotype in mice treated with anti-μ antibody, *Eur. J. Immunol.* **10**:159–163.

20. Janeway, C. A., Jr., Bert, D. L., and Shen, F.-W., 1980, Cell cooperation during *in vivo* anti-hapten antibody responses. V. Two synergistic Lyt-1$^+$23$^-$ helper T cells with distinctive specificities, *Eur. J. Immunol.* **10**:231–236.

21. Kelsoe, G., Isaak, D., and Cerny, J., 1980. Thymic requirement for cyclical idiotypic and reciprocal anti-idiotypic immune responses to a T-independent antigen, *J. Exp. Med.* **151**:289–300.

22. L'Age-Stehr, J., Tuchmann, H., Gershon, R. K., and Cantor, H., 1980, Stimulation of regulatory T cell circuits by Ig-associated structures on activated B cells, *Eur. J. Immunol.* **10**:21–26.

23. L'Age-Stehr, J., 1981, Priming of T helper cells by antigen-activated B cells: B cell-primed Lyt-1$^+$ helper cells are restricted to cooperate with B cells expressing the IgV_H phenotype of the priming B cells, *J. Exp. Med.* **153**:1236–1245.

24. Nutt, N., Haber, J., and Wortis, H. H., 1981, Influence of Igh-linked gene products on the generation of T helper cells in the response to sheep erythrocytes, *J. Exp. Med.* **153**:1225–1235.

25. Seman, M., and Morisset, J., 1981, Analysis of T clones provide evidence of two distinct populations of helper T cells (Th1 and Th2) one of them participating to the isotypic regulation of the antibody response, *J. Supramol. Struct. Cell Biochem. Suppl.* **5**:86.

26. Rosenberg, Y. J., and Asofsky, R., 1981, T cell regulation of isotype expression: The requirement for a second Ig-specific helper T cell population for the induction of IgG responses, *Eur. J. Immunol.* **11**:705–710.

27. Cerny, J., and Caulfield, M. J., 1981, Stimulation of specific antibody-forming cells in antigen-primed nude mice by the adoptive transfer of syngeneic anti-idiotypic T cells, *J. Immunol.* **126:**2262–2266.
28. Jayaraman, S., Swierkosz, J. E., and Bellone, C. J., 1982, T cell replacing factor substitutes for an I-J⁺ idiotype-specific T helper cell, *J. Exp. Med.* **155:**641–646.
29. Yamauchi, K., Chao, N., Murphy, D. B., and Gershon, R. K., 1982, Molecular composition of an antigen-specific Ly1 T suppressor inducer factor: One molecule binds antigen and is I-J⁻; another is I-J⁺, does not bind antigen, and imparts an Igh-variable region-linked restriction, *J. Exp. Med.* **155:**655–664.
30. Flood, P. M., Yamauchi, K., Singer, A., and Gershon, R. K., 1982, Homologies between cell interaction molecules controlled by major histocompatibility complex and Igh-V-linked genes that T cells use for communication: Tandem "adaptive" differentiation of producer and acceptor cells, *J. Exp. Med.* **156:**1390–1397.
31. McDougal, J. S., Shen, F.-W., Cort, S. P., and Bard, J., 1982, Two Ly1 T helper cell subsets distinguished by Qa1 phenotype: The priming environment determines whether one or both subsets will be generated, *J. Exp. Med.* **155:**831–838.
32. Rohrer, J. W., Gershon, R. K., Lynch, R. G., and Kemp, J. D., 1983, The enhancement of B lymphocyte secretory differentiation by an Ly1⁺,2⁻; Qa-1⁺ helper T cell subset, that sees both antigen and determinants on immunoglobulin, *J. Mol. Cell. Immunol.* **1:**50–61.
33. Flood, P. M., Janeway, C. A., Jr., and Gershon, R. K., 1984, B cell deprived mice are deficient in an I-J⁺ subset of T cells required for suppression, *J. Mol. Cell. Immunol.* (in press).
34. Rohrer, J. W., and Janeway, C. A., Jr., 1984, Absence of a helper cell subset in B cell deficient mice, submitted for publication.
35. Mitchison, N. A., 1971, The carrier effect in the secondary response to hapten–protein conjugates. II. Cellular cooperation. *Eur. J. Immunol.* **1:**18–27.
36. Singer, A., Morrisey, P. H., Hathcock, K. S., Ahmed, A., Scher, I., and Hodes, R. I., 1981, Role of the major histocompatibility complex in T cell activation of B cell subpopulations: Lyb 5⁺ and Lyb 5⁻ B cell subpopulations differ in their requirements for major histocompatibility complex-restricted T cell recognition, *J. Exp. Med.* **154:**501–516.
37. Singer, A., Asano, Y., Shigeta, M., Hathcock, K. S., Ahmed, A., Rathman, C. G., and Hodes, R. I., 1982, Distinct B cell subpopulations differ in their genetic requirements for activation by T helper cells, *Immunol. Rev.* **64:**137–160.
38. Melchers, F., Anderson, J., Lernhardt, W., and Schreir, M. H., 1980, H-2-unrestricted polyclonal maturation without replication of small B cells induced by antigen-activated T cell help factors, *Eur. J. Immunol.* **10:**679–685.
39. Julius, M. H., Chiller, J. M., and Sidman, C. L., 1982, Major histocompatibility complex-restricted cellular interactions determining B cell activation, *Eur. J. Immunol.* **12:**627–633.
40. Ratcliffe, M. J., and Julius, M. H., 1982, H-2-restricted T–B interactions involved in polyspecific B cell responses mediated by soluble antigen, *Eur. J. Immunol.* **12:**634–641.
41. Kishimoto, T., and Ishizaka, K., 1973, Regulation of antibody response *in vitro.* VI. Carrier-specific helper cells for IgG and IgE antibody response, *J. Immunol.* **111:**720–732.
42. Janeway, C. A., Jr., Sakato, N., and Eisen, H. N., 1975, Recognition of immunoglobulin idiotypes by thymus-derived lymphocytes, *Proc. Natl. Acad. Sci. USA* **74:**2357–2360.
43. Sakato, N., Janeway, C. A., Jr., and Eisen, H. N., 1977, Immune response of BALB/c mice to the idiotype of T15 and other myeloma proteins of BALB/c origin: Implications for an immune network and antibody multispecificity, *Cold Spring Harbor Symp. Quant. Biol.* **41:**719–724.
44. Cosenza, H., Julius, M. H., and Augustin, A. A., 1977, Idiotypes as variable region markers: Analogies between receptors on phosphorylcholine-specific T and B lymphocytes, *Immunol. Rev.* **34:**3–33.
45. Eichmann, K., Falk, I., and Rajewsky, K., 1978, Recognition of idiotypes in lymphocyte interactions. II. Antigen-independent cooperation between T and B lymphocytes that possess similar and complementary idiotypes, *Eur. J. Immunol.* **8:**853–857.
46. Pierce, S. K., Speck, N. A., Gleason, K., Gearhart, P. J., and Kohler, H., 1981, BALB/c T cells have the potential to recognize the TEPC 15 prototype antibody and its somatic variants, *J. Exp. Med.* **154:**1178–1187.
47. Jorgensen, T., and Hannestad, K., 1982, Helper T cell recognition of the variable domains of a mouse myeloma protein (315): Effect of the major histocompatibility complex and domain conformation, *J. Exp. Med.* **155:**1587–1596.

48. Kawahara, D. J., Marrack, P., and Kappler, J., 1982, Helper T cells specific for a VH determinant(s) are under H-2 linked Ir gene control, *Fed. Proc.* **41:**366.
49. Dunn, E. D., Jones, F., III, and Bottomly, K. Ly1 T cells that bind specifically to the TEPC 15 myeloma protein augment T15 idiotype production in *in vitro* anti-phosphorylcholine antibody responses, submitted for publication.
50. Paul, W. E., and Bona, C., 1982, Regulatory idiotypes and immune networks: A hypothesis, *Immunol. Today* **3:**230–234.
51. Bottomly, K., and Mosier, D. E., 1980, Analogous dual specificity of helper T cells cooperating in the generation of clonally restricted antibody responses, in: *Strategies of Immune Regulation* (E. E. Sercarz and A. J. Cunningham, eds.), Academic Press, New York, pp. 487–492.
52. Bottomly, K., 1981, Activation of the idiotypic network: Environmental and regulatory influences, in: *Immunoglobulin Idiotypes* (C. A. Janeway, Jr., E. E. Sercarz, and H. Wigzell, eds.), Academic Press, New York, pp. 517–532.
53. Jones, B., and Janeway, C. A., Jr., 1981, Cooperative interaction of B lymphocytes with antigen-specific helper T lymphocytes is MHC restricted, *Nature* **292:**547–549.
54. Bottomly, K., Jones, B., Kaye, J., and Jones, F., III, Subpopulations of B cells distinguished by cell surface expression of Ia antigens: Correlation of Ia and idiotype during activation by cloned, Ia restricted T cells, *J. Exp. Med.* **158:**265–279.
55. Bottomly, K., and Jones, F., III, 1981, Idiotype dominance manifested during a T-dependent anti-phosphorylcholine response requires a distinct helper T cell, in: *B Lymphocytes in the Immune Response: Function, Developmental, and Interactive Properties* (N. Klinman, D. E. Mosier, I. Scher, and F. S. Vitetta, eds.), Elsevier/North-Holland, Amsterdam, pp. 415–421.
56. Lee, W., Cosenza, H., and Kohler, H., 1974, Clonal restriction of the immune response to phosphorylcholine, *Nature* **247:**55–56.
57. Claflin, J. L., and Cubberley, M., 1978, Clonal nature of the immune response to phosphorylcholine. VI. Molecular uniformity of a single idiotype among BALB/c mice, *J. Immunol.* **121:**1410–1415.
58. Janeway, C. A., Jr., Lerner, E. A., Conrad, P. J., and Jones, B., 1982, The precision of self and non-self major histocompatibility complex encoded antigen recognition by cloned T cells, *Behring Inst. Mitt.* **70:**200–221.
59. Mond, J. J., Lieberman, R. L., Inman, J. K., Mosier, D. E., and Paul, W. E., 1977, Inability of mice with a defect in B-lymphocyte maturation to respond to phosphorylcholine on immunogenic carriers, *J. Exp. Med.* **146:**1138–1142.
60. Kenny, J., Guelde, G., Claflin, J., and Scher, I., 1981, Altered idiotype responses to phosphorylcholine in mice bearing an X-linked immune defect, *J. Immunol.* **127:**1629–1633.
61. Sachs, D. H., and Cone, J. L., 1973, A mouse B cell alloantigen determined by genes linked to the major histocompatibility complex, *J. Exp. Med.* **138:**1289–1304.
62. Mond, J. J., Kessler, S., Finkelman, F., Paul, W. E. and Scher, I., 1980, Heterogeneity of Ia expression on normal B cells, neonatal B cells and on cells from B cell-defective CBA/N mice, *J. Immunol.* **12:**1675–1682.
63. Press, J. L., Strober, S., and Klinman, N. R., 1977, Characterization of B cell subpopulations by velocity sedimentation, surface Ia antigens and immune function, *Eur. J. Immunol.* **7:**329–335.
64. Greenstein, J. L., Lord, E. M., Horan, P., Kappler, J. W., and Marrack, P., 1981, Functional subsets of B cells defined by quantitative differences in surface I-A, *J. Immunol.* **126:**2419–2423.
65. Huber, B. T., 1979, Antigenic marker on a functional subpopulation of B cells, controlled by the IA subregion of the H-2 gene complex, *Proc. Natl. Acad. Sci. USA* **76:**3460–3463.
66. Henry, C., Chan, E. L., and Kodlin, D., 1977, Expression and function of I-region products on immunocompetent cells. II. I-region products in T–B interaction, *J. Immunol.* **119:**744–748.
67. Matis, L. A., Jones, P. P., Murphy, D. B., Hedrick, J. M., Lerner, E. A., Janeway, C. A., Jr., McNicholas, J. M., and Schwartz, R. H., 1982, Immune response gene function correlates with the expression of an Ia antigen. II. A quantitative deficiency in A$_e$:E complex expression causes a corresponding defect in antigen-presenting cell function, *J. Exp. Med.* **155:**508–523.
68. Cosenza, H., Julius, M., and Augustin, A., 1977, Idiotypes as variable region markers: Analogies between receptors on phosphorylcholine-specific T and B lymphocytes, *Immunol. Rev.* **34:**3–33.
69. Gearhart, P. J., Sigal, N. H., and Klinman, N. R., 1975, Heterogeneity of the BALB/c anti-phosphorylcholine antibody response at the precursor cell level, *J. Exp. Med.* **141:**56–71.

70. Bottomly, K., and Mosier, D. E., 1981, Antigen-specific helper T cells required for dominant idiotype expression are not H-2 restricted, *J. Exp. Med.* **154**:411–421.
71. Bottomly, K., and Maurer, P. H., 1980, Antigen-specific helper T cells required for dominant production of an idiotype (ThId) are not under immune response (Ir) gene control, *J. Exp. Med.* **152**:1571–1582.
72. Quintans, J., and Cosenza, H., 1976, Antibody response to phosphorylcholine *in vitro*. II. Analaysis of T dependent and T independent responses, *Eur. J. Immunol.* **6**:359–366.
73. Mond, J. J., Mongini, P. K., Sieckmann, D., and Paul, W. E., 1980, Role of T lymphocytes in the response to TNP-AECM-Ficoll, *J. Immunol.* **125**:1066–1070.
74. Sieckmann, D. G., 1980, The use of anti-immunoglobulins to induce a signal for cell division in B-lymphocytes via their membrane IgM and IgD, *Immunol. Rev.* **52**:181–196.
75. Mond, J. J. Seghal, E., King, J., and Finkelman, F. D., 1981, Increased expression of I-region-associated antigen (Ia) on B cells after crosslinking of surface immunoglobulin, *J. Immunol.* **127**:881–888.
76. Claflin, J. L., and Davie, J. M., 1974, Clonal nature of the immune response to phosphorylcholine. IV. idiotypic uniformity of binding site-associated antigenic determinants among mouse anti-phosphorylcholine antibodies, *J. Exp. Med.* **140**:673–686.
77. Lieberman, R., Potter, M., Humphrey, W., and Chien, C. C., 1976, Idiotypes of insulin-binding antibodies and myeloma proteins controlled by genes linked to the allotype locus of the mouse, *J. Immunol.* **117**:2105–2111.
78. Dzierzak, E. A., and Janeway, C. A., Jr., 1981, Expression of an idiotype (Id-460) during *in vitro* anti-dinitrophenyl antibody responses. III. Detection of Id-460 in normal serum that does not bind dinitrophenyl, *J. Exp. Med.* **154**:1442–1454.
79. Wysocki, L. J., and Sato, V. L., 1981, The strain A anti-*p*-azobenzene-arsonate major cross-reactive idiotypic family includes members with no reactivity toward p-azophenylarsonate, *Eur. J. Immunol.* **11**:832–839.
80. Hornbeck, P. V., and Lewis, G. K., 1983, Idiotype connectance in the immune system. I. Expression of a cross-reactive idiotope on induced anti-p-azophenylarsonate antibodies and on endogenous antibodies not specific for arsonate, *J. Exp. Med.* **157**:1116–1135.
81. Briles, D. E., Nahm, M., Schroer, K., Davie, J., Baker, P., Kearney, J., and Barletta, R., 1981, Anti-phosphocholine antibodies found in normal mouse serum are protective against intravenous infection with type 3 *Streptococcus pneumoniae, J. Exp. Med.* **153**:694–699.
82. Briles, D. E., Forman, C., Hudak, S., and Claflin, J. L., 1982, Antiphosphorylcholine antibodies of the T15 idiotype are optimally protective against *Streptococcus pneumoniae, J. Exp. Med.* **156**:1177–1185.

24

Autologous Idiotope-Specific T Cells in Regulation of Antibody Response

JAN CERNY

1. Introduction: Search for Autochthonous* Network Regulation

The existence of autologous anti-idiotypic (anti-Id) lymphocytes—both B and T cells—has been convincingly demonstrated using various experimental manipulations described elsewhere in this volume. When they are activated with an appropriate probe (e.g., Id-bearing molecules or cells), the anti-Id cells and their products display a strong regulatory effect on the immune response of lymphocytes bearing the corresponding Id. Whether the anti-Id response is an autochthonous process that occurs within the system without any manipulation is less certain. This assumption, which is the cornerstone of the network hypothesis of immune self-regulation,[1] has been questioned by several investigators.[2,3] Does lymphocyte stimulation with *antigen* always induce a complementary anti-Id reaction? How important is this autochthonous anti-Id response for regulation of the first response? What is the internal mechanism of activation of anti-Id clones? In this chapter we will try to strenghten the case for anti-Id self-regulation by providing experimental data in answer to the aforementioned questions.

First, let us review the evidence for autochthonous anti-Id antibody. Although the production of autochthonous anti-Id antibody was demonstrated in mice hyperimmunized with *S. pneumoniae* R36A strain vaccine more than 10 years ago,[4] the search for its immunoregulatory role in several systems has yielded controversial results. Goidl, Schrater, and co-workers have claimed that such antibody is responsible for the rapid decline and the termination of the primary response to TNP-Ficoll.[5,6] The evidence is based on the "hapten augmentation" of TNP-specific PFC. When the plaque assay is performed with splenocytes from a later stage of anti-TNP response, an addition of a small amount of TNP

---

*Autochthonous process is that initiated within the system without an outside experimental manipulation.

JAN CERNY • Department of Microbiology, University of Texas Medical Branch, Galveston, Texas 77550.

into the assay increases the number of TNP-specific plaques. The PFC are presumably blocked by autochthonous anti-Id antibody, which is displaced by the hapten.

Using a more direct methodology, Hiernaux et al. studied the anti-Id antibody-forming cells in the course of primary response to levan using a plaque assay with Id-coupled red blood cells.[7] Euthymic mice immunized with levan produced anti-Id PFC in the spleen, whereas nude mice did not. Yet the numbers and the kinetics of Id-bearing (Id⁺) antilevan PFC were comparable in both euthymic and nude mice. It appeared that the autochthonous anti-Id antibody-producing cells (which were outnumbered by the antilevan PFC 200 : 1) had no detectable effect on the early course of the antigen-driven, Id⁺ antibody response. A similar conclusion can be drawn from the studies of Rodkey on anti-Id serum antibody produced by rabbits hyperimmunized with *M. lactodycecus*.[8,9] Sera of those rabbits contained self-reactive antibodies to private Id; however, only one third of the immunized animals developed anti-Id and there was no apparent difference in the response to the antigen between the positive and the negative rabbits.

Concurrently with this work we have focused on the cellular rather than humoral aspects of autochthonous anti-Id response. The results described in the next section provide evidence for an immunoregulatory role of self-reacting T cells.

2. Experimental Model

The antibody response to phosphocholine (PC) was generated *in vivo* or in lymphocyte cultures with a vaccine made from *S. pneumoniae* R36A strain (Pn). The main characteristics of the response were reviewed thoroughly by Köhler.[10] The murine PC-reactive B cells form three distinct Id families designated M603, M511, and T15. A unique situation has arisen in the BALB/c strain in that all (> 90%) of the anti-PC antibody is made by the T15⁺ B cells. However, when the T15⁺ clones are suppressed by neonatal injection of anti-T15 antibody, they are replaced by other T15⁻ clones (presumably those of the M603 and M111 families, but that has not been well established) later in the life of the mice.[11]

The object of our experiments was the regulation of T15 Id-bearing B cells. The prototype T15 immunoglobulin is the PC-reactive myeloma protein of BALB/c origin, TEPC15. We have used this protein to study the activation of anti-T15 lymphocytes (by binding of [¹²⁵I]-TEPC15), to enrich for anti-T15 T cells (by panning on TEPC15-coated plates), and to activate anti-T15 T-suppressor cells (with TEPC15–antigen complexes).

Like other Ids, T15 is a complex of several non-cross-reacting idiotopic determinants detectable with monoclonal antibodies. The TEPC15 molecule may carry 6 to 12 distinct idiotopes some of which are paratopic and others are not.[12,13] Some T15 idiotopes are "private" for BALB/c while others are frequently expressed in other strains.[14] The T15 clones are idiotopically heterogeneous even in BALB/c, i.e., a given clone belonging to the T15 family expresses some but not all idiotopes of the TEPC15 prototype molecule.[13,15] One of the goals of our work has been to find out if the autologous T cells distinguish between the serologically defined sets of idiotopes (i.e., idiograms) of the T15 family.

The anti-PC response has been measured by PFC assay using red cells coupled either with PnC, the cell wall polysaccharide from Pn, or with the PC hapten. Both types of plaques are inhibitable with 10^{-6} to 10^{-7} M of free PC chloride. The idiotopic profile of the response has been determined by plaque inhibition with various monoclonal anti-idi-otopes.[14] Thus, the proportion of PFC expressing a given idiotope is the fraction (%) of total plaques inhibitable with the corresponding anti-idiotopic antibody. The results in this chapter will deal with the expression of three idiotopes: B36-82, AB1-2, and MaId5-4.[12,13,16] The total T15$^+$ PFC were defined by a conventional rabbit or mouse antiserum against TEPC15 protein.

3. Cyclical Activation of PC-Specific, T15$^+$ B Cells by Anti-T15 T Cells

The antibody response of BALB/c mice to a single immunization with Pn is a cyclical process. Antibody PFC in the spleen appear in distinct peaks at about 7-day intervals.[17] Such a cyclical course of primary antibody response is commonly observed with various antigens and in different animals species (reviewed in Ref. 18). We wished to determine if the antigen-driven PFC response is accompanied by autochthonous anti-Id response *in situ*. As the anti-Pn response in BALB/c mice is composed exclusively of lymphocyte clones sharing the same Id, T15, the putative autochthonous anti-Id response would always be directed against T15 which is represented by the TEPC15 myeloma protein. To detect that response, we utilized a radioimmunoassay whereby splenocytes from Pn-immunized mice were incubated with [^{125}I]-TEPC15. The amount of bound radioactivity was considered to be a measure of the total population of cells with receptors for T15, i.e., anti-T15 cells, regardless of their class or function.

We observed that the cyclical production of splenic T15$^+$ PFC after a single injection of Pn was accompanied by a cyclical expansion (or activation) of anti-T15 cells in the spleen.[17,19] When the two curves were superimposed (Fig. 1), it appeared that the early rise of anti-T15 activity occurred with, if not earlier than, the increase of T15$^+$ PFC. After that, the two curves oscillated in a near reciprocal manner, the anti-Id response peaking at the time of PFC declining and vice versa.

Both the cycling of the anti-Pn response and the development of an autochthonous anti-Id response appeared to be thymus-dependent, for they were absent from congenitally thymus-deficient (nude) mice[19] (Fig. 2). Nude mice responded to Pn with a single peak of T15$^+$ PFC that was comparable to the first PFC peak of Pn-immunized euthymic lit-termates ($nu/+$ or $+/+$) both in kinetics and in magnitude. However, the second PFC peak did not occur in the spleen of nude mice, and no anti-Id response was detectable. Implantation of syngeneic thymus glands in nude mice prior to immunization reconstituted both the cycling and the autochthonous anti-Id response.[19]

These results showed that an autochthonous anti-Id response is (1) T-dependent and may involve effector T cells, and (2) may be causally linked with cycling of PFC. Could the initial expansion of antibody-forming, T15$^+$ B cells activate anti-T15 T cells (peak on day 10) which, in turn, stimulate the second cycle of PFC (peak on day 12)? The possibility was tested in an adoptive transfer experiment[20] (Fig. 2). Euthymic mice (= prospective donors) and nude mice (= prospective recipients) were immunized with Pn. When the primary response subsided on day 9, the splenic T cells from euthymic mice were purified on nylon wool columns and transferred into half of the nude recipients; the other half served as a control. The level of Pn-specific PFC in the spleen was monitored daily after the T cell transfer. As shown in Fig. 3, the nude recipients of T cells developed a second peak of

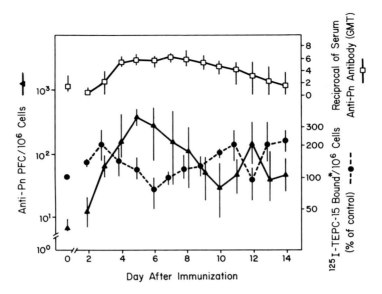

FIGURE 1. Groups of three to five BALB/c mice were injected i.p. with 20 μg of Pn vaccine 2 to 14 days before removal of their spleens. Aliquots containing 10^6 viable splenic lymphocytes were assayed for anti-Pn PFC (▲) and specific binding of $[^{125}I]$-TEPC15 myeloma protein (●). Serum, collected at the time of splenectomy, was assayed for anti-Pn antibody by passive hemagglutination of antigen-coated SRBC (□). Each symbol represents the mean of four experiments (12–15 mice). The vertical bars indicate the range of those experiments. For determination of $[^{125}I]$-TEPC15 binding, ascitic fluid from BALB/c mice bearing the plasmacytomas TEPC15, MOPC315, or McPC603 was recovered and purified by $(NH_4)_zSO_4$ precipitation and gel (Sephadex G-200) filtration. Each purified protein was tested for its capacity to hemagglutinate Pn- or TNP-coated SRBC. Iodination was with radioiodinated Bolton–Hunter reagent (NEN), 5 mg protein/mCi ^{125}I. Iodinated proteins were equivalent to nonlabeled proteins in their ability to hemagglutinate. To determine the optimal concentration of radioligand, spleen cells from BALB/c mice injected with TEPC15 protein and then allowed to rest for 2 months were incubated with 10-fold dilutions of $[^{125}I]$-TEPC15 or $[^{125}I]$-MOPC315 0.1–100 μg protein. Saturation occurred at $\simeq 1$ μg for both proteins. Inhibition of binding (68–75%) occurred in the presence of 100 μg cold homologous ligand but not with the heterologous ligand or bovine serum albumin. To measure T15 binding, duplicate tubes containing 10^6 cells in 0.1 ml of ice-cold Hanks' balanced salt solution containing 2% FCS were incubated at 4°C for 10–12 hr with $\simeq 1$ μg (0.05 ml) of labeled TEPC15, MOPC315, or McPC603. The cells were then washed three times in cold Hanks' containing 10% FCS and the radioactivity of the cell pellet was determined as cpm. Variation within duplicates was routinely less than 15%. Specific TEPC15 binding is defined as: (cpm bound $[^{125}I]$-TEPC15) − (cpm bound $[^{125}I]$-MOPC315 or $[^{125}I]$-McPC603). In any single experiment, specific TEPC15 binding was computed by the subtraction of only one of the control proteins. Because the cpm of bound MOPC315 or McPC603 remains constant throughout the 14-day experimental period, both serve equally well as specificity controls. The specific TEPC15 binding is then expressed as percent of binding by spleen cells from the control group of unimmunized mice (control = 100%).

T15$^+$ anti-Pn PFC on day 12 (i.e., 3 days after the T cell transfer) whereas the control groups did not. The T cells that induce the second cycle of PFC have receptors for the T15 Id as shown by panning on TEPC15-coated dishes: the nonadherent cell fraction lost the ability to induce PFC upon the adoptive transfer whereas the adherent fraction was enriched for this activity (Table I).

An important aspect of this "antigen-independent" triggering of PFC by T cells is that the recipient must be primed with the antigen between 9 and 14 days prior to the cell

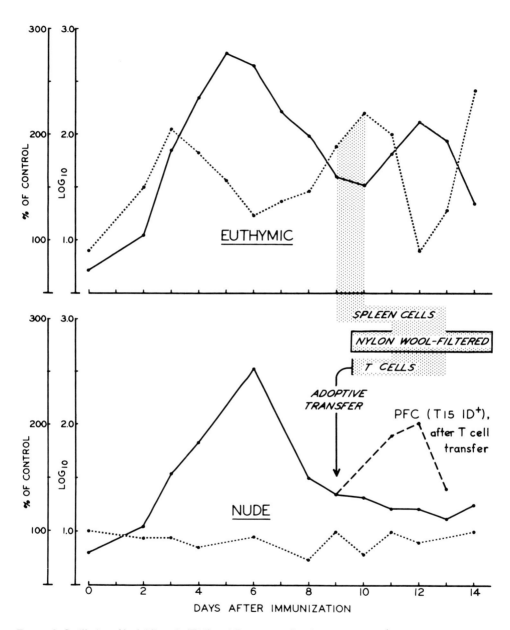

FIGURE 2. Oscillation of both idiotypic (T15) anti-Pn response [log (anti-Pn PFC/10^6 cells)] (———) and anti-T15 response [^{125}I-TEPC-15 bound/10^6 cells (% of control)] (-----) in euthymic mice and lack of it in nude mice. The experiment on adoptive transfer of T cells is shown schematically (see text for details).

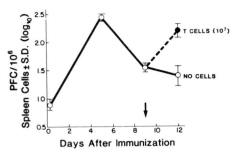

FIGURE 3. The induction of a second cycle of anti-Pn PFC in nude mice by adoptively transferred T cells. Nude mice were immunized with 20 μg Pn on day 0. The specific primary response in the spleen was determined by PFC assay on day 5 and day 9. On that day, a parallel group of nude mice received 15 $\times$ 10^6 splenic T cells (arrow) from BALB/c donors primed with Pn 9 days before. The number of Pn-specific plaques in the recipients increased to 164 $\pm$ 365 PFC/10^6 splenocytes on day 12 (i.e., 3 days after the T-cell transfer) ($\bullet$), whereas the PFC level in the nude mice that did not receive any cells remained at 28 PFC/10^6 splenocytes ($\circ$). Each point represents the mean from a group of four to seven mice with S.D. indicated by the vertical bars.

transfer.[20] An injection of T cells into normal, unprimed recipients primed 21 days or longer failed to induce the second cycle of PFC (Table II). These results were reproduced *in vitro* using cultures of splenic B cells from Pn-primed (-10 days) mice. The Pn-specific, T15$^+$ PFC response was triggered *either* with the antigen (Pn) or with anti-Id T cells isolated from the spleen of syngeneic donors. In contrast, B cells from unprimed mice responded to Pn but not to the addition of anti-Id T cells.[18] Similar results were obtained earlier by Eichmann *et al.*[21]

Our interpretation of the data has been that anti-Id T cells may interact with antigen-primed Id$^+$ B cells, but not with resting B cells, in a manner that reactivates the lymphocytes into a new round of antibody synthesis. It may be that the priming with antigen induces a transient change in the B cells that is recognized by the T cells. A similar concept has been suggested by Thomas and Calderon.[22]

We have shown that autologous anti-Id T cells do indeed regulate the antigen-driven

TABLE I

Adoptive Transfer of T Cells Not Adherent to Myeloma Protein-Coated Dishes

Expt.	T cells ($\times 10^{-6}$), from dishes coated with[a]	PnC-specific PFC/10^6 spleen cells (day 3 after T cell transfer)
A	MOPC315 (15) (control)	2.37 $\pm$ 0.15 (248)
	TEPC15 (15)	1.54 $\pm$ 0.38 (50)*
B	None (control)	1.80 $\pm$ 0.07 (64)
	Untreated (20)	2.10 $\pm$ 0.18 (136)*
	McPC603 (20)	2.11 $\pm$ 0.17 (124)*
	TEPC15 (20)	1.76 $\pm$ 0.24 (63)
C	None (control)	1.16 $\pm$ 0.31 (19)
	Untreated (20)	1.85 $\pm$ 0.13 (73)*
	McPC603 (20)	1.78 $\pm$ 0.13 (63)*
	TEPC15 (20)	1.43 $\pm$ 0.17 (25)

[a]T cells were prepared from the spleens of BALB/c mice primed with Pn on day -9 previously; they were injected either untreated or after adsorption to plastic dishes coated with the indicated myeloma proteins. Cells that were nonadherent (or loosely adherent) were harvested and injected into Pn-primed (day -9) nude recipients.
*The difference between experimental and control groups is significant at $p < 0.01$.

TABLE II

The Requirement of Antigen Priming of the Recipient Mice for the Induction of Specific PFC by Adoptively Transferred T cells

Expt.	Recipients primed with[a]	T cells ($\times 10^{-6}$)[b]	PFC/10^6 spleen cells, specific for:[c]	
			PnC	TNP
A	Pn	None (control)	1.61 ± 0.06 (42)	NT[d]
		Pn-primed (20)	2.02 ± 0.20 (114)*	NT
	Unprimed	None	0.48 ± 0.35 (4.2)	NT
		Pn-primed (20)	0.62 ± 0.14 (4.4)	NT
B	Pn	None (control)	1.16 ± 0.27 (17)	0.98 ± 0.35 (18)
		Pn-primed (15)	2.07 ± 0.11 (122)*	1.15 ± 0.28 (18)
	Unprimed	None	0.61 ± 0.18 (4.5)	1.39 ± 0.29 (31)
		Pn-primed (15)	0.46 ± 0.30 (3.4)	1.51 ± 0.42 (44)
	TNP-LPS	None	0.51 ± 0.23 (3.7)	2.16 ± 0.19 (158)
		Pn-primed (20)	0.39 ± 0.17 (2.7)	2.38 ± 0.37 (151)
C	Pn + TNP-	None (control)	1.46 ± 0.12 (30)	1.44 ± 0.30 (32)
	LPS	TNP-LPS-primed (20)	1.80 ± 0.09 (63)	2.02 ± 0.12 (107)

[a] Nude mice were injected i.p. with 20 μg of Pn vaccine or with 10μg of TNP-LPS (or both), 9 days before the adoptive transfer.
[b] T cells were obtained from BALB/c mice primed 9 days before with Pn (20 μg) or TNP-LPS (10 μg).
[c] Plaque-forming cells were enumerated on day 3 after the T-cell administration by using PnC-burro RBC or TNP-burro RBC as indicator cells.
[d] NT, not tested.
*The difference between experimental and control groups is significant at $p < 0.01$.

B-cell response. However, the regulation appears to be a late effect in that the anti-Id clones interact with the Id$^+$ clones only after the latter had completed the first round of antibody synthesis. A comparison of PFC curves in Fig. 2 shows that the first peak in nude mice which did not produce a measurable anti-Id response is very similar to the first peak in euthymic mice which did develop the autochthonous anti-Id response. It is as if the early anti-Id activity had no immunoregulatory function, a conclusion reached also by Hiernaux et al.[7] We have recently reinvestigated this puzzle in studies on anti-Pn response and T15 expression in the C57BL/6 strain. The data suggest that the role of anti-Id T cells during the first peak of anti-Pn response may be to select (by suppression or help) various clones of B cells expressing different Ids.[54] The curve of total Pn-specific PFC in C57BL/6 that peaks on day 5 to 6 and then declines is, in fact, a sum of overlapping curves representing distinct PFC populations with different idiograms. Two T15 idiotopes, AB1-2, and MaId5-4, were essentially undetectable on PFC on day 3, became highly expressed on day 5 (up to 90% PFC were idiotope-positive, and then diminished again by day 12 after immunization Table III. We isolated splenic T cells from immunized mice, at those intervals (days 3, 5, and 12), and added them into cultures of naive, syngeneic B cells. The mixed cultures were stimulated with Pn and the idiotopic profile of the response was determined (Table IV). It turned out that the immune T cells modulated the readout response according to their origin. T cells from day 2 inhibited idiotope expression, those from day 5 enhanced idiotope expression, and those from day 12 were, again, inhibitory. The regulation was idiotope-specific, as neither of the T-cell populations had a substantial effect on the *total* PFC response of the B cells. I assume that when B cells bearing the T15 Id (AB1-2 and MaId5-4) are suppressed by T cells, there is a "compensatory" activation of other B-cell clones expressing different idiotypes, and *vice versa*. These data suggest that distinct

Table III

Changes of T15 Idiotope Expression during a Primary Anti-Pn Response in C57BL/6 Mice

PC-specific PFC in the spleen		Days after immunization with Pn		
		3	5	12
Total		4,560 (±1,827)	20,000 (±8,390)	3,180 (±1,130)
AB1-2 Id$^+$	positive animals^a	1/5	5/5	3/5
	PFC^b	35%	75% (±20)	50% (±35)
MaId5-4Id$^+$	positive animals^a	2/5	5/5	3/5
	PFC^b	42%	80% (±15)	65% (±28)

^{a}Number of mice which expressed the given Id (positive/total). The negative animals were those in which the PFC were not significantly inhibited by addition of the appropriate anti-Id antibody.
^{b}Percent of PFC inhibitable with anti-Id (mean from positive animals ± S.D.). The variability is not shown for day 3 when only one and two mice expressed AB1-2 and MaId5-4, respectively.

phenotypes of Id-specific T-cell subsets are activated at various stages of antigen-driven antibody response and that such T cells may select B-cell populations with different idiotypes by help or suppression.

4. Mechanisms of Activation of Anti-Id T Cells: Antigen–Antibody Complex

The Id$^+$ and anti-Id lymphocyte clones exist in an equilibrium until the introduction of the antigen. It is not known what change in the antigen-reactive cells (and their Id$^+$ receptors) constitutes the signal for expansion and activation of anti-Id cells. The studies of Klaus on production of anti-Id antibodies against Id$^+$ myeloma proteins demonstrated

Table IV

Activation of Anti-Id Suppressor and Helper-T Cells during Primary Antibody Response: Assay for the T-Cell Activity in a Cell Culture System

Normal B cells (10^6) stimulated with Pn *in vitro:* T cells added^a (2 × 10^5)	PC-specific PFC			Effect on Id expression	Lyt phenotypes of the T cells^b
	Total/wells (mean ± S.D.)	ID-positive PFC (%)			
		AB1-2	Mid5-4		
None	150 ± 19	33 ± 6	18 ± 4		
T-d.2	255 ± 30	4 ± 3	0	suppression	1$^+$2$^+$
T-d.5	217 ± 20	45 ± 5	54 ± 6	enhancement	1$^+$2$^-$
T-d.12	128 ± 18	10 ± 7	28 ± 15	suppression	1$^-$2$^+$

^{a}Splenic T cells were isolated by panning from mice (pool of 2-3 animals) immunized with Pn on days 2, 5 or 12 previously. The T cells were added into the cultures of normal (unprimed) splenic B cells with Pn as antigen. PC-specific PFC were enumerated after a 4-day stimulation *in vitro*.
^{b}T cells were pre-treated with mouse antibodies to Lyt-1.2 or Lyt-2.2 (from F.-W. Shen, Memorial Sloan-Kettering Cancer Center, New York) plus rabbit complement. The column shows which treatment abolished the effect of T cells on Id expression. Thus, a treatment with either anti-Lyt-1 or anti-Lyt-2 plus C abolished the apparent suppression of Id expression by day 2-T cells, etcetera.

the peculiar autoimmunogenicity of immune complexes.[23] Mice immunized with a soluble myeloma protein developed little if any anti-Id antibody whereas animals injected with a preformed complex of the myeloma protein and the specific antigen produced high titers of antibody against the Id portion of the complex. These results lend support to the speculation of Singer and Williams on the immunogenicity of "altered idiotype."[24] They proposed that an Id becomes autoimmunogenic only after a configurational "change" of the variable region upon its interaction with the epitope.

Klaus' results prompted us to investigate the possibility of activation of anti-T15 cells with complexes of TEPC15 proteins and PnC, an antigen bearing the PC epitope. We used an *in vitro* system in which normal BALB/c splenic lymphocytes were incubated with the immune complex for 2 days, washed, and transferred into a second culture system containing fresh responder cells and Pn. An ability of the "immune complex-educated" cells to modulate the anti-PnC response was determined by the changes in numbers of specific PFC generated in the readout culture.[25] A typical result is shown in Table V. Lymphocytes which were "educated" with either TEPC15 (= Id) or PnC (= antigen) alone were unable to modulate the response to Pn (as compared to the effect of cells that were simply incubated in the culture medium) whereas the cells exposed to the TEPC15–PnC complex were strongly immunosuppressive. The suppression appeared to be specific for the anti-PnC response (Table V). The experiment was repeated using purified T cells. After a 2-day incubation of the T cells with the immune complex, a positive selection procedure was used to obtain T cells free of immune complex (carryover of the immune complex into the readout culture would cause a direct suppression of the response and might lead to false results). As shown in Table VI, the doubly purified cells were able to suppress the anti-PnC response, specifically.

The T cells educated with the immune complex have increased binding capacity for the [^{125}I]-TEPC15 and the binding could be specifically inhibited with cold TEPC15 but not with MOPC315, a different IgA myeloma protein (Fig. 4). This suggested that the immune complex has induced the expression of receptors on T cells for T15 or an expansion of cells bearing Id receptors, and that the T-suppressor cells (Ts) may be anti-idiotypic. The notion was confirmed by comparing the effect of Ts on T15$^+$ and T15$^-$ syn-

TABLE V

Induction of Specific "Suppressor Cells" With Antigen–Antibody Complexes[a]

Cells added (2 × 10^6/culture) after induction with:	PFC per culture specific for:			
	PnC	% of control	TNP	% of control
Medium	293 ± 22	(control)	4548 ± 920	(control)
TEPC15 (60 μg)	384 ± 71	131	6340 ± 560	139
PnC (6 μg)	253 ± 44	86	5200 ± 312	114
TEPC15–PnC (20 μg)	50 ± 23	17	3872 ± 1040	85

[a]BALB/c spleen cells were incubated in Marbrook vessels in medium alone or with the indicated reagent. After 2 days, the cells were harvested, washed twice, and added to Marbrook vessels together with fresh BALB/c spleen cells (10^7) and stimulated with 10^6 bacteria from a Pn vaccine and with TNP-BA. After 5 days, the number of direct PFC per culture was determined.

TABLE VI
Specific Suppressor T Cells Induced by TEPC15-PnC Complexes

Day -2^a	Day 0^b	Day 5 Specific PFC/culture vs.:	
Preincubation of T cells with:	Positive selection for T cells	PnC	SRBC
Medium	−	817 ± 126	ND^c
	+	590 ± 55	
TEPC15–PnC	−	185 ± 23	ND
	+	158 ± 36	3730 ± 316

^{a}T cells (BALB/c spleen cells not adherent to RAMIg plates) were cultured in Marbrook vessels (10^7/culture) in medium alone or with 50 μg/culture of TEPC15–PnC complexes.
^{b}On day 0, the cells were harvested and treated with a murine monoclonal antibody (anti-Thy-1.2) and then added to RAMIg plates. After 1 hr at 4°C, the nonadherent cells were removed. After the plates were washed five times, the adherent cells were collected and compared with unselected cells for suppressor cell activity by adding 10^6 cells from each group to Marbrook vessels containing 10^7 fresh BALB/c spleen cells together with either S RBC or Pn vaccine. Direct PFC were assayed on day 5 using S RBC or PnC-coated S RBC as indicator cells in the PFC assay.
^{c}ND, not determined.

geneic (BALB/c) responder cells. The T15$^-$ lymphocytes were obtained from mice neonatally injected with anti-T15 antibody; the B cells from these mice respond to Pn very well but they lack all recognized T15-related determinants.[26] As shown in Fig. 5, the Ts generated with T15–PnC complex inhibited the anti-PnC response of T15$^+$ responder cells (in a dose-dependent manner) but they had no measurable effect on the response of T15$^-$ cells.

Our data show that anti-Id T cells (at least those with suppressor phenotype) are activated by Id born on antibody molecules complexed with antigen, much more efficiently than with Id on native antibody. It is reasonable to speculate that this anti-Id response will be directed against nonparatopic idiotopic determinants rather than the idiotopes within the paratope because the latter should be blocked by the antigen. The increase "immunogenicity" of complexed idiotopes could be due to the lattice formation; the complex may be visualized as a multivalent idiotope that is more efficient in cross-linking the anti-idiotopic receptors on T cells than the divalent soluble immunoglobulin molecule. It may also be that the nonparatopic idiotopic idiotope is altered by an allosteric mechanism from the paratope–antigen interaction, as previously suggested,[24] but this concept presents some theoretical difficulties as noted in the discussion.

5. Autologous Anti-Id T Cells Recognize Distinct Idiotopes Defined by Monoclonal Antibodies

The Id of an immunoglobulin molecule consists of several distinct non-cross-reacting determinants, idiotopes. The T15 Id on TEPC15 protein may carry more than eight idiotopes defined with a panel of anti-T15 monoclonal antibodies.[12–14,16] The data in this section indirectly show that there are subsets of autologous T cells specific for individual idiotopes of T15 and that these cells can regulate the expression of different idiotope-bearing B cells independently of one another.

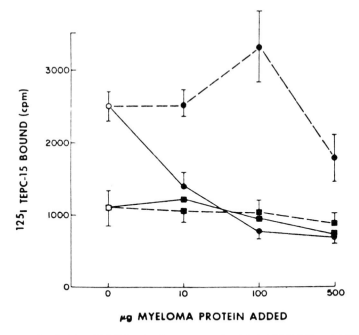

FIGURE 4. Binding of radiolabeled TEPC15 in the presence of unlabeled TEPC15 or MOPC315 myeloma proteins. BALB/c T cells were incubated with 50 μg/culture of TEPC15–PnC complexes (○) or with medium alone (□) for 2 days. The T cells were then positively selected as described in Table VI and incubated overnight at 4°C with 5 μg [^{125}I]-TEPC15 in the presence of the indicated amount of unlabeled TEPC15 (———) or MOPC315 (-----). The cells were washed four times and then the radioactivity associated with the cell pellet was determined. Each point represents the mean of four cultures ± S.D.

FIGURE 5. Assay of immune complex-induced Ts on normal (T15$^+$) or T15-suppressed (T15$^-$) BALB/c mice. BALB/c T cells (10^7/culture) were cultured with TEPC15–PnC complexes (●) (50 μg/culture) or medium (■) in Marbrook vessels. After 2 days, T cells were positively selected as described in Table VI and added to fresh responder spleen cells from normal (———) or T15-suppressed (-----) BALB/c mice. Direct PFC were assayed on day 5. PFC from the normal BALB/c control cultures could be inhibited by 73% by incorporating AB1-2 monoclonal anti-T15 antibody into the plaquing mixture whereas PFC from the T15-suppressed mice were not inhibited by AB1-2.

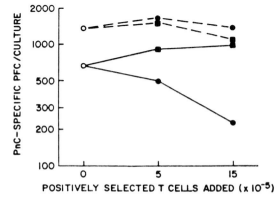

The experiments employed BALB/c mice injected with a monoclonal anti-T15 antibody at birth. Such treatment has a profound effect on the response of the animals to PC antigens and previously it has been used in studies on network regulation in several laboratories.[11,17–30] The only novelty of our experiments has been the use of monoclonal anti-T15 antibodies rather than conventional antisera for both the treatment and the assessment of the idiotopic spectrum of the anti-PC response.[26] BALB/c mice were injected with the monoclonal anti-T15 antibody MaId5-4 (20 ug/mouse) within 24 hr after birth. The response of the splenic lymphocytes from these mice to Pn *in vitro* was studied when the animals reached the age of 2 to 5 months. As seen in Table VII, the spleen cells from adult, neonatally injected mice responded to Pn immunization as well as cells from control littermates except that the PFC did not express T15 idiotopes. Neonatal treatment with MaId5-4 antibody suppressed the expression of the corresponding idiotope as well as two other idiotopes, AB1-2 and B36-82. When we eliminated T cells from the lymphocyte suspension of MaId5-4-suppressed donors and stimulated the remaining B cells with Pn, the PFC generated in these cultures expressed no MaId5-4 idiotope, but they occasionally did express near-normal levels of either B36-82 or both B36-82 and AB1-2 (Table VII, Expts. 2, 3). This result prompted us to set up cultures containing reciprocal mixtures of T and B cells from normal (n) and MaId5-4-suppressed mice (s). Results of several experiments are shown in Table VIII. T cells from idiotope-suppressed donors (Ts) inhibited the expression of the target determinant, MaId5-4, in *all* cultures of Pn-stimulated, normal B cells (Bn) Occasionally, the Ts also inhibited the expression of either AB1-2 or B36-82, or both; this pattern has varied from one experiment to another. In other words, there were distinct suppressor cells for the three T15 idiotopes and a given Ts pool might contain a subset specific for one idiotope but not for another. B cells from suppressed mice cocultured with normal T cells were never able to express the MaId5-4 but did occasionally express

TABLE VII

Expression of AB1-2 and B36-82 T15 Idiotopes by Splenocytes and B Cells for MaId5-4-Suppressed Mice

Expt.	Cells in culture with Pn[a]	PC-specific PFC (total/10^6 cells)	PFC (%) positive for:[b]		
			MaId5-4	AB1-2	B36-82
1	Splenocytes	408 ± 68	<20	NT[c]	<20
	B Cells	63 ± 8	<20	NT	79
2	Splenocytes	450 ± 106	<20	<20	<20
	B Cells	84 ± 7	<20	<20	70
3	Splenocytes	339 ± 15	<20	<20	<20
	B cells	150 ± 10	<20	75	68
4	Splenocytes	207 ± 20	<20	<20	<20
	B cells	36 ± 14	<20	<20	<20

[a]All cells were from neonatally suppressed mice.
[b]Proportion of plaques inhibitable by the respective monoclonal anti-idiotopic antibody. The amount of protein required for maximum plaque inhibition was [c]NT, not tested.

TABLE VIII

The Role of T Cells in Control of AB1-2 and B36-82 Idiotope Expression in Mice Suppressed with MaId5-4 Anti-Idiotopic-Antibody

Expt.	Cells in culture with Pn[a]	PC-specific PFC (total/10^6 cells)	PFC (%) positive for:[b]		
			MaId5-4	AB1-2	B36-82
1	Bn + Tn	158 ± 17	70	55	NT[c]
	Bn + Ts	153 ± 12	<20	<20	NT
	Bs + Tn	65 ± 2	<20	50	NT
	Bs + Ts	53 ± 6	<20	<20	NT
2	Bn + Tn	138 ± 14	60	60	47
	Bn + Ts	140 ± 18	<20	73	38
	Bs + Tn	170 ± 21	<20	NT	<20
	Bs + Ts	135 ± 7	<20	NT	<20
3	Bn + Tn	198 ± 24	75	89	88
	Bn + Ts	177 ± 18	39	69	64
	Bs + Tn	126 ± 12	<20	43	57
	Bs + Ts	108 ± 3	<20	<20	<20
4	Bn + Tn	310 ± 12	82	81	84
	Bn + Ts	206 ± 20	<20	32	48
	Bs + Tn	105 ± 3	<20	35	<20
	Bs + Ts	141 ± 23	<20	<20	<20

[a]Cultures contained 10^6 lymphocytes/well, either whole spleen cell suspension or splenic B-cell fraction (= B) obtained by cytotoxic treatment with anti-Thy-1.2 monoclonal antibody and complement. T cells (T) were obtained as nonadherent fraction of splenocytes panned on dishes coated with a goat anti-mouse immunoglobulin antiserum. Mixed cultures contained 10^6 B and 3×10^5 T cells. Lymphocytes were obtained from either neonatally suppressed mice (s) or normal, age-matched controls (n).

[b]Proportion of plaques inhibitable by the respective monoclonal anti-idiotope antibody. The amount of protein required for maximum plaque inhibition was determined previously.

[c]NT, not tested.

the other idiotopes (Table VIII). This supports the notion that the neonatal administration of MaId5-4 antibody induced both central tolerance (functional B-cell paralysis) and active Ts specific for MaId5-4 idiotope, as well as cosuppression of at least two other idiotopic determinants of the T15 family which appear to involve either an active suppression by idiotope-specific T cells or, less frequently, a central tolerance. The relative contribution of the mechanisms of cosuppression may vary from one animal to another.

Our results are very similar to those of Kelsoe *et al.* who have studied the effect of passively administered monoclonal anti-idiotopic antibodies on the expression of idiotopes of the B1-8 family in the response of C57BL/6 mice to nitrophenylacetyl.[31] They, too, found an independent modulation of different idiotopic determinants within the family, they showed the participation of idiotope-specific T cells in the process, and they also found that mice suppressed with antibody to one idiotope (Ac38) may develop suppressor T cells for another idiotope (Ac166). This phenomenon of cosuppression that has been seen in both laboratories is schematically depicted in Fig. 6 using our data. We speculate that when the anti-MaId5-4 (M) antibody reacts with the corresponding idiotope on the B-cell receptor

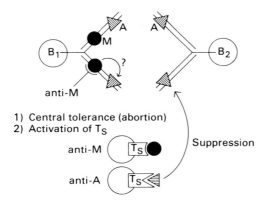

FIGURE 6. Schematic interpretation of the "cosuppression" phenomenon. Neonatal injection of monoclonal antibody against the idiotopic determinant M (anti-M) induces a central tolerance in clone B_1 as well as T-suppressor cells (Ts) specific for M. In addition, the interaction of anti-M with the target determinant causes a change (?) in the expression of an adjacent but distinct determinant A which, in turn, leads to activation of anti-A Ts. The latter inhibit the clone B_2 that expresses the determinant A only.

(B_1), a conformational change occurs (allosteric mechanism?) in the adjacent region of the molecule bearing another idiotope, AB1-2 (A). The change is recognized by T cells and leads to triggering of AB1-2-specific Ts which can, once activated, react with "unchanged" AB1-2 expressed on other lymphocyte clones (B_2) which do not share the target determinant, MaId5-4. The target clone (M^+,A^+) is suppressed (functionally paralyzed) by the direct action of anti-M, and the M-specific Ts are activated but not required for the suppression of M^+ cells. On the other hand, the suppression of M^-,A^+ clones will depend on active Ts.

Another piece of evidence for separate T cells which recognize distinct idiotopes and which can regulate the idiotope-positive B-cell clones independently of one another has come from experiments on idiotope expression in different inbred strains of mice described in the next section.

6. Genetics of the T-Cell-Mediated Control of Idiotope Expression

The expression of an Id by murine B cells is regulated by genes in both Ig[32–34] and H-2 loci.[35,36] The lack of expression of an Id in the antibody response of a given mouse strain may be either due to the absence of the appropriate V gene[37] or due to a supression of the Id^+ B cells by the complementary anti-Id clones.[38,39] The obvious regulatory mechanism that comes to mind are anti-Id T cells. In general, T cells tend to recognize various epitopes in context with specific self gene products. Perhaps the anti-Id T cells recognize the idiotypic determinants in context of products of the Ig or MHC alleles.

Our studies on the possible T-dependence of idiotope expression have been carried out in cultures of lymphocytes from various strains of mice.[40] Splenocytes, splenic B cells, or B cells supplemented with syngeneic T lymphocytes were stimulated with Pn and the expression of individual idiotopes of the T15 family on Pc-specific antibody-forming cells was monitored with monoclonal anti-idiotopic antibodies. We have shown previously that among the idiotopes present on the PC-reactive TEPC15 myeloma, some determinants are fairly private for BALB/c strains whereas others are frequently expressed in both BALB/c and C57BL/6 mice[14] (Table IX). Three of these "common" idiotopes were chosen for the genetic studies, namely AB1-2, MaId5-4 and B36-82.

In BALB/c mice (Table X), the elimination of T cells did not change the expression

TABLE IX

Expression of T15 Idiotopes on Pn-Receptive Spleen Cells of BALB/c and C57BL/6 Mice as Determined by Inhibition with Monoclonal Anti-Idiotopic Antibodies[a]

	Antibody		Hapten inhibition[b]		BALB/c				C57BL/6			
					PFC inhibition		Suppression of primary response		PFC inhibition		Suppression of primary response	
Group	Clone	Ig class	Pc-chloride	PC-KLH	Positive animals[c]	Mean (range)[d]	Positive animals[c]	Mean (range)[e]	Positive animals[c]	Mean (range)[d]	Positive animals[e]	Mean (range)[e]
I	AB1-2[f]	γ1	−	+	12/12	82 (65–100)	12/12	84 (65–100)	19/24	70 (33–100)	16/24	57 (32–80)
	MaId5-4[g]	γ1	−	+	10/10	83 (80–100)	10/10	91 (80–100)	18/19	61 (29–90)	19/19	78 (38–95)
	B36-82[h]	μ	−	30	11/11	81 (65–100)	10/10	78 (65–100)	19/19	72 (44–99)	19/23	62 (28–95)
	B39-38[h]	γ1	−	−	2/3	50 (48–52)	2/3	80 (70–90)	0/7	−	0/4	−
	B36-69[h]	γ1	10^{-5}	10			2/2	82 (75–90)	0/3	−	0/3	−
II	B36-75[h]	γ1	10^{-3}	20	7/11	53 (33–67)	8/10	62 (35–80)	7/22	40 (24–48)	14/24	49 (30–80)
	B24-50[h]	γ2b	−	−	6/9	60 (40–80)	5/8	55 (25–70)	3/19	45 (29–62)	12/23	47 (30–75)
	B24-44[h]	γ1	10^{-5}	1	6/11	57 (44–78)	NT		3/19	38 (27–44)	3/16	52 (35–76)

[a] The inhibition of differentiated PFC and the suppression of induction of primary anti-Pn response are described in the text.
[b] Concentration of antigen (moles of PC-chloride, μg/ml of PC-KLH) required for 50% inhibition of binding of [^{125}I]-HOPC8 to anti-idiotopes. The information on AB1-2 and MaId5-4 is only qualitative (+ or −).
[c] The number of animals with inhibitable lymphocytes/total tested. NT, not tested.
[d] Mean (percent) of inhibitable PFC, calculated only from positive individuals (≥ 20% inhibition). Range indicates lowest and highest individual values (percent inhibition).
[e] Mean (percent) of inhibitable fraction of anti-Pn response; includes positive individuals(≥ 25% inhibition) only.
[f] Ref. 12.
[g] C. Heusser (personal communication).
[h] Ref. 13.

TABLE X

T-Cell-Independent Expression of T15 By B Cells from BALB/C

		PC-specific PFC			
Pn-stimulated responder cells (10⁶/well)	Added to cultures	Total[a]	Proportion expressing:[b]		
			AB1-2	MaId5-4	B36-82
Spleen	−	162	68%	80%	>85%
B cells[c]	−	51	72%	70%	>85%
	T cells[d] (2 × 10⁵)	150	75%	74%	>85%

[a] PFC/well, mean from quadruplicate cultures. Standard error was ≤20% of the means.
[b] Percent plaques inhibitable by a given anti-idiotopic antibody.
[c] B cells were prepared by repeated treatment of splenocytes with a monoclonal anti-Thy-1.2 antibody and complement.
[d] Nonadherent cell fraction from plates coated with a goat anti-mouse immunoglobulin antiserum. Prepared from the same splenocytes pool as the B cells.

of AB1-2, MaId5-4, or B36-82 by Pn-stimulated B cells *in vitro* even though the magnitude of the response was significantly reduced compared to the cultures of splenocytes. The magnitude of the B-cell response was restored by addition of syngeneic T cells; however, the idiotopic profile of the response remained the same.

Quite different results were obtained with lymphocytes from other inbred mice. In DBA/2 (Table XI), Pn-stimulated splenocytes produced PFC expressing all three idiotopes. Two of the idiotopes, AB1-2 and MaId5-4, disappeared from the response following depletion of T cells, whereas the B36-82 remained unchanged. Syngeneic T cells restored the idiotopic profile of the response. Thus, it appears that B cells expressing AB1-2 or MaID5-4 idiotopes of T15, but not those bearing B36-82, are absolutely T helper-dependent in DBA/2 mice although their expression is T-independent in BALB/c mice. Results obtained with C57BL/6 lymphocytes (Table XII) are similar to those in DBA/2; however, in this case the expression of AB1-2 and MaId5-4 appears to be under Ts regulation as the removal and addition of T cells respectively enhanced and inhibited the expression of B cells bearing those idiotopes. Again, the third T15 idiotope, B36-82, was expressed equally well in all types of Pn-stimulated cultures of C57BL/6 lymphocytes.

Naturally occurring anti-Id Ts cells were first shown by Bona and Paul.[41] Our results demonstrate that the T-cell regulation is specific for various idiotopic determinants comprising an Id and that the recognition of idiotope develops in the context of the self environment. It is this context which determines whether an idiotope-bearing B lymphocyte is actively suppressed or amplified (helped).

7. Discussion and Conclusions

This chapter describes several properties of autologous anti-idiotopic T cells and their autochthonous immunoregulatory potential. The discussion will concentrate on the following points: (1) the fine specificity of self-reacting T cells, (2) the genetics of idiotope-specific T cells, (3) the autochthonous mechanisms of their activation, and (4) the regulation of antigen-driven B cells by anti-idiotopic cells.

1. It appears that the autologous T cells can recognize the discrete, non-cross-reacting, idiotopic determinants defined by monoclonal anti-idiotopic antibodies. This would argue

TABLE XI
T Cell Depletion Abolishes the Expression of Some T15 Idiotopes by B Cells from DBA/2[a]

Pn-stimulated responder cells (10^6/well)	Added to cultures	Pc-specific PFC			
			Proportion expressing:		
		Total	AB1-2	MaId5-4	B36-82
Spleen	—	190	38%	58%	75%
B cells	—	84	<15%[b]	<15%	>85%
	T cells (2×10^5)	168	47%	51%	>85%

[a]See Table X footnotes.
[b]Inhibition by <15% is considered not significant (= idiotope not expressed).

TABLE XII

Effect of T Cells on T15 Profile of the Anti-PC Response of Lymphocytes from C57BL/6^a

Pn-stimulated responder cells (10^6/well)	Added to cultures	PC-specific PFC			
		Total	Proportion expressing:		
			AB1-2	MaId5-4	B36-82
Spleen	—	122	27%	32%	84%
B cells	—	80	>85%	75%	83%
	T cells (2×10^5)	116	42%	28%	>85%

^{a}See Table X footnotes.

that the repertoires of anti-idiotopic T cells and B cells are similar. However, the evidence for that is only circumstantial, since idiotopes have not been isolated and their interaction with T cells cannot be measured directly. The argument is based on the observation that the T cells can regulate—suppress or help—the B cells that express different idiotopic determinants *independently of each other*. This has been observed in studies on idiotope expression by B cells from different inbred strains (Section 6) as well as in BALB/c mice that were immunosuppressed with monoclonal anti-idiotopic antibody (Section 5). Nonetheless, in some instances the neonatal treatment with a monoclonal anti-idiotope produced T cells which suppressed the expression of the corresponding (target) idiotope as well as another, non-cross-reacting idiotopic determinant. To interpret this so called "cosuppression" we have proposed[26,40] that two distinct populations of Ts have been induced, one of which is specific for the target idiotope and a second with specificity for an *adjacent* but serologically distinct idiotope (Fig. 6). There is a bias in this interpretation. Since the two putative idiotope-specific T-cell subsets cannot be separated physically, we cannot exclude the possibility that there are Ts involved in the "cosuppression" that cross-react with both idiotopes.

The model shown in Fig. 6 has something in common with the concept of "altered idiotype" that was proposed to explain why antigen–antibody complexes activate anti-idiotopic Ts (Section 4). Both models assume that a T cell with idiotope-specific receptor recognizes, and is activated by a change in the idiotopic expression following an interaction of a ligand—an anti-idiotopic antibody or antigen—with another portion of the immunoglobulin molecule. Once activated, the Ts obviously recognizes and binds to the idiotope on intact (unaltered) immunoglobulin. Thus, the proposed allosteric "change" in the idiotopic expression would have to be such that it would enhance the immunogenicity of the idiotope but not its fine epitopic specificity. Speculations on how this might be possible are futile as little is known about the structure of idiotopes or the T-cell receptor.

2. The effect of the *H-2* gene complex on Id expression has been demonstrated[35,36] but the mechanism of that regulation is not known. Recently, Yamamoto *et al.* demonstrated that Id-specific cytotoxic T lymphocytes (CTL) generated against myeloma cells (M104E) are restricted by products of *H-2* allele on the target cells.[42] Their experimental system does not allow the distinction between CTL specific for idiotopes within the M104E Id; however, it is reasonable to assume that different idiotope-specific T cells—like those specific for conventional epitopes—will have different *H-2* restriction patterns. This would

provide a rational explanation for the role of T cells in regulation of an idiotopic expression in different strains of mice as observed in our studies (Section 6). The genes involved in the apparent T-cell self-regulation of idiotope in our system have not yet been mapped; however, our preliminary studies do imply some role for the *H-2*. The expression of AB1-2, by C57BL/6 *(H-2^b)* PC-reactive lymphocytes was consistently increased following the removal of T cells but this was not the case with cogenic B10D2 *(H-2^d)* cells which frequently showed a loss of idiotopes upon T-cell depletion.[43] I speculate that a given idiotope recognized in junction with one allelic H-2 product activates Ts whereas in junction with another allele, the same idiotope may activate T-helper or amplified cells.

Obviously, this simplistic view does not explain all results. There must be another explanation for the unique behavior of BALB/c antibody-forming cells which express both AB1-2 and MAId5-4 regardless of the presence of T cells (Table X) or for the fact that one T15 idiotope, B36-82, appears to be expressed in all inbred strains tested, independent of any detectable T-cell control (Tables IX–XII). More importantly, the speculation may have little bearing on the *Ig* locus-dependent Id expression which appears to be due to the preferential linkage of *IgV* genes with a particular *IgC* gene in a given inbred mouse strain. In order to postulate another mechanism, namely, an active regulation of idiotope expression governed by allotype genes, one would have to assume that T cells recognize idiotopes in association with the products of *Ig* loci. Experimental support for *Ig*-restricted T cells comes from studies on hapten-specific delayed-type hypersensitivity,[44,45] from experiments with helper cells in B-cell suppressed mice,[46] and, most directly, from the work of Juy *et al.* who showed that the M460 Id-specific Ts cells recognize the Id in conjunction with products of *IgH*.[47] The two mechanisms—*H-2* restricted and *Ig*-restricted—could regulate the idiotopic expression of different levels. Cancro *et al.* have found an effect of *H-2* on T15$^+$ B-cell precursor frequency while the *Ig* locus regulated the amount of T15 produced after immunization.[35]

3. Evidence was presented for an autochthonous anti-Id reaction in the course of primary antibody response. The self-reaction is thymus-dependent and involves anti-Id T cells. The mechanism of the autochthonous activation of complementary clones is not known. Richter[48] has tried to explain it in the quantitative terms of cell population dynamics. In his model, the expansion of antigen-driven, Id$^+$ clones represents a signal for activation and expansion of the complementary anti-Id clones. Thus, the network signal would be generated by a disturbance of the balance between complementary clones which presumably exist in the "naive" state, prior to the antigen administration.[1] However, this simple model is not consistent with the early appearance of anti-Id response as measured experimentally. Figures 1 and 2 show that in mice immunized with Pn, the increased activity (expansion?) of cells with receptors for T15 occurred concurrently with, if not prior to, the increase of T15$^+$, Pn-reactive cells. Similarly, Hiernaux *et al.*[7] observed the emergence of anti-Id PFC 1 day *prior to* the Id$^+$ PFC in the spleen of mice immunized with bacterial lipopolysaccharide. To explain this paradox, we[49] speculate that the preimmune balance of complementary clones and their receptor molecules is disturbed as soon as the antigen enters the system and forms complexes with the paratope of Id$^+$ molecules (immunoglobulins and T-cell receptors). This "removal" of Id$^+$ molecules from the balanced pool may represent an early signal for the activation of anti-Id cell clones. Furthermore, the complexes may have "super-antigenic" properties toward the anti-Id clones. Our data on induction of anti-T15 Ts cells with TEPC15–PnC complexes (Section 4) support the con-

cept. It may be that the character of the complex—its size and ratio of antibody to antigen— may influence the phenotype (i.e., help or suppression) of the anti-Id T cell.

4. The autochthonous anti-Id response has a major regulatory effect on the antigen-driven responses. We have shown that it is involved in the repeated activation of B cells and thereby in the periodic cycling of the primary immune response. The autochthonous activation of anti-idiotopic T cells seems to be also involved in sequential switching of idiotopically distinct clones in the course of immune response, by the mechanism of help or suppression. An important, even critical point in these network regulations appears to be a qualitative change in the antigen-driven, Id-bearing cells with respect to their interaction with the regulatory clones. We have shown that the autologous anti-idiotopic T cells would trigger the antibody production in memory B cells but not in virgin, unprimed ones (Ref. 20 and Section 3) and that the idiotope-specific Ts cells that appear, transiently in the course of the primary response, would inhibit the naive, unstimulated idiotope-positive B cells but not antigen-primed B cells expressing the same idiotope. These observations are consistent with the increasing amount of data showing that antigen-activated (memory?) B cells are qualitatively different from the naive cells so far as their regulation is concerned.[22,50–53] Particularly revealing are the experiments of Thomas and Calderon[22,52] suggesting that antigen-primed B cells become refractory to suppression by T cells and, furthermore, may recruit a Ts population that acts on the virgin, not yet activated B cells. The concept helps to understand the fine tuning of the Id network in which the interaction between complementary clones must fulfill the momentary needs of the immune system.

ACKNOWLEDGMENT. I thank Dr. Garnett Kelsoe for critical evaluation of the manuscript and for valuable contribution to the discussion.

References

1. Jerne, N. K., 1974, Towards a network theory of the immune system, *Ann. Immunol. (Inst. Pasteur)* **125C**:373–389.
2. Cohn, M., 1981, Conversations with Niels Kaj Jerne on immune regulation: Associative versus network recognition, *Cell. Immunol.* **61**:425–436.
3. Morrison, C., and Coeshott, C., 1981, Is idiotypic regulation the real thing? *Immunol. Today* **2**:121–122.
4. Kluskens, L., and Kohler, H., 1974, Regulation of immune response by autogenous antibody against receptor, *Proc. Natl. Acad. Sci. USA* **71**:5083–5087.
5. Schratter, A. F., Goidl, E. A., Thorbecke, G. J., and Siskind, G. W., 1979, Production of auto-anti-idiotypic antibody during the normal response to TNP-Ficoll. I. Occurrence in AKR/J and BALB/c mice of hapten-augmentable, anti-TNP plaque forming cells and their accelerated appearance in recipients of immune spleen cells, *J. Exp. Med.* **150**:138–153.
6. Goidl, E. A., Schrater, A. F., Siskind, G. W., and Thorbecke, G. J., 1979, Production of auto-anti-idiotypic antibody during the normal immune response of TNP-Ficoll. II. Hapten-reversible inhibition of anti-TNP plaque forming cells by immune serum as an assay for auto-anti-idiotypic antibody, *J. Exp. Med.* **150**:154–165.
7. Hiernaux, J. R., Chiang, J., Baker, P. J., DeLisi, C., and Prescott, B., 1982, Lack of involvement of auto-anti-idiotypic antibody in the regulation of oscillations and tolerance in the antibody response to levan, *Cell. Immunol.* **67**:334–345.
8. Brown, J. C., and Rodkey, L. S., 1979, Autoregulation of an antibody response *via* network-induced auto-antiidiotype, *J. Exp. Med.* **150**:67–85.

9. Binion, S. B., and Rodkey, L. S., 1982, Naturally induced auto-anti-idiotypic antibodies: Induction by identical idiotopes in some members of an outbred rabbit family, *J. Exp. Med.* **156**:860–872.

10. Köhler, H., 1975, The response to phosphorylcholine: Dissecting an immune system, *Transplant. Rev.* **27**:24–56.

11. Augustin, A., and Cosenza, H., 1976, Expression of new idiotypes following neonatal idiotypic suppression of a dominant clone, *Eur. J. Immunol.* **6**:497–501.

12. Hammerling, G. J., and Wallich, R., 1980, Monoclonal anti-idiotypes as a probe for the analysis of the diversity of anti-phosphorylcholine antibodies, in: *Protides of Biological Fluids,* Volume 28 (H. Peters, ed.), Pergamon Press, Elmsford, N. Y., pp. 569–574.

13. Kearney, J. F., Barletta, R., Quare, Z. A., and Quintans, J., 1981, Monochlonal versus heterogenous anti-H-8 antibodies in the analysis of the anti-phosphorylcholine response in BALB/c mice, *Eur. J. Immunol.* **11**:877–883.

14. Cerny, J., Wallich, R., and Hammerling, G. J., 1982, Analysis of T15 idiotypes by monoclonal antibodies: Variability of idiotopic expression on phosphorylcholine-specific lymphocytes from individual inbred mice, *J. Immunol.* **128**:1885–1891.

15. Berek, C., 1982, Modulation of immune response by anti-idiotopic antibodies, in: *Idiotypes—Antigens on the Inside* (I. Westen-Schnurr ed.), Editiones "Roche," Basle, pp. 159–164.

16. Heusser, C. H., Poskocil, S., and Julius, M. H., 1980, A major idiotype (T15-MI-2) on T15-positive B and T cells, *Immunobiology* **157**:227.

17. Kelsoe, G., and Cerny, J., 1979, Reciprocal expansion of idiotypic and anti-idiotypic clones following antigen stimulation, *Nature* **279**:333–334.

18. Cerny, J., 1982, The role of anti-idiotypic T cells in the cyclical course of an antibody response, in: *Regulation of Immune Response Dynamics,* Volume I (C. DeLisi and J. R. J. Hiernaux, eds.), CRC Press, Boca Raton, pp. 59–74.

19. Kelsoe, G., Isaak, D., and Cerny, J., 1980, Thymic requirement for cyclical idiotypic and reciprocal anti-idiotypic immune response to a T-independent antigen, *J. Exp. Med.* **151**:289–300.

20. Cerny, J., and Caulfield, M. J., 1981, Stimulation of specific antibody-forming cells in antigen-primed nude mice by the adoptive transfer of syngeneic anti-idiotypic T cells, *J. Immunol.* **126**:2262–2266.

21. Eichmann, K., Falk, I., and Rajewsky, K., 1978, Recognition of idiotypes in lymphocyte interactions, II. Antigen-independent cooperation between T and B cells that possess similar and complementary idiotypes, *Eur. J. Immunol.* **8**:853–857.

22. Thomas, D. B., and Calderon, R. A., 1982, Cyclic changes in helper/suppressor function during the immune response, in: *Regulation of Immune Response Dynamics,* Volume II (C. DeLisi and J. R. J. Hiernaux, eds.), CRC Press, Boca Raton, pp. 63–78.

23. Klaus, G. G. B., 1978, Antigen–antibody complexes elicit anti-idiotypic antibodies to self-idiotopes, *Nature* **272**:265–266.

24. Singer, D. E., and Williams, R. M., 1978, Hypothesis: Altered idiotype induces immune suppression, *Cell. Immunol.* **39**:1–4.

25. Caulfield M. J., Luce, K. J., Proffitt, M. R., and Cerny, J., 1983, Induction of idiotype-specific suppressor T cells with antigen–antibody complex. *J. Exp. Med.* **157**:1713–1725.

26. Cerny, J., Cronkhite, R., and Heusser, C., 1983, Antibody response of mice following neonatal treatment with a monoclonal anti-receptor antibody: Evidence for B cell tolerance and T suppressor cells specific for different idiotopic determinants, *Eur. J. Immunol.* **13**:244–248.

27. Fung, J. J., and Kohler, H., 1980, Immune response to phosphorylcholine. VII. Functional evidence for three separate B-cell subpopulations responding to T1 and TD PC-antigens, *J. Immunol.* **125**:640–646. Heusser, C., 1982, On the mechanism of anti-idiotype induced suppression in the T15 system, in: *Idiotypes—Antigen on the Inside* (I. Westen-Schnurr, ed.), Editiones "Roche," Basel, pp. 165–176.

29. Strayer, D. S., Lee, W. M. F., Rowly, D. A., and Kohler, H., 1975, Anti-receptors antibody. II. Induction of long-term unresponsiveness in neonatal mice, *J. Immunol.* **114**:728–733.

30. DuClos, T. W., and Kim, B. S., 1977, Suppressor T cells: Presence in mice rendered tolerant by neonatal treatment with anti-receptor antibody or antigen, *J. Immunol.* **119**:1769–1772.

31. Kelsoe, G., Takemori, T., Reth, M., and Rajewsky, K., 1981, Generation of specific regulatory T cells with monoclonal anti-idiotype antibody: Induction of suppressor T cells, in: *The Proceedings of the 2nd International Conference on B Lymphocytes and the Immune Response* (N. Klinman, D. Mosier, I. Scher, and E. Vitetta, eds.), Elsevier/North-Holland, Amsterdam, pp. 423–431.

32. Lieberman, R. M., Potter, M., Mushinski, E., Humphrey, W., and Rudikoff, S., 1974, Genetics of a new IgV$_H$ (T15 idiotype) marker in the mouse regulating natural antibody to phosphorylcholine, *J. Exp. Med.* **139**:983–1001.
33. Pawlak, L. L., Mushinski, E. B., Nisonoff, A., and Potter, M., 1973, Evidence for the linkage of the *IgC$_H$* locus to a gene controlling the idiotypic specificity of anti-*p*-azophenylarsonate antibodies in strain A mice, *J. Exp. Med.* **137**:22–31.
34. Mäkelä, O., and Karjalainen, K., 1977, Inherited immunoglobulin idiotypes of the mouse, *Immunol. Rev.* **34**:119–138.
35. Cancro, P. M., Sigal, N. H., and Klinman, N. R., 1978, Differential expression of an equivalent clonotype among BALB/c and C57BL/6 mice, *J. Exp. Med.* **147**:1–12.
36. Babu, V. M., and Maurer, P. H., 1981, The expression of anti-poly (LGlu60, LPhe40) idiotypic determinants dictated by the gene products in the major histocompatibility complex, *J. Exp. Med.* **154**:649–658.
37. Siekevitz, M., Gefter, M. L., Brodeur, P., Riblet, R., and Marshak-Rothstein, A., 1982, The genetic basis of antibody production: The dominant anti-arsonate idiotype response of the strain A mouse, *Eur. J. Immunol.* **12**:1023–1032.
38. Wikler, M., Demeur, C., Dewasame, G., and Urbain, J., 1980, Immunoregulatory role of maternal idiotypes, *J. Exp. Med.* **152**:1024–1035.
39. Primi, D., Juy, D., and Cazenave, P.-A., 1981, Induction and regulation of silent idiotype clones, *Eur. J. Immunol.* **11**:393–398.
40. Cerny, J., and Cronkhite, R., 1983, An independent regulation of distinct idiotopes of the T15 idiotype by autologous T cells, *Ann. NY Acad. Sci.* **148**:31–34.
41. Bona, C., and Paul, W. E., 1979, Cellular basis of regulation of expression of idiotype. I. T-suppressor cells specific for MOPC 460 idiotype regulate the expression of cells secreting anti-TNP antibodies bearing 460 idiotype, *J. Exp. Med.* **149**:592–600.
42. Yamamoto, H., Bitoh, S., Torii, M., and Fujimoto, S., 1983, Idiotype-specific T lymphocytes. I. Regulation of antibody production by idiotype-specific H-2-restricted T lymphocytes, *J. Immunol.* **130**:1038–1042.
43. Cronkhite, R., Tabbara, K., and Cerny, J., 1983, Genetic control of expression of distinct idiotopes (Id) within T15 is mediated by specific T cells, *Fed. Proc.* **42**:703.
44. Weinberger, J. Z., Benacerraf, B., and Dorf, M., 1980, Hapten-specific T cell response to 4-hydroxy-3-nitrophenyl acetyl. III. Interaction of effector suppressor T cells is restricted by H-2 and Igh-V genes, *J. Exp. Med.* **151**:1413–1423.
45. Jayaraman, S., and Bellone, C. J., 1982, Hapten-specific responses to the phenyltrimethylamino hapten. II. Regulation of delayed hypersensitivity by genetically restricted, anti-idiotypic suppressor T cells induced by nonvalent antigen L-tyrosine-p-azaphenyltrimethylammonium, *Eur. J. Immunol.* **12**:278–284.
46. Bottomly, K., Janeway, C. A., Jr., Mathieson, B. J., and Mosier, D. E., 1980, Absence of antigen-specific helper T cell required for the expression of the T15 idiotype in mice treated with anti-μ antibody, *Eur. J. Immunol.* **10**:159–163.
47. Juy, D., Primi, D., Sanchez, D., and Cazenave, P.-A., 1982, Idiotype regulation: Evidence for the involvement of Igh-C-restricted T cells in the M-460 idiotype suppressive pathway, *Euro. J. Immunol.* **12**:24–29.
48. Richter, P. H., 1975, A network theory of the immune system, *Eur. J. Immunol.* **5**:350–354.
49. Cerny, J., and Kelsoe, G., 1984, Priority of the anti-idiotypic response after antigen administration: artifact or an intriguing network mechanism?, *Immunol. Today* **5**:61–63.
50. Calkins, C. E., Orbach-Arbouys, S., Stutman, O., and Gershon, R. K., 1976, Cell interactions in the suppression of *in vitro* antibody response, *J. Exp. Med.* **143**:1421–1428.
51. L'Age-Stehr, J., Teichmann, H., Gershon, R. K., and Cantor, H., 1980, Stimulation of regulatory T-cell circuits by Ig-associated structures on activated B cells, *Eur. J. Immunol.* **10**:21–26.
52. Thomas, D.B., and Calderon, R. A., 1982, T helper cells change their Ly-1,2 phenotype during an immune response, *Eur. J. Immunol.* **12**:16–23.
53. Shimamura, T., Hashimoto, K., and Sasaki, S., 1982, Feedback suppression of the immune response *in vivo*. I. Immune B cells induce antigen-specific suppressor T cells, *Cell. Immunol.* **68**:104–113.
54. Cerny, J., 1984, Immune regulation by autologous anti-idiotopic (anti-Id) T cells: Rapid changes of the phenotype of anti-Id T cells during a primary antibody response, *J. Cell. Biochem.* **Suppl. 8A** (in press).

25

Idiotype Regulation in the Antibody Response to Phosphocholine

Antigen Selection of B-Lymphocyte Subsets with Differential Idiotype Expression?

D. E. MOSIER AND ANN J. FEENEY

1. Introduction

The antibody response to many natural or experimental antigens is often dominated by a single family of immunoglobulin molecules directly encoded by or derived from a single germ-line variable-region gene.[1-3] This is the case even though a number of alternative antibodies with apparent specificity for the same antigen can be produced.[4-7] The essential question we wish to address concerns the mechanism by which one gene product is selected from many for expression in the antibody response. If we assume that all V genes have an equal opportunity for expression at the pre-B-cell level, then a given B-cell clone must be expanded to become dominant either by *antigen selection* or by a *regulatory* system that can distinguish one V region from another, i.e., an idiotypic network.[8] While both types of regulatory mechanisms could operate simultaneously, we wish to present in this chapter some recent observations that lead us to emphasize the importance of antigen selection acting on distinct emerging B-cell subpopulations in explaining the idiotype composition of the murine antiphosphocholine (anti-PC) response.

Antigen selection as a model for clonotype regulation has only a few important precepts. When developing B lymphocytes express membrane immunoglobulin of a given V-region composition, a given B cell can be positively selected if it binds an available antigen with sufficient affinity *and* the B cell has reached a state of maturation when clonal expansion can be initiated. Alternatively, negative selection or clonal abortion can occur if antigen

---

D. E. MOSIER AND ANN J. FEENEY • Institute for Cancer Research, Philadelphia, Pennsylvania 19111.

is bound with high affinity at a sufficiently immature stage of B-cell development.[9-11] The important considerations for the positive selection of a given clonotype therefore are the presence of an appropriate antigen and the conditions necessary for B-cell expansion. What is important but difficult to ascertain in this type of model is the potential set of selecting antigens available, namely, how many variable regions are expressed that never encounter their antigen and what is the pressure for maintaining such V genes in the germ line?

The alternative view is that a set of anti-idiotypic elements (T cells and/or anti-idiotypic antibodies) selectively regulates different clones of B lymphocytes by recognizing V-region determinants and augmenting or suppressing a particular clone.[5,12-26] The network theory[8] proposes that many V regions are "internal images" of foreign antigens and, in essence, have the same selective potential suggested above for nominal antigens. While much work has addressed and partially supported this theory, many fundamental questions remain. Do the idiotypic determinants identified on immunoglobulin variable regions by heteroantisera, alloantisera, or monoclonal antibodies play an important role in the regulation of antibody responses in intact animals? Are idiotypic determinants (idiotopes) recognized both by autoantibodies and T cells, or does the specificity of these two potential regulatory elements differ? When auto-anti-idiotope antibody responses can be detected, are they invariably dependent upon helper T cells and, if so, what are the "carrier" determinants? How connected is the "immune network" and how likely is it that one antibody will recognize another simultaneously produced antibody? What comes first in ontogeny, the idiotype or the anti-idiotype? These (and many other) questions can be asked about the importance of self-recognition of idiotopes for the regulation of antibody production

We will attempt to review in this chapter evidence generated by our laboratory as well as by other workers that bears on these questions. This is not intended to be an extensive review, and interested readers are referred to other articles (Refs. 12, 13, 25–27, and this volume). Our main goal is to restrict some current hypotheses regarding idiotypic regulation and to introduce some alternative hypotheses compatible with most existing data. Many of the points we will emphasize in the model to be presented have been made independently by Kenny and his colleagues.[28,29] Our data are similar and have led us to similar conclusions.

2. The Nature of the Model System, the Antibody Response to PC

Much work on idiotype regulation has focused on the antibody response to PC in mice, beginning with the early demonstration by Cosenza and Köhler[30] that A/He anti-TEPC15 antibodies would inhibit the anti-PC response of BALB/c mice. We now know that the anti-PC response of most inbred mouse strains is remarkably homogeneous, although somatic variants do occur (see elsewhere in this volume). Three related families of anti-PC antibodies have been identified.[4] These are generally encoded by one germline V_H segment, several D segments, one J_H segment (J_H1), one of three V_K segments (V_K8, M603; V_K22, T15; or V_K24, M511), and one J_K (J_K5)[31,32] The families are designated T15, 603, and 511 as the use of different L chains is their most distinctive feature. The three families may be distinguished by heterologous anti-idiotype sera (Table I) or isoelectric focusing of isolated L chains.[4] Diversity within and between families seems to occur by somatic mutation and alterations in the D segment.[33] Thus, one important feature of

TABLE I
Rabbit Anti-Idiotype Sera Distinguish Three Mouse Anti-PC Antibody Families

	$\mu g/ml$ of IgM anti-PC hybridoma protein[a] required to inhibit by 50% binding of[^{125}I] anti-PC to anti-idiotype		
Inhibitor H chain L chain	T15 T15	T15 511	T15 603
Anti-idiotype			
Anti-T15	0.334	>1000	>1000
Anti-511	>1000	0.824	>1000
Anti-603	>1000	>1000	0.521

[a]Hybridoma proteins were HPCM2, HPCM27, and 180.6B6 and were kindly donated by P.Gearhart or L. Claflin.

this model system for the study of regulation is that the inherited germline basis of anti-PC antibody responses is known.

Antibodies of the T15 family dominate the IgM anti-PC responses of most strains of mice to many PC-containing antigens,[34-36] e.g., R36A *S. pneumoniae* or PC-keyhole limpet hemocyanin (PC-KLH). These anti-PC antibodies are encoded by the V1 V_H segment in BALB/c mice[1] (or its equivalent in other strains[57] and a V_K22 V_L segment and comprise 60–95% of the anti-PC response. Anti-PC antibodies of the 603 or 511 family emerge after immunization with *Proteus morganii*[38] or in IgG antibodies following hyperimmunization with PC-KLH.[39] The T15, 511, and 603 families do not differ significantly in their binding affinity for free PC although fine-specificity differences are detectable with PC analogs.[40,41] However, natural antigen selection may favor T15 dominance of the anti-PC response. For example, Briles *et al.*[42] have shown that IgM hybridoma anti-PC antibodies bearing the T15 idiotype are 8 times more effective at protecting BALB/c mice from a lethal *S. pneumoniae* infection than 603$^+$ antibodies and 30 times more effective than 511$^+$ antibodies. Antibodies of the T15 family also are more effective than 511$^+$ or 603$^+$ anti-PC antibodies at binding *S. pneumoniae* polysaccharide.[40] Since the anti-PC response is directed against a ubiquitous antigenic determinant in nature, if antigen selection can play a role in determining which anti-PC clonotypes (families) are expressed, it will.

3. Regulation of Anti-PC Responses

If clones of B lymphocytes expressing either T15, 511, or 603 anti-PC antibodies emerge in similar numbers at the same time during ontogeny (an assumption discussed below), then some form of regulatory event must intervene during postnatal development because most "primary" (first *experimental* antigen exposure) anti-PC responses are T15-dominant in adult mice.[34] The central question is, what is the nature of this regulation? One or more mechanisms, acting independently or in concert, can be envisioned as shaping the anti-PC response. These include: (1) the timing, duration, and intensity of initial antigen exposure, (2) the maternal transfer (pre- or postnatal) of anti-PC antibodies and/or anti-idiotype antibodies. (3) the generation of regulatory T cells (helper or suppressor) that differentially affect specific anti-PC clonotypes, and (4) the generation of auto-anti-idiotype antibodies that selectively allow T15-bearing clones to emerge. A similar set of influences can be postulated if the three anti-PC clonotypes emerge at different times in ontogeny (as might happen, for example, if there were ordered V_K gene rearrangement), but the timing of clonotype appearance might be an important factor in activating one or more of the regulatory pathways.

3.1. Suppression

It has been demonstrated that neonatal administration of small quantities of anti-T15 antibodies leads to profound and long-lasting suppression of the entire anti-PC antibody response,[43] and that eventual recovery of responsiveness to PC begins with T15⁻ clones.[44] Neonatal administration of PC yields similar results.[24,45] Thus, early encounter of emerging B cells with antigen or anti-idiotype sets in motion a *long-lasting* suppressive mechanism that remains obscure despite many studies. Some groups[24,46,47] propose that T lymphocytes maintain the suppression while others[48-50] have observed such suppression in *nu/nu* mice and suggest that anti-idiotype antibody or antigen is sufficient for regulation. The specificity of the suppressive mechanism is uncertain since T15 V_H determinants are shared by all three anti-PC antibody families. Nonetheless, it is clear that neonatal exposure to antigen or anti-idiotype must induce a self-sustaining mechanism that limits the expression of anti-PC B cells for many months.

Administration of anti-T15 antibodies to adult BALB/c mice results in the *short-term* (2–3 weeks) suppression of anti-PC responses.[43] We[16] and others[51] have shown that injection of a protein antigen and anti-idiotype (e.g., KLH and anti-T15) leads to the generation of suppressor T cells capable of suppressing the response to PC-KLH, but *not* PC-fowl γ-globulin. As shown in Table II, this suppression of secondary adoptive transfer anti-PC responses is caused by Lyt-2⁺ suppressor T cells. The mechanism of induction and activation (upon adoptive transfer) of these anti-idiotype-induced suppressor T cells is complex and most probably involves multiple cell populations. It is clear that anti-idiotype can

TABLE II

Injection of KLH and Anti-Idiotype Leads to the Generation of Suppressor T-Cells for the PC-KLH Antibody Response

PC-primed B cells + KLH-primed T cells from:	Antigen	IgM (IgG) PFC/spleen[a]
Normal BALB/c	PC-KLH	32,800
Anti-T15-treated BALB/c	PC-KLH	7,200
Normal + anti-T15-treated	PC-KLH	17,100
Lyt-1 anti-T15-treated	PC-KLH	38,700
Normal + Lyt-1 anti-T15-treated	PC-KLH	41,900
Normal	TNP-KLH	6,300 (11,100)
Anti-T15-treated	TNP-KLH	4,800 (15,300)

[a] 5×10^6 T-cell-depleted B cells plus 4×10^6 KLH-primed T cells were injected intravenously into syngeneic irradiated recipients with antigen and the direct (IgM) or indirect (IgG) plaque-forming cell response measured with PC- or TNP-coupled sheep erythrocytes 8 days later.

induce a persistent regulation of anti-PC antibody formation that is mediated by suppressor T cells. The population of Lyt-2 cells responsible for suppression may include two sub-populations, one that recognizes KLH and another that has specificity for an epitope on PC-binding antibodies. These two postulated T cells may synergize for suppression. The anti-idiotype pretreatment of T-cell donors in these experiments may activate PC-specific B cells (environmentally primed?) that are further stimulated by KLH priming, via "bystander" help,[52–54] to synthesize anti-PC antibodies in small amounts. This anti-PC antibody may induce suppressor T cells via a feedback suppression loop.[55] The KLH priming may induce both help and suppression as has been demonstrated in *in vivo* systems by Herzenberg *et al.*[56] In the presence of PC-KLH, both suppressors would be activated and the anti-PC response would be depressed. What is not clear in these experiments is whether or not anti-T15 antibody had any effect that would not have been achieved with an appropriate dose of PC-containing antigen.

3.2. Help

Some of the above experiments suggested the presence of T cells that were primed by anti-idiotype and could augment anti-PC responses.[16] Positive effects of anti-idiotype treatment have been reported in several systems, beginning with the experiments of Eichmann.[57] We have evaluated the contribution of T-helper cells (Lyt-1$^+$2$^-$) to anti-PC responses in general, and the expression of T15, 503, and 511 idiotypes in particular, in a series of experiments.[16,58–60a] The main question posed in these experiments is the contribution of circulating idiotype levels to the generation of T-helper cells that augment the production of the idiotype. Mice with X-linked immune deficiency of the CBA/N strain produce very low primary anti-PC antibody responses. They are profoundly deficient in preimmune T15 levels,[61] while having near-normal 511 and 603 idiotype expression (A. J. Feeney and D. E. Mosier, unpublished observations). If circulating T15$^+$ anti-PC antibody is required to generate T-helper cells that promote T15 dominance, then CBA/N × BALB/c F$_1$ male T cells should be less effective than CBA/N × BALB/c F$_1$ female T cells in supporting a T15-dominated anti-PC response. This experiment involves KLH-priming F$_1$ male and F$_1$ female T-cell donors, purifying their T cells, and adding them to PC-primed B cells from F$_1$ female mice, adoptively transferring the cell mixture with PC-KLH to irradiated F$_1$ female recipients, and measuring anti-PC responses and idiotype levels 8 days later. We originally reported[15] that F$_1$ male T cells were defective in their ability to support a T15-idiotype-positive IgM anti-PC response. Subsequent experiments by other workers[28,62] and in our laboratory[60a] suggest that there is *not* an important difference in the ability of F$_1$ male or F$_1$ female primed T cells to support the T15$^+$ anti-PC response. A representative recent experiment is summarized in Table III. We would conclude that preexisting idiotype levels have little or no influence on the generation of T-cell help that is reflected in the idiotypic composition of the anti-PC response. The question of the existence or activation requirements of T-helper cells specific for idiotype is not addressed in these experiments except for the inference that, if such T cells are necessary for T15-dominant anti-PC responses, they exist in both *xid*-bearing and normal mice and they are independent of preimmunization circulating T15 levels.

Table III
KLH-Primed T Cells From Low-T15 CBA/N × BALB/c F_1 Male Mice Provide Similar Helper T-Cell Function as KLH-Primed T Cells from High-T15 F_1 Female Mice

	5×10^6 PC-primed F_1 female B cells plus 2 $\times 10^6$ KLH-primed T cells from:	
Assay	F_1 male	F_1 female
IgM anti-PC PFC/spleen	91,997	94,673
% anti-T15 inhibitable	97%	98%
% anti-511 inhibitable	0%	4%
IgG anti-PC PFC/spleen	165,053	101,462
% anti-T15 inhibitable[a]	12%	15%
% anti-511 inhibitable	16%	21%
Anti-T15 protein A PFC/spleen	108,271	104,271
Anti-511 protein A PFC/spleen	32,082	29,708

[a]Much of the secondary IgG anti-PC-KLH response consists of antibody that binds NPPC with much higher affinity than PC [as originally reported by Chang et al.[77]] and probably does not bear either T15, 511, or 603 idiotype. We find that most of the 511$^+$ PC-binding antibody in these experiments is IgG1 (our unpublished data).

We have also undertaken another set of experiments concerning whether the quality of T-cell help derived from CBA/N × BALB/c F_1 male mice differs from that derived from normal F_1 female littermates. Long-term KLH-specific, H-2-restricted T-cell lines were generated according to the protocol of Augustin et al.[63] using either F_1 male or female lymph node donors. These two T-cell lines supported an *in vitro* TNP-KLH response equally. The response was similar whether the unprimed B cells (plus antigen-presenting cells) came from defective F_1 male mice or normal F_1 females, i.e., these lines could provide help for the "Lyb-5$^-$" subpopulation of B cells.* Both T-cell lines also supported the *in vitro* primary response to PC-KLH, but in this case only F_1 female B cells generated an anti-PC response. This response was dominated by T15-idiotype-positive IgM antibody (see Table IV) and the T–B-cell collaboration necessary for this response was H-2-restricted (data not shown). Therefore, T-cell lines from *xid* or normal mice can collaborate with normal (probably Lyb-5$^+$) B cells in an H-2-restricted fashion to generate a T15-dominant anti-PC response. It should be noted that this result differs from the prediction of Singer et al.[66] that T-cell–Lyb-5$^+$ B-cell interactions should not be MHC-restricted. We cannot rule out the coexistence of *two* helper cell subsets in these long-term lines (e.g., Ref. 67), so these experiments do not rule out a role for an auxiliary idiotype-specific T-helper cell such as we have previously proposed.[59]

*Anti-Lyb-5[64] is a difficult-to-prepare alloantiserum that is cytotoxic for about 50% of normal B cells in an appropriate strain of mouse, so a normal splenic B-cell population contains roughly equal numbers of Lyb-5$^-$ and Lyb-5$^+$ B cells. CBA/N mice lack the Lyb-5$^+$ population by definition (they are used in anti-Lyb-5 preparation), so their B cells are often used as a source of "Lyb-5$^-$" B cells. We will continue this terminology even though it has recently been shown that CBA/N cells are *not* equivalent to the normal Lyb-5$^-$ subpopulation.[65]

These results do point out an alternative hypothesis that may explain *apparent* idiotype-specific help. Since CBA/N mice do not make T15$^+$ responses, but can make anti-PC responses to PC-KLH or *P. morganii* (Refs. 29, 68, and our unpublished results), one could propose that "Lyb-5$^-$" B cells are devoid of T15$^+$ precursors. If the converse were also true (i.e., a predominance of T15$^+$ precursors in the Lyb-5$^+$ population), then any T-cell help that preferentially acts on the Lyb-5$^+$ subset of B cells would have the effect of increasing T15 expression relative to the 511 or 603 idiotypes. (A similar proposal has been made by Kenny *et al.*[28]) Likewise, any help that preferentially activates "Lyb-5$^-$" B cells should increase 511 and 603 expression. The expression of these idiotypes also is related to heavy-chain class (see Table III and Refs. 29, 69); IgM antibodies are T15-dominant while the 511 idiotype is associated with IgG responses. The proposed differential expression of anti-PC clonotypes among B-cell subsets raises many questions about the regulation of clonotype emergence, some of which we will deal with below.

3.3. Regulation of Anti-PC Clonotype Expression

We have sought evidence that T lymphocytes have any positive or negative influence on the expression of the three anti-PC clonotypes used in most mouse strains. We have examined in detail the anti-PC antibody responses of athymic BALB/c *nu/nu* mice. The assumption is that the absence of mature, conventional T cells in these mice should alter the pattern of idiotype expression if such cells normally regulate clonotype emergency and/or expansion. We have immunized *nu/nu* mice with *S. pneumoniae* R36A and extensively analyzed the resulting serum anti-PC antibodies for idiotype expression. Some representative results are summarized in Table V. The major increase in anti-PC antibody after R36A immunization is T15-idiotype-positive in both nude and normal mice, and the main effect of the *nu/nu* mutation is an overall decrease in the magnitude of anti-PC responses. Thus, the nominally T-independent response to R36A can be augmented by T cells, but there is no suggestion that the absence of T cells in *nu/nu* mice causes any shift in relative T15-idiotype expression. [If cryptic T cells, e.g., NK cells or B' cells (Lyt-1, sIg$^+$ cells),[70,71] can regulate B-cell development, then nude mice, which have these cell types,

TABLE IV
KLH-Specific, H-2-Restricted T-Helper Cell Lines From CBA/N × BALB/c F₁ Male or F₁ Female Mice Provide Equal Help for the in Vitro PC-KLH Response

T-helper line from:[a]	PFC/10^6 cultured cells versus		
	PC-SRBC	PC-SRBC + anti-T-15	Anti-T15 + protein A SRBC
F₁ male + PC-KLH	1501	12 (99% T15$^+$)	2728
F₁ female + PC-KLH	1927	45 (98% T15$^+$)	3778
PC-KLH alone (no T cells)	10	0	10

[a]5 × 10⁴ KLH-specific T cells were added to 5 × 10⁵ (CBA/N × BALB/c)F₁ female unprimed spleen cells and plaque-forming cells measured after 5 days of culture. Similar results were obtained in other experiments using T-depleted spleen as a source of responding B cells. "Reverse" plaque assay with anti-T15 and protein A SRBC measures both IgM and IgG T15$^+$ anti-PC PFC.

TABLE V
Response of BALB/c nu/nu or nu/+ Mice to S. Pneumoniae R36A Immunization

	Serum Idiotype Levels (μg/ml)		
	T15	511	603
nu/nu (N = 11)			
Preimmune	8.7 $\pm$ 1.7	28 $\pm$ 4.6	19.2 $\pm$ 2.3
Immune	127 $\pm$ 42	30 $\pm$ 1.6	39 $\pm$ 5.4
Increment	118 $\pm$ 41	2 $\pm$ 3	21 $\pm$ 5.2
	(84%)	(1%)	(15%)
nu/+ (N = 12)			
Preimmune	9 $\pm$ 1.3	27 $\pm$ 24	12.3 $\pm$ 1.5
Immune	446 $\pm$ 70	69 $\pm$ 15	94 $\pm$ 22
Increment	437 $\pm$ 70	42 $\pm$ 13	83 $\pm$ 24
	(78%)	(7%)	(15%)

might be similar to normal littermates.] Moreover, T15 dominance in this experimental system is unlikely to be due to T15-specific helper T cells. Rather, the T15-dominant anti-PC response can be explained by one of two nonexclusive mechanisms—the preferential stimulation by R36A of T15$^+$ precursors because they bind antigen with higher avidity[40,42] and/or the selective activation of the Lyb-5$^+$ B-cell subset (See Section 3.4). These experiments would seem to rule out an important regulatory role not only for T cells but also for T-dependent anti-idiotype antibody. Since the only evidence available[72] suggests that anti-idiotype production is indeed T-dependent, then the role of T cells in the natural regulation of anti-PC clonotype expression becomes more doubtful. This is not to say that under some experimental condition T cells cannot influence idiotype expression, but simply that we fail to find compelling evidence that they make a major contribution to clonotype regulation under normal circumstances.

3.4. B-Lymphocyte Ontogeny, Subset Differentiation, and Selective Expression of Different Idiotypes

It is well documented that the response to different antigenic determinants first appears at different times in ontogeny.[73] The ability to produce anti-PC antibody is first detected relatively late, at about 1 week of age in mice.[74] The antibody response to other environmental antigens such as $\alpha 1 \rightarrow 3$ dextran and levan also appears late in ontogeny.[21,75] We have previously provided evidence that there is another major shift in immune responsiveness that takes place between 1 and 2 weeks after birth; the response to T-independent 1 antigens such as TNP-*B. abortus* is present from birth whereas the antibody response to T-independent 2 antigens such as TNP-Ficoll appears later in normal mice and never develops in *xid* mice.[76] This pattern of ontogeny has been explained by the early appearance of Lyb-5$^-$ B cells followed by the subsequent differentiation of Lyb-5$^+$ B lymphocytes. The adult anti-PC response seems to be segregated between a T15-idiotype-positive IgM response of Lyb-5$^+$ B cells and a 511- or 603-idiotype-positive IgG response of "Lyb-5$^-$" B cells. [The secondary IgG response to PC-KLH also contains many antibodies specific for PC + X determinants on PC-KLH that probably do not bear T15, 511, or 603 idiotypic markers (Refs. 29, 77, and our unpublished observations); we are excluding such antibodies from consideration in these arguments.] How can these observations in the adult be explained by considering the neonatal emergence of anti-PC clonotypes?

We propose that an important event in regulating the expression (*not* the generation) of the emerging anti-PC repertoire is the appearance of the Lyb-5$^+$ subset of B lymphocytes. We suggest [in concurrence with Wicker *et al.*[29] and N. Klinman (personal communication)] that the first B cells with anti-PC specificity are within the Lyb-5$^-$ subset, that these early B cells express T15, 511, and 603 idiotypes in a relatively equal and fixed ratio, and that these B cells are both unresponsive to T-independent PC antigens and highly susceptible to tolerance induction[10,78] in the absence of substantial T-cell help. The T15 clonotype is even more susceptible to tolerance induction than 511 or 603 clones because of its presumed higher avidity for environmental PC antigens.[40,42] Thus, when one manages to activate early PC precursors, e.g., with PC-LPS,[79] the response is *not* T15-dominant. At about 1 week of age, the Lyb-5$^+$ subset of B cells appears and expresses the T15, 511, and 603 idiotypes in similar proportion to the Lyb-5$^-$ subset. The Lyb-5$^+$ subset *is* responsive to T-independent forms of PC (which predominate in nature) and the T15 clonotype is selectively expanded for the same reason it is depleted in the Lyb-5$^-$ subset, because it is the best antigen binder. *Antigen selection* is therefore postulated to be a critical factor in establishing the adult balance of clonotype expression, as has been suggested by Thompson and Cancro.[80] The ratio of T15$^+$ to 511/603$^+$ antibodies in the adult can be influenced by the conditions of T-cell help, since Lyb-5$^-$ and Lyb-5$^+$ B cells seem to differ[66] in their susceptibility both to T cells and to helper factors. However, these T-cell influences are suggested to have little or no role in the initial shaping of the anti-PC repertoire (in agreement with our observations in nude mice). The major feature of this model is that it gives germline variable regions important for the survival of the species *two* chances to emerge and it absolves T cells of the responsibility of generating an anti-idiotypic repertoire during early ontogeny. The Lyb-5$^+$ subset also rapidly produces IgM and IgG3 anti-PC antibodies[81] that are highly effective against pathogenic PC-containing organisms.[82]

This model is as important for what it does *not* invoke as for what is postulated. Neither T cells specific for idiotypes nor anti-idiotype antibodies are postulated to play an important role in shaping the neonatal anti-PC response. Maternal transmission of anti-idiotype antibodies has been shown to influence clonotype expression in other systems[75,83] and can be shown under experimental conditions to influence the anti-PC repertoire (A. J. Feeney and D. E. Mosier, unpublished observations), but our view would be that antigen selection is more likely than anti-idiotype selection, and that both would have similar effects on emerging B cells. Helper and suppressor T cells with nominal specificity for "regulatory idiotopes"[25] may play a role in controlling ongoing adult anti-PC responses, but demonstration of their specificity must be stringent since any T cell with selective effects on either the Lyb-5$^-$ or the Lyb-5$^+$ subset could appear to be "specific" for a given idiotope. While T cells that proliferate when exposed to PC-binding antibodies have been demonstrated,[84] it is important to note that the fine specificity of such T cells is not for the observed anti-PC families but for some broadly shared determinant common to all anti-PC antibodies. These T cells would thus be of little value in the differential regulation of the major anti-

PC clonotypes. The final question then becomes, if we grant that anti-idiotypic regulation *can* occur, *does* it often play an important role?

References

1. Crews, S., Griffin, J., Huang, H., Calame, K., and Hood, L., 1981, A single V_H gene segment encodes the immune response to phosphorylcholine: Somatic mutation is correlated with the class of the antibody, *Cell* **25**:59.
2. Bothwell, A. L. M., Paskind, M., Reth, M., Imanishi-Kari, T., Rajewsky, K., and Baltimore, D., 1981, Heavy chain variable region contribution to the NP^b family of antibodies: Somatic mutation evident in a $\gamma 2_a$ variable region, *Cell* **24**:625.
3. Siekevitz, M., Gefter, M. L., Brodeur, P., Riblet, R., and Marshak-Rothstein, A., 1982, The genetic basis of antibody productions: The dominant anti-arsonate idiotype response of the strain A mouse, *Eur. J. Immunol.* **12**:1023.
4. Claflin, J. L., 1976, Uniformity in the clonal repertoire of the immune response to phosphorylcholine in mice, *Eur. J. Immunol.* **6**:669.
5. Nisonoff, A., Ju, S.-T., and Owen, F. L., 1977, Studies of structure and immunosuppression of a cross-reactive idiotype in strain A mice, *Immunol. Rev.* **34**:89.
6. Mäkelä, O., and Karjalainen, K., 1977, Inherited immunoglobulin idiotypes of the mouse, *Immunol. Rev.* **34**:119.
7. Weigert, M., and Riblet, R., 1978, The genetic control of antibody variable regions in the mouse, *Springer Semin. Immunopathol.* **1**:33.
8. Jerne, N. K., 1974, Towards a network theory of the immune system, *Ann. Immunol. (Inst. Pasteur)* **125C**:373.
9. Metcalf, E. S., and Klinman, N. R., 1977, *In vitro* tolerance induction of bone marrow cells: A marker for B cell maturation, *J. Immunol.* **118**:2111.
10. Metcalf, E. S., Sigal, N. H., and Klinman, N. R., 1977, *In vitro* tolerance induction of neonatal murine B cells as a probe for the study of B-cell diversification, *J. Exp. Med.* **145**:1382.
11. Nossal, G. J. V., and Pike, B. L., 1975, Evidence for the clonal abortion theory of B-lymphocyte tolerance, *J. Exp. Med.* **141**:904.
12. Kelsoe, G., Reth, M., and Rajewsky, K., 1980, Control of idiotype expression by monoclonal anti-idiotope antibodies, *Immunol. Rev.* **52**:75.
13. Eichmann, K., 1978, Expression and function of idiotypes on lymphocytes, *Adv. Immunol.* **26**:195.
14. Cosenza, H., Julius, M. H., and Augustin, A. A., 1977, Idiotypes as variable region markers: Analogies between receptors on phosphorylcholine-specific T and B lymphocytes, *Immunol. Rev.* **34**:3.
15. Bottomly, K., and Mosier, D. E., 1979, Mice whose B cells cannot produce the T15 idiotype also lack an antigen-specific helper T cell required for T15 expression, *J. Exp. Med.* **150**:1399.
16. Bottomly, K., Mathieson, B. J., and Mosier, D. E., 1978, Anti-idiotype induced regulation of helper cell function for the response to phosphorylcholine in adult BALB/c mice, *J. Exp. Med.* **148**:1216.
17. Woodland, R., and Cantor, H., 1978, Idiotype-specific T helper cells are required to induce idiotype-positive B memory cells to secrete antibody, *Eur. J. Immunol.* **8**:600.
18. Rowley, D. A., Köhler, H., Schreiber, H., Kaye, S. T., and Lorbach, I., 1976, Suppression by autogenous complementary idiotype: The priority of the first response, *J. Exp. Med.* **144**:946.
19. Cazenave, P. A., 1977, Idiotypic–anti-idiotypic regulation of antibody synthesis in rabbits, *Proc. Natl. Acad. Sci. USA* **74**:5122.
20. Urbain, J. Wikler, M., Fraussen, J. D., and Collignon, C., 1977, Idiotypic regulation of the immune system by the induction of antibodies against anti-idiotypic antibodies, *Proc. Natl. Acad. Sci. USA* **74**:5126.
21. Bona, C., Lieberman, R., Chien, C. C., Mond, J., House, S., Green, I., and Paul, W. E., 1978, Immune response to levan. I. Kinetics and ontogeny of anti-levan and anti-inulin antibody response and of expression of cross-reactive idiotype, *J. Immunol.* **120**:1436.
22. Bona, C., and Paul, W. E., 1979, Cellular basis of regulation of expression of idiotype. I. T-suppressor cells specific for MOPC 460 idiotype regulate the expression of cells secreting anti-TNP antibodies bearing 460 idiotype, *J. Exp. Med.* **149**:592.

23. Lewis, G. K., and Goodman, J. W., 1978, Purification of functional, determinant-specific, idiotype-bearing murine T cells, *J. Exp. Med.* **148**:915.
24. DuClos, T. W., and Kim, B. S., 1977, Suppressor T cells: Presence in mice rendered tolerant by neonatal treatment with anti-receptor antibody or antigen, *J. Immunol.* **119**:1769.
25. Paul, W. E., and Bona, C., 1982, Regulatory idiotopes and immune networks: A hypothesis, *Immunol. Today* **3**:230.
26. Sercarz, E. E., and Metzger, D. W., 1980, Epitope-specific and idiotype-specific cellular interactions in a model protein antigen system, *Springer Semin. Immunopathol.* **3**:145.
27. Rudikoff, S., 1983, Immunoglobulin structure–function correlates: Antigen binding and idiotypes, *Contemp. Top. Mol. Immunol.* **9**:169.
28. Kenny, J. J., Wicker, L. S., Guelde, G., and Scher, I., 1982, Regulation of T15 idiotype dominance. I. Mice expressing the *xid* immune defect provide normal help to T15$^+$ B cell precursors, *J. Immunol.* **129**:1534.
29. Wicker, L. S., Guelde, G., Scher, I., and Kenny, J. J., 1982, Antibodies from the Lyb-5$^-$ B cell subset predominate in the secondary IgG response to phosphocholine, *J. Immunol.* **129**:950.
30. Cosenza, H., and Köhler, H., 1972, Specific suppression of the antibody response by antibodies to receptors, *Proc. Natl. Acad. Sci. USA* **69**:2701.
31. Rudikoff, S., and Potter, M., 1976, Size differences among immunoglobulin heavy chains from phosphorylcholine-binding proteins, *Proc. Natl. Acad. Sci. USA* **73**:2109.
32. Kwan, S.-P., Rudikoff, S., Seidman, J. G., Leder, P., and Scharff, M. D., 1981, Nucleic acid and protein sequences of phosphocholine-binding light chains, *J. Exp. Med.* **153**:1366.
33. Clarke, S. H., Claflin, J. L., Potter, M., and Rudikoff, S., 1982, Polymorphisms in antiphosphocholine antibodies reflecting evolution of immunoglobulin families, *J. Exp. Med.* **157**:98.
34. Sher, A., and Cohn, M., 1972, Inheritance of an idiotype associated with the immune response of inbred mice to phosphorylcholine, *Eur. J. Immunol.* **2**:319.
35. Cosenza, H., and Köhler, H., 1972, Specific inhibition of plaque formation to phosphorylcholine by antibody against antibody, *Science* **176**:1027.
36. Claflin, J. L., and Davie, J. M., 1974, Clonal nature of the immune response to phosphorylcholine. III. Species-specific binding characteristics of rodent anti-phosphorylcholine antibodies, *J. Exp. Med.* **113**:1678.
37. Claflin, J. L., and Rudikoff, S., 1979, Structural evidence for a polymorphic or allelic form of the heavy chain variable region, *J. Immunol.* **122**:1402.
38. Williams, K. R., and Claflin, J. L., 1980, Clonotypes of anti-phosphocholine antibodies induced with *Proteus morganii* (Potter). I. Structural and idiotypic similarities in a diverse repertoire, *J. Immunol.* **125**:2429.
39. Wolfe, J., and Claflin, J. L., 1980, Clonal nature of the immune response to phosphocholine. IX. Heterogeneity among antibodies bearing M511 idiotypic determinants, *J. Immunol.* **125**:2397.
40. Andres, C. M., Maddalena, A., Hudak, S., Young, N. M., and Claflin, J. L., 1981, Anti-phosphocholine hybridoma antibodies. II. Functional analysis of binding sites within these antibody families, *J. Exp. Med.* **154**:1584.
41. Leon, M., and Young, N. M., 1971, Specificity for phosphorylcholine of six murine myeloma proteins reactive with pneumococcus C polysaccharide and β-lipoprotein, *Biochemistry* **10**:1424.
42. Briles, D. E., Forman, C., Hudak, S., and Claflin, J. L., 1983, Antiphosphorylcholine antibodies of the T15 idiotype are optimally protective against *Streptococcus pneumoniae*, *J. Exp. Med.* **156**:1177.
43. Strayer, D. S., Cosenza, H., Lee, W. M. F., Rowley, D. A., and Köhler, H., 1974, Neonatal tolerance induced by antibody against antigen-specific receptor, *Science* **186**:640.
44. Augustin, A., and Cosenza, H., 1976, Expression of new idiotypes following neonatal suppression of a dominant clone, *Eur. J. Immunol.* **6**:497.
45. Etlinger, H. M., and Heusser, C. H., 1982, Expression of a distinct B cell clonotype profile after recovery from antigen-induced unresponsiveness, *Eur. J. Immunol.* **12**:530.
46. Kim, B. S., and Greenberg, J. A., 1981, Mechanisms of idiotype suppression. IV. Functional neutralization in mixtures of idiotype-specific suppressor and hapten-specific suppressor T cells, *J. Exp. Med.* **154**:809.
47. Fung, J., and Köhler, H., 1980, Mechanism of neonatal idiotype supression. II. Alterations in the T cell compartment suppress the maturation of B cell precursors, *J. Immunol.* **125**:2489.

48. Heusser, C. H., Etlinger, H. M., and Julius, M. H., 1983, Thymus-independent induction and antigen-dependent recovery of idiotype-specific suppression, *Cell. Immunol.* **76**:148.
49. Etlinger, H. M., and Heusser, C. H., 1983, Alteration of immunologic function through early ontogenetic experiences: Selective inactivation of T15-positive B cells in neonatal mice is related to receptor avidity and is independent of thymus function, *Eur. J. Immunol.* **13**:180.
50. Kim, B. S., and Hopkins, W. J., 1978, Tolerance rendered by neonatal treatment with anti-idiotypic antibodies: Induction and maintenance in athymic mice, *Cell. Immunol.* **35**:460.
51. Ward, K., Cantor, H., and Boyse, E. A., 1977, Clonally-restricted interactions among T and B cell subclasses, in: *Immune System: Genetics and Regulation* (E. Sercarz, L. A. Herzenberg, and C. F. Fox, eds.), Academic Press, New York, p. 397.
52. Marrack (Hunter), P. C., and Kappler, J. W., 1975, Antigen-specific and nonspecific mediators of T cell/B cell cooperation. I. Evidence for their production by different T cells, *J. Immunol.* **114**:1116.
53. Tada, T., Takemori, T., Ikumura, K., Nonaka, M., and Tokuhisa, T., 1978, Two distinct types of helper T cells involved in the secondary antibody response: Independent and synergistic effects of Ia$^-$ and Ia$^+$ helper T cells, *J. Exp. Med.* **147**:446.
54. Janeway, C. A., Jr., Bert, D. L., and Shen, F.-W., 1980, Cell cooperation during *in vivo* anti-hapten antibody responses. V. Two synergistic Ly-1$^+$23$^-$ helper T cells with distinctive specificities, *Eur. J. Immunol.* **10**:231.
55. Eardley, D. D., Hugenberger, J., McVay-Boudreau, L., Shen, F.-W., Gershon, R. W., and Cantor, H., 1978, Immunoregulatory circuits amont T-cell sets. I. T-helper cells induce other T-cell sets to exert feedback inhibition, *J. Exp. Med.* **147**:1106.
56. Herzenberg, L. A., Tokuhisa, T., Parks, D. R., and Herzenberg, L. A., 1982, Epitope-specific regulation. II. A bistable, Igh-restricted regulatory mechanism central to immunologic memory, *J. Exp. Med.* **155**:1741.
57. Eichmann, K., 1974, Idiotypic suppression. I. Influence of the dose and of the effector function of anti-idiotypic antibody on the production of an idiotype, *Eur. J. Immunol.* **4**:296.
58. Bottomly, K., Janeway, C. A., Jr., Mathieson, B. J., and Mosier, D. E., 1980, Absence of an antigen-specific helper T cell required for the expression of the T15 idiotype in mice treated with anti-μ antibody, *Eur. J. Immunol.* **10**:159.
59. Bottomly, K., and Mosier, D. E., 1980, Analogous dual specificity of helper T cells cooperating in the generation of clonally-restricted antibody responses, in: *Strategies for Immune Regulation* (E. E. Sercarz and A. Cunningham, eds.), Academic Press, New York, pp. 487–492.
60. Bottomly, K., and Mosier, D. E., 1981, Antigen specific helper T cells required for dominant idiotype expression are not H-2 restricted, *J. Exp. Med.* **154**:411.
60a. Feeney, A. J., and D. E. Mosier, 1984, Helper-T lymphocytes from *xid* and normal mice support anti-phosphocholine antibody response with equivalent T15, 511, and 603 idiotypic composition, submitted for publication.
61. Mond, J. J., Lieberman, R. L., Inman, J. K., Mosier, D. E., and Paul, W. E., 1977, Inability of mice with a defect in B-lymphocyte maturation to respond to phosphorylcholine on immunogenic carriers, *J. Exp. Med.* **146**:1138.
62. Quintáns, J., Quan, Z. A., and Arias, M. A., 1982, Mice with the *xid* defect have helper cells for T15 idiotype dominant anti-phosphorylcholine primary and secondary plaque-forming cell responses, *J. Exp. Med.* **155**:1245.
63. Augustin, A. A., Julius, M. H., and Cosenza, H., 1979, Antigen-specific stimulation and trans-stimulation of T cells in long-term culture, *Eur. J. Immunol.* **9**:665.
64. Ahmed, A., Scher, I., Sharrow, S. O., Smith, A. H., Paul, W. E., Sachs, D. H., and Sell, K. W., 1977, B-lymphocyte heterogeneity: Development and characterization of an alloantiserum which distinguishes B-lymphocyte differentiation alloantigens, *J. Exp. Med.* **145**:101.
65. Ono, S., Yaffee, L. J., Ryan, J. L., and Singer, A., 1983, Functional heterogeneity of the Lyb-5$^-$ B cell subpopulation: Mutant *xid* B cells and normal Lyb-5$^-$ B cells differ in their responsiveness to phenol-extracted lipopolysaccharide, *J. Immunol.* **130**:2014.
66. Singer, A., Asano, Y., Shigeta, M., Hathcock, K. S., Ahmed, A., Fathman, C. G., and Hodes, R. J., 1982, Distinct B cell subpopulations differ in their genetic requirements for activation by T helper cells, *Immunol. Rev.* **64**:137.

67. Imperiale, M. J., Faherty, D. A., Sproviero, J. F., and Zauderer, M., 1982, Functionally distinct helper T cells enriched under different culture conditions cooperate with different B cells, *J. Immunol.* **129**:1843.
68. Clough, E. R., Levy, D. A., and Cebra, J. J., 1981, CBA/N × BALB/cJ F₁ male and female mice can be primed to express quantitatively equivalent secondary anti-phosphocholine responses, *J. Immunol.* **126**:387.
69. Chang, S. P., and Rittenberg, M. R., 1981, Immunologic memory to phosphorylcholine *in vitro*. I. Asymmetric expression of clonal dominance, *J. Immunol.* **126**:975.
70. Kiessling, R., and Wigzell, H., 1979, An analysis of the murine NK cell as to structure, function and biological relevance, *Immunol. Rev.* **44**:165.
71. Okumura, K., Hayakawa, K., and Tada, T., 1982, Cell-to-cell interaction controlled by immunoglobulin genes: Role of Thy-1⁻, Lyt-1⁺, Ig⁺ (B′) cell in allotype-restricted antibody production, *J. Exp. Med.* **156**:443.
72. Cosenza, H., Augustin, A. A., and Julius, M. H., 1977, Induction and characterization of "autologous" anti-idiotypic antibodies, *Eur. J. Immunol.* **7**:273.
73. Klinman, N. R., Sigal, N. H., Metcalf, E. S., Pierce, S. K., and Gearhart, P. J., 1977, The interplay of evolution and environment in B-cell diversification, *Cold Spring Harbor Symp. Quant. Biol.* **41**:165.
74. Sigal, N. H., Gearhart, P. J., Press, J. L., and Klinman, N. R., 1976, Late acquisition of a germ line antibody specificity, *Nature* **259**:51.
75. Weiler, I. J., Weiler, E., Sprenger, R., and Cosenza, H., 1977, Idiotype suppression by maternal influence, *Eur. J. Immunol.* **7**:592.
76. Mosier, D. E., Mond, J. J., and Goldings, E. A., 1977, The ontogeny of thymic independent antibody responses *in vitro* in normal mice and mice with an X-linked B cell defect, *J. Immunol.* **119**:1874.
77. Chang, S. P., Brown, M., and Rittenberg, M. B., 1982, Immunologic memory to phosphorylcholine. II. PC-KLH induces two antibody populations that dominate different isotypes, *J. Immunol.* **128**:702.
78. Metcalf, E. S., Scher, I., and Klinman, N. R., 1980, Susceptibility to *in vitro* tolerance induction of adult B cells from mice with an X-linked B cell defect, *J. Exp. Med.* **151**:486.
79. Fung, J., and Köhler, H., 1980, Mechanism of neonatal idiotype suppression. I. State of the suppressed B cell, *J. Immunol.* **125**:1998.
80. Thompson, M. A., and Cancro, M. P., 1982, Dynamics of B-cell repertoire formation: Normal patterns of clonal turnover are altered by ligand interaction, *J. Immunol.* **129**:2372.
81. Slack, J., Der-Balian, G. P., Nahm, M., and Davie, J. M., 1980, Subclass restriction of murine antibodies. II. The IgG plaque-forming cell response of thymus-dependent type 1 and 2 antigens in normal mice and mice expressing an X-linked immunodeficiency, *J. Exp. Med.* **151**:853.
82. Briles, D. E., Claflin, J. L., Schroer, K., and Forman, C., 1981, Mouse IgG₃ antibodies are highly protective against infection with *Streptococcus pneumoniae, Nature* **294**:88.
83. Olson, J. C., and Leslie, G. A., 1981, Inheritance patterns of idiotype expressions: Maternal–fetal immune regulatory networks, *Immunogenetics* **13**:39.
84. Gleason, K., Pierce, S., and Köhler, H., 1981, Generation of idiotypic-specific T cell help through network perturbation, *J. Exp. Med.* **153**:924.

26

Auto-Anti-Idiotype Production during the Response to Antigen

G. JEANETTE THORBECKE AND GREGORY W. SISKIND

1. Introduction

Jerne, [1] building on earlier observations on the existence of idiotypic determinants related to the antigen combining sites of human myeloma proteins[2] and rabbit antibodies,[3] proposed that the immune system is self-regulated by a network of idiotype–anti-idiotype (Id–anti-Id) interactions. Numerous studies have documented biological effects of passively administered heterologous anti-Id consistent with predictions based on the Jerne network hypothesis.[1] An important advance was the observation that anti-Id can be induced in animals which are genetically identical to the donor of the immunizing antibody.[4-6] This was crucial in establishing that this form of autoimmune response can occur. However, the ultimate testing of Jerne's hypothesis must include the demonstration of spontaneous auto-anti-Id production following antigen administration and a regulatory influence of such autoantibody. Evidence is accumulating that T cells may also express Id-like determinants[7-14] and that V_H-restricted receptor–antireceptor circuits are activated during an immune response and serve important regulatory functions. T–T-cell interactions are dealt with in other chapters of this volume. In addition, specific immune B cells are known to induce suppressor activity which is T cell mediated, in some cases shown to be V_H-restricted and likely to be anti-Id in specificity.[15,16] In most of the reports on suppressor cell circuits, secretion of auto-anti-Id by the B cells is not regarded as the mechanism of suppression. In the present discussion we will focus on humoral auto-anti-Id of which the immunoglobulin nature has been established and we will primarily consider auto-anti-Id produced "spontaneously" during the response to antigen.

G. JEANETTE THORBECKE • Department of Pathology, New York University School of Medicine, New York, New York 10016.   GREGORY W. SISKIND • Division of Allergy and Immunology, Department of Medicine, Cornell University Medical College, New York, New York 10021.
Support: AG-04980 and AI-11694, NIH, DHHS.

417

2. Demonstration of Auto-Anti-Id Production

The earliest report of the production of auto-anti-Id antibody following antigen administration appeared in 1974 when Kluskens and Kohler[17] documented the appearance of autoantibodies against the T15 Id in BALB/c mice hyperimmunized with *S. pneumoniae* R36A vaccine. They demonstrated this antibody by agglutination of T15-coated SRBC and clearly established its anti-Id specificity. In subsequent studies Cosenza[18] was able to demonstrate anti-Id PFC and follow the kinetics of their appearance. After these initial observations spontaneous autologous anti-Id antibody production during the course of an immune response to antigen has been described for haptens,[19,20] proteins,[21] polysaccharide antigens,[22,23] SRBC,[24] and auto- and alloantigens,[25–28] including Ids themselves.[29]

Two general approaches have been employed to detect serum anti-Id: (1) direct binding to Id$^+$ antibody detected by hemagglutination,[17] radioimmunoassay,[5,6,21] or enzyme-linked immunosorbent assay (ELISA)[30]; and (2) hapten-reversible inhibition of antibody secretion detected in a PFC assay.[31] Finally, cells whose secretion of antibody has been down-regulated *in vivo* by the binding of auto-anti-Id have been detected by the demonstration of an increased number of PFC in the presence of low concentrations of hapten or after brief preincubation of cells with hapten (hapten augmentation of plaque formation[20]). The validity, advantages and disadvantages, and technical problems associated with the use of hapten augmentation of plaque formation as an assay for auto-anti-Id-inhibited potential antibody-secreting cells have been discussed in detail[32] and will therefore not be considered here. Using such assays, auto-anti-Id production has been demonstrated in mice,[17] rabbits,[5,33] rats,[27] chickens,[33] and humans.[21,34–36] Auto-anti-Id-secreting cells have also been detected as PFC using Id-coated erythrocytes as targets.[18]

In addition to the evidence which shows auto-anti-Id production during the response to antigen, it has been demonstrated that injection of Id bearing immunoglobulin can lead not only to production of anti-Id (Ab$_2$) but also to appearance in the serum of antibody directed to Ab$_2$, i.e., Ab$_3$. This represents an interesting form of auto-anti-Id production, supporting the concept that an Id-specific network can be activated.[29] Furthermore, the recent preparation of monoclonal Ab$_3$ from spleen cells of mice immunized with pneumococcal vaccine shows that the progression from Ab$_2$ to Ab$_3$ can follow the immunization with antigen.[37]

3. Properties of Auto-Anti-Id

3.1. Role of Antigen

Auto-anti-Id production has been observed following immunization with a variety of antigens including RBC,[24,38] proteins,[21,25,39] hapten–protein conjugates,[32,40] polysaccharides,[17,22,23,41] polysaccharide conjugates,[18,32] hapten–*B. abortus* conjugates,[33] and chemically reactive haptens.[19] It thus appears that the nature of the antigen and its thymic dependence is not critical for the activation of the network. It is likely that the degree of immunogenicity of the antigen is important since immune complexes are known to be particularly effective in inducing anti-Id responses.[4] Binion and Rodkey[42] suggest that the expression of a particular germline is of importance in the induction of regulatory auto-anti-Id. Since the presence of a dominant public Id greatly facilitates the application of techniques required for the detection of anti-Id, it is difficult to defend a definitive conclusion about this point.

3.2. T-Cell Dependence of Auto-Anti-Id Production

Since the antigen (Id) which induces auto-anti-Id production is a protein, the response would be expected to be T cell dependent. This dependence is most readily demonstrated using T-independent (TI) antigens. We have shown that both nude (athymic) mice and irradiated thymectomized mice reconstituted with bone marrow fail to produce auto-anti-Id during the immune response to TNP-Ficoll.[43] Similar observations were subsequently reported in the T15 Id response to R36 *S. pneumoniae* by Kelsoe *et al.*[41] and by Hiernaux *et al.*[44] in the E109 Id response to levan. Several reports suggest that Id-specific helper cells are important in promoting the production of Id.[45–52] However, the specificity of the helper cell required for the production of auto-anti-Id has not been established.

3.3. Kinetics of Auto-Anti-Id Response and Id–Anti-Id Cycling

In general auto-anti-Id appears after the Id but relatively early during the immune response. For example, following TNP-Ficoll injection of mice, anti-TNP PFC peak approximately on day 3–4 while hapten-augmentable PFC are first detectable on day 5.[20] In the T15 Id system auto-anti-Id PFC appear approximately 3 days after the peak of the secondary antiphosphorylcholine response.[18] The observation that the auto-anti-Id PFC response is higher in the secondary than in the primary response to *S. pneumoniae*[18] is consistent with findings of Goidl *et al.*[40] who report a high incidence, and more rapid occurrence of hapten-augmentable PFC in the secondary than in the primary response to TNP-Ficoll. Thus, the auto-anti-Id response to a TI antigen has the classical characteristics of a secondary immune response. In contrast, the incidence and kinetics of appearance of hapten-augmentable PFC during the primary and secondary responses to the T-dependent (TD) antigen TNP-BGG are indistinguishable. However, the optimal concentration of hapten required to detect hapten-augmentable PFC is considerably lower in the secondary response to TNP-BGG than in the primary response (10^{-10} M TNP-EACA as compared with 10^{-8} M). These observations are consistent with the known marked heterogeneity of the antibody response to TNP-proteins and the increased affinity of the antibody produced during the secondary response to these antigens. The increased affinity suggests that different clones are stimulated early in the secondary as compared with early in the primary response. Thus, the anti-Id produced in the secondary response to TNP-BGG may in effect be a primary response to a different Id. The higher affinity (for TNP) of the antibody-secreting cells in the secondary response accounts for the ability of lower concentrations of hapten to be effective in competing with anti-Id antibody for binding to cell surface Id.[40]

During the primary response to *S. pneumoniae,* Cosenza[18] observed a peak anti-pneumococcal polysaccharide PFC response on day 5 followed by an anti-T15 Id PFC response which peaked on day 8. It is of interest that this antipneumococcal pattern of Id and anti-Id production was also observed by Kelsoe and Cerny[53] who described a cycling of antipneumococcal PFC and T15 Id-binding cells. Cycling of Id and anti-Id production was also described in the response of mice to bacterial levan[44] and thus may represent a general phenomenon at least in responses to polysaccharide antigens.

3.4. Isotype of Auto-Anti-Id

The earliest auto-anti-Id detected by Cosenza[18] during the primary response consisted of IgM antibody since it was detected as direct PFC. Most analyses of sera have identified the auto-anti-Id as IgG.[30,54,55] In our own studies[54] the auto-anti-Id detected 1 week after injection of TNP-Ficoll and 3 weeks after TNP-*B. abortus* tended to belong to the IgG2a and IgG2b isotypes. In the human[21,35] the auto-anti-Id detected so far has also been identified as IgG.

3.5. Effect of Age on the Auto-Anti-Id Response

Although the antibody responses of aged mice are generally of low magnitude, their auto-anti-Id responses appear to be disproportionately high, rapid in onset, and less T dependent[56–58] than in young mice. This has been observed with both TD and TI antigens. The enhanced auto-anti-Id response of aged mice can be detected both serologically (by an ELISA) and as an increased incidence of hapten-augmentable PFC. In fact, the auto-anti-Id response of aged mice has properties more typical of a secondary than of a primary response, as if repeated exposure to environmental and self antigens had primed the animal for auto-anti-Id responses.

In a further analysis of the cellular basis for this phenomenon[57] it has been found that the increased auto-anti-Id response of aged mice is an inherent property of splenic B-cell population since irradiated mice reconstituted with splenic B cells from aged donors produce a high incidence of hapten-augmentable PFC. In contrast, bone marrow from aged donors fails to transfer a high hapten-augmentable PFC response. It appears that peripheral T cells regulate this effect since irradiated mice reconstituted with bone marrow from young or old donors together with splenic T cells from old donors produce a high hapten-augmentable PFC response while recipients of splenic T cells from young donors produce a low incidence of hapten-augmentable PFC regardless of the age of the bone marrow donor. Thus, if life-long contact with environmental antigens is responsible for shifts in the Id network, then the long-lived peripheral T-cell population appears to act as a repository for this information, presumably via Id–anti-Id interactions with B cells arising from the bone marrow.

3.6. Auto-Anti-Id as Internal Image

The possibility that anti-Id can be an "image" of the epitope has been discussed extensively by Nisonoff and Lamoyi.[59] An auto-anti-Id may thus be an *internal* image of an epitope on an antigen. Such an anti-Id, rather than reacting with a specific Id, would react with all antibodies (paratopes) reactive with that epitope since it is structurally mimicking that antigenic determinant. If antibody to a hormone were to mimic the spatial configuration of a receptor, anti-Id could act as an antireceptor antibody and be difficult to distinguish from an autoantibody to that receptor.[60,67]

4. Regulation of Immune Response by Auto-Anti-Id

Network theories postulate that the immune system is regulated via Id–anti-Id interactions.[1] That heterologous anti-Id can down-regulate or stimulate Id expression has been firmly established (reviewed in Ref. 68). This suggests that auto-anti-Id could have similar regulatory influences. A number of observations consistent with this view have been reported and are discussed below.

4.1. Influence of Auto-anti-Id on the Quantity and Quality of the Humoral Immune Response

The observation[20] that addition of hapten to an immune cell suspension can at times increase the number of detectable antibody-secreting cells (hapten-augmentable PFC) implies that down-regulation of antibody secretion by mature B cells occurs *in vivo*. Since such hapten-augmentable PFC are mainly seen after the peak of the primary antibody response it is likely that, in part, the decrease in antibody-secreting cells is due to regulatory effects of auto-anti-Id. Nude (athymic) mice which do not produce auto-anti-Id show a reduced rate of decrease in PFC as compared with euthymic congenic mice.[43] Similarly, the inverse relationship between the production of Id and auto-anti-Id[26,44,53] implies an *in vivo* down-regulating effect of auto-anti-Id. However, it should be emphasized that there still is a relatively rapid decrease in PFC within a few days after the peak of the primary response to TNP-Ficoll in nude mice[43,69] and that in some systems the cycling of antibody production persists in nude mice.[44] Thus, auto-anti-Id does not appear to be an essential factor in causing the decrease in antibody synthesis late in the primary response.

Since down-regulation by anti-Id is necessarily Id specific (except when anti-Id is an internal image of the antigen) the production of anti-Id probably not only affects the quantity but also the quality of the antibody response. Thus, changes in Id expression with time during the immune response could, to some extent, be a consequence of auto-anti-Id down regulation. The possibility that auto-anti-Id contributes to the known tendency to shift toward high-affinity antibody production during the immune response[70,71] has not yet been evaluated. Recent findings indicate that mice also tend to produce different Ids in response to the same hapten on different carriers.[54,72–75] In our own studies with TNP conjugates[54] we could not determine with certainty whether the difference between responses to TNP-Ficoll and TNP-protein conjugates was qualitative or merely quantitative. It was, however, clear that individual mice of a single inbred strain differed at least quantitatively in Id expression following immunization with a single TNP conjugate. In considering differences in Id expression one must bear in mind that many antihapten immune responses, such as the anti-DNP response, are highly heterogeneous.[71] We have obtained a minimal estimate that at least 12 anti-DNP antibodies of different affinities are required to account for the shape of hapten-binding curves of immune serum[76] and many more clones are probably involved in these responses. Shifts in clonal expression are also implied by observations of changes in antibody affinity with time.[70,71,76,77] In view of this marked heterogeneity, the occurrence of variability in Id expression with time after antigen injection or upon immunization with a hapten conjugated to different carriers is not surprising.

Differences in Id expression during the immune response to haptens on TD and TI carriers appear to be particularly marked.[54,72,73] It is conceivable that such differences reflect actual paratope differences since hapten is presumably recognized in combination with some part of the carrier structure. In addition, however, there may be some delineation of Id expression among B-cell subpopulations. It is possible that the Lyb-5$^+$ B-cell population, which is the predominant or only one responding to TNP-Ficoll, differs sufficiently from the Lyb-5$^-$ population to be stimulated to expand by totally different environmental antigens. As a result, the B-cell populations which are ready to respond upon introduction of a TI conjugate have a different V^H repertoire than the population responding to a TD one. Differential representation of κ and λ light chains in anti-DNP antibodies of mice responding to TD and TI antigens has also been reported.[78] It is also of interest to note that differences in Id repertoire are exhibited even by polyclonally activated B cells *in vitro* depending on the B-cell mitogen used for their activation.[79] The possible role of auto-anti-Id production in mediating the control of Id repertoire expression by different B-cell subpopulations cannot be evaluated from data available at this time.

It is theoretically possible to explain the persistence of certain immune responses as due to Ab$_2$ stimulating Ab$_1$ production and *vice versa,* i.e., the establishment of a steady state which is self-maintained in the absence of antigen at the Id–anti-Id level of interaction as suggested by Jerne.[1] This provides a powerful adaptive mechanism by which the organism can record and maintain an inventory of its interactions with its environment. These interactions most likely occur at both T- and B-cell levels.

It is of interest to consider why anti-Id might differ from antigen in its effects on cells. Studies by Eichmann[80] suggest that at least part of the effect of anti-Id on cells might be dependent on its isotype. Indeed, in view of the wealth of literature which suggests that interaction with the Fc receptor on the B-cell surface, particularly by ligands which also bind to surface immunoglobulin,[81–83] delivers a down-regulatory signal to the cell, the isotype influence is not surprising. For instance, it is known that suppression by immune complexes and by passive antibody is dependent, at least in part, on the presence of the Fc portion of the immunoglobulin molecule.[84] Down-regulation of Id production by heterologous anti-Id is also Fc dependent.[80,85] Furthermore, the relative ease of B-cell tolerance induction with certain immunoglobulins appears to be Fc related,[86–88] as is the ability of immature B cells to be primed for a high-affinity secondary response.[89] The importance of cross-linking Fc receptors and surface immunoglobulin in providing an inhibiting signal to B cells was clearly demonstrated by Phillips and Parker (83) who studied the activation of B cells by F(ab')$_2$ fragments of anti-μ and lymphokines. This activation was prevented by intact anti-μ, but not by rabbit anti-μ complexed to staphylococcal protein A in which the Fc was blocked nor by antigen–antibody complexes which did not interact with surface immunoglobulin. Therefore, it is likely that the effect of auto-anti-Id on both B and T cells will depend on (1) the isotope of the anti-Id, (2) the availability of costimulatory molecules, and (3) the state of differentiation of the lymphoid cell population.[90–92]

4.2. Regulatory Role of Auto-Anti-Id on the Cellular Immune Response

Antisera known to contain auto-anti-Id specific for anti-TNP antibody[19,93] and auto-anti-Id-containing eluates, prepared by incubating TNP-Ficoll immune spleen cells with hapten[94], have been shown to modulate cellular immunity. Inhibition of delayed hypersensitivity could be demonstrated in two ways: (1) by incubation of cells used for transfer of contact sensitivity with auto-anti-Id with or without complement[19,95] and (2) by injection of auto-anti-Id at the time of sensitization for contact sensitivity *in vivo*.[94] Since the auto-anti-Id-containing antisera employed by Sy *et al.*[19] were obtained from animals which had been painted with DNCB, it appears that auto-anti-Id is produced during contact sensitization and can influence the course of the immune response. The consequence of this influence is hard to predict since a similarly induced auto-anti-Id was shown by Asherson *et al.*[93] to inhibit the down-regulating activity of suppressor effector cells on contact sensitivity.

In a totally different system Forstrom *et al.*[96] obtained a monoclonal antibody which exhibited anti-Id properties from mice immunized with a methylcholanthrene-induced sarcoma. It was capable of inducing delayed hypersensitivity to the sarcoma in an antigen-specific and allotype-restricted manner and did not bind to the sarcoma cells. The authors postulated that the so-called "unblocking" antibodies in tumor immune mice may represent auto-anti-Id.

4.3. Oral Immunization

It has been suggested that one of the factors contributing to the unresponsiveness resulting from oral presentation of antigen is the production of auto-anti-Id. Kagnoff[38] described a suppressive activity in the sera of SRBC-fed mice which bore immunoglobulin determinants and in some cases did not bind to antigen, suggesting that either an auto-anti-Id or an immune complex mediated the effect. Jackson and Mestecky[39] observed the appearance of anti-Id-containing plasma cells in the spleens and mucosal tissues of rabbits given antigen both orally and intravenously. In our laboratory the incidence of hapten-augmentable PFC during the immune response to intravenously injected TI antigens was found to be much higher in rabbits which had previously been fed with antigen than in controls.[97] Although the down-regulating role of auto-anti-Id following oral administration of antigen is difficult to evaluate, it is clear that this route of antigen presentation may lead to the appearance of Id–anti-Id complexes in the serum. This has been documented in man by Cunningham-Rundles[35] who found immune complexes consisting of anticasein antibody and auto-anti-Id in sera of IgA-deficient subjects. Immune complexes of casein–anticasein were proposed as the inducers of the auto-anti-Id. While it is clear that immune complexes are very efficient in inducing anti-Id[4] there is no compelling evidence that they are essential for its induction.

4.4. Possible Importance of Auto-Anti-Id in the Maternal–Fetal Relationship

Since immature B cells are exquisitely sensitive to the suppressive effects of anti-Id[92], auto-anti-Id transferred from mother to fetus would be expected to modulate Id expression by the offspring in a manner distinct from anticipated Id inheritence patterns. Such a non-genetic influence on the pattern of Id expression has been demonstrated in studies by Olson and Leslie[98] who suggest that the effects might be mediated by auto-anti-Id.

The relatively low percentage of multiparous women who produce antibody specific for the paternal contribution to their offsprings' HLA antigens is surprising.[99] Recent studies by Suciu-Foca et al.[100] suggest that this may be due to the production of auto-anti-Id to Ids reactive with these HLA antigens. They found putative auto-anti-Id, which specifically inhibited the antipaternal HLA activity of autologous sera, in all parous women studied.

4.5. Possible Role of Auto-Anti-Id in Immunologic Tolerance

Binz and Wigzell[7] demonstrated that stimulation of anti-Id activity can bring about a state of homograft tolerance. Resistance to graft-versus-host disease on the basis of auto-anti-Id production was described by McKearn et al.[101] It is possible that self tolerance, as well as neonatally induced tolerance to a foreign antigen, may in some cases be due to auto-anti-Id production. However, the relatively normal development of agammaglobulinemic chickens and humans, and the possibility of inducing tolerance in agammaglobulinemic chickens[102,103] suggest that humoral auto-anti-Id cannot be essential for self tolerance.

Although auto-anti-Id is produced during the immune response to dextran and suppresses the secondary response it is not found in neonatally tolerized mice.[104] Wood et al.[104] conclude that a B-cell response to dextran is required for the induction of auto-anti-Id and that therefore, in partial but not in complete tolerance, auto-anti-Id might contribute to the unresponsive state to TI antigens.

5. Relevance of Auto-Anti-Id to Disease

5.1. Production of Immune Complexes

The simultaneous production of Id and auto-anti-Id can lead to the presence of circulating immune complexes as well as the deposition of complexes in the tissues, in particular the kidneys. The animal model in which complexes of Id and anti-Id have been demonstrated in both the circulation and tissues is the T15 Id system.[105,106] Injection of LPS, a polyclonal B-cell activator, into BALB/c mice leads to the simultaneous production of T15 Id and auto-anti-Id. Since these immune complexes are produced without injection of specific antigen the findings suggest that one pathway to the production of immune complexes and tissue damage in human disease may be via polyclonal B-cell activation. It is interesting to note in this regard that many of the immune complex diseases are associated with polyclonal hypergammaglobulinemia. The presence of Id–anti-Id complexes has also been suggested in sera of some patients with mixed cryoglobulinemia.[107] Id–anti-Id complexes have also been observed during hyperimmunization of rabbits with *M. lysodeikticus* vaccine. These complexes precipitated upon dilution of the sera.[55] In man, as was already discussed above, immune complexes of anticasein and anti-Id were found in sera of IgA-deficient individuals presumably in response to ingested milk protein.[35]

If the increased auto-anti-Id in aged mice is a general phenomenon, then one would expect Id–anti-Id complexes to be prevalent in the sera of the aged. Such complexes might in turn stimulate the production of rheumatoid factor, the incidence of which is known to increase with age.[108,109]

5.2. Production of Auto-Anti-Id in the Response to Autoantigens

Auto-anti-Id specific for antibodies to a number of different autoantigens including erythrocytes,[28] DNA,[34,36] and the acetylcholine receptor[110] have been described. In addition, auto-anti-Id, which reacts with the insulin receptor and thereby has insulin-like activity, is produced in mice immunized with heterologous insulin.[111] Autoantibodies with similar ability to interact with the insulin receptor, but which were not clearly identified as anti-Id, were detected in the serum of patients with juvenile-onset diabetes.[112]

Thus, in addition to the nonspecific effects of auto-anti-Id via immune complex production, such antibodies can have both positive and negative immunologically specific influences on autoimmune disease. If the auto-anti-Id (internal image of an autoantigen) interacts with a cell surface receptor, it may disrupt normal homeostasis by activating cells inappropriately or by competing with the normal ligand (hormone), thereby blocking activation of the cells. Furthermore, depending on the isotype, concentration, and other properties of the auto-anti-Id and of the host, such antibodies could down-regulate or stimulate autoantibody production.

The occurrence of hapten-augmentable PFC and the cyclic shifts in Id and anti-Id discussed above strongly suggest a regulatory function for auto-anti-Id. Responses of restricted heterogeneity, such as the response to an autoantigen is likely to be, should be easier to down-regulate than a highly heterogeneous response. While the production of an internal image of the antigen might create complications, auto-anti-Id would usually be expected to depress autoantibody production. If auto-anti-Id, perhaps by cross-linking Fc receptors and surface immunoglobulin, contributes to the maintenance of self tolerance, then the development of autoimmunity would be favored by: (1) decreased auto-anti-Id production or (2) reduced sensitivity of immunocytes to down-regulation. Some evidence for both of these predisposing conditions has been observed in autoimmune-prone mouse strains. NZB mice have been reported to lack hapten-augmentable PFC during the immune response to TNP-Ficoll.[32] In addition, B cells of NZB mice have been shown to be resistant to the down-regulatory effects of anti-μ.[113] (R. T. Woodland, personal communication). If, as we have suggested,[114] cross-linking is important, defects in Fc receptors would also lead to resistance to down-regulation. Indeed, an HLA-linked defect in Fc receptor function has been observed in patients with dermatitis herpetiformis and systemic lupus erythematosus.[115,116]

5.3. Potential Applications in Immune Modulation

Stimulation of auto-anti-Id production might, in some circumstances, have a therapeutically desirable effect. (1) In the case of Id-bearing lymphomas, an immunotoxin prepared by coupling a toxic molecule such as ricin to a heterologous anti-Id has been shown to have a therapeutic effect.[117] Clearly, prolonged treatment with heterologous antibody can lead to many complications (e.g., serum sickness or anaphylaxis). On the other hand, if a method could be found to stimulate appropriate auto-anti-Id production, possibly by use of modified tumor cells, adjuvants, or by hybridomas prepared from autologous lymphoid cells, these immunological complications would be avoided. (2) Down-regulation of autoantibody production by promotion of auto-anti-Id production might have a beneficial effect on the course of autoimmune disease. The potential feasibility of such an approach is suggested by the ability of Neilson and Phillips[118] to prevent the induction of experimental interstitial nephritis by pretreating the rats with tubular antigen-reactive T lymphoblasts so as to induce anti-Id antibodies. In humans, the approach of Schwartz et al.[119] of "immunizing" lymphoid cells in vitro to produce putative Id-bearing immunocytes for use in induction of anti-Id, might be applicable. (3) Since some anti-Id specific for anti-hormone antibodies have been shown to possess hormone-like activity,[61,63,66] it is theoretically possible to stimulate an autologous immunoglobulin which could replace a hormone in a deficiency state. (4) In some experimental systems, suppressor cells prevent effective tumor immunity. If such suppressor cells are Id-bearing, then stimulation of auto-anti-Id might change the balance in favor of tumor rejection. The possibility of modifying humoral Id expression by inactivating suppressor T cells with anti-Id has been demonstrated by Bona et al.[120] in the mouse MOPC460 Id system. (5) As discussed above, tolerance to allografts can be due to auto-anti-Id reactivity.[7] This could potentially provide a useful model for prevention of allograft rejection. Thus, considerations of autologous network interactions lead to a variety of theoretical approaches to modulating the immune system in a therapeutically beneficial manner.

ACKNOWLEDGMENT. The research described in this chapter was supported by grants AG-04980 and AI-11694 from the National Institutes of Health, Department of Health and Human Services.

References

1. Jerne, N. K., 1974, Towards a network theory of the immune system, Ann. Immunol. (Inst. Pasteur) 125C:373.
2. Kunkel, H. G., Mannik, M., and Williams, R. C., 1963, Individual antigenic specificity of isolated antibodies, Science 140:1218.
3. Oudin, J., and Michel, M., 1963, Une nouvelle forme d'allotypie des globulins γ du serum de lapin, apparemment liée et a la specificite anticorps, C.R. Acad. Sci. 257:805.
4. Klaus, G. G. B., 1978, Antigen–antibody complexes elicit anti-idiotypic antibodies to self-idiotypes, Nature 272:265.
5. Rodkey, L. S., 1974, Studies of idiotypic antibodies: Production and characterization of autoantiidiotypic antisera, J. Exp. Med. 139:712.
6. Rodkey, L. S., 1976, Studies of idiotypic antibodies: Reactions of isologous and autologous anti-idiotypic antibodies with the same antibody preparations, J. Immunol. 117:986.

7. Binz, H., and Wigzell, H., 1977, Antigen-binding idiotypic T-lymphocyte receptors, in: *Contemporary Topics in Immunobiology*, Vol. 7 (O. Stutman, ed.), Plenum Press, New York, pp. 113–177.
8. Bach, B. A., Greene, M. I., Benacerraf, B., and Nisonoff, A., 1979, Mechanisms of regulation of cell-mediated immunity. IV Azobenzenearsonate-specific suppressor factor(s) bear cross-reactive idiotypic determinants the expression of which is linked to the heavy-chain allotype linkage group of genes. *J. Exp. Med.* **149**:1084.
9. Rajewsky, K., and Eichmann, K., 1977, Antigen receptors of T helper cells, in: *Contemporary Topics in Immunobiology*, Vol. 7 (O. Stutman, ed.), Plenum Press, New York, pp 69–112.
10. Ertl, H. C. J., Greene, M. I., Noseworthy, J. H., Fields, B. N., Nepom, J. T., Spriggs, D. R., and Finberg, R. W., 1982, Identification of idiotypic receptors on reovirus-specific cytolytic T cells, *Proc. Natl. Acad. Sci. USA* **79**:7479.
11. Cerny, J., Heusser, C., Wallich, R., Hammerling, G. J., and Eardley, D. D., 1982, Immunoglobulin idiotopes expressed by T cells. I. Expression of distinct idiotopes detected by monoclonal antibodies on antigen-specific suppressor T cells, *J. Exp. Med.* **156**:719.
12. Infante, A. J., Infante, P. D., Gillis, S., and Fathman, C. G., 1982, Definition of T cell idiotypes using anti-idiotypic antisera produced by immunization with T cell clones, *J. Exp. Med.* **155**:1100.
13. Nadler, P. I., Miller, G. G., Sachs, D. H., and Hodes, R. J., 1982, The expression and functional involvement of nuclease-specific idiotype on nuclease-primed helper T cells, *Eur. J. Immunol.* **12**:113.
14. Binz, H., Fenner, M., Frei, D., and Wigzell, H., 1983, Two independent receptors allow selective target lysis by T cell clones, *J. Exp. Med.* **157**:1252.
15. L'Age Stehr, J., 1980, Priming of T helper cells by antigen-activated B cells: B cell-primed Lyt-1$^+$ helper cells are restricted to cooperate with B cells expressing the IgvH phenotype of the priming B cells, *J. Exp. Med.* **153**:1236.
16. Zubler, R. H., Benacerraf, B., and Germain, R. N., 1980, Feedback suppression of the immune response in vitro. II. IgV$_H$-restricted antibody dependent suppression, *J. Exp. Med.* **151**:681.
17. Kluskens, L., and Köhler, H., 1974, Regulation of immune response by autogenous antibody against receptor, *Proc. Natl. Acad. Sci. USA* **71**:5083.
18. Cosenza, H., 1976, Detection of anti-idiotype reactive cells in the response to phosphyrylcholine, *Eur. J. Immunol.* **6**:114.
19. Sy, M.-S., Moorhead, J. W., and Claman, H. N., 1979, Regulation of cell mediated immunity by antibodies: Possible role of anti-receptor antibodies in the regulation of contact sensitivity to DNFB in mice, *J. Immunol.* **123**:2593.
20. Schrater, A. F., Goidl, E. A., Thorbecke, G. J., and Siskind, G. W., 1979, Production of auto-anti-idiotypic antibody during the normal immune response to TNP-Ficoll. I. Occurrence in AKR/J and BALB/c mice of hapten-augmentable, anti-TNP plaque-forming cells and their accelerated appearance in recipients of immune spleen cells, *J. Exp. Med.* **150**:138.
21. Geha, R. S., 1982, Presence of auto-anti-idiotypic antibody during the normal human immune response to tetanus toxoid antigen, *J. Immunol.* **129**:139.
22. Fernandez, C., and Möller, G., 1979, Antigen-induced strain-specific autoantiidiotypic antibodies modulate the immune response to dextran B 512, *Proc. Natl. Acad. Sci. USA* **76**:5944.
23. Bona, C., Lieberman, R., Chien, C. C., Mond, J. S., House, S., Green, I., and Paul, W. E., 1978, Immune response to levan. I. Kinetics and ontogeny of anti-levan and anti-inulin antibody response and of expression of cross-reactive idiotype, *J. Immunol.* **120**:1436.
24. Bankert, R. B., and Pressman, D., 1976, Receptor-blocking factor present in immune serum resembling auto-anti-idiotype antibody, *J. Immunol.* **117**:457.
25. Rodkey, L. S., and Adler, F. L., 1983, Regulation of natural anti-allotype antibody responses by idiotype network-induced autoanti-idiotypic antibodies, *J. Exp. Med.* **157**:1920.
26. Courand, P.-O., Lü, B.-Z., and Strosberg, A. D., 1983, Cyclical antiidiotypic response to anti-hormone antibodies due to neutralization by autologous anti-antiidiotype antibodies that bind hormone, *J. Exp. Med.* **157**:1369.
27. McKearn, T. J., Stuart, F. P., and Fitch, F. W., 1974, Anti-idiotypic antibody in rat transplantation immunity. I. Production of anti-idiotypic antibody in animals repeatedly immunized with alloantigens, *J. Immunol.* **113**:1876.
28. Cohen, P. L., and Eisenberg, R. A., 1982, Anti-idiotypic antibodies to the Coombs antibody in NZB F$_1$ mice, *J. Exp. Med.* **156**:173.
29. Bona, C. A., Heber-Katz, E., and Paul, W. E., 1981, Idiotype–anti-idiotype regulation. I. Immunization

with a levan-binding myeloma protein leads to the appearances of auto-anti-(anti-idiotype) antibodies and to the activation of silent clones, *J. Exp. Med.* **153:**951.

30. Cowdery, J. S., and Steinberg, A. D., 1981, Serum antibody-binding antibodies produced during a primary antibody response, *J. Immunol.* **126:**2136.

31. Goidl, E. A., Schrater, A. F., Siskind, G. W., and Thorbecke, G. J., 1979, Production of auto-anti-idiotypic antibody during the normal immune response to TNP-Ficoll. II. Hapten-reversible inhibition of anti-TNP plaque-forming cells by immune serum as an assay for auto anti-idiotypic antibody, *J. Exp. Med.* **150:**154.

32. Goidl, E. A., Hayama, T., Shepherd, G. M., Siskind, G. W., and Thorbecke, G. J., 1983, Production of auto-anti-idiotypic antibody during the normal immune response. VI. Hapten augmentation of plaque formation and hapten-reversible inhibition of plaque formation as assays for anti-idiotype antibody, *J. Immunol. Methods* **58:**1.

33. Siskind, G. W., Bhogal, B. S., Gibbons, J. J., Weksler, M. E., Thorbecke, G. J., and Goidl, E. A., 1983, Regulation of the anti-TNP response by anti-idiotype antibodies, *Ann. NY Acad. Sci.* **418:**26.

34. Abdou, N. I., Wall, H., and Clancy, J., Jr., 1981, The network theory in autoimmunity: *In vitro* modulation of DNA-binding cells by antiidiotypic antibody present in inactive lupus sera, *J. Clin. Immunol.* **1:**234.

35. Cunningham-Rundles, C., 1982, Naturally occurring autologous anti-idiotypic antibodies: Participation in immune complex formation in selective IgA deficiency, *J. Exp. Med.* **155:**711.

36. Zouali, M., and Eyquem, A., 1983, Expression of anti-idiotypic clones against auto-anti-DNA antibodies in normal individuals, *Cell. Immunol.* **76:**137.

37. Pollok, B. A., Brown, A. S., and Kearney, J. F., 1982, Structural and biological properties of a monoclonal auto-anti-(anti-idiotype) antibody, *Nature* **299:**447.

38. Kagnoff, M. F., 1978, Effects of antigen-feeding on intestinal and systemic immune responses. III. Antigen-specific serum-mediated suppression of humoral antibody responses after antigen feeding, *Cell. Immunol.* **40:**186.

39. Jackson, S., and Mestecky, J., 1981, Oral-parenteral immunization leads to the appearance of IgG auto-anti-idiotypic cells in mucosal tissues, *Cell. Immunol.* **60:**498.

40. Goidl, E. A., Schrater, A. F., Thorbecke, G. J., and Siskind, G. W., 1980, Production of auto-anti-idiotypic antibody during the normal immune response. IV. Studies of the primary and secondary responses to thymus-dependent and -independent antigens, *Eur. J. Immunol.* **10:**810.

41. Kelsoe, G., Isaak, D., and Cerny, J., 1980, Thymic requirement for cyclical idiotypic and reciprocal anti-idiotypic immune responses to a T-independent antigen, *J. Exp. Med.* **151:**289.

42. Binion, S. B., and Rodkey, L. S., 1982, Naturally induced auto-anti-idiotypic antibodies: Induction by identical idiotopes in some members of an outbred rabbit family, *J. Exp. Med.* **156:**860.

43. Schrater, A. F., Goidl, E. A., Thorbecke, G. J., and Siskind, G. W., 1979, Production of auto-anti-idiotypic antibody during the normal response to TNP-Ficoll. III. Absence in *nu/nu* mice: Evidence for T cell dependence of the anti-idiotypic antibody response, *J. Exp. Med.* **150:**808.

44. Hiernaux, J. R., Chiang, J., Baker, P. J., Delisi, C., and Prescott, B., 1982, Lack of involvement of auto-anti-idiotypic antibody in the regulation of oscillations and tolerance in the antibody response to levan, *Cell. Immunol.* **67:**334.

45. Julius, M. H., Augustin, A. A., and Cosenza, H., 1977, Recognition of a naturally occurring idiotype by autologous T cells, *Nature* **265:**251.

46. Adorini, L., Harvey, M., and Sercarz, E. E., 1979, The fine specificity of regulatory T cells. IV. Idiotypic complementarity and antigen-bridging interactions in the anti-lysozyme response, *Eur. J. Immunol.* **9:**906.

47. Rubenstein, L. J., Yeh, M., and Bona, C. A., 1982, Idiotype–anti-idiotype network. II. Activation of silent clones by treatment at birth with idiotypes is associated with the expansion of idiotype-specific helper T cells, *J. Exp. Med.* **156:**506.

48. Jayaraman, S., and Bellone, C. J., 1982, Hapten-specific responses to the phenyltrimethylamino hapten. I. Evidence for idiotype–anti-idiotype interactions in delayed-type hypersensitivity in mice, *Eur. J. Immunol.* **12:**272.

49. Woodland, R., and Cantor, H., 1978, Idiotype-specific T helper cells are required to induce idiotype-positive B memory cells to secrete antibody, *Eur. J. Immunol.* **8:**600.

50. Hetzelberger, D., and Eichmann, K., 1978, Recognition of idiotypes in lymphocyte interactions. I. Idiotypic selectivity in the cooperation between T and B lymphocytes, *Eur. J. Immunol.* **8:**846.

51. Eichmann, K., Falk, I., and Rajewsky, K., 1978, Recognition of idiotypes in lymphocyte interactions. II.

Antigen-independent cooperation between T and B lymphocytes that possess similar and complimentary idiotypes, *Eur. J. Immunol.* **8**:853.

52. Bottomly, K., and Mosier, D. E., 1981, Antigen-specific helper T cells required for dominant idiotype expression are not H-2 restricted, *J. Exp. Med.* **154**:411.

53. Kelsoe, G., and Cerny, J., 1979, Reciprocal expansions of idiotypic and anti-idiotypic clones following antigen stimulation, *Nature* **279**:333.

54. Goidl, E. A., Samarut, C., Schneider-Gadicke, A., Hochwald, N. L., Thorbecke, G. J., and Siskind, G. W., 1984, Production of auto-anti-idiotypic antibody during the normal immune response. IX. Characteristics of the auto-anti-idiotype antibody and its production, *Cell. Immunol.* **85**:25.

55. Brown, J. C., and Rodkey, L. S., 1979, Autoregulation of an antibody response via network-induced auto-anti-idiotype, *J. Exp. Med.* **150**:67.

56. Goidl, E. A., Thorbecke, G. J., Weksler, M. E., and Siskind, G. W., 1980, Production of auto-anti-idiotypic antibody during the normal immune response. V. Changes in the auto-anti-idiotypic antibody response and the idiotype repertoire associated with aging, *Proc. Natl. Acad. Sci. USA* **77**:6788.

57. Goidl, E. A., Choy, J., Gibbons, J. J., Weksler, M. E., Thorbecke, G. J., and Siskind, G. W., 1983, Production of auto-antiidiotypic antibody during the normal immune response. VII. Analysis of the cellular basis for the increased auto-antiidiotype antibody production by aged mice, *J. Exp. Med.* **157**:1635.

58. Szewczuk, M. R., and Campbell, R. J., 1980, Loss of immune competence with age may be due to auto-anti-idiotypic antibody regulation, *Nature* **286**:164.

59. Nisonoff, A., and Lamoyi, E., 1981, Hypothesis implications of the presence of an internal image of the antigen in anti-idiotypic antibodies: Possible applications to vaccine production, *Clin. Immunol. Immunopathol.* **21**:397.

60. Sege, K., and Peterson, P. A., 1978, Use of anti-idiotypic antibodies as cell-surface receptor probes, *Proc. Natl. Acad. Sci. USA* **75**:2443.

61. Shechter, Y., Elias, D., Maron, R., and Cohen, I. R., 1983, Mice immunized to insulin develop antibody to the insulin receptor, *J. Cell. Biochem.* **21**:179.

62. Marasco, W. A., and Becker, E. L., 1982, Anti-idiotype as antibody against the formyl peptide chemotaxis receptor of the neutrophil, *J. Immunol.* **128**:963.

63. Islam, M. N., Pepper, B. M., Briones-Urbina, R., and Farid, N. R., 1983, Biological activity of anti-thyrotropin anti-idiotypic antibody, *Eur. J. Immunol.* **13**:57.

64. Lefvert, A.-K., James, R. W., Alliod, C., and Fulpius, B. W., 1982, A monoclonal anti-idiotypic antibody against anti-receptor antibodies from myasthenic sera, *Eur. J. Immunol.* **12**:790.

65. Wassermann, N. H., Penn, A. S., Freimuth, P. I., Treptow, N., Wentzel, S., Cleveland, W. L., and Erlanger, B. F., 1982, Anti-idiotypic route to anti-acetylcholine receptor antibodies and experimental myasthenia gravis, *Proc. Natl. Acad. Sci. USA* **79**:4810.

66. Schreiber, A. B., Couraud, P. O., Andre, C., Vray, B., and Strosberg, A. D., 1980, Anti-alprenolol anti-idiotypic antibodies bind to β-adrenergic receptors and modulate catecholamine-sensitive adenylate cyclase, *Proc. Natl. Acad. Sci. USA* **77**:7385.

67. Homcy, C. J., Rockson, S. G., and Haber, E., 1982, An antiidiotypic antibody that recognizes the β-adrenergic receptor, *J. Clin. Invest.* **69**:1147.

68. Nisonoff, A., and Bangasser, S. A., 1975, Immunological suppression of idiotypic specificities, *Transplant. Rev.* **27**:100.

69. Cowdery, J. S., and Steinberg, A. D., 1982, Regulation of primary thymus-independent, anti-hapten responses of normal and autoimmune mice by synegeneic antibody, *J. Immunol.* **129**:1250.

70. Eisen, H. N., and Siskind, G. W., 1964, Variations in affinities of antibodies during the immune response, *Biochemistry* **3**:996.

71. Siskind, G. W., and Benacerraf, B., 1969, Cell selection by antigen in the immune response, *Adv. Immunol.* **10**:1.

72. Conger, J. D., Lewis, G. K., and Goodman, J. W., 1981, Idiotype profile of an immune response. I. Contrasts in idiotypic dominance between primary and secondary responses and between IgM and IgG plaque-forming cells, *J. Exp. Med.* **153**:1173.

73. Conger, J. D., Lamoyi, E., Lewis, G. K., Nisonoff, A., and Goodman, J. W., 1983, Idiotype profile of an immune response. II. Reversal of the relative dominance of major and minor cross-reacting idiotypes in arsonate-specific T-independent responses, *J. Exp. Med.* **158**:438.

74. Chang, S. P., and Rittenberg, M. B., 1981, Immunologic memory to phosphorycholine in vitro. I. Asymmetric expression of clonal dominance, *J. Immunol.* **126**:975.

75. Kenny, J. J., Guelde, G., Claflin, J. L., and Scher, I., 1981, Altered idiotype response to phosphocholine in mice bearing an X-linked immune defect, *J. Immunol.* **127:**1629.
76. Werblin, T. P., and Siskind, G. W., 1972, Distribution of antibody affinities: Technique of measurement, *Immunochemistry* **9:**987.
77. Werblin, T. P., Kim, Y. T., Quagliata, F., and Siskind, G. W., 1973, Studies on the control of antibody synthesis. III. Changes in heterogeneity of antibody affinity during the course of the immune response, *Immunology* **24:**477.
78. Burkly, L. C., Zaugg, R., Eisen, H. N., and Wortis, H. H., 1982, Influence on the nude and X-linked immune deficiency genes on expression of κ and λ light chains, *Eur. J. Immunol.* **12:**1033.
79. Primi, D., Mami, F., Le Guern, C., and Cazenave, P.-A., 1982, The relationship between variable region determinants and antigen specificity on mitogen reactive B cell subsets, *J. Exp. Med.* **156:**924.
80. Eichmann, K., 1974, Idiotype suppression. I. Influence of the dose and of the effector functions of anti-idiotypic antibody on the production of an idiotype, *Eur. J. Immunol.* **4:**296.
81. Kölsch, E., Oberbarnscheidt, J., Bruner, K., and Heuer, J., 1980, The Fc-receptor: Its role in the transmission of differentiation signals, *Immunol. Rev.* **49:**61.
82. Parker, D. C., 1980, Induction and suppression of polyclonal antibody responses by anti-Ig reagents and antigen-nonspecific helper factors: A comparison of the effects of anti-Fab, anti-IgM, and anti-IgD on murine B cells, *Immunol. Rev.* **52:**115.
83. Phillips, N. E., and Parker, D. C., 1983, Fc dependent inhibition of mouse B cell activation by whole anti-μ antibodies, *J. Immunol.* **130:**602.
84. Kappler, J. W., Vander Hoven, A., Dharmarajan, U., and Hoffman, M., 1973, Regulation of the immune response. IV. Antibody-mediated suppression of the immune response to haptens and heterologous erythrocyte antigens *in vitro*, *J. Immunol.* **111:**1228.
85. Pawlak, L. L., Hart, D. A., and Nisonoff, A., 1973, Requirements for prolonged suppression of an idiotypic specificity in adult mice, *J. Exp. Med.* **137:**1442.
86. Borel, Y., Golan, D. T., Kilham, L., and Borel, H., 1976, Carrier determined tolerance with various subclasses of murine myeloma IgG, *J. Immunol.* **116:**854.
87. Waldschmidt, T. J., Borel, Y., and Vitetta, E. S., 1983, The use of haptenated immunoglobulins to induce B-cell tolerance *in vitro*. The roles of hapten density and the Fc portion of the immunoglobulin carrier, *J. Immunol.* **131:**2204.
88. Szewczuk, M. R., Sherr, D. H., Cornacchia, A., Kim, Y. T., and Siskind, G. W., 1979, Ontogeny of B-lymphocyte function. XI. The secondary response by neonatal and adult B cell populations to different T-dependent antigens, *J. Immunol.* **122:**1294.
89. Szewczuk, M. R., and Siskind, G. W., 1977, Ontogeny of B-lymphocyte function. III. *In vivo* and *in vitro* studies on the ease of tolerance induction in B lymphocytes from fetal, neonatal, and adult mice, *J. Exp. Med.* **145:**1590.
90. Sigal, N. H., Pickard, A. R., Metcalf, E. S., Gearhart, P. J., and Klinman, N. R., 1977, Expression of phosphorylcholine-specific B cells during murine development, *J. Exp. Med.* **146:**933.
91. Kim, B. S., and Hubchak, S., 1981, Compensation for idiotype suppression. I. Acquirement of ability to compensate for TEPC-15 idiotype suppression in mice during the early neonatal period, *Eur. J. Immunol.* **11:**428.
92. Massey, P. B., and Kim, B. S., 1981, Mechanisms of idiotype suppression. III. Relative resistance of PBA-induced anti-phosphorylcholine responses to *in vitro* idiotype suppression, *J. Immunol.* **127:**199.
93. Asherson, G. L., Zembala, M., Gautam, S. C., and Watkins, M. C., 1982, Control of suppressor cell activity: Auto anti-idiotype B cells produced by painting with picryl chloride inhibit the T-suppressor cell which blocks the efferent stage of contact sensitivity, *Cell. Immunol.* **70:**160.
94. Shepherd, G. M., Gibbons, J. J., Siskind, G. W., Thorbecke, G. J., and Goidl, E. A., Production of auto-anti-idiotypic antibody during the normal immune response. VIII. Effect of auto-anti-idiotypic antibody on contact sensitivity, submitted for publication.
95. Moorhead, J. W., 1982, Antigen receptors on murine T lymphocytes in contact sensitivity. III. Mechanism of negative feedback regulation by auto-anti-idiotypic antibody, *J. Exp. Med.* **155:**820.
96. Forstrom, J. W., Nelson, K. A., Nepom, G. T., Hellström, I., and Hellström, K. E., 1983, Immunization to a syngeneic sarcoma by a monoclonal auto-anti-idiotypic antibody. *Nature* **303:**627.
97. Bhogal, B. S., Jacobson, E. B., Siskind, J. W., and Thorbecke, G. J., 1984, Factors affecting auto-anti-idiotypic antibody production in chickens and rabbits, in: Proceedings of the Workshop on the Assessment of the Chemical Regulation of Immunity in Veterinary Medicine (in press).

98. Olson, J. C., and Leslie, G. A., 1981, Inheritance patterns of idiotype expression: Maternal–fetal immune regulatory networks, *Immunogenetics* **13**:39.

99. Opelz, G., and Terasaki, P. I., 1977, Studies on the strength of HLA antigens in related donor kidney transplants, *Transplantation* **24**:106.

100. Suciu-Foca, N., Reed, E., Rohowsky, C., Kung, P., and King, D. W., 1983, Anti-idiotypic antibodies to anti-HLA receptors induced by pregnancy, *Proc. Natl. Acad. Sci. USA* **80**:830.

101. McKearn, T. J., Hamada, Y., Stuart, F. P., and Fitch, F. W., 1974, Anti-receptor antibody and resistance to graft-versus-host disease, *Nature* **251**:648.

102. Rouse, B. T., and Warner, N. L., 1972, Induction of T cell tolerance in agammaglobulinemic chickens, *Eur. J. Immunol.* **2**:102.

103. Grebenau, M.D., and Thorbecke, G. J., 1978, T cell tolerance in the chicken. I. Parameters affecting tolerance induction to human γ-globulin in agammaglobulinemic and normal chickens, *J. Immunol.* **120**:1046.

104. Wood, C., Fernandez, C., and Möller, G., 1982, Ontogenic development of the suppressed secondary response to native dextran, *Scand. J. Immunol.* **16**:287.

105. Rose, L. M., Goldman, M., and Lambert, P.-H., 1982, The production of anti-idiotypic antibodies and of idiotype–anti-idiotype immune complexes after polyclonal activation induced by bacterial LPS, *J. Immunol.* **128**:2126.

106. Goldman, M., Rose, L. M., Hochmann, A., and Lambert, P. H., 1982, Deposition of idiotype–anti-idiotype immune complexes in renal glomeruli after polyclonal B cell activation, *J. Exp. Med.* **155**:1385.

107. Geltner, D., Franklin, E. C., and Frangione, B., 1980, Antiidiotypic activity in the IgM fractions of mixed cryoglobulins, *J. Immunol.* **125**:1530.

108. Hallgren, H. M., Buckley, C. E., Gilbertsen, V. A., and Yunis, E. J., 1973, Lymphocyte phytohemagglutinin responsiveness, immunoglobulins and autoantibodies in aging humans, *J. Immunol.* **111**:1101.

109. Van Snick, J. L., and Masson, P. L., 1980, Incidence and specificities of IgA and IgM anti-IgG autoantibodies in various mouse strains and colonies, *J. Exp. Med.* **151**:45.

110. Dwyer, D. S., Bradley, R. J., Urquhart, C. K., and Kearney, J. F., 1983, Naturally occurring anti-idiotypic antobodies in myasthenia gravis patients, *Nature* **301**:611.

111. Shechter, Y., Maron, R., Elias, D., and Cohen, I. R., 1982, Auto-antibodies to insulin receptor spontaneously develop as anti-idiotypes in mice immunized with insulin, *Science* **216**:542.

112. Maron, R., Elias, D., deJongh, B. M., Bruining, C. J., van Rood, J. J., Shechter, Y., and Cohen, I. R., 1983, Autoantibodies to the insulin receptor in juvenile onset insulin-dependent diabetes, *Nature* **303**:817.

113. Kincade, P. W., Jyonouchi, H., Landreth, K. S., and Lee, G., 1982, B-lymphocyte precursors in immunodeficient, autoimmune and anemic mice, *Immunol. Rev.* **64**:81.

114. Thorbecke, G. J., Bhogal, B. S., and Siskind, G. W., 1984, Possible mechanism for down-regulation of auto-antibody production by auto-anti-idiotype, *Immunol. Today* **5**:92.

115. Frank, M. M., Hamburger, M. I., Lawley, T. J., Kimberly, R. P., and Plotz, P. H., 1979, Defective reticuloendothelial system Fc-receptor function in systemic lupus erythematosus, *N. Engl. J. Med.* **300**:518.

116. Lawley, T. J., Hall, R. P., Fauci, A. S., Katz, S. I., Hamburger, M. I., and Frank, M. M., 1981, Defective Fc receptor functions associated with the HLA-B8/DRw3 haplotype, *N. Engl. J. Med.* **304**:185.

117. Vitetta, E. S., Krolick, K. A., and Uhr, J. W., 1982, Neoplastic B cells as targets for antibody-ricin A chain immunotoxins, *Immunol. Rev.* **62**:159.

118. Neilson, E. G., and Phillips, S. M., 1982, Suppression of interstitial nephritis by auto-anti-idiotypic immunity, *J. Exp. Med.* **155**:179.

119. Schwartz, M., Novick, D., Givol, D., and Fuchs, S., 1978, Induction of anti-idiotypic antibodies by immunization with syngeneic spleen cells educated with acetylcholine receptor, *Nature* **273**:543.

120. Bona, C. A., Heber-Katz, E., and Paul, W. E., 1981, Idiotype–anti-idiotype regulation. I. Immunization with a levan-binding myeloma protein leads to the appearance of auto-anti-(anti-idiotype) antibodies and to the activation of silent clones, *J. Exp. Med.* **153**:951.

PART IV
STRUCTURES ON T CELLS

27

Suppressor T-Cell Hybridoma with a Receptor Recognizing KLH-Specific Suppressor Factor

Masaru Taniguchi, Izumi Takei, Takayuki Sumida, Masamoto Kanno, Masatoshi Tagawa, and Toshihiro Ito

1. Introduction

Immune responses are known to be regulated by complicated interactions of T-cell subsets that play different functional roles.[1-6] In our previous studies of the cellular mechanisms in the suppression of antibody response, at least three functionally distinct subsets of suppressor T cells, i.e., suppressor T cells producing antigen-specific factor (TsF), suppressor T cells with acceptor site for TsF (acceptor T cell), and effector-suppressor T cells, were found to be involved in the regulatory T-cell interactions.[1] The initial step of suppressor T cell interaction is a process of activation of acceptor T cells by an antigen-specific TsF. The effector-suppressor T cells are then generated under the influence of activated acceptor T cells. Therefore, antigen-specific TsF mediates the regulatory T-cell interaction in which no direct cell contact is necessary. Moreover, antigen-specific TsF seems not to be an effector-suppressor molecule but rather a molecule whose function is to activate other subsets of suppressor T cells. In this sense, the antigen-specific TsF appears to work as a device to recognize antigens and also to communicate with other T cells.

It is thus important to characterize the functional and biochemical structures of T-cell recognition, or the mechanisms of regulatory T-cell interactions. In this respect, recently

Masaru Taniguchi, Izumi Takei, Takayuki Sumida, Masamoto Kanno, Masatoshi Tagawa, and Toshihiro Ito • Department of Immunology, School of Medicine, Chiba University, Chiba, 280 Japan.

developed technology to establish monoclonal functional T-cell lines, such as T-cell hybridomas or TCGF-dependent T-cell clones, permits us to characterize T-cell-mediated functions at the biochemical and molecular levels.

2. The Organization of Monoclonal KLH-Specific Suppressor T-Cell Factors

Our previous functional and biochemical studies on the suppressor factor derived from a T-cell hybridoma specific for KLH have demonstrated its important characteristics[7–13]:

1. The antigen-specific suppressor T-cell factor (KLH-TsF) possesses the ability to bind to the native relevant antigen (KLH), but not to irrelevant antigens (i.e., OVA or *Ascaris* extract), suggesting that the TsF carries specific antigen-binding affinity just like immunoglobulins. Neither constant-region determinants nor the Fab portion of immunoglobulins were, however, demonstrated on TsF.

2. The TsF was found to be composed of two distinct polypeptide chains: one is the heavy chain (45,000 daltons) with an antigen-binding moiety and constant-region determinants unique to suppressor T cells and their factors. The constant-region determinants on the antigen-binding heavy chain could be detected by conventional and monoclonal antibodies made by the *Igh* allotype-congenic pair of mice (BALB/c anti-CB-20), because BALB/c anti-CB-20 antibody absorbed TsF derived from *Igh^b* mice, such as C57Bl/6, CB-20, CWB, and BAB-14 mice, but not those from mice of other Igh allotypes, e.g., BALB/c (*Igh^a*), C3H (*Igh^j*), C3H.SW (*Igh^j*), etc. The other molecule is the light chain (28,000 daltons) the determinants of which can be detected by conventional or monoclonal antibodies raised in B10.A(5R) and B10.A(3R) combinations [BR10.A(5R) anti-B10.A(3R)].

3. Suppressor activity could be obtained either in the cell-free extracts of hybridoma cells as the cellular form of TsF or in the ascites from hybridoma-bearing mice as the secreted form of TsF. Usually, cell-free extracts from the suppressor T-cell hybridoma contain three distinct types of suppressor molecules: the heavy chain, the light chain, and the combined form of the heavy and light chains of TsF. This was deduced from the following experimental results. Suppressor activity in the extracts was completely absorbed by an immunosorbent column composed of either the antigen, the anti-heavy-chain (BALB/c anti-CB-20), or the anti-light-chain of TsF [B10.A(5R) anti-B10.A(3R)]. However, mixing the filtrates from the antigen and the anti-light-chain columns or those of the anti-heavy-chain and the anti-light-chain columns, neither of which manifests any suppressor effect by itself, reconstituted significant suppressor function. The results suggest that cell-free extracts contain free heavy or light chains, and that mixing these free heavy and light chains reconstitutes the suppressor function. The presence of the combined form of the heavy and light chains in the extracts is indicated by the fact that suppressor activity is fully recovered in the eluate of the extracts from the antigen or the antibody columns. Therefore, the combined form of the two chains in the extracts seems to be composed of heavy and light chains, linked in noncovalent association. It is also conceivable that a state of equilibrium exists between the associated and the dissociated forms of TsF in the extract.

On the other hand, the reconstitution of suppressor activity observed after mixing the extracted TsF filtrates from the anti-heavy and anti-light chain columns was not observed when the secreted TsF was used. However, the secreted TsF had a composition distinct from the extracted factor. In fact, the reduction of the secreted TsF with dithiothreitol (DTT) splits the molecule into two distinct chains. The heavy and light chains isolated after cleavage of the secreted TsF, which displayed no suppressor activity by themselves, could reconstitute suppressor function only when both were combined. It was suggested that the heavy and light chains of TsF are independently synthesized and are covalently associated with disulfide bonds when they are secreted.

4. The heavy or light chain by itself could not express any functional activity. However, as the mixture of the two polypeptide chains reconstituted the active suppressor molecule, it is apparent that both heavy and light chains of the factor are required for the functional expression of TsF.

5. Molecular genetic studies have clearly shown that two distinct mRNAs with different sizes encode the light and heavy chains of KLH-TsF, respectively. 11 S mRNA directs synthesis of the light chain bearing I-J determinants detected by monoclonal B10.A(5R) anti-B10.A(3R). Similarly, 13S or 18.5 S mRNAs code for the two heavy chains of TsF with different molecular sizes carrying constant-region determinants defined by monoclonal BALB/c anti-CB-20. The heavy or light chain of the 13 S or 11 S mRNA-translation product per se showed no biological activity. On the other hand, when the heavy and light chains were mixed, the antigen-specific suppressor activity was successfully recovered.

6. In terms of the biological role of the heavy chain of TsF, it seems to determine the antigen specificity of TsF, since the isolated heavy chain or the 13 S mRNA translation product per se does have the ability to bind native antigen KLH. Moreover, the antigen specificity of TsF could be converted by interchanging the heavy chain having different antigen-binding activity. The functional role of the light chain of TsF relates to its activity as the element determining the genetic restriction specificity of TsF. In fact, the mixture of the heavy chain of 13 S mRNA translation products and the light chain isolated from C3H ($H\text{-}2^k$) mice suppressed the antibody response of C3H mice which carry the same $H\text{-}2$ haplotypes as those of the light chain, but not that of C57BL/6 ($H\text{-}2^b$) or BALB/c ($H\text{-}2^d$). Similarly, when the light chain obtained from C57BL/6 ($H\text{-}2^b$) mice was mixed with the heavy chain of the 13 S mRNA products, the mixture only acted on the response of C57BL/6 mice but not on that of mice having different $H\text{-}2$ haplotypes. It is apparent that the light chain of TsF determines the genetic restriction specificity in the regulatory T-cell interactions and also that identity of the light-chain and the responding-cell $H\text{-}2$ haplotypes is necessary for the expression of TsF function. Taken collectively, KLH-TsF, as described here, is composed of two distinct polypeptide chains mediating antigen-specific and $H\text{-}2$-restricted regulatory functions.

Despite the above-mentioned results, there are several reports demonstrating that isolated T-cell receptors or suppressor factors with antigen-binding capacity are composed of a single chain (approximately 70 kd). Some of the molecules are easy to degrade into two chains of 45 and 25 kd. Fresno et al.,[14] in fact, demonstrated that SRBC-specific TsF could be digested by papain into 45- and 25-kd molecules. The 45-kd molecule expressed nonspecific suppressor activity, while the 25-kd molecule possessed antigen-binding activity. It is most likely that several distinct suppressor molecules may operate in different stages of the suppressor pathways.

3. Characteristics of a Suppressor Hybridoma Which Accepts the KLH-Specific Suppressor T-Cell Factor

Our previous studies have shown that Lyt-1^+2^+ acceptor-suppressor T cells play an important role in the suppression of antibody response.[1] In the first step of the suppressor pathway, the two-chain suppressor factor produced by Lyt-2^+ T cells activates Lyt-1^+2^+ acceptor T cells. The acceptor T cells have been demonstrated by the absorption of TsF activity with Lyt-1^+2^+ T cells and by the loss of TsF function after treatment of acceptor T cells with anti-Lyt-1 or anti-Lyt-2 antiserum and complement. In the second step of the suppressor pathway, the activated Lyt-1^+2^+ acceptor T cells generate new effector–suppressor T cells (Ts^e) that directly suppress the responses mounted by B cells and helper T cells. This indicated that the two-chain TsF is not an effector molecule but works as a signal to activate other suppressor T cells. Similar observations have been demonstrated in the GAT- or ABA (azobenzenearsonate)-specific suppressor systems reported by Germain et al.[5] and Sy et al.[6] Sy et al. demonstrated that administration of ABA-coupled syngeneic spleen cells in A/J mice results in the generation of suppressor T cells that exhibit specific binding to ABA. The Ts$_1$ bears the antigen-binding structure, shares idiotypic determinants with the major cross-reactive idiotype (CRI) of the anti-ABA antibodies of A/J mice, and also produces a soluble idiotype-positive suppressor factor (TsF$_1$). They also found that TsF$_1$ acts on second-order antigen-specific Lyt-1^+2^+ suppressor T cells (Ts$_2$) bearing anti-idiotypic receptor to induce the effector type of Lyt-2^+ suppressor T cells (Ts$_3$). Germain et al. also demonstrated that administration of GAT-specific suppressor factor from nonresponder animals to responder mice 7 days before in vitro antigen challenge could elicit second-order antigen-specific Lyt-1^+2^+ suppressor T cells. Thus, it is suggested that the induction of effector–suppressor T cells by the initial regulatory signal (TsF) through activation of Lyt-1^+2^+ acceptor T cells is a general phenomenon. Taken collectively with the results mentioned above, the soluble suppressor T-cell factor seems to serve as a communication device among subsets of suppressor T cells in the regulation of immune response, and the acceptor T cell appears to behave as an amplifier of suppressor signals.

Among several suppressor T-cell hybridomas with distinct functional activities established by the fusion of BW5147 and C57BL/6 KLH-primed suppressor T cells enriched with KLH-coated Petri dishes, the hybridoma cell line 34S-281 was found to act as an acceptor T cell of the intermediary type in KLH-specific antibody formation.[15] The hybridoma cells do not express active suppressor activity by themselves but possess the receptor for KLH-specific TsF. This was determined because the activities of the conventional or monoclonal KLH-TsF were specifically absorbed with 34S-281 (acceptor hybridoma) but not with BW5147 cells. In this respect, the acceptor hybridoma seems to have similar properties of acceptor T cells observed in various suppressor systems as mentioned above. It is, therefore, apparent that the acceptor hybridoma is useful in characterizing the mechanisms of TsF–acceptor T-cell interactions in the regulation of immune responses.

The acceptor hybridoma was found to produce antigen-specific factor capable of suppressing the anti-DNP-KLH responses only after it was stimulated with monoclonal or conventional "KLH-TsF." The experimental protocol for the activation of acceptor hybridoma cells is illustrated in Fig. 1. The hybridoma cells were incubated with KLH-specific monoclonal TsF for 1 hr on ice in the absence of the relevant antigen, KLH. The incubated cells were washed and further cultured in fresh medium. To detect the activity of the acti-

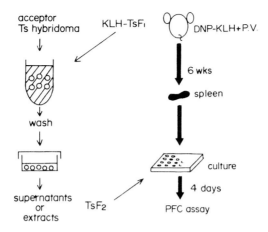

FIGURE 1. Protocol for the activation of the acceptor hybridoma.

vated acceptor hybridoma cells, the culture supernatants or the cell-free extracts were collected at various time intervals after stimulation, and were tested for their activity in the secondary anti-DNP IgG responses. As control, untreated hybridoma cells were cultured under the same conditions as the experimental groups. The results are shown in Table I. The acceptor hybridoma was stimulated by monoclonal KLH-TsF and started to produce TsF 8 hr after stimulation. No suppressor activity was obtained by the culture supernatants or the cell-free extracts from the unstimulated acceptor hybridoma. The production of new TsF from the activated acceptor hybridoma continued up to 17 days or more. It is likely that the monoclonal KLH-TsF per se works as a signal to activate the acceptor hybridoma in the resting state without the process of an antigen-bridging interaction.

The immunochemical properties of the newly produced suppressor factor from the activated acceptor hybridoma are: (1) the new suppressor factor, like KLH-TsF of the two-

TABLE I

Activation of the Acceptor Hybridoma with
Monoclonal KLH-TsF

Time after activation (hr)	Anti-DNP IgG PFC Culture supernatants from[a]	
	Activated	Unactivated
—	3930	3930
4	3380	4200
8	1330	3630
16	1090	3400

[a]The culture supernatants from the acceptor hybridomas unactivated or activated with monoclonal KLH-TsF were harvested at different time intervals and tested for their activity in the in vitro anti-DNP IgG PFC response of spleen cells primed with DNP-KLH.

chain type, inhibits all antibody responses to DNP-KLH in an antigen-specific fashion, and (2) the new suppressor factor, unlike KLH-TsF, does not have the ability to bind native antigen KLH, regardless of its KLH-specific suppressor function. It is thus strongly suggested that the newly induced suppressor factor seems to have an anti-idiotypic structure for the KLH-binding two-chain factor.

The presence of the anti-idiotypic structure on the new suppressor factor or on the acceptor hybridoma was also suggested by data indicating that the acceptor hybridoma cells were killed by mouse anti-KLH antisera but not by mouse anti-OVA antisera (Fig. 2). The cytotoxic activity of the anti-KLH antisera observed on the acceptor hybridoma cells seemed to be specific, because the antisera could not kill the BW5147 thymoma cell line, which is a parental cell line for the acceptor-suppressor hybridoma. The results suggested that the acceptor hybridoma possesses an anti-idiotypic receptor complementary to the structures on the KLH-TsF, and also that the idiotype-like structure of KLH-TsF seems to be shared with that of the anti-KLH antibody. Although no major CRI on anti-KLH antibodies have so far been reported, it is important to understand the biological roles of the acceptor T cells with an anti-idiotypic receptor on the KLH-specific antibody response. This will be discussed in Section 6.

4. Activation of Acceptor Hybridoma with KLH-Specific Suppressor Factor

As the acceptor hybridoma bearing complementary receptor for KLH-TsF was found to be directly stimulated by monoclonal or conventional KLH-TsF in the absence of relevant antigen, the activation mechanisms of suppressor T cells via idiotype–anti-idiotype-like interactions was investigated. For this purpose, the acceptor hybridoma was incubated with monoclonal KLH-TsF or conventional TsF of thymocyte extract obtained from mice

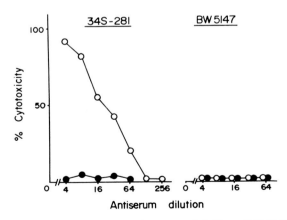

FIGURE 2. The cytoxicity of anti-KLH antiserum on the acceptor hybridoma (34S-281) bearing a receptor for KLH-TsF. Antiserum dilutions × 10^2. (○) C57BL/6 anti-KLH (●) C57BL/6 anti-OVA.

(C57BL/6, C3H, or BALB/c) primed with antigen (i.e., KLH or OVA). The hybridoma cells activated were further cultured in fresh medium for 12 hr. The activity in the culture supernatants or the cell-free extracts was tested in the *in vitro* secondary response. Only monoclonal and conventional KLH-specific suppressor factors derived from C57BL/6 mice (C57BL/6 KLH-TsF) stimulated the acceptor hybridoma, while no significant stimulatory effect was obtained by C57BL/6 OVA-TsF, C3H KLH-TsF, or BALB/c OVA-TsF (Table II). As the acceptor hybridoma was derived by the fusion of C57BL/6 KLH-primed splenic T cells, the identity of both KLH specificity and genetic specificity between TsF and acceptor hybridoma is required for activation of the acceptor hybridoma. Moreover, the two polypeptide chains that compose KLH-TsF were demonstrated to mediate antigen-specific and genetically restricted suppressor function. Therefore, the acceptor site may have the complementary structures for both chains of TsF.

Further experiments were designed to investigate the events that generate the genetic specificity required in the TsF–acceptor interaction. For this purpose, the involvement of the *H-2* gene complex in the generation of the genetic specificity of TsF was studied, because the I-J molecule which is a light chain of TsF seems to work as an element to mediate the genetic specificity, and because our previous studies have also suggested that the identity of *H-2* haplotypes between the light chains of TsF and the responding cells is required for the expression of TsF activity.

The acceptor hybridoma cells were stimulated by conventional KLH-primed thymocyte extracts obtained from various mice strains with different *H-2* haplotypes, such as C57BL/6 (H-2^b), B10.A(3R) (H-2^{i3}), B10.A(5R) (H-2^{i5}), B10.A(2R) (H-2^{h2}), and A/WySn (H-2^a). As shown in Table III, KLH-TsF derived from C57BL/6 and B10.A(3R) but not from B10.A(5R), B10.A(2R), or A/WySn mice could stimulate the acceptor hybridoma. As the genetic difference between B10.A(3R) and B10.A(5R) is found to be only the *I-J*, the genetic restriction shown in the TsF–acceptor interaction seems to be governed by the *I-J*.

The *I-J* subregion is defined as a chromosomal segment encompassing the *Ia-4* locus with the crossover positions in strains B10.A(5R) and B10.A(3R) forming regional boundaries (Fig. 3). The recombinants are derived from a cross between A/WySn and C57BL/10 and carry the chromosomal segment of A/WySn origin, which is extended from the intra-*H-2* recombinant points to somewhere to the right of the *H-2D*. The left side of the extra-*H-2* in both B10.A(3R) and B10.A(5R) mice originates from C57BL/10 mice. However, the extra-*H-2* (right) end of the inserted chromosomal segment is totally unknown. It is therefore possible that the genes coding for the I-J molecule are present not only within the intra-*H-2* complex, but also on the right side of the chromosomal segment, which can be either the A/WySn or the C57BL/10 type.

Recombinant B10.A(2R), which arose in the same series of the back crossing that produced B10.A(3R) and B10.A(5R), should have inherited the chromosomal segment to the right of the *H-2D* from the parental C57BL/10 and the inserted chromosome to the left of the *H-2S* from A/WySn. A/WySn and B10.A(2R) strains are κ type at the *I-J* subregion, and the right-side end of chromosome 17 in these mice should represent the respective parental type. The experimental data described here, however, demonstrated that the suppressor factor derived from B10.A(2R) and A/WySn mice could not stimulate the C57BL/6-derived acceptor hybridoma, strongly indicating that the genes coding for the

TABLE II

*Requirement of Antigenic and Genetic-
Restriction Specificities of TsF in the
Stimulation of the Acceptor Hybridoma*

Acceptor hybridoma stimulated with TsF[a]	Anti-DNP IgG PFC/culture
—	6848
None	6432
Hybridoma (34S-18)	1760
KLH-C57BL/6	2272
OVA-C57BL/6	7648
KLH-C3H	6880
OVA-BALB/c	6912

[a]Cell-free extracts obtained from KLH-TsF-producing hybridoma (34S-18) or from thymocytes of mice primed with high doses of KLH or OVA were incubated with the acceptor hybridoma. The activity in the extracts of the activated hybridoma was tested in the *in vitro* anti-DNP PFC responses of C57BL/6 spleen cells primed with DNP-KLH.

elements that determine the genetic restriction specificity should be present in the intra-*H-2* gene complex. However, recent molecular genetic studies on the *I-J* subregion genes reported by Steinmetz *et al.*[16] have demonstrated the possibility that the *I-J* subregion is not encoded between *I-A* and *I-E* subregions of the *I* region of the *H-2* complex. Thus, it would appear that the genes coding for the I-J molecule on the light chain of the suppressor factor have not been precisely mapped.

The previous studies have shown that two different signals, i.e., antigen specificity and genetic specificity, are essential in the activation of the acceptor hybridoma. Furthermore,

TABLE III

*Activation of the Acceptor Hybridoma with KLH-TsF Derived
from Thymus Extracts of Various Strains of Mice*

Acceptor hybridoma stimulated with KLH-TsF[a] derived from	I-J haplotype	Anti-DNP IgG PFC/culture
Control	—	1530
Not activated	—	1770
C57BL/6[b]	b	730
B10.A(3R)	b	450
B10.A(5R)	k	1310
B10.A(2R)	k	1520
A/WySn	k	1440

[a]The KLH-specific TsF in thymocyte extracts used in this experiment has been demonstrated to exhibit antigen-specific suppression of PFC responses in the appropriate recipients.
[b]Monoclonal KLH-TsF derived from hybridoma cells.

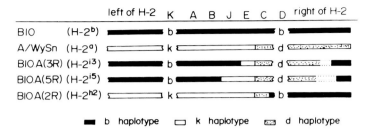

FIGURE 3. Origins of chromosomal segments containing the *H-2* complex of the recombinant mouse strains. The *I-J* subregion is mapped between *I-A* and *I-E* subregions. However, molecular genetic studies by Steinmetz *et al.* have suggested the possibility that the *I-J* subregion is not present at this position.

it is also suggested that antigen specificity is mediated by the heavy chain, whereas the light chain (I-J molecule) determines the genetic restriction specificity. In order to confirm that the two signals are mediated by the two chains of TsF, the mRNAs coding for the light and heavy chains of KLH-TsF were translated in *Xenopus laevis* oocytes. The translated free light and heavy chains of TsF were used for activation of the acceptor hybridoma.

For this purpose, total RNA was isolated from 10^9 cultured hybridoma cells by the guanidine/cesium chloride methods as originally described by Chirgwin *et al.*[17] Poly(A) RNAs were purified by chromatography on oligo(dT)-cellulose. Usually, 50–100 μg of mRNA was obtained from 10^9 cells. The mRNA purified was further fractionated in size by 5–22% sucrose density gradient centrifugation. The fractionated mRNAs were injected into *X. laevis* oocytes. The heavy and light chains translated in oocytes were detected by cytotoxic inhibition assay using monoclonal BALB/c anti-CB-20 for detection of the heavy chain and monoclonal B10.A(5R) anti-B10.A(3R) for detection of the light chain of TsF. The results were that 11 S mRNA directs synthesis of the light chain, whereas 13 S and 18.5 S mRNAs encode the heavy chain of TsF.[13] Furthermore, the heavy and light chains of the translation products per se do not exert any functional activity, whereas the combination of heavy and light chains reconstitutes the active suppressor molecule to express the antigen-specific and genetically restricted suppressor activity when the translation products are added to the culture of spleen cells primed with DNP-KLH.[13]

By using these active components of *in vitro* mRNA translation products, we tried to stimulate the acceptor hybridomas to determine whether both heavy and light chains are necessary for constructing biological signals for the stimulation of the acceptor hybridomas. In this experiment, the acceptor hybridomas were incubated with either 11 S or 13 S mRNA products or both for 1 hr on ice. The cells reacted were washed and further cultivated in fresh medium. The cell-free extract or the culture supernatant of the activated acceptor hybridoma cells was tested for suppressor activity. The results are shown in Table IV. Either the 11 S or the 13 S mRNA translation products could not activate the acceptor hybridomas, whereas the mixture of one-half volume of the 11 S and 13 S mRNA products successfully reconstituted the active suppressor factor to stimulate the acceptor hybridomas. It is thus clear that the two distinct signals mediated by the heavy and light chains of TsF lead to the stimulation of the acceptor T cells in the resting state.

TABLE IV
Stimulation of Acceptor T-Cell Hybridoma with Heavy and Light Chains of TsF-mRNA Translation Products[a]

Acceptor cells stimulated with	Anti-DNP IgG PFC/culture
—	3300
None	3200
Monoclonal KLH-TsF	953
11 S mRNA translates	3327
13 S mRNA translates	3512
11 S + 13 S mRNA translates	887

[a]The acceptor hybridoma was stimulated with monoclonal KLH-TsF or translation products of the fractionated mRNAs obtained from KLH-TsF-producing hybridoma cells. The activity in the extracts of the activated acceptor hybridoma was tested in the *in vitro* anti-DNP IgG PFC response.

5. Biochemical and Molecular Events of the Activation of the Acceptor Hybridoma

Molecular events in the activation of suppressor T cells were investigated by using activated and nonactivated acceptor hybridoma cells. Total RNAs were isolated by the guanidine/cesium chloride methods from the acceptor hybridoma before or after stimulation with KLH-TsF. The mRNAs were further purified from the total RNA fraction by chromatography on oligo(dT)-cellulose. For detection of suppressor activities in the translation product, the purified mRNAs obtained from the activated or the nonactivated hybridoma cells were injected into *X. laevis* oocytes. The activity of the translation products was tested in the *in vitro* secondary anti-DNP PFC response to DNP-KLH. As shown in Table V, suppressor activity was only obtained in the translation products of mRNAs derived from the activated hybridoma cells, while no significant effect was observed by the mRNA translation products of nonactivated hybridoma cells. The findings are quite consistent with the data demonstrating that the activated acceptor hybridoma produced new suppressor factor after activation with KLH-specific TsF of the two-chain type.

TABLE V
Biological Activity of Translation Products of mRNAs Obtained from Activated or Unactivated Acceptor Hybridoma Cells[a]

Material added to culture	mRNAs from acceptor hybridoma	Anti-DNP IgG PFC/culture
—	—	2950
mRNA products	Unactivated	3150
mRNA products	Activated	700
Oocyte extracts	—	2590

[a]The same amounts of mRNAs purified from activated or unactivated acceptor hybridoma were injected into *X. laevis* oocytes. The translation products were added to the culture at a concentration of 0.3 μl oocyte extracts (10 cells in 300 μl)/ml.

To characterize the biochemical events resulting after activation, mRNAs which are the same material as used in the functional assays were translated *in vitro* in a rabbit reticulocyte lysate system in the presence of [^{35}S]methionine. The internally labeled translation products were analyzed by a high-resolution two-dimensional electrophoresis procedure combining isoelectric focusing (using a mixture of 1 volume of pH 3.5–10 Ampholines and 1 volume of pH 5–7 Ampholines) and SDS slab gel electrophoresis (12% polyacrylamide) as described by O'Farrell.[18] The gels are run until the dye front reaches the bottom of the gel, dried, and then exposed to X-ray film. The radioactive protein spots in the two autoradiograms obtained from nonactivated and activated hybridoma cells were compared. About 200 protein spots with different intensities of radioactivity and various sizes were resolved by this method. Among the spots in the radiogram of the activated cells, about 10 spots were newly produced after activation, because they were not present in the autoradiogram of the nonactivated hybridoma cells. It is therefore apparent that the protein spots are derived from the events of the stimulation. This may not always, however, mean that the spots newly developed are directly related to the suppressor factor newly produced by the activated acceptor hybridoma. In any event, the activated hybridoma cells are very helpful in focusing on the functional proteins produced after activation and in searching for the genes coding for the proteins related to the suppressor molecules.

6. Discussion

Our previous studies on the KLH-specific suppressor system have shown that KLH-TsF acts on a subset of suppressor T cells, such as acceptor T cells, in a process by which effector-precursor cells are stimulated to become effector-suppressor T cells. In this respect, KLH-TsF serves as a signal for activating suppressor pathways and consequently for enhancing suppressor activity. The amplification mechanisms mediated by the TsF and acceptor T cells have also been demonstrated by others. The intermediary cells of the acceptor T cell type they described bear the anti-idiotypic receptor for the idiotypic determinants expressed on suppressor T cells and their factors, and this idiotypic structure is similar to that of the major CRI on the antibodies. In our present studies on the "KLH-specific" acceptor hybridoma, we have also demonstrated that the acceptor hybridoma cells have the anti-idiotypic (complementary) receptor for the KLH-TsF. The presence of anti-idiotypic receptor on the acceptor hybridoma cells has been demonstrated by the following experimental data:

1. The acceptor hybridoma is able to absorb KLH-TsF.
2. The acceptor hybridoma in the resting state is activated by KLH-TsF in the absence of relevant antigen KLH and starts to produce new KLH-specific suppressor factor.
3. The new suppressor factor produced inhibits the antibody response in KLH-specific fashion, despite its inability to bind to the native antigen column.
4. The KLH specificity of TsF is essential for the activation of the acceptor T-cell hybridoma.
5. The acceptor hybridoma cell is specifically killed by conventional anti-KLH but not by anti-OVA antisera.

Based on the above evidence, it is most likely that the acceptor hybridoma described here, like anti-idiotypic acceptor T cells in other systems, possesses the anti-idiotypic receptor for KLH-TsF. Moreover, the idiotypic determinant on monoclonal KLH-TsF seems to be shared with some of the anti-KLH antibodies, because the acceptor hybridoma with complementary structure for KLH-TsF was killed by conventional anti-KLH.

It is believed that the antigen KLH equally stimulates a variety of anti-KLH clones so that no major idiotype has been found on the anti-KLH antibodies. Therefore, the KLH system in C57BL/6 mice is apparently distinct from the GAT, GT, or ABA systems, in which these antigens stimulate only limited specific clones in a particular animal. However, little is understood about the idiotypes on T cells specific for conventional antigens.

In any event, all cells of acceptor-suppressor T-cell types detected in various systems seem to be anti-idiotypic. If so, the question to be asked is why the particular repertoire limitation observed in T cells is dictated even in the conventional antigen systems. One possibility is that the family of suppressor T cells recognizes only the limited epitopes on the conventional antigens (i.e., epitopes for suppressor cells as mentioned by E. Sercarz). In that case, the suppressor T cells and their factors will bear a predominant idiotype, whereas B cells or antibodies can recognize whole epitopes on the KLH molecule so that no major idiotype is detected at the anti-KLH antibody level. Thus idiotype–anti-idiotype-like interactions appear to operate exclusively at T-cell levels. In fact, monoclonal KLH-TsF recognizing only one of the epitopes on the KLH molecules or the monoclonal anti-idiotypic TsF derived from the activated acceptor hybridoma suppresses all antibody responses against total epitopes on KLH macromolecules in an antigen-specific fashion. It is strongly suggested that in the immune systems against conventional antigens, e.g., KLH, idiotype–anti-idiotype regulatory interactions predominantly operate at T-cell levels and may play decisive roles in the homeostatic regulation of the immune response.

ACKNOWLEDGMENT. We wish to express our gratitude to Miss Hisano Nakajima for her excellent secretarial assistance.

References

1. Taniguchi, M., and Tokuhisa, T., 1980, Cellular consequences in the suppression of antibody response by the antigen-specific suppressor T cell factor, *J. Exp. Med.* **151:**517–527.
2. Waltenbaugh, C., Thèze, J., Kapp, J. A., and Benacerraf, B., 1977, Immunosuppressive factor(s) specific for L-glutamic acid^{50}-L-tyrosine^{50} (GT). III. Generation of suppressor T cells by a suppressive extract derived from GT-primed lymphoid cells, *J. Exp. Med.* **146:**970–985.
3. Eardley, D. D., Kemp, J., Shen, F. W., Cantor, H., and Gershon, R. K., 1979, Immunoregulatory circuits among T cell sets: Effect of mode of immunization on determining which Ly1 T cell will be activated, *J. Immunol.* **122:**1663–1665.
4. Dorf, M. E., Okuda, K., and Minami, M., 1982, Dissection of a suppressor cell cascade, *Curr. Top. Microbiol. Immunol.* **100:**61–67.
5. Germain, R. N., Thèze, J., Waltenbaugh, C., Dorf, M. E., and Benacerraf, B., 1978, Antigen specific T cell mediated suppression. II. In vitro induction of I-J coded L-glutamic acid^{50}-L-tyrosine^{50} (GT)-specific T cell suppressor factor (GT-TsF) of suppressor T cells (Ts$_2$) bearing distinct I-J determinants, *J. Immunol.* **121:**602–607.
6. Sy, M.-S., Dietz, M. H., Germain, R. N., Benacerraf, B., and Greene, M. I., 1980, Antigen- and receptor-driven regulatory mechanisms. IV. Idiotype-bearing I-J$^+$ suppressor T cell factors induced second-order suppressor T cells which express anti-idiotypic receptors, *J. Exp. Med.* **151:**1183–1195.

7. Taniguchi, M., Saito, T., and Tada, T., 1979, Antigen-specific suppressive factor produced by a transplantable I-J bearing T cell hybridoma, *Nature* **278**:555–558.
8. Taniguchi, M., Takei, I., and Tada, T., 1980, Functional and molecular organization of an antigen-specific suppressor factor derived from a T cell hybridoma, *Nature* **283**:227–228.
9. Saito, T., and Taniguchi, M., 1983, Chemical features of an antigen-specific suppressor T cell factor composed of two polypeptide chains, submitted *J. Mol. Cell. Immunol.* (in press).
10. Tokuhisa, T., Komatsu, Y., Uchida, Y., and Taniguchi, M., 1982, Monoclonal antibodies specific for the constant region of the T cell antigen-receptors, *J. Exp. Med.* **156**:888–897.
11. Kanno, M., Kobayashi, S., Tokuhisa, T., Takei, I., Shinohara, N., and Taniguchi, M., 1981, Monoclonal antibodies that recognize the product controlled by a gene in the I-J subregion of the mouse H-2 complex, *J. Exp. Med.* **154**:1290–1304.
12. Taniguchi, M., Saito, T., Takei, I., and Tokuhisa, T., 1981, Presence of interchain S-S bonds between two gene products that compose the secreted form of an antigen-specific suppressor factor, *J. Exp. Med.* **153**:1672–1677.
13. Taniguchi, M., Tokuhisa, T., Kanno, M., Yaoita, Y., Shimizu, A., and Honjo, T., 1982, Reconstitution of an antigen-specific suppressor activity with the translation products of mRNA coding for the antigen-binding and the I-J bearing molecules, *Nature* **298**:172–174.
14. Fresno, M., McVay-Boudreau, L. and Cantor, H., 1982, Antigen-specific T lymphocyte clones. III. Papain splits purified T suppressor molecules into two functional domains, *J. Exp. Med.* **155**:981–993.
15. Taniguchi, M., Takei, I., Saito, T., and Tokuhisa, T., 1981, Activation of an acceptor T cell hybridoma by a V_H I-J$^+$ monoclonal suppressor factor, in: *Immunoglobulin idiotypes* (C. A. Janeway, Jr., E. E. Sercarz, and H. Wigzell, eds.), Academic Press, New York, pp. 397–406.
16. Steinmetz, M., Minard, K., Hovath, S., McNicholas, J., Frelinger, J., Wake, C., Long, E., Mach, B., and Hood, L., 1982, A molecular map of the immune response region from the major histocompatibility complex of the mouse, *Nature* **300**:35–42.
17. Chirgwin, J. M., Prezybyla, A. E., MacDonald, R. J., and Rutter, W. J., 1979, Isolation of biochemically active ribonucleic acid from sucroses enriched in ribonuclease, *Biochemistry* **18**:5294–5299.
18. O'Farrell, P. H., 1975, High resolution two dimensional electrophoresis of proteins, *J. Biol. Chem.* **250**:4007–4021.

28

Role of Idiotypes in the (4-Hydroxy-3-Nitrophenyl)Acetyl (NP)-Specific Suppressor T-Cell Pathway

David H. Sherr, Michael J. Onyon, and Martin E. Dorf

1. Role of Idiotype-Related Determinants in T-Cell Regulation

It has recently become evident that modulation of the immune response can be effected by regulatory elements which recognize unique idiotypic determinants associated with the binding site of antibody molecules. For example, injection of mice with antigen[1] or idiotypic antibodies[2] results in the production of autoantibody specific for predominant idiotypic determinants. Injection of anti-idiotypic antibodies may similarly result in the appearance of idiotypic antibody.[3] These data support the hypothesis first proposed by Jerne predicting the participation of complementary idiotypic–anti-idiotypic antibodies in the regulation of the immune response.[4]

Since some T lymphocytes bear antigen-binding receptors which appear to share idiotypic determinants with B-cell populations,[5] it would be predicted that recognition of idiotypic determinants is also important for interactions among T-cell subsets. Indeed, it now has been shown in several systems that injection of antigen,[6-10] anti-idiotypic antibodies,[11,12] or idiotype-bearing antibodies[13-15] may result in the appearance of idiotypic or anti-idiotypic suppressor or helper T lymphocytes. It appears then that recognition of predominant idiotype-related determinants expresssed on antigen-reactive T lymphocytes is involved in induction and/or activation of regulatory T cells.

The requirement for recognition of predominant idiotype-related determinants for T-cell communication is underscored in systems in which multiple T-cell interactions occur. In one such system we have studied the idiotype-dependent regulation of B-cell and T-cell

David H. Sherr, Michael J. Onyon, and Martin E. Dorf • Department of Pathology, Harvard Medical School, Boston, Massachusetts 02115.

responses to the (4-hydroxy-3-nitrophenyl)acetyl (NP) hapten. When coupled to T-dependent or T-independent carriers, this hapten elicits a relatively restricted primary antibody response characterized by a family of NP-specific idiotypically related antibodies.[16,17] The idiotypic determinants, detected by standard idiotype analysis, identify V_H NP^b gene products which are encoded by genes within the $Igh-1^b$ heavy-chain linkage group and are collectively referred to as the NP^b idiotype family. NP^b idiotype-positive antibody predominantly expresses the λ light chain. The presence of NP^b determinants is generally, but not exclusively, associated with a heteroclitic response, i.e., the ability of anti-NP antibodies to bind the related hapten (4-hydroxy-5-iodo-3-nitrophenyl)acetyl (NIP) with greater affinity than the immunizing NP hapten. The expression of NP^b idiotype-bearing antibodies in serum is paralleled by the appearance of NP^b idiotype-bearing B cells in the spleen.[18] These NP^b idiotype-bearing B cells can be detected in the spleens of Igh^b-bearing mice primed with T-dependent (NP-KLH, NP-GLA) or relatively T-independent (NP-*Brucella abortus*, NP-Ficoll) NP conjugates by the ability of NP^b idiotype-specific antibodies from guinea pigs to specifically inhibit plaque formation. The presence of NP^b idiotype-bearing B-cell clones can similarly be determined following *in vitro* challenge of NP-primed splenocytes.[18-21]

T-cell-mediated contact sensitivity (CS) responses have been studied by priming mice subcutaneously with NP-coupled cells or with the reactive compound NP-*O*-succinimide (NP-*O*-Su) and challenging in one footpad 5–6 days later with NP-coupled spleen cells or NP-*O*-Su. NP-specific footpad swelling can be measured 24 hr later.[22-24] The ability of T cells from NP-*O*-Su-primed Igh^b mice but not mice expressing the Igh^j allotype to cross-react with the NP hapten [22] suggests that the fine specificity of the T-cell receptors may be related to the heteroclicity of anti-NP antibodies. However, several differences in the strain distribution of NP-induced NP-elicited CS and B-cell responses suggest that the genes which control T- and B-cell responses are distinct.[23]

Using both the T-cell-mediated CS and the B-cell-mediated PFC responses, we have characterized an intricate suppressor T-cell cascade capable of modulating NP-specific responses.[16-24] This suppressor T-cell pathway involves three interacting T-cell subsets and is activated by the intravenous injection of NP-modified syngeneic spleen cells. The first T-cell population detected, termed Ts^i or Ts_1, functions only when added early in the immune response (induction phase) and bears an NP^b idiotype-related NP-specific surface receptor. Its ability to work only when added in the induction phase reflects the temporal requirement for this T-cell population to induce second-order Ts cells, called Ts^e or Ts_2. This latter population suppresses NP-specific responses when added within 24 hr of assay of plaque formation or footpad swelling (effector phase). The Ts_2 population bears anti-idiotypic receptors and interacts with a third T-cell population (Ts_3). The Ts_3 population is induced, but not activated, by immunization with NP conjugates. This NP-binding, T-cell subset also bears an NP^b idiotype-related receptor and probably reflects the effector population in the suppressor pathway. It is in the context of this Ts cell pathway that the role of the NP^b idiotype in regulation of immune responses will be discussed.

2. Idiotype-Related Determinants Present on NP-Specific Ts_1 Cells

The ability of NP-coupled syngeneic spleen cells to induce antigen-specific Ts cells was first demonstrated by Weinberger *et al.* in a delayed-type hypersensitivity system.[25]

It was shown that the spleens of mice injected 7 days previously with NP-coupled syngeneic spleen cells contained an NP-binding T-cell population capable of suppressing DTH-mediated footpad swelling to NP only when these cells were added in the induction phase of the response. This T-cell population, then called Ts^i, adheres to NP-BSA-coated petri dishes. Furthermore, treatment of T cells from NP spleen-treated Igh^b mice with anti-NP^b idiotype antiserum plus complement abrogates the transfer of NP-specific suppression to normal, syngeneic C57BL/6 or SJL recipients. It should be noted that NP-specific antibodies from SJL mice are nonheteroclitic and express only a fraction of the NP^b idiotypic family presumably because of a λ_1-light-chain defect.[26] The presence of readily detectable NP^b-related idiotypic determinants on SJL Ts^i required for functional suppression again suggests that the NP^b-related idiotypic determinants present on Ts^i, subsequently referred to as Ts_1 cells, do not correlate with the set of idiotypic determinants present on immunoglobulin molecules. The results imply that T-cell and B-cell-derived idiotypic receptors are distinct.

In a related system, splenic T cells from NP spleen-treated mice (Ts^i or Ts_1) were shown to specifically suppress the *in vivo* PFC response to T-dependent or T-independent forms of NP conjugates when transferred to normal, syngeneic recipients.[18] In this system, the percent of NP-specific PFC which expressed NP^b determinants was determined by addition of microliter quantities of NP^b idiotype-specific antiserum to the plaquing mixture. While the idiotype content of the PFC response from control mice ranged from 30 to 50% of the total NP-specific PFC response, the idiotype level in recipients of Ts cells was 0%. The complete suppression of NP^b idiotype-bearing B-cell clones correlated well with a 30–50% suppression of the magnitude of the response. Thus, suppression induced with NP-modified spleen cells preferentially affects NP^b idiotype-bearing B cells as well as the T-cell-mediated CS response of Igh^b mice.

To further analyze this induction-phase Ts population, NP-binding splenic T cells from NP spleen-treated mice were fused with BW5147 thymoma cells according to standard procedures.[27] The HAT-resistant cell lines were screened for determinants detected with anti-I-J alloantisera generally found on Ts cells and for NP^b idiotype-related cell surface markers. Culture supernatants were then tested for their ability to suppress CS and/or *in vitro* NP-specific PFC responses. Two NP-specific Ts hybridomas derived from CKB mice and one from C57BL/6 mice were identified. As with the heterogeneous Ts^i population from which they were derived, these hybridomas were shown to suppress only when added in the induction phase of the responses.[27–28] Suppressor factors detected in supernatants of hybridoma cultures were shown to resemble the cell surface receptors of heterogeneous Ts^i cells in that the factors bound to and could be eluted from NP-BSA or anti-NP^b-coupled immunosorbent columns.[28] Furthermore, the cell-free membrane fraction derived from Ts_1 hybridoma cells mediated specific suppressor activity,[29] adding additional support to the concept that these suppressor factors represent a soluble form of the membrane receptor.

3. NP^b Idiotype-Dependent Induction of Ts_2 Cells

In order to determine how induction-phase Ts_1 cells can recruit other T-cell subsets, supernatants from the Ts_1 hybridomas described above were injected into normal syngeneic recipients. Four days later spleen cells from these recipients were shown to have suppressive activity in both the CS and the *in vitro* PFC systems.[27] Unlike Ts_1 cells with which they were induced, these second-order Ts cells (Ts_2) were capable of suppressing NP-specific responses when added in the effector phase of the response. Effector-phase Ts_2 cells can also be generated by *in vitro* incubation of Ts_1 hybridoma supernatants with normal, syngeneic spleen cells.[19] The data indicate that the requirement for addition of Ts_1 cells to responder animals in the induction phase represents the temporal requirement for a Ts_1-derived factor (TsF_1) to induce second-order Ts cells (Ts_2).

Since the cellular interaction molecule derived from Ts_1 hybridoma cells (TsF_1) expressed NP^b idiotype-related determinants [30] and since the overall effect of the suppression of the PFC response was the preferential down-regulation of NP^b idiotype-bearing B-cell clones, [18-19] it seemed possible that recognition of these determinants was required for the proper interaction between Ts populations. Since idiotypic determinants are linked to the immunoglobulin heavy-chain locus, it was possible to test this hypothesis by investigating the possible requirement for Igh allotype homology between the TsF_1 donor and the Ts_2 donor. In the CS system it was shown that C57BL/6-derived TsF_1 failed to manifest suppression in B.C-8 *(Igh^a)* recipients.[27] Thus, there is an apparent Igh restriction in the action of TsF_1. This restriction can be further mapped to the *Igh-V* region since C57BL/6-derived TsF_1 suppresses NP responses in C.B-20 *(Igh-V^b, Igh-C^b)* but not in congenic BAB/14 *(Igh-V^a, Igh-C^b)* mice.[27]

This type of restriction may be a function of a restriction between the TsF_1 and Ts_2 which it induces and/or between the Ts_2 population and its target cell population. Further experimentation revealed that the apparent Igh restriction was not a reflection of the inability of TsF_1 to induce Ts_2 cells in Igh-incompatible recipients but rather the inability of Ts_2 cells induced with and specific for determinants present on Igh-incompatible TsF_1 to recognize target cells which do not express these same Igh-linked determinants. For example, injection of B6-derived (Igh^b) TsF_1 into C3H (Igh^j) mice did not result in suppression of CS responses in Igh-incompatible C3H recipients.[27] However, suppression was observed when spleen cells from the above C3H mice that had received TsF_1 were transferred to Igh^b-bearing CKB or B10.BR recipients during the effector phase of the response. On the basis of this type of data the apparent requirement for Igh homology between the TsF_1 donor and the Ts_2 producer was shown to be a "pseudogenetic" restriction.[27] The implication of this conclusion is that recognition of Igh-linked NP^b-related idiotypic determinants is required for communication between Ts_1 cells and Ts_2 cells and between Ts_2 cells and their target population. This conclusion is further supported by the Igh restriction observed between Ts_2 cells generated by injection of syngeneic TsF_1 or by 4-day culture of Ts_1 cells with normal spleen and the primed recipients of the Ts_2 cells for immune suppression of CS or PFC responses.[19,27]

Since the Ts_2 cell population was shown to be restricted by Igh-linked genes in both T- and B-cell-mediated responses, it was predicted that these suppressor cells specifically recognized Igh-linked, NP^b-related idiotypic determinants. This prediction was substantiated by the demonstration that Ts_2 effector-phase Ts cells, which were induced *in vitro* by 4-day culture of Ts_1-containing spleen cells with normal cells, could specifically bind to and be recovered from culture dishes coated with NP^b-bearing anti-NP antibody.[19,20]

Since idiotypic systems may be composed of a family of idiotypically related but non-identical molecules,[17,31] it was important to determine whether T-cell receptors recognize the same repertoire of NP^b idiotypic determinants as anti-idiotypic antiserum. For this purpose, the ability of effector-phase suppressor cells (Ts_2) to bind monoclonal anti-NP antibodies bearing different levels of NP^b idiotypic determinants was studied in the PFC system.[20] Ts cells were fractionated on petri dishes coated either with N, 4C2, or 6100.15 monoclonal murine anti-NP antibody. Each of these monoclonal anti-NP antibodies is of the IgM class and Igh^b allotype but differs with respect to light-chain class, carrying the λ_2, κ, and λ_1 chains, respectively. Molecular genetic analysis indicates that the N and 6100.15 antibodies express the same germline V_H and J_H genes but use different D_H genes (S.-T. Ju, personal communication). Adherent and nonadherent T-cell populations were then tested for their ability to suppress when added in the effector phase of an *in vitro* PFC response. The data indicate that TS activity can be detected in the N antibody-adherent and to a lesser extent in the N antibody-nonadherent fraction. Thus, Ts$_2$ cells represent a heterogeneous population only a portion of which recognizes NP^b-related idiotypic determinants present on N antibody. In contrast, all of the suppressive activity was detected in the 4C2 antibody-nonadherent fraction. This result is not surprising since this monoclonal antibody does not express serologically detectable NP^b determinants.[20] Of greatest importance is the finding that all of the suppressor activity was recovered in the 6100.15 antibody-nonadherent fraction. This antibody expresses the predominant, serologically detected NP^b idiotypic determinants and, by serologic analysis, shares NP^b idiotypic determinants with the N antibody. From these experiments we concluded that Ts$_2$ cells did not recognize the predominant, serologically detected NP^b idiotypic determinants. The implication is that this T-cell population interacts with other T-cell populations by recognition of determinants expressing only a minor fraction of NP^b-related idiotypic determinants expressed on anti-NP antibody and detected by serologic analyses. This interpretation further underscores the differences between T- and B-cell idiotypes. In this regard, the reactivity of certain anti-idiotypic antisera with T-cell receptors which apparently lack the light chain required for expression of predominant, serologically detected idiotypic determinants[37] may be attributable to serologically minor idiotypic determinants which may not require conventional light chains for idiotype expression that are expressed on T-cell receptors. Similarly, the presence of NP^b-related idiotypic determinants on T cells from SJL mice which have a λ_1-light-chain defect[25] may represent these serologically minor subsets of determinants expressed on T cells and on the SJL-derived N hybridoma antibody. Thus, idiotypic determinants present on T cells appear related but not identical to those expressed on B cells and immunoglobulins. Furthermore, it is not clear whether T- and B-cell idiotypes are encoded by the same set of germ-line genes. Recent data suggest that V_H genes may not be expressed in T cells.[38]

Finally, the specificity of suppressor factors from fusion products of BW5147 thymoma and NP^b idiotype-binding Ts$_2$ cells was studied. As expected from the genetic and specificity studies performed on the heterogeneous Ts$_2$ population, the Ts$_2$ was shown to specifically bind to and be eluted from NP^b idiotype-coupled immunosorbent columns when tested in the CS system.[32]

4. NP^b Idiotype-Related Determinants Present on Third-Order (Ts$_3$) Suppressor Cells

Although the effector-phase Ts$_2$ cell population or factors derived from Ts$_2$ hybridomas were specific for Igh-linked NP^b-related idiotypic determinants and the overall effect of the suppression was idiotype-specific in the PFC system, there was no direct evidence proving that the Ts$_2$ was the final effector cell population in the suppressor pathway. In fact, the inability of Ts$_2$ cells to recognize serologically predominant NP^b determinants may be interpreted as evidence against the direct interaction of Ts$_2$ cells with NP-specific B cells. To address this question the effector-phase suppressor cell population (Ts^e, subsequently termed Ts$_2$) was transferred to normal or cyclophosphamide-treated recipients in the effector phase of the CS response.[24] Cyclophosphamide treatment has been shown to inhibit Ts activity. In these experiments, it was shown that Ts$_2$-containing spleen cell populations did not effect suppression when transferred to cyclophosphamide-treated primed recipients. Furthermore, Ts$_2$ cells did not suppress when transferred to normal recipients with anti-I-J antisera plus complement-treated, NP-primed responder cells.[24] Taken together, the data suggest that in the CS system, the Ts$_2$ effector-phase cells require a third cell type which reacts with anti-I-J serum and is cyclophosphamide-sensitive in order to mediate suppressive activity. These results were extended to the PFC system with the demonstration that Ts$_2$ cells, induced by the subculture of Ts$_1$-containing populations with normal cells, were ineffective when added to cultures of anti-I-J (but not NMS) plus complement-treated, NP-KLH-primed responder cells.[21] The suppressive activity mediated by Ts$_2$ cells was restored by addition of T cells from NP-KLH, but not TNP-KLH, primed donors to responder populations depleted of I-J-bearing T cells. With this reconstitution protocol it was shown that the third-order Ts population (Ts$_3$) specifically bound to and could be recovered from NP-BSA-coated petri dishes. Since the Ts$_3$ population specifically bound NP and was activated by anti-NP^b idiotypic Ts$_2$ cells, it would be expected that Ts$_3$ cells express NP^b-related idiotypic determinants. This conclusion was validated by the demonstration that treatment of Ts$_3$ cells with guinea pig anti-NP^b idiotype antiserum plus complement ablated suppressive activity in the reconstitution protocol described above.

In order to further characterize the Ts$_3$ population, splenic T cells from NP-KLH- or NP-O-Su-primed mice were fused with BW5147 tumor cells. Supernatants from HAT-resistant hybridoma cultures were tested for NP-specific suppressive activity when added in the effector phase of the CS or *in vitro* PFC response. Several hybridoma supernatants were shown to be capable of specific immune suppression.[28,33] Immunochemical characterization of these Ts$_3$ factors (TsF$_3$) in both CS and *in vitro* PFC systems revealed that these TsF$_3$, like the heterogeneous Ts$_3$ population from which they were derived, bound NP and expressed NP^b-related idiotypic determinants. Furthermore, the TsF$_3$ exists as a disulfide-linked two-chain structure. One chain binds NP and the other reacts with anti-I-J alloantisera.[28,34]

Hybridoma TsF$_3$ is similar to TsF$_1$ in that both bind NP, express I-J-encoded and NP^b-related idiotypic determinants, and are capable of affecting both CS and PFC responses.[28,33] However, like the parent populations, these factors can be distinguished on the basis of kinetics of suppression and their ability to induce effector-phase suppressor cell populations.[28,33] In addition, TsF$_3$, but not TsF$_1$, is capable of directly suppressing *in vitro* B-cell resonses to a T-independent antigen (NP-BA) in the absence of Thy-1.2-bearing T cells, supporting the notion that this molecule represents an effector factor in the suppressor pathway.[28]

In the CS system it has been shown that suppression effected by TsF$_3$ is restricted both by *H-2*-encoded and by *Igh*-linked genes.[33] For example, B6-Ts$_3$-8 TsF$_3$, derived from C57BL/6 spleen cells (*H-2^b, Igh^b*), suppresses CS responses of CWB (*H-2^b, Igh^b*) mice but fails to function in either B10.WB (*H-2^j, Igh^b*) or C3H.SW (*H-2^b, Igh^j*) mice.

Interestingly, the *H-2* restriction maps to the *I-J* subregion. Since the same B6-Ts$_3$-8 TsF$_3$ can specifically suppress *in vitro* PFC responses in the effector phase, its genetic restrictions in the PFC system were studied. Responder cells were obtained from C57BL/6 or B10.BR (*H-2^k*, *Igh^b*) mice primed 4 weeks previously with NP-KLH. 7.5 × 10^6 primed or unprimed splenic responder cells were challenged *in vitro* with 100 ng NP-Ficoll or, as a specificity control, 2 × 10^6 SRBC. Four days later, 40 μl of supernatant from BW5147 or B6-Ts$_3$-8 cell cultures was added to the responder cultures and the direct NP- or SRBC-specific PFC responses assayed 1 day later. The data presented in Table I substantiate previous work demonstrating the ability of B6-Ts$_3$-8 supernatants to specifically suppress the NP response when added in the effector phase of the PFC response. In the same series of experiments, however, B6-Ts$_3$-8 supernatants were significantly less effective when added to B10.BR responder cells. Thus, at least an *H-2* preference if not a complete restriction on activity of TsF$_3$ exists. These data are consistent with those obtained in the CS system.[33]

To investigate a possible Igh-linked restriction on TsF$_3$, similar experiments were performed with responder cells from NP-KLH-primed B.C-8 *(H-2^b, Igh^a)* and B6.Igh^e *(H-2^b, Igh^n)* mice. The data in Table II indicate that C57BL/6-derived B6-Ts$_3$-8 supernatants can consistently suppress the *in vitro* PFC response of Igh-congenic B.C-8 and B6.Igh^e mice. It should be noted that the large standard error and the slightly reduced mean suppression observed in B6.Igh^e mice is attributable to one out of six experiments in which no suppression was observed. Thus, in the *in vitro* PFC system, the TsF$_3$ activity is restricted by *H-2*, but is not restricted by genes linked to the *Igh* locus. These results are in contrast to those previously obtained in the CS system.[33] This discrepancy may be a function either of different mechanisms of interaction of TsF$_3$ with target B or T cells involved in contact sensitivity cells or of differences resulting from *in vivo* injection or *in vitro* addition of the factor. In either case, it should be noted that the lack of Igh restriction for TsF$_3$ is the only difference observed to date between the Ts cell pathway as described

TABLE I

H-2 Restriction on the Activity of B6-Ts$_3$-8 Suppresor Factor in Vitro^a

Strain	NP-specific		SRBC-specific	
	Direct PFC/ control culture $\overset{\times}{\div}$ log S.E.^{b}	Normalized percent suppression with TsF$_3$ ± S.E.^{c} (No. of experiments)	Direct PFC/ control culture $\overset{\times}{\div}$ log S.E.	Normalized percent suppression with TsF$_3$ ± S.E. (No. of experiments)
C57BL/6 (*H-2^b*)	1320 $\overset{\times}{\div}$ 1.4	71 ± 13 (11)	3750 $\overset{\times}{\div}$ 1.5	4 ± 3 (4)
B10.BR (*H-2^k*)	1350 $\overset{\times}{\div}$ 1.3	21 ± 12* (11)	NT	NT

^{a}C57BL/6 and B10.BR mice were immunized with 200 μg NP-KLH in pertussis adjuvant. Four weeks later 7.5 × 10^6 spleen cells from these or unprimed donors were cultured together with 100 ng NP-Ficoll or 2 × 10^6 SRBC, respectively. Four days later 40 μl supernatant from cultures of BW5147 thymoma (control) or C57BL/6-derived B60-Ts$_3$−8 hybridoma (TsF$_3$) was added to cultures. One day later cultures were assayed for direct NP- or SRBC-specific PFC responses.
^{b}Geometric mean $\overset{\times}{\div}$ log S.E.
^{c}Arithmetic mean ± S.E. An asterisk indicates a significant drop in suppression relative to 71 ± 13, $p < 0.02$.

Table II
Lack of Igh Restriction of B6-Ts₃-8 Suppresor Factor in Vitro[a]

Strain	Direct PFC response/ control culture $\overset{\times}{\div}$ log S.E.	Normalized percent suppression with $TsF_3 \pm$ S.E. (No. of experiments)
C57BL/6 $(Igh\text{-}1^b)$	1400 $\overset{\times}{\div}$ 1.3	73 $\pm$ 10 (18)
B.C-8 $(Igh\text{-}1^a)$	710 $\overset{\times}{\div}$ 1.8	85 $\pm$ 9 (4)
B6.Igh^e $(Igh\text{-}1^n)$	1660 $\overset{\times}{\div}$ 1.3	46 $\pm$ 24 (6)

[a]See Table I footnotes.

in the CS and PFC systems. Preliminary data suggest that the Igh restrictions noted in the CS system may reflect additional cellular interactions required between TsF_3 and cells in the host

5. Preferential Suppression of NP^b-Bearing, High-Affinity B-Cell Populations *in Vivo*

If the suppressor pathway preferentially affects NP^b idiotype-bearing B cells *in vivo* and *in vitro,* and the final effector cell, Ts_3, is specific for NP, then it might be postulated that suppression is attributable to the preferential inactivation of high-affinity NP^b-bearing B cells by complexes of TsF_3 and NP antigen. Consistant with this hypothesis is the lack of Igh restrictions observed for TsF_3. To determine if the suppressor pathway preferentially affects NP^b idiotype-bearing, high-affinity B cells, spleen cells from control or NP spleen-treated mice (containing Ts_1 cells) were adoptively transferred to normal recipients. Recipients were then immunized with NP-Ficoll and assayed for the magnitude, NP^b idiotype content, and affinity of the direct NP-specific PFC responses 7 days later. A population of high-affinity B cells was arbitrarily defined as the percent of the total, NP-specific PFC that were inhibitable with a relatively low concentration of free hapten inhibitor, 10^{-4} M NP-caproic acid. As previously reported, the magnitude of the response to NP-Ficoll is only modestly reduced upon transfer of suppressor cells (Table III). However, the percent NP^b-positive B cells, as defined by PFC inhibition with this particular NP^b idiotype-specific guinea pig antiserum, was significantly reduced from 24% in controls to 0% in suppressor cell recipients. At the same time the percentage of the total PFC which falls into the highest affinity category, i.e., inhibitable with 10^{-4} M NP hapten, is significantly reduced from 34% to 19% ($p < 0.02$). These data suggest that suppression preferentially affects NP^b-bearing as well as high-affinity B-cell populations. In order to determine if NP^b idiotype-bearing B cells were also of high affinity, the percent high-affinity B cells remaining after inhibition of control PFC with anti-NP^b antiserum was determined. The data indicate that while 34% of the total control population is of high affinity, only 15% ($p < 0.02$) of the non-NP^b-bearing B cells fall into this high-affinity category (Table III).

TABLE III

Preferential Suppression of High-Affinity, NP^b-Bearing B-Cell Subsets in a Primary NP-Specific PFC Response[a]

Spleen cells transferred (No. of mice)	Direct NP-specific PFC/spleen[b]	Percent PFC inhibited[c]	Percent PFC inhibited[d]	Percent PFC inhibited[e]
Control (27)	$7550 \overset{\times}{\div} 1.1$	24 ± 3	34 ± 4	15 ± 4
Suppressor (24)	$6090 \overset{\times}{\div} 1.1$	0 ± 4	19 ± 4	NT

[a] Untreated or NP-conjugated spleen cells were injected i.v. into normal syngeneic mice. Seven days later 3×10^7 spleen cells from these mice were transferred to normal recipients and these mice were immunized with 50 μg NP-Ficoll. Seven days later the direct splenic NP-specific PFC responses were assayed. NP^b idiotype levels were determined by PFC inhibition with guinea pig anti-NP^b idiotype antiserum. The affinity of the PFC response was determined by PFC inhibition with 0.3×10^{-3} to 10^{-5} M NP-caproic acid added in half log increments.
[b] Geometric mean of PFC response $\overset{\times}{\div}$ log S.E.
[c] Arithmetic mean of percent PFC inhibited with 40 μl anti-NP^b antiserum $\pm$ S.E. The suppressed group is significantly different relative to 24 ± 3, $p < 0.002$.
[d] Arithmetic mean of percent PFC inhibited with $\leq 10^{-4}$ M NP hapten $\pm$ S.E. The data represent significant differences, $p < 0.02$.
[e] Arithmetic mean of percent PFC inhibited with $\leq 10^{-4}$ M NP hapten in the presence of anti-NP^b antiserum $\pm$ S.E. The data represent significant differences relative to the control value of 34 ± 4, $p < 0.03$.

The data are consistent with the hypothesis that high-affinity B-cell subpopulations express NP^b idiotypic determinants.

If suppression is truly affinity-dependent and not NP^b idiotype-specific per se, then it would be predicted that suppression of high-affinity, NP-specific populations would be manifest even in the absence of NP^b idiotype-bearing B cells. To test this hypothesis, suppression of high-affinity B-cell populations induced by secondary immunization with the T-dependent antigen NP-BGG was studied. As reported by others for serum antibodies, the secondary B-cell response is characterized by a very heterogeneous κ-bearing anti-NP response[35] with few NP^b idiotype-bearing B cells (Table IV). Despite this, the percentage of the total NP-specific PFC population falling into an arbitrarily defined high-affinity category, i.e., inhibited with $\leq 10^{-6}$ M NP-caproic acid, significantly decreases from 57% to 35% ($p < 0.004$) after transfer of suppressor cells. Identical results are obtained if the high-affinity population is defined as percentage of the total PFC population inhibitable with $\leq 0.3 \times 10^{-6}$ M or 10^{-7} M NP hapten (data not shown). The suppression of approximately 22% (57% minus 35%) of this high-affinity subpopulation may account for the slight suppression of the magnitude of the response. This suppression can be seen to be antigen-specific since no effect on either the magnitude or the percent high-affinity PFC in a secondary TNP-BGG response was demonstrated. The data are consistant with the hypothesis that suppression in this system preferentially affects NP^b-related idiotype-bearing, high-affinity B-cell subpopulations. The final mechanism of suppression may then represent preferential inhibition of high-affinity (NP^b-bearing) B-cell clones by a complex of TsF_3 and NP antigen. Preferential suppression of high-affinity B-cell subsets in the NP system appears similar to the mechanism of suppression reported elsewhere.[36]

TABLE IV

Preferential Suppression of High-Affinity NP^b-Negative B Cells in a Secondary NP-Specific PFC Response[a]

Spleen cells transferred	Indirect NP-specific PFC		Indirect TNP-specific PFC	
	PFC/spleen $\overset{\times}{\div}$ log S.E.[b] (No. of mice)	Percent PFC inhibited[c]	PFC/ spleen $\overset{\times}{\div}$ log S.E. (No. of mice)	Percent PFC[c]
Control	15,200 $\overset{\times}{\div}$ 1.2 (18)	57 ± 4	3100 $\overset{\times}{\div}$ 1.2 (14)	27 ± 6
Suppressor	12,000 $\overset{\times}{\div}$ 1.3 (16)	35 ± 5	3400 $\overset{\times}{\div}$ 1.2 (14)	24 ± 4

[a]C57BL/6 mice received 3×10^7 spleen cells from control or NP spleen-injected mice and were immunized with 200 μg NP_{12}-BGG or TNP_{14}-BGG in pertussis adjuvant. Fourteen days later mice received a second i.v. injection of spleen cells from normal or NP spleen-treated donors and were challenged with 200 μg NP-BGG or TNP-BGG in saline. Ten days later mice were assayed for indirect, splenic NP- or TNP-specific PFC responses. The affinity of the PFC responses was determined by the addition of from 10^{-5} to 10^{-7} M NP- or TNP-caproic acid in half log increments. NP-specific indirect PFC were inhibited $-15 \pm 9\%$ when anti-NP^b antiserum was added, confirming the lack of NP^b idiotype-bearing B cells in the secondary, *in vivo* B-cell response.
[b]Geometric mean $\overset{\times}{\div}$ log S.E.
[c]Arithmetic mean of PFC inhibited with $\leq 10^{-6}$ M NP hapten $\pm$ S.E. The data represent a significant difference, $p < 0.004$.

References

1. Schrater, A., Goidl, E., Thorbecke, G., and Siskind, G., 1979, Production of auto-anti-idiotypic antibody during the normal immmune response to TNP-Ficoll, *J. Exp. Med.* **150**:138.
2. Bona, C., Heber-Katz, E., and Paul, W., 1981, Idiotype–anti-idiotype regulation. I. Immunization with a levan-binding myeloma protein leads to the appearance of auto-anti-(anti-id) antibodies and to the activation of silent clones, *J. Exp. Med.* **153**:951–967.
3. Eichmann, K., and Rajewsky, K., 1975, Induction of T and B cell immunity by anti-idiotypic antibody, *Eur. J. Immunol.* **5**:661.
4. Jerne, N.-K., 1974, Towards a network theory of the immune system, *Ann. Immunol. (Inst. Pasteur)* **125C**:373–389.
5. Binz, H., and Wigzell, H., 1976, Shared idiotypic determinants of B and T lymphocytes reactive against the same antigenic determinants. V. Biochemical and serological characteristics of naturally occurring soluble antigen-binding T-lymphocyte-derived molecules, *Scand. J. Immunol.* **5**:559–571.
6. Woodland, R., and Cantor, H., 1978, Idiotype-specific T helper cells are required to induce idiotype-positive B memory cells to secrete antibody, *Eur. J. Immunol.* **8**:600.
7. Bottomly, K., Mathieson, B. J., and Mosier, D. E., 1978, Anti-idiotype induced regulation of helper cell function for the response to phosphorylcholine in adult BALB/c mice, *J. Exp. Med.* **148**:1216–1227.
8. Pierce, S. K., Speck, N. A., Gleason, K., Gearhart, P. J., and Kohler, H., 1981, BALB/c T cells have the potential to recognize the TEPC 15 prototype antibody and its somatic variants, *J. Exp. Med.* **154**:1178–1187.
9. Alevy, Y. G., and Bellone, C. J., 1980, Anti-phenyltrimethylamino immunity in mice: L-Tyrosine-p-azophenyltrimethylammonium-induced suppressor T cells selectively inhibit the expression of B-cell clones bearing a cross-reactive idiotype, *J. Exp. Med.* **151**:528.
10. Gorczynski, R., Khomasurya, B., Kennedy, M., Macrae, S., and Cunningham, A., 1980, Individual-specific

(idiotypic) T-B cell interactions regulating the production of anti-TNP Ab. II. Development of id-specific helper and suppressor T cells within mice making an immune respoonse, *Eur. J. Immunol.* **10**:781.

11. Eichmann, K., 1975, Idiotype suppression. II. Amplification of a suppressor T cell with anti-idiotypic activity, *Eur. J. Immunol.* **5**:511.

12. Sy, M.S., Bach B. A., Dohi, Y., Nisonoff, A., Benacerraf, B., and Greene, M. I. 1979, Antigen and receptor stimulated regulatory mechanisms. I. Induction of suppresor T cells with anti-idiotypic antibodies, *J. Exp. Med.* **150**:1216.

13. Dohi, Y., and Nisonoff, A., 1979, Suppression of idiotype and generation of suppressor T cells with idiotype conjugated thymocytes, *J. Exp. Med.* **150**:909.

14. Abbas, A. K., Burakoff, S. J., Gefter, M. L., and Greene, M. I., 1980, T lymphocyte mediated suppression of myeloma function in vitro. III. Regulation of antibody production in hybrid myeloma cells by T lymphocyutes, *J. Exp. Med.* **152**:968.

15. Rubinstein, L. J., Yeh, M., and Bona, C. A., 1982, Idiotype–anti-idiotype network. II. Activation of silent clones by treatment at birth with idiotypes is associated with the expansion of idiotype-specific helper T cells, *J. Exp. Med.* **156**:506–521.

16. Imanishi, T., and Mäkelä, O., 1975, Inheritance of antibody specificity. II. Anti-(4-hydroxy-5-bromo-3-nitrophenyl) acetyl in the mouse, *J. Exp. Med.* **141**:840–854.

17. Reth, M., Imanishi-Kari, T., and Rajewsky, K., 1979, Analysis of the repertoire of anti-(4-hydroxy-3-nitrophenyl) acetyl (NP) antibodies in C57BL/6 mice by cell fusion. II. Characterization of idiotopes by monoclonal anti-idiotope antibodies, *Eur. J. Immunol.* **9**:100–1013.

18. Sherr, D. H., Ju, S.-T., Weinberger, J. Z., Benacerraf, B., and Dorf, M. E., 1981, Hapten-specific T cell responses to 4-hydroxy-34-nitrophenyl acetyl. VII. Idiotype specific suppression of plaque forming cell responses, *J. Exp. Med.* **153**:640–652.

19. Sherr, D. H., and Dorf, M. E., 1981, Hapten specific T cell responses to 4-hydroxy-3-nitrophenyl acetyl. IX. Characterization of idiotype specific effector phase suppressor cells on plaque forming cell responses in vitro, *J. Exp. Med.* **153**:1445–1456.

20. Sherr, D. H., Ju, S.-T., and Dorf, M. E., 1981, Hapten specific T cell responses to 4-hydroxy-3-nitro-phenyl acetyl. XII. Fine specificity of anti-idiotypic suppresor T cells (Ts2), *J. Exp. Med.* **154**:1382-1 389.

21. Sherr, D. H., and Dorf, M. E., 1982, Hapten specific T cell responses to 4-hydroxy-3-nitrophenyl acetyl. XIII. Characterization of a third order T cell (Ts3) involved in suppression of in vitro PFC responses, *J. Immunol.* **128**:1261–1266.

22. Sunday, M. E., Weinberger, J. Z., Benacerraf, B., and Dorf, M. E., 1980, Hapten-specific T cell responses to 4-hydroxy-3-nitrophenyl acetyl. IV. Specificity of cutaneous sensitivity responses, *J. Immunol.* **125**:1601–1605.

23. Sunday, M. E., Benacerraf, B., and Dorf, M. E., 1980, Hapten-specific responses to 4-hydroxy-3-nitro-phenyl acetyl. VI. Evidence for different T cell receptors in cells which mediate H-2I-restricted and H-2D-restricted cutaneous sensitivty responses, *J. Exp. Med.* **152**:1554–1562.

24. Sunday, M. E., Benacerraf, B., and Dorf, M. E., 1981, Hapten specific T cell responses to 4-hydroxy-3-nitrophenyl acetyl. VIII. Suppressor cell pathways in cutaneous sensitivity responses, *J. Exp. Med.* **153**:811–822.

25. Weinberger, J. Z., Germain, R. N., Ju, S.-T., Greene, M. I., Benacerraf, B., and Dorf, M. E., 1979, Hapten-specific T-cell responses to 4-hydroxy-3-nitrophenyl acetyl. II. Demonstration of idiotypic determinants on suppressor T cells, *J. Exp. Med.* **150**:761–776.

26. Gechler, W., Faversham, J., and Cohn, M., 1978, On a regulatory gene controlling the expresssion of murine λ-light chain, *J. Exp. Med.* **148**:1122–1136.

27. Okuda, K., Minami, M., Sherr, D. H., and Dorf, M. E., 1981, Hapten-specific T cell responses to 4-hydroxy-3-nitrophenyl acetyl. XI. Pseudogenetic restrictions of hybridoma suppressor factors, *J. Exp. Med.* **154**:468–479.

28. Sherr, D. H., Minami, M., Okuda, K., and Dorf, M. E., 1983, Analysis of T cell hybridomas. III. Distinctions between two types of hapten specific suppressor factors which affect plaque-forming cell responses, *J. Exp. Med.* **157**:515–529.

29. Dorf, M. E., Okuda, K., and Minami, M., 1982, Dissection of a suppressor cell cascade, *Curr. Top. Microbiol. Immunol.* **100**:61–67.

30. Okuda, K., Minami, M., Ju, S.-T., and Dorf, M. E., 1981, Functional association of idiotypic and I-J determinants on the antigen receptor of suppressor T cells, *Proc. Natl. Acad. Sci. USA* **78**:4557–4561.

31. Ju, S.-T., Pierres, M., Waltenbaugh, C., Germain, R. N., Benacerraf, B., and Dorf, M. E., 1979, Idiotypic analysis of monoclonal antibodies to poly-(Glu^{60}Ala^{30}Tyr^{10}), *Proc. Natl. Acad. Sci. USA* **76**:2942–2946.
32. Minami, M., Okuda, K., Furusawa, S., Benacerraf, B., and Dorf, M. E., 1981, Analysis of T cell hybridomas. I. Characterization of H-2 and Igh restricted monoclonal suppressor factors, *J. Exp. Med.* **154**:1390–1402.
33. Okuda, K., Minami, M., Furusawa, S., and Dorf, M. E., 1981, Analysis of T cell hybridomas. II. Comparisons among three distinct types of monoclonal suppressor factors, *J. Exp. Med.* **154**:1838–1851.
34. Furusawa, S., Minami, M., Sherr, D. H., and Dorf, M. E., 1984, Analysis of the suppressor T cell cascade with products derived from T cell hybridomas, in: *Cell Fusion* (R. F. Beers, Jr. and E. G. Basset, eds.), Raven Press, New York, pp. 299–311
35. Mäkelä, O., and Karjalainen, K., 1978, A Mendelian idiotype is demonstrable in the heteroclitic anti-NP antibodies of the mouse, *Eur. J. Immunol.* **8**:105–112.
36. Takemori, T., and Tada, T., 1974, Selective roles of thymus-derived lymphocytes in the antibody response. II. Preferential suppression of high affinity antibody-forming cells by carrier-primed suppressor T cells, *J. Exp. Med.* **140**:253–266.
37. Krawinkel, U., Cramer, M., Imanishi-Kari, T., Jack, R. S., Rajwesky, K., and Mäkelä, O., 1977, Isolated hapten-binding receptors of sensitized lymphocytes. I. Receptors from nylon wool-enriched mouse T lymphocytes lack serological markers of immunoglobulin constant domains but express heavy chain variable portions, *Eur. J. Immunol.* **7**:556–573.
38. Nakanishi, K., Sugimura, K., Yaunta, Y., Maeda, K., Kashiwamura, S. I., Honjo, T., and Kishimoto, T., 1982, A T15-idiotype-positive T suppressor hybridoma does not use the T15 V$_H$ gene segment, *Proc. Natl. Acad. Sci. USA* **79**:6984.

29

Differential Expression of *Igh-1*-Linked T-Cell Alloantigens

Antigen Receptors or Evolutionary Rudiments of Immunoglobulin Genes?

FRANCES L. OWEN

1. Introduction

The relationship between antigen receptors on T and B cells has long been debated.[1-3] Immunoglobulin on the surface of B cells clearly acts as an antigen recognition structure[4] and may also be a key to the differentiation of an IgM-bearing early B cell[5] to a cell population expressing both IgM and IgD.[6-7] T- and B-cell receptors may closely resemble one another in that at least part of the polypeptide chain coding for antigenic specificity of each cell type carries determinants cross-reactive with the major serum idiotypes (reviewed in Ref. 8). Although the V_H gene products expressed on T and B cells may overlap,[9,10] the fine specificity of the repertoire may not be identical.[11,12] The constant-region markers (isotypes) on B cells have never been found to be expressed on the surface of T cells.[13]

One must hypothesize that T and B cells share a common cellular origin in order to share some genes coding for V_H determinants. Diversification may occur very easily in the lineage of T–B differentiation so that each cell line (T or B) can then continue to modify and expand its V_H germline gene repertoire separately. Recently, B cells have been shown to rearrange pieces of their immunoglobulin genes during early development.[14,15] Mature, functioning B cells rearrange their V_H genes adjacent to the appropriate constant-region gene, a mechanism well documented for the μ gene.[16] Each μ gene actually consists of a "minigene" for each domain separated by intervening sequences.[17] Recently, it has been

FRANCES L. OWEN • Department of Pathology and Cancer Research Center, Tufts University School of Medicine, Boston, Massachusetts 02111.

found that thymus cells, largely a pool of very early undifferentiated prothymocytes,[18] and T-lymphoid lines[19] synthesize RNA which encodes some segments of the μ chain. This has been used as an argument that T cells utilize IgM as antigen reeptors. An alternative interpretation is that the cells used for these studies represent intermediate steps in the differentiation pathway speculated above. It is unlikely that translocation of V_H genes in T-cell precursors takes place in an analogous way to the B-cell gene segments [14,15]. However, it is possible that there is a separate V_H gene complex for T cells teleomeric to Igh-1, and that the μ gene in T cells is intact, but quiescent (Fig. 1). The T-cell genes could be translocated next to a characteristic constant-region gene without perturbing the germ-line sequence of B-cell products. Occasional aberrant T cells might make a nonfunctional μ-related product.

In order to fulfill the model outlined above, T cells would be required to have a set of unique and previously undefined constant-region genes. A group of T-cell-specific structural products which may be constant-region determinants for T-cell antigen binding have been described in this laboratory. These antigens are coded for by a new gene complex on chromosome 12 (Fig. 2).[20,21] The proximity of this gene complex to the immunoglobulin genes suggests the genetic mechanisms regulating expression of T-cell gene products may be similar to those for the immunoglobulin isotypes.

If antigen recognition by the T cell requires a macromolecular complex rather than a single polypeptide chain,[22] then any one of the required structural products could be encoded on chromosome 12. This would explain the apparent mapping of genes coding for "T-cell idiotypes" to chromosome 12 in the face of data suggesting this chromosome is not exclusively responsible for antigen binding.[23] It is possible that more than one species of antigen-binding chain could be represented in the antigen recognition complex and that each could utilize a separate gene pool. If any one of those polypeptides was inactivated, then antigen-binding function would be lost. An effective way of inactivating single polypeptides without destroying others has been to make T-cell hybrids with antigen-binding function and to look for sublines which had lost specific identifiable chromosomes.[23] Loss of chromosome 12 with retention of antigen binding could eliminate this chromosome from participation in antigen binding. However, loss of antigen binding and retention of chromosome 12 could not eliminate the possibility that a separate polypeptide encoded on another chromosome is required in addition to chromosome 12 for optimal antigen binding. A second way to selectively inactivate a single polypeptide would be by using a monoclonal antibody to block that structure. If antigen recognition involves a complex structure, then blocking of any of the polypeptides involved would prevent biological function.

Alternatively, there may be two groups of antigen receptors for T cells. One type of receptor could code for antigen binding by alloreactive T cells[24,25] and a second, genetically unrelated type could participate in antigen recognition by suppressor T-cell subsets or their secreted products.[26-28] Since the requirements for antigen binding by suppressor cells and helper cells are so different, it is not unreasonable to assume these functional subsets may have evolved at different times in development and that separate gene pools code for these discrepant receptors.

This chapter reviews the evidence suggesting that there is an evolutionary relationship between the gene products encoded in the T region and immunoglobulins. The major question of interest is whether these determinants are part of an antigen receptor mechanism or only rudiments of an evolutionary system related to the immunoglobulin genes and now nonfunctional in T cells.

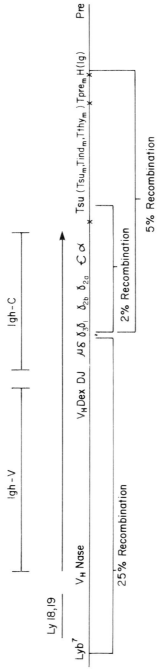

FIGURE 1. Map of chromosome 12; a gene cluster encodes Tsu, Tind, Tthy, and Tpre.

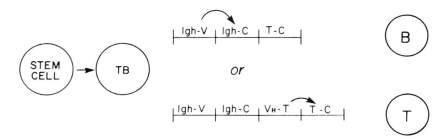

FIGURE 2. Schemata for the diversification of T and B cells.

2. Genetic Analysis

2.1. Monoclonal Antibodies

Monoclonal antibodies specific for T-cell surface antigens have been raised.[29] These antibodies recognize the products of a cluster of tightly linked genes on chromosome 12[20,21] encoded in a new region tentatively named *IgT-C*.[30] The gene cluster encodes a minimum of three products, separable using classical genetic analysis; physiological studies suggest that a minimum of four separate gene products are encoded in this region. These antigens, named Tpre, Tind, Tsu, and Tthy, are surface markers for subpopulations of T cells. The nomenclature was based on the following rationale: anti-Tsu antiserum had been defined[31] as recognizing an antigen linked to Igh-1 on Lyt-1.2-bearing suppressor cells. Monoclonal anti-Tsu most closely mimics the specificity of the original antiserum. Anti-Tind recognizes an antigen on Lyt-1.2-bearing cells which regulate the immune response.[32] Recently, this antigen has been shown to be present on a clone of *augmenting* T cells[33] and on the antigen-specific product of that clone.[27,28] Cells which have helper function have not been found to express this antigen.[34] Monoclonal anti-Tthy recognizes an antigen preferentially expressed on thymocytes.[35–37] Monoclonal anti-Tpre recognizes a prethymic hemopoietic cell which overlaps the adult lymphoid T lineage.[38,39] Tpre is expressed on cells in fetal liver from days 13–16 and on thymocytes from day 15 of gestation through adult life. This cell population may or may not be analogous to a unipotential stem cell for T-lymphocyte lineage.[39]

2.2. Mapping Using Recombinant Strains of Mice

Evidence that the antigens described above are products of separate genes stems from mapping studies using recombinant inbred strains of mice and commercially available inbred strains.[20,21] Monoclonal anti-Tpre, Tthy, Tsu, and Tind have been used to map these respective antigens. The genes coding for this group of antigens have been localized to chromosome 12 by using a panel of 32 recombinant lines with known recombination events between immunoglobulin and prealbumin. Recombination between *Tpre* and the cluster encoding Tthy, Tind, and Tsu occurred in one of these strains (1/32 lines); data from this recombination suggest the gene which codes for Tpre must lie closer to prealbumin than those encoding Tthy, Tind, and Tsu. No recombination between *Tthy, Tind,* and *Tsu* was documented; these genes were not ordered with respect to immunoglobulin. The map of this region presents these antigens (Tthy, Tind, Tsu) in random order and Tpre in its mapped position relative to the other three antigens and to prealbumin (Fig. 2).

Tpre can be separated by recombination in the CB13632 mouse leading to the conclusion that it is the product of a unique gene. Although *Tthy, Tind,* and *Tsu* could not be separated in these lines, evidence for evolutionary recombination is seen by looking at a panel of commercial strains (Table I). NIH Swiss and C3H/HeJ strains show recombination between *Thy/Tind* and *Tsu* and between *Thy/Tind* and *Tpre.*[21,30] These data suggest that there are a minimum of three genes; one codes for Tsu, a second for Tpre, and a third for Tthy and/or Tind. Tthy and Tind could be modified products of the same gene, although the physiological distribution of Tthy and Tind shows these two antigens can be expressed on separate cells. Tthy is expressed on early thymocytes; Tind is preferentially expressed on antigen-activated lymph node cells. Tthy and Tind are, however, expressed on a similar population of thymocytes and are occasionally expressed on the same T-cell hybrids (Section 2.4). In ontogeny Tthy and Tind appear very close to the same time. Developmental studies (Section 4.2) suggest the cell expressing Tthy could be a precursor for those expressing Tind. Many of our monoclonal anti-T-cell antibodies react with both Tthy and Tind.[34] These observations suggest Tind and Tthy are closely related molecules, possibly with shared homology.

The recombination events in this region are reminiscent of the pattern of recombination documented for the immunoglobulin allotypes.[42] Experimental recombination has

TABLE I
Expression of Allelic Forms of Tpre, Tthy, Tind, and Tsu in Inbred Strains of Mice[a]

Strain	Igh-1[a]	IgT-C			
		Tsu[b]	Tind[c]	Tthy[d]	Tpre[e]
C.AL-20	d	d	d	d	d
AKR/J	d	d	d	d	d
NZB	e	d	d	d	d
A/J	e	d	d	d	d
BALB/c	a	—	—	—	—
C3H/HeJW	j	—	d	d	—
C3H/HeJ	j	—	d	d	—
NIH Swiss		—	d	d	—
CBA/Tufts	j	—	—	—	—
C57BL/6J	b	—	—	—	—
CB.20	b	—	—	—	—
SWR/J	c	—	—	—	—
HRS/J		—	—	—	—
MRL/LPR		—	—	—	—
MRL/++		—	—	—	—

[a]Table taken from Ref. 21.

never been shown to occur between genes coding for the different isotypes of immunoglogulin. However, recombination between allelic forms (allotypic markers) of each isotype has been observed in many inbred strains.

In summary, the gene cluster for these T-cell alloantigens is a tight linkage group. A minimum of three genes have been documented. Because Tpre can be separated by recombination, it is possible that this antigen has a functionally unrelated biological role and is simply linked to the complex.

2.3. Allelic Forms of T-Cell Antigens

The monoclonal antibodies specific for these antigens recognize presumed alleles of Tpre, Tthy, Tind, and Tsu. Strains expressing the d allele are shown in Table I. Antibodies were raised in BALB/c animals $(Igh-1^a)$ against T cells of C.AL-20 animals $(Igh-1^d)$. The BALB/c and C.AL-20 animals differ from one another in a segment of Chromosome 12 which includes the immunoglobulin genes, the T cluster, a histocompatibility marker (HIIg) and excludes Ly-16 (originally named Ly-18[41]) and prealbumin. Because antigens similar to Tsu have been detected using monoclonal BALB/c $(Igh-1^a)$ anti-CB.20 $(Igh-1^b)$ antibodies,[26,42] it seems likely that there are at least three alleles of the Tsu gene, Tsu^a (BALB/c), Tsu^d (C.AL-20), and Tsu^b (CB.20). The polymorphisms in this region could be as extensive as those for the immunoglobulin genes.

2.4. Somatic Cell Hybrids as a Genetic Tool

Hybrid cells made with BW5147 (AKR origin, $Igh-1^d$) and *adult* C.AL-20 $(Igh-1^d)$ immune lymph node were used to study expression of antigens encoded in this linkage group.[36] A panel of 26 hybrid lines were generated (Table II).[38] No line expressed Tind or Tsu simultaneously, leading to the conclusion that the cells which bear these antigens belong to separate developmental lineages. In contrast, many hybrids coexpress Tthy and either Tind or Tsu. Although BW5147 does not express any of these antigens, it originated from a strain which has the genetic information to code for this allele. Transcomplementation could occur so that genes not expressed in BW5147, but originating from that cell, may be expressed in the hybrid. It is, therefore, not possible to determine the origin of the gene coding for Tthy in these cells because both partners in the hybrid have the $Igh-1^d$ genotype.

Fetal and adult T-cell hybrids show a very different pattern of expression of these antigens. Lines originating from fusion of BW5147 with *fetal liver* of day 12 or day 19 gestation express all four antigens in this series simultaneously (Table II).[38] The cells expressing Tpre can be detected on normal tissue from days 13–16 gestation in fetal liver,[37] prior to detection of cells expressing Tthy, Tind, or Tsu, all postnatal markers.[36] It is possible that a common precursor for these cells exists in fetal liver. One hybrid FBL 12-3, originating from fusion between day 12 fetal liver and P.3U1, yielded a line with similar expression of all four of these T-cell antigens and Thy-1.2. Since P.3U1 originated from BALB/c $(Igh-1^a)$ it is improbable that complementation from the fusion partner could account for this aberrant simultaneous expression of Tpre, Tthy, Tind, and Tsu.

TABLE II
Adult versus Fetal Expression of Antigen in Somatic Cell Hybrids

Normal tissue	HAT-sensitive line	Hybrid line	Marker expressed				
			Tpre	Tthy	Tind	Tsu	Thy-1.2
		Fetal lines[a]					
Fetal liver							
Day 19	BW5147	FTL 19-5	+	+	+	+	+
Day 12	BW5147	FTL 12-3	+	+	+	+	+
	P.3U1	FBL 12-3	+	+	+	+	+
		Adult lines[b]					
			Tpre	Tthy[d]	Tind[d]	Tsu[d]	Thy-1.2
Immune lymph node	BW5147	JTφ3	ND	−	+	−	−
		JTφ4	ND	−	−	+	−
		JTφ6	ND	+	−	−	+
		JTφ7	ND	−	+	−	−
		JTφ8	ND	+	−	−	−
		JTφ9	ND	+	−	+	+
		JTφ11	ND	−	+	−	+
		JTφ13	ND	−	−	+	+
		JTφ14	ND	−	−	+	−
		JTφ15	ND	+	−	−	−
		JTφ16	ND	+	+	−	−
		JPD	ND	−	−	+	−
		JPE	ND	+	+	−	+
		JTφ19	ND	+	−	+	−
		JTφ21	ND	−	−	+	+
		JTφ22	ND	+	−	−	−
		JTφ23	ND	−	−	+	−
		JTφ24	ND	+	−	−	−
		JTφ26	ND	+	−	−	−
		JTφg27	ND	−	−	+	−
		JTφ28	ND	−	+	−	+
		JTφ30	ND	+	−	−	−
		JTφ31	ND	+	−	+	−

[a]Data summarized from Ref. 38.
[b]Data summarized from Ref. 36.

One must consider at what time in gestation commitment of developing cells takes place so that adult cells express only one of these antigens.

Active gene repression in the adult and/or gene deletion could account for the observation that adult cells express only one antigen while fetal hybrids coexpress four or more antigens in the same series. This observation is in marked contrast to what we know about regulation of the immunoglobulin genes. Early, pre-B cells rearrange the V_H gene segments as a commitment step prior to the ability to detect any of the other immunoglobulin isotypes. Each isotype, with the exception of IgM and IgD, is encoded by a separate gene, translated and transcribed as separate entities. Cells have not been described which simultaneously express multiple isotypes, with the exception of IgM and IgG. IgM and IgD may be coexpressed because these genes are cotranscribed.[15] Our data with the fetal liver hybrids may suggest that long transcripts of several genes could be made or that there are separate initiation sites for each gene. If these were the case, then adult cells would have to have an exogenous signal to prevent coexpression. Perhaps growth factors, known to be necessary for maturation of functional cells, may play a regulatory role in determining commitment to expression of one or more of these genes.

The more trivial explanation for multiple antigen expression in these hybrids is that fetal hybrids are a result of trisomatic hybrids. This seems unlikely since Tind and Tsu cannot be detected in early fetal tissues of the normal animal.[37]

2.5. How Many Genes Are in the *IgT-C* Linkage Group?

The distance between *IgA* and *Tsu* on chromosome 12, estimated by classical recombination studies,[20,21] could be as great at 4 map units; there is enough distance between α and *Tsu* to code for hundreds of genes. The prediction of multiple additional genes in this region is dependent on the identity of the cell which expresses the gene product encoded in this region which is detected on very early developing T cells (Tpre). If one assumes that these antigens are requisite for antigen recognition, then all cells in the same developmental lineage should use related structures for antigen binding. If the cell bearing Tpre is a unipotential precursor for the T-lymphoid lineage, then all T cells should express determinants encoded in this linkage group. If, however, Tpre is a marker on a precursor cell for only the suppressor/regulatory cell lineage, then only T cells in the suppressor lineage need have antigens encoded in this linkage group. We have observed that Tpre, Tthy, Tind, and Tsu are not expressed on functional helper effector cells for antibody responses or on cytolytic T-effector cells.[34] The majority of mature T cells apparently express none of these determinants. The question of whether other cell types (Th, Tc) express as yet undescribed antigens linked to Tsu is being pursued.

3. Relationship to Antigen-Binding Products of T Cells

3.1. Alloantiserum Anti-Tsu Blocks Antigen Binding

The alloantiserum anti-Tsu was raised in BALB/c mice by immunizing them with C.AL-20 T cells activated with concanavalin A.[31] The resultant antiserum was specific for C.AL-20 cells and could be used *in vivo* to activate suppressor cells which were Igh-V restricted.[45] The antiserum selectively blocked[31] the interaction of anti-idiotype-specific C.AL-20 Ts$_2$ cells[44] with their target idiotype coated on RBC.[45] The antiserum did not block lymph node cell proliferation in response to KLH-TNP (unpublished observation), did not block cytolytic T cells at the effector level,[34] did not block MLR reactivity,[34] and did not block generation of cytolytic cells *in vtiro* (unpublished observation).

Alloantiserum anti-Tsu could have had antibodies specific for all the antigens in this linkage group (Tpre, Tthy, Tind, and Tsu) because it was made in BALB/c AnN animals against C.AL-20 Con A blasts. If cytotoxic or helper cells expressed these antigens, one would have expected the antiserum to block those functional assays.

3.2. Monoclonal Antibodies Do Not Block Allo-Restricted Recognition

Monoclonal antibodies specific for Tthy, Tind, Tsu, and Tpre were generated in the same strain combination used to generate anti-Tsu alloantiserum. None of these monoclonal antibodies, or a cocktail of the same, block cell proliferation *in vitro* (PETLES assay[30]), MLR reactions, or cytotoxic T cells.[34]

3.3. Monoclonal Anti-Tind Binds Antigen-Specific Factor

Monoclonal anti-Tind has been shown to react with an antigen-specific T-cell factor from the monoclonal line FL10, a T-cell hybrid with augmenting functional activity.[27,28] The line releases a factor which binds to KLH and augments the secondary PFC response for TNP.[33] Monoclonal anti-Tind antibody insolubilized on Sepharose retains the biological activity of the antigen-specific factor; monoclonal anti-I-A_t also retains this activity. Elution of the columns and simultaneous use of the material retained by anti-Tind and Anti-I-A_t is required to recover functional activity.

These results suggest complementation between products of two chromosomes (17 encoding I-A_t) and (12 encoding Tind) is required for antigen binding by a cell-free product. If these data can be extrapolated to an antigen-binding receptor model, then one might speculate that a molecular complex would be required for recognition. Alternatively, it is possible that these determinants are expressed on the factors destined for secretion and are not an intrinsic part of the antigen recognition structure.

The major difficulties in demonstrating surface expression of these antigens with fluoresceinated antibodies and the fluorescence-activated cell sorter, and the need to amplify these antigens with indirect antibodies in order to use them with complement, suggest that these surface determinants are low density/surface area. It is possible that factors, not anchored in the membrane, express these antigens which are only transiently expressed on the cell surface. The latter possibility must be considered since we have only been able to show expression of these antigens on regulatory cells which are known to release factors mediating their function.

3.4. Are Antigens on Cytotoxic and Helper Cells Related Structures?

3.4.1. Search for Anti-Th

An attempt was made to produce anti-Th antibodies by immunizing BALB/c animals with C.AL-20 T cells from immune lymph node. Monoclonal antibodies originating from a BALB/c recipient spleen cell fusion with P.3U1 were screened for inhibition of helper function for plaque assays and for inhibition of T-cell proliferation. An antibody-releasing line was selected, anti-Tep, which modestly inhibited early T-cell proliferation of immune node cells. Pursuit of the antibody specificity suggested the cell population expressing this antigen was not characteristic of the majority of helper T cells in normal animals (J. Bissette, unpublished data). The antibody must recognize either a small subset of proliferating cells or a regulatory cell for that response.

3.4.2. Search for Anti-Tc

Alloantiserum against Tc was produced by immunizing CB.20 mice with BALB/c cytotoxic T cells (A. Finnegan, Ph.D. thesis, Tufts University). The resultant antibodies recognized an antigen linked to Igh-1 on cytotoxic T cells but not MLR proliferating T cells specific for the same antigen.[43] Mapping studies showed the antigen recognized by the antibody was linked closely to the *Igh-V* genes more than to the *IgT-C* cluster.[41] This antigen was named Ly-18[41] and is not part of the cluster of genes including *Tind*, *Tsu*, and *Tthy*.

4. Evolutionary Similarities Between the T-cell Products and *Igh-1*

4.1. Position of the Genes Relative to Immunoglobulin

This region of chromosome 12 encodes a cluster of genes which are preferentially expressed on T cells. There are some striking similarities with the gene products encoded by the cluster of immunoglobulin genes. First, the position of the genes coding for T-cell antigens is not greater than 4 map units removed from *Igh-1*, the cluster of immunoglobulin constant-region genes.[40] This group of genes lies closer to the constant-region genes than do the variable-region genes. Although other genes which regulate B-cell differentiation are known to be linked to *Igh-1*,[41,46] the recombination frequency with respect to immunoglobulin is 25%, implying a map distance of approximately 25 units. The close proximity of these genes and the immunoglobulin genes might suggest an intimate relationship. Such a relationship between the class I *MHC* genes and *TLA*, a linked locus,[47] had been documented.[48]

4.2. Conservation in Order of Expression of T-Cell Gene Products

The T-cell alloantigens in this linkage group are expressed sequentially in ontogeny. Tpre appears in fetal liver on days 13–16, then in fetal thymus on day 15.[37] In contrast, Tthy appears on day 1 of neonatal life, Tind on days 2–3, and Tsu appears later on days 5–6 of neonatal life (Fig. 3).[36]

Surprisingly, this ontological expression parallels the order of expression of the same antigens on developing organs.[36] Tpre is expressed in the bone marrow on a cell which is Thy-1.2$^-$. Tthy is also expressed in bone marrow, but on a cell which is Thy-1.2$^+$. Both Tpre and Tthy are expressed in thymus on both cortisone-resistant and -sensitive thymocytes. BSA sedimentation separates a low-density cell in thymus which is Tthy$^-$, Tsu$^+$, Tind,$^+$ Tthy-1.2$^+$, and H-2$^+$. Resting cells in spleen express Tind and Tsu with low surface density per cell. Antigen-activated lymph node cells express Tind and Tsu with either a higher frequency and/or density per cell.

The only antigen in this linkage group expressed in the nude animal (AKR nu^{str}/nu^{str}) is Tpre; marrow cells in the nude express this marker with a higher density per cell than do spleen cells of the same animal.[38]

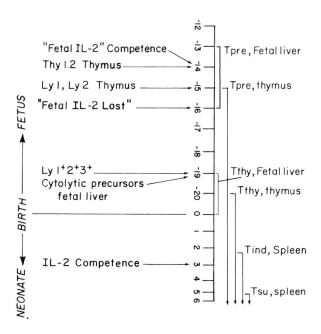

FIGURE 3. Developmental expression of T-cell antigens encoded by genes linked to *Igh-1*.

In vivo administration of monoclonal anti-Tthy to resting animals from birth to adult life has been used to develop an animal model where the cells expressing Tthy are depleted.[49] The cells expressing Tind and Tsu also do not appear. This suggests a developmental relationship between the cells which express Tthy, Tind, and Tsu. The cell bearing Tthy must either be the direct precursor for cells expressing Tthy, Tind, and Tsu or are cells required for the development of the latter two cell types. One obvious requirement step might be the release of IL-2, known to be a factor in maturation of T-cell precursors in nude animals to functional cytolytic T cells.[50] Similarities in the size and properties of the reported precursor pool of thymocytes for IL-2-producing cells[51] led to speculation that the Tthy-bearing cell might be a precursor for the IL-2-producing cells. This hypothesis was tested by quantitatively measuring the amount of IL-2 produced per spleen cell in C.AL-20 animals pretreated with monoclonal anti-Tthy^d or anti-Tthy^a antibodies.[37] The IL-2 responses of anti-Tthy^d, anti-Tthy^a, and untreated mice were indistinguishable. Therefore, the cell expresing Tthy could not be the sole precursor for those releasing IL-2. The model is consistent with a developmental pathway in which the cells expressing Tthy develop prior to those expressing Tind and Tsu. A possible precursorial role is indicated.

The parallel between the order of expression of Tpre, Tthy, Tind, and Tsu in ontogeny and in functional lymphoid organ development is reminiscent of the parallel between B-cell development and the appearance of the immunoglobulin isotypes. Pre-B cells in fetal liver are believed to express cytoplasmic μ chain prior to synthesis of light chain.[52] As cells mature, surface IgM, then IgD and, later, the other immunoglobulin isotypes appear.[53] The order of appearance in ontogeny[54] and on developing antigen-competent B cells[55] is the same order as that in which the genes lie on chromosome 12 (IgM, IgD, IgG3, IgG1, IgG2b, IgG2a, IgA).[56] Control mechanisms for expression of T-cell gene products and B-cell isotypes are suggested by the conservation in expression of products of each group of genes.

4.3. Isotypic Expression of T-Cell Gene Products

4.3.1. Evidence for Isotypes

Monoclonal anti-Tind binds to a T-cell antigen-specific factor, T-augmenting factor (TaF) (Section 3.3). The antibody which recognizes Tsu alloantigenic determinants does not recognize this factor. This suggests that Tind and Tsu antigenic determinants are not encoded by the same polypeptide chains. Products of closely linked genes which are expressed exclusively on separate antigen-binding polypeptides would suggest an isotypic organization for T-cell antigen-binding proteins. Although no stable line releasing a factor expressing Tsu has been identified, to confirm this hypothesis, the data are consistent with this model.

4.3.2. Why Would Isotypes Be Retained in Evolution?

If suppressor cell interaction from multiple cell types (Ts_1, Ts_2, Ts_3, Ts_{pre}) regulates immunoglobulin synthesis, then the factors which interact may have functional capabilities separable from their antigen-binding specificity. The "constant portion" of those molecules could have effector functions which help to mediate the immune response.

5. Conclusion

A new cluster of genes on chromosome 12 have been described. There are some similarities between the products of genes in this linkage group and the immunoglobulin genes. It is possible that these T-cell-specific genes and the immunoglobulin genes arose from duplication of a common primordial gene. The close proximity of the two gene clusters, some similarities in control of expression of both groups of genes on lymphoid cells, and an association with antigen-binding products suggest an evolutionary relationship. The immunoglobulin gene complex may have developed as a host defense mechanism. A second related group of T-cell genes could have arisen as a duplication, positively selected for in evolution by a need to regulate the levels of immunoglobulin produced in response to a single antigen. Under these circumstances one might select for a cell population which had suppressor and/or augmenting function for immunoglobulin synthesis. If this recognition mechanism for a specific cell population developed as a late evolutionary modification, then all the genes in the complex could be restricted to "suppressor-like" cells.

Cells which recognize alloantigens can be found in phylogeny[57] prior to the ability of vertebrates to produce IgM[58] and in ontogeny[59] prior to a recognizable μ chain.[54] Alloreactive T cells may be the most primitive antigen recognition mechanism of animals. If gene banks (V genes) determining antigenic specificity of alloreactive T cells evolved prior to the V_κ, V_λ, and V_H genes of immunoglobulins, it is not unreasonable that they should be encoded elsewhere in the chromosome. V_κ, V_λ, and V_H gene pools for immunoglobulins are not closely related at a genetic level and are coded for by clusters encoded on separate chromosomes. If alloreactive structures develop prior to immunoglobulin genes and suppressor T-cell receptors develop after the immunoglobin genes, then alloreactive T-helper or cytotoxic T cells and suppressor T cells need not have identical variable-region gene pools. In fact, separate gene clusters on different chromosomes may encode two different T-cell receptors. Recent molecular studies with the genomic clone for the β chain of the T-cell receptor on cytotoxic and helper T cells[60] support this concept. Hybrid cells that function as suppressor cells do not rearrange this gene,[61] implying that their recognition structure must use a different gene product.

An alternative possibility must be considered. T cells which regulate the immune response may express determinants encoded in this region of chromosome 12, but at a site discrete from the antigen receptor mechanism. The T-cell alloantigens may mark cellular differentiation and be nonfunctional rudiments of a system not deleted by evolution. It has been documented that these antigens are represented at characteristic stages in lymphoid development. A role as antigen receptor *has not been proven*. Current efforts are focused on studying T-cell clones to discriminate between these models.

ACKNOWLEDGMENT. Supported by ROI-15262 from the National Institutes of Health. The author is the recipient of Research Career Development Award KO3 AI-00546.

References

1. Marchalonis, J. J., Atwell, J. L., and Cone, R. E., 1972, Isolation of surface immunoglobulin for lymphocytes from human and murine thymus, *Nature (New Biol.)* **235**:240–242.
2. Vitetta, E. S., and Urh, J. W., 1973, Synthesis, biochemistry and dynamics of all surface Ig on lymphocytes, *Fed. Proc.* **32**:35–40.
3. Merrill, J. E., and Ashman, R. F., 1979, Changes in receptor isotype and T/B ratio in an antigen-binding cell after *in vitro* immunization, *J. Immunol.* **123**:434–441.
4. Roelants, G., Forni, L., and Pernis, B., 1972, Blocking and redistribution of antigen receptors on T and B lymphocytes by anti-immunoglobulin antibody, *J. Exp. Med.* **137**:1060–1077.
5. Siden, E. T., Baltimore, D., Clark, D., and Rosenberg, N., 1979, Immunoglobulin synthesis by lymphoid cells transformed *in vitro* by Abelson murine leukemia virus, *Cell* **16**:389–396.
6. Vitetta, E. S., and Urh, J. W., 1975, Immunoglobulin receptors revisited, *Science* **189**:964–968.
7. Black, S. J., Vanderloo, W., Loken, M. R., and Herzenberg, L. A., 1978, Expression of IgG by murine lymphocytes: Loss of surface IgD indicates maturation of memory B cells, *J. Exp. Med.* **147**:984–996.
8. Eichmann, K., 1978, Idiotypes on T and B cells, *Adv. Immunol.* **26**:195–320.
9. Eichmann, K., and Rajewsky, K., 1975, Induction of T and B cell immunity by anti-idiotypic antibody, *Eur. J. Immunol.* **5**:661–666.
10. Mozes, E., and Haimovich, J., 1979, Antigen specific T-cell helper factor crossreacts idiotypically with antibodies of the same specificity, *Nature* **278**:56–57.
11. Krawinkel, U., Cramer, M., Melchers, I., Imanishi-Kari, T., and Rajewsky, K., 1978, Isolated hapten-binding receptors of sensitized lymphocytes. III. Evidence for idiotypic restriction of T cell receptors, *J. Exp. Med.* **147**:1341–1347.
12. Binz, H., Frischknecht, H., Shen, F. W., and Wigzell, H., 1979, Idiotypic determinants on T-cell subpopulations, *J. Exp. Med.* **149**:910–922.
13. Krawinkel, U., and Rajewsky, K., 1976, Specific enrichment of antigen binding receptors from sensitized lymphocytes, *Eur. J. Immunol.* **6**:529–536.

14. Tonegawa, S., Maxam, A. M., Tizard, R., Bernard, O., and Gilbert, W., 1978, Sequence of a mouse germ-line gene for a variable region of an immunoglobulin light chain, *Proc. Natl. Acad. Sci. USA* **75**:1485–1489.

15. Tonegawa, S., 1983, Somatic generation of antibody diversity, *Nature* **302**:575–581.

16. Early, P. W., Davis, M. M., Kaback, D. B., Davidson, N., and Hood, L., 1979, Immunoglobulin heavy chain gene organization in mice: Analysis of a myeloma genomic clone containing variable and α constant regions, *Proc. Natl. Acad. Sci. USA* **76**:857–861.

17. Corey, S., and Adams, J. M., 1980, Deletions are associated with somatic rearrangement of immunoglobulin heavy chain genes, *Cell* **19**:37–51.

18. Putnam, D., Clagett, J., and Storb, U., 1980, Immunoglobulin synthesis by T cells: Quantitiative and qualitative aspects, *J. Immunol.* **124**:902–912.

19. Kemp, D. J., Harris, A. M., Cory, S., and Adams, J. M., 1980, Expression of the immunoglobulin $C\mu$ gene in mouse T and B lymphoid and myeloid cells lines, *Proc. Natl. Acad. Sci. USA* **77**:2876–2880.

20. Owen, F. L., Riblet, R., and Taylor, B., 1981, The suppressor cell alloantigen Tsu^d maps near immunoglobulin allotype genes and may be a heavy chain constant-region marker on a T cell receptor, *J. Exp. Med.* **153**:801–810.

21. Owen, F. L., and Riblet, R., 1984, Tpre, Tthy, Tind and Tsu map as a tight linkage group on chromosome 12 using IgH strains of mice, *J. Exp. Med.* **159**:313–317.

22. Reinherz, E. L., Meuer, S. C., and Schlossman, S. F., 1983, The delineation of antigen receptors on human T lymphocytes, *Immunol. Today* **4**:5–9.

23. Marrack, P., and Kappler, J., 1983, Use of somatic cell genetics to study chromosomes contributing to antigen plus I recognition by T cell hybridomas, *J. Exp. Med.* **157**:404–418.

24. Haskins, K., Kubo, R., White, J., Pigeon, M., Kappler, J., and Marrack, P., 1983, The major histocompatibility complex-restricted antigen receptor on T cells. I. Isolation with a monoclonal antibody, *J. Exp. Med.* **157**:1149–1169.

25. Meuer, S. C., Fitzgerald, K. A., Hussey, R. E., Hodgdon, J. D., Schlossman, S. F., and Reinherz, E. L., 1983, Clonotypic structures involved in antigen specific human T cell function: Relationship to the T3 molecular complex, *J. Exp. Med.* **157**:705–729.

26. Takeshi, T., Komatsu, Y., Uchida, Y., and Taniguchi, M., 1982, Monoclonal alloantibodies specific for the constant region of T cell antigen receptors, *J. Exp. Med.* **156**:888–897.

27. Nakajima, P. B., Ochi, A., Owen, F. L., and Tada, T., 1983, The presence of IgT-C and I-A subregion encoded determinants on distinct chains of monoclonal antigen-specific augmenting factors derived from a T cell hybridoma, *J. Exp. Med.* **157**:2110–2120.

28. Miyatani, S., Hiramatsu, K., Nakajima, P. B., Owen, F. L., and Tada, T., 1983, Structural analysis of antigen-specific Ia-bearing regulatory T cell factors: Gel electrophoretic analysis of the antigen-specific augmenting T cell factor, *Proc. Natl. Acad. Sci. USA* **80**:6336–6340.

29. Owen, F. L., and Spurll, G. M., 1981, The T cell constant region gene family: Preliminary characterization of cell surface antigens by immunoprecipitation with alloantisera and monoclonal antibodies, in: *Immunoglobulin Idiotypes: Proceedings of the ICN–UCLA Symposium*, Volume 20 (C. A. Janeway, Jr., E. E. Sercarz, H. Wigzell, and F. Fox, eds.), New York, pp. 419–428.

30. Owen, F. L., 1983, T cell alloantigens encoded by the IgT-C region of chromosome 12 in the mouse, *Adv. Immunol.* **34**:1–37.

31. Owen, F. L., Finnegan, A., Gates, E. R., and Gottlieb, P. D., 1979, I. A mature T lymphocyte subpopulation marker closely linked to the Ig-1 allotype C_H locus, *Eur. J. Immunol.* **9**:948–955.

32. Spurll, G. M., and Owen, F. L., 1981, A family of T cell alloantigens linked to Igh-1, *Nature* **293**:742–746.

33. Hiramatsu, K., Ochi, A., Miyatoni, S., Segawa, A., and Tada, T., 1982, Monoclonal antibodies against unique I-region genes products expressed only on mature functional T cells, *Nature* **296**:666–668.

34. Spurll, G. M., Frye, M., Riendeau, L., Finnegan, A., and Owen, F. L., 1984, Biological specificity of a panel of 12 monoclonal antibodies raised in Igh-1 allotype congenic mice against products of the IgT-C region, in preparation.

35. Owen, F. L., Spurll, G. M., and Pangeas, E., 1982, Tthy^d, a new thymocytes alloantigen linked to Igh-1: Implications for a switch mechanism for T cell antigen receptors, *J. Exp. Med.* **154**:52–60.

36. Owen, F. L., 1982, Products of the IgT-C region are maturational markers for T cells: Sequence of isotype appearance in immunocompetent cells parallels ontogenetic appearance, *J. Exp. Med.* **156**:703–718.

37. Owen, F. L., Riendeau, L., and Keesee, S. K., 1984, Fetal splenic IL-2 competence precedes expression of Tpre and Tthy in fetal thymus, in preparation.
38. Owen, F. L., 1983, Tpre, a new alloantigen encoded in the IgT-C region of chromosome 12, is expressed on nude bone marrow and fetal T cells, *J. Exp. Med.* **157**:419–432.
39. Basch, R. S., and Kadish, J. L., 1977, Thymocyte precursors, II. Properties of the precursors, *J. Exp. Med.* **145**:405–411.
40. Greene, M. C., 1977, Genetic nomenclature for the immunoglobulin loci of the mouse, *Immunogenetics* **8**:890-97.
41. Finnegan, A., and Owen, F. L., 1981, Ly-18, a new alloantigen present on cytotoxic T cells controlled by genes linked to the *Igh-V_a* locus, *J. Immunol.* **127**:1947–1953.
42. Aihara, Y., Tadokoro, I., Katoh, K., Minami, M., and Okuda, K., 1983, T cell allotypic determinants encoded by genes linked to the immunoglobulin heavy chain locus. I. Establishment of monoclonal antibodies against allotypic determinants, *J. Immunol.* **130**:2920–2925.
43. Owen, F. L., Riblet, R., and Gottlieb, P. D., 1982, T suppressor cells activated by anti-Tsu^d serum are Igh-V restricted, *Eur. J. Immunol;.* **12**:94–97.
44. Nisonoff, A., Ju, S.-T., and Owen, F. L., 1977, Studies of structure and immunosuppresion of a cross-reactive idiotype in strain A mice, *Immunol. Rev.* **34**:89–118.
45. Owen, F. L., and Nisonoff, A., 1978, Contribution of the erythrocyte matrix to the formation of rosettes by idiotype specific lymphocytes, *Cell. Immunol.* **37**:243–253.
46. Subbaro, B. A., Ahmad, W. E., Paul, I., Schur, R., Lieberman, R., and Mosier, D. W., 1979, Lyb-7, a new B cell alloantigen controlled by genes linked to the *IgC_H* locus, *J. Immunol.* **122**:2279–2285.
47. Hood, L., Steinmetz, M., and Malissen, B., 1983, Genes of the major histocompatibility complex of the mouse, *Annu. Rev. Immunol.* **1**:529–568.
48. Winoto, A., Steinmetz, M., and Hood, L., 1983, Genetic mapping in the major histocompatibility complex by restriction enzyme site polymorphisms; most mouse class I genes map to the TLA complex, *Proc. Natl. Acad. Sci. USA* **80**:3425–3429.
49. Keesee, S. K., and Owen, F. L., 1983, Modulation of Tthy^d alloantigen expression in the neonatal mouse: The Tthy^d bearing thymocyte is a precursor for the peripheral cells expressing Tsu^d and Tind^d, *J. Exp. Med.* **157**:86–97.
50. Hunig, T., and Bevan, M., 1980, The specificty of cytotoxic T cells from anthymic mice, *J. Exp. Med.* **152**:688–702.
51. Ceredig, R. A., Glasebrook, L., and MacDonald, H. R., 1982, Phenotypic and functional properties of murine thymocytes. I. Precursors of cytolytic T lymphocytes and interleukin 2-producing cells are all contained within a subpopulation of mature thymocytes, *J. Exp. Med.* **155**:358–367.
52. Baltimore, D., Rosenberg, N., and Witte, O. N., 1978, Transformation of immature lymphoid cells by Abelson murine leukemia virus, *Immunol. Ref.* **48**:3–22.
53. Lawton, A. R., Asofsky, R., Hylton, M. B., and Cooper, M. D., 1972, Suppression of immunoglobulin class synthesis in mice. I. Effects of treatment with antibody to μ chain, *J. Exp. Med.* **135**:277–297.
54. Kearney, J. F., Cooper, M. D., Klein, J., Abney, E. R., Parkhouse, R. M. E., and Lawton, A. R., 1977, Ontogeny of Ia and IgD and IgM bearing B cells in mice, *J. Exp. Med.* **146**:297–301.
55. Black, S. J., Van der Loo, W., Loken, M. R., and Herzenberg, L. A., 1978, Expression of IgD by murine lymphocytes: Loss of surface IgD indicates maturation of memory B cells, *J. Exp. Med.* **147**:984–1006.
56. Honjo, T., and Katavka, T., 1978, Organization of immunoglobulin heavy chain genes and allelic deletion model. *Proc. Natl. Acad. Sci. USA* **75**:2140–2149.
57. Scofield, V. L., Schlumpberger, J. M., West, L. A., and Weissman, I. L., 1982, Protochordate allorecognition is controlled by a MHC-like gene system, *Nature* **295**:499–503.
58. Clem, L. W., 1971, Phylogeny of immunoglobulin structure and function, *J. Biol. Chem.* **246**:9–15.
59. Owen, J. J. T., Jordan, R. K., Robinson, J. H., Singh, U., and Willcox, H. N. A., 1977, *In vitro* studies on the generation of lymphocyte diversity, *Cold Spring Harbor Symp. Quant. Biol.* **41**:129–137.
60. Hedrick, S. M., Cohen, D. I., Nielsen, E. A., and Davis, M. M., 1984, Isolation of cDNA clones encoding T-cell specific membrane associated proteins, *Nature* **308**:149.
61. Hendrick, S. et al. P.N.A.S. in press.

30
Mechanisms of Idiotypic Control of the Antibody Repertoire

KLAUS RAJEWSKY

1. Introduction

The coexistence in the immune system of antibodies and anti-antibodies (idiotypes and anti-idiotypes) is the basis of Jerne's network hypothesis[1] which postulates that idiotypic interactions of antibodies are a main regulatory principle in the immune system. Since Köhler and Milstein developed their hybridization technique for the isolation of cell lines secreting antibodies of predefined specificity,[2] it was possible to isolate antibodies and anti-antibodies from any given inbred mouse strain and to test with these reagents the network hypothesis in a straightforward way. This approach has been used by a number of laboratories and much of that work is discussed throughout this volume and has also recently been reviewed.[3] In the present chapter, I shall summarize the work of this laboratory on this subject and point out the mechanisms of idiotypic control which have emerged from it. The main question asked is whether the idiotypic network controls the functional antibody repertoire. If so, what are the rules of that control, and does the network contribute to the maintenance of a diverse repertoire, to immunological memory and to the guarantee of self tolerance? In the course of the discussion it will become obvious that T cells play a crucial role in idiotypic regulation as has also been suggested by experimental evidence obtained by others.[3] T and B cells might thus communicate via idiotypic interactions and this might lead to the idiotypic similarities of T- and B-cell receptors as they have been observed in many experimental systems.

KLAUS RAJEWSKY • Institute for Genetics, University of Cologne, D-5000 Cologne 41, Federal Republic of Germany.

2. Model System: The NP^b Antibody Family

2.1. History

Our model system is based on the original work of Imanishi and Mäkelä, who showed that the primary antibody response of mice carrying the Igh^b haplotype to the hapten (4-hydroxy-3-nitrophenyl)acetyl (NP) is restricted in that the antibodies display a peculiar fine specificity of hapten binding which is inherited as a Mendelian trait in linkage with the heavy-chain locus.[4,5] In subsequent work of Mäkelä's and our own group it was found that these antibodies could be idiotypically defined as the so-called NP^b idiotype[6,7] and bore λ light chains.[6,8] Through the isolation of monoclonal anti-NP antibodies it also became clear that despite the restrictions in terms of fine specificity of hapten binding, idiotype, and light-chain class, the primary anti-NP response consists of a large family of closely related, but structurally distinct antibodies.[8,9] We have called this family the NP^b antibody family.

2.2. Genetic and Structural Basis

Through the analysis of cDNA from hybridomas secreting individual antibodies of the NP^b antibody family and of germline V_H genes it became clear that the V regions of a large fraction of the NP^b antibody family is encoded by a single germline V_H gene *(V186.2)*, several D and J_H genes, and, of course, the $V_\lambda 1$ and $J_\lambda 1$ genes[10,11] (see also Ref. 3 in which sequences communicated to us by A. L. M. Bothwell, M. Paskind, and D. Baltimore and H. Sakano and K. Karjalainen are quoted. Further sequence data are contained in a paper by Dildrop, *et al.*[11a]) To date, all of six independent anti-NP antibodies have been found to express the $V186.2$ V_H gene. Although it is quite possible that, as in the case of other "major" idiotypes (see, for example, the Ars idiotype in this volume), other V_H genes also contribute to the response, it would thus appear that a single V_H and a single V_L gene control most of the primary anti-NP response in Igh^b mice. These genes may or may not carry somatic point mutations.[10,11]

2.3. Idiotopes of the NP^b Antibody Family

2.3.1. Definition of NP^b Idiotopes by Monoclonal Anti-Idiotope Antibodies against the Germline-Encoded Anti-NP Antibody B1-8

Idiotopes of the NP family were defined by raising monoclonal anti-idiotope antibodies against a prototype NP^b antibody, namely antibody B1-8[9] whose V regions are fully germline encoded. The anti-idiotopes were of either allogeneic[12] or isogeneic[13] origin. Analysis of the anti-idiotope antibodies on a variety of monoclonal anti-NP antibodies and on anti-NP serum antibodies indicated that they all recognize distinct (although possibly overlapping) idiotypic determinants[9,13−17] and that some of these determinants appear to be close to or in the hapten-binding site (free hapten inhibits anti-idiotope binding to idiotope), whereas others are more distant from it (inhibition of the idiotypic interaction by hapten–carrier complexes, but not by free hapten).[12,13] The structural basis of the B1-8 idiotopes will not be discussed further in the present context. There is clear evidence that most of these idiotopes are complex structures controlled by amino acids in several segments of the variable regions of heavy and light chains.[3,16]

2.3.2. Expression of NP^b Idiotopes in the NP^b Antibody Family

All idiotopes defined on antibody B1-8 are regularly expressed in primary anti-NP antibodies of mice carrying the Igh^b haplotype, e.g., C57BL/6 mice.[12–15,18a] However, the situation is complex in two respects. First, each anti-idiotope antibody appears to detect a set of idiotopes which differ from each other in terms of their affinity for the anti-idiotope. This had already been observed at the level of monoclonal anti-NP antibodies.[12] In practice this leads to problems in the quantitative determination of idiotope-bearing antibodies in the serum. In a direct binding assay (where idiotope-bearing antibodies are detected with an ^{125}I-labeled anti-λ1 antibody on anti-idiotope-coated plastic plates and the concentrations determined by comparison with a standard curve obtained with antibody B1-8[15,18]), lower values are obtained as compared to an absorption assay in which idiotope-bearing antibodies are determined as the fraction of anti-NP antibodies that binds to insolubilized anti-idiotope antibody.[15,17,19] In the former assay the values obtained range from 5 to 10% of the total λ-chain-bearing anti-NP response, depending on the idiotope measured; in the latter they range from 10 to 50%.[15,17–19]

Second, the NP^b idiotopes defined on antibody B1-8 can be found in molecular association like an antibody B1-8 or, in certain cases, expressed independently of each other.[12–14] Absorption analysis has permitted us to define within the NP^b antibody family subsets of antibodies which carry characteristic patterns of idiotopes.[15,19a,20] In Table I four such subsets are listed. Subsets $a1$ and $a2$ resemble antibody B1-8 closely in terms of their idiotopes. Subsets b and c each carry only one B1-8 idiotope. Absorption analysis has dem-

TABLE I
Subsets of Primary Anti-NP Antibodies Bearing B1-8 Idiotopes

		Idiotope^b				
Antibody subset^a	Prototype antibody	Ac38	A39-40	A6-24	Ac146	A25-9
$a1$	B1-8^c	+^{d}	+	+	+	+
$a2$	—	+	+	+	+	—
b	B1-48^c	+	—	—	—	—
c	—	—	+	—	—	—

^{a}Idiotypically defined subsets of anti-NP antibodies regularly expressed in primary anti-NP responses of C57BL/6 mice.
^{b}Defined by monoclonal anti-idiotope antibodies raised against antibody B1-8.[12,13] The anti-idiotope antibodies bear the same designation as the idiotope they recognize, i.e., antibody Ac38 binds to idiotope Ac38, etc. The anti-idiotope antibodies Ac38 and Ac146 are κ-chain-bearing IgG1 proteins of CBA origin. Antibodies A6-24 (IgG2a,κ), A39-40 (IgG1,κ), and A25-9 (IgG1,κ) are of C57BL/6 origin.
^{c}Monoclonal NP-binding antibodies isolated from the primary anti-NP response of C57BL/6 mice. Both antibodies bear λ1 light chains as most primary C57BL/6 anti-NP antibodies and express the same germ-line-encoded V genes. They differ from each other in D and J and in heavy-chain isotype.[3,9]
^{d}"+" means that antibodies bind to anti-idiotope-coated plastic (as detected by radiolabeled anti-λ1 antibodies) and can be absorbed on insolubilized anti-idiotope. "−" means that antibodies are negative in both respects.

onstrated that the idiotopes represented in subsets *a1* and *a2* but not in subsets *b* and *c* occur in anti-NP serum antibodies mostly in molecular association and also in association with the idiotopes characteristic of subsets *b* and *c*[19a] although exceptions to this rule exist in about one out of five antisera.[13] We also know that the idiotope expressed in subset *b* (idiotope Ac38) binds to the corresponding anti-idiotope with an average avidity similar to that of antibody B1-8.[18a] In the case of subset *c* a similar analysis has not yet been done. The subsets in Table I are important since, as shall be discussed below, they differ from each other drastically in their sensitivity to regulation by the monoclonal anti-idiotope antibodies.

2.3.3. Expression of NP^b Idiotopes in the Total Antibody Population

Are the NP^b idiotopes also expressed in non-NP-binding antibodies? In order to answer this question we immunized mice with various anti-idiotope antibodies cross-linked to KLH, following the device of Cazenave and colleagues[21] and Urbain and colleagues.[22] We then analyzed the idiotypic and antigen-binding properties of the resulting idiotope-bearing antibodies.[14,17,19] Our experimental system offers a special advantage here in that idiotope-bearing antibodies (antibody $3I\beta$)[19,23] can be distinguished from anti-anti-idiotypes (antibody 3α) by their light-chain class, since NP^b idiotopes either require the λ chain for their expression or are lost when the B1-8 heavy chain is combined with a κ chain (Ref. 16; C. Kappen, M. Reth, and K. Rajewsky, in preparation). Antibodies of the α type, on the other hand, would be expected to bear κ light chains as do 95% of murine immunoglobulin molecules. The notion that λ-chain-bearing antibodies obtained in this system upon immunization with anti-idiotope represent idiotope-bearing antibodies has gained strong support from a recent molecular analysis of such antibodies obtained in monoclonal form after immunization with the anti-idiotope Ac38. All 10 antibodies analyzed expressed a V_H gene cross-hybridizing with the *V186.2* gene expressed in antibody B1-8. In four cases the V_H region was sequenced and found to be closely related to that of antibody B1-8.[11a]

Table II shows some properties of anti-idiotope-induced λ1-chain-bearing serum antibodies of C57BL/6 origin. Obviously, different results are obtained with different anti-

TABLE II
Idiotope-Bearing Antibodies Induced by Anti-Idiotope Antibody

Immunization with[a]	λ1-chain-bearing antibodies (μg/ml)[a]			
	Ac38$^+$	Ac146$^+$	A6-24$^+$	NP-binding
Ac38-KLH	233 (1.5)[b]	4.0 (4.3)[c]	20 (2.6)	18.8 (2.2)
A6-24-KLH	18.2 (2.7)	17.0 (1.7)	92.2 (1.2)	14.8 (2.1)
Ac146-KLH	1.5 (3.2)	1.8 (3.6)[c]	ND[d]	2.4 (3.3)

[a]C57BL/6 mice (5–6 animals/group) were immunized with anti-idiotope antibody (Ac38, A6-24, or Ac146) coupled to KLH and bled 4 weeks later. Idiotope-bearing and NP-binding antibodies carrying the λ1 light chain were titrated in a radioimmunoassay. The titration was standardized with the monoclonal anti-NP antibody B1-8. The antibody titers were corrected by subtracting the titers of antibodies in the sera of KLH-primed animals. Data from Ref. 17.
[b]Geometric means of titers determined in individual sera with standard deviations.
[c]83–90% of the antibodies bearing idiotope Ac146 absorb to NP-Sepharose.[17]
[d]ND, Not determined.

idiotopes. Thus, idiotopes Ac38 and A6-24 are mostly expressed on non-NP-binding molecules whereas idiotope Ac146 appears largely associated with NP-binding specificity. Furthermore, only part of the Ac38- and A6-24-bearing antibodies coexpress other B1-8 idiotopes, whereas idiotope Ac146 is largely associated with idiotope Ac38. These results are fully compatible with the data in Table I, concerning the idiotypically defined subsets of NP^b antibodies. One might also note that the anti-idiotope antibody Ac146 (recognizing idiotope Ac146) behaves in these experiments as an "internal image"[23] of the NP hapten. However, the antibody can surely not carry a perfect internal image since many anti-NP antibodies lack idiotope Ac146. In fact, idiotope Ac146 is inherited as a genetic marker linked to the *Igh* locus and is not expressed in Igh^a or Igh^j mice, although the latter animals exhibit a good λ1-chain-bearing anti-NP response.[17,19] This problem has been discussed in more detail elsewhere.[3,17,19]

In summary of this section, B1-8 idiotopes are partly restricted to the NP^b antibody family (e.g., idiotope Ac146) and partly also expressed on non-NP-binding antibodies. These results are confirmed by the idiotypic analysis of LPS-reactive B cells.[17,32]

3. Why Does the NP^b Family Dominate in the Anti-NP Response?

The dominance of "major idiotypes" in antibody responses against certain simple antigenic determinants has led to various speculations concerning the possible reasons of this phenomenon. It seems to us most striking in this context that all major idiotypes so far analyzed at the molecular level have turned out to be encoded by just a few antibody structural genes in the germ line (reviewed in Ref. 3). One might therefore think that in a first approximation idiotypic dominance simply reflects the expression of these (few) antibody structural genes which happen to be present in the germ line and which encode antibodies of the required specificity. Although this simple concept may not apply in all cases, the experimental evidence supports it, with certain limitations (see below), in the case of the NP^b antibody family.

With respect to λ-chain dominance, the V regions of murine λ chains appear to contribute efficiently to the binding of nitrophenyl compounds because of their particular primary structure[24-26] which exhibits little variability.[27] The notion that λ-chain-bearing antibodies are selected in primary anti-NP responses merely on the basis of affinity to the NP hapten is further supported by recent results suggesting that upon stimulation with NP-LPS both κ- and λ-chain-bearing NP-binding precursor cells are activated, but that the products of the latter exhibit a higher affinity for the hapten than those of the former (F. Smith, A. Cumano, and K. Rajewsky, in preparation). κ-chain-bearing anti-NP antibodies with a high affinity have only been observed in hyperimmune responses[9] and may represent selected somatic mutants. In line with these results, λ-light-chain dominance was also found in the response of nude mice to NP-Ficoll and in adoptive primary anti-NP responses in irradiated hosts, mediated by cloned, carrier-specific T-helper cells.[28,29] This argues against the idea (see Ref. 3) that T cells specific for the constant region of λ chains or for idiotopes controlled by λ chains might be responsible for λ-chain dominance in the anti-NP response.

With respect to the dominant expression of the *V186.2* gene in the heavy chain of antibodies of the NP^b family, sequence comparison of NP-binding and non-NP-binding λ-chain-bearing antibodies has permitted the identification of five residues in the V_H region which appear to play a key role in NP binding.[26] These residues have so far been found collectively only in the $V186.2$ sequence and not in any of the closely related V_H genes in the same family.[3,10] Significantly, BALB/c mice appear to use a different V_H gene in their primary anti-NP response, but that gene shares four of the five "key" residues with the C57BL/6 gene.[30] It should also be pointed out in this context that the structural analysis of anti-idiotope-induced hybridomas (see Ref. 11a) argues against the idea that the $V186.2$ gene is more frequently rearranged in B cells than other V_H genes, a suspicion one might have had in view of the fact that the same V_H gene also controls most of the anti-GAT response in C57BL/6 mice.[31]

Taken together, the available evidence is compatible with the view that of all germ-line genes, the V_λ and $V186.2$ genes, together with suitable D and J elements, encode the best-fitting anti-NP antibodies emerging from the germline. This provides a simple genetic basis for the dominance of the NP^b antibody family in the primary anti-NP response. However, it should be stressed that this does not speak to the question whether *within* the family of anti-NP antibodies in which V_λ and $V186.2$ are expressed, certain antibody subsets are selected on grounds other than the hierarchy of NP-binding affinities. In fact, as will be discussed in section 4, there is suggestive evidence that certain subsets of NP^b antibodies are specifically controlled by T cells in the frame of the idiotypic network. Since the frequencies of LPS-reactive B cells expressing NP^b idiotopes were found to be identical in B-cell populations from adult or newborn spleens or in B cells generated from bone marrow pre-B cells *in vitro*,[32] we think that T-cell-controlled idiotypic selection of B cells (see Section 4) sets in after the B cells generated in the bone marrow have arrived in the periphery.

4. Antibody-Mediated Control of the Idiotypic Repertoire

4.1. Long-Lasting Enhancement and Suppression of Idiotype Expression by Anti-Idiotope Antibodies

The availability of monoclonal anti-idiotope antibodies allows one to assay their regulatory properties in an immunochemically well-defined way and under quasi-physiological conditions. We have used the monoclonal anti-idiotopes listed in Table I in order to continue a line of research initiated in our laboratory several years ago,[33,34] namely the investigation of the effect of small doses of anti-idiotypic antibodies applied in native form, on the expression of the target idiotype in later immune responses.

The results of these experiments, as far as they have been published,[14,15,18,35,36] can be summarized as follows:

1. Nanogram doses of anti-idiotope antibodies, applied to adult mice, lead to the enhancement of the expression of the target idiotope in subsequent anti-NP responses, even several months after anti-idiotope administration.
2. Microgram doses suppress idiotope expression, and again the effect is long-lasting. Suppression is also observed, when the antibody is injected into newborn animals.
3. The regulatory effects do not require a disparity of the injected anti-idiotope and the immunoglobulin of the recipients in terms of allotype.

4. The regulatory effects are seen most strikingly, but not exclusively, at the level of IgG (as opposed to IgM) antibodies.
5. The regulatory effects appear to variable extents also at the level of NP^b idiotopes other than the target idiotope. However, the effects are specific in that the total λ-chain-bearing anti-NP response is not or is only marginally affected.

Recently, a few further points have been established and can be added to the list:

6. The duration of neonatally induced suppression depends on the dose of the injected anti-idiotope. Recovery from suppression sets in when the concentration of anti-idiotope in the animal has fallen below the microgram range.[18a,36a]
7. Anti-idiotopes of the IgG1, IgG2a, IgG2b, and IgE class have similar regulatory properties with respect to both idiotype enhancement and suppression in the adult mouse.[19a] This result contrasts with earlier data,[18,37] but appears indisputable, since isotype switch variants of anti-idiotope antibodies (hence identical in idiotope-binding specificity) were used in the experiments in a syngeneic situation. Both these conditions were not fulfilled in the earlier work.
8. Surprisingly, both enhancement and suppression by the anti-idiotope antibodies are most strongly expressed at the level of certain subsets of idiotypically defined anti-NP antibodies. Of the subsets listed in Table II, *a1* and *a2* are preferentially affected, and these subsets can apparently be regulated by any anti-idiotope recognizing an idiotope on these subsets.[19a,20]

We conclude from these experiments that anti-idiotope antibodies have striking regulatory functions in a situation mimicking closely physiological conditions. They enhance or suppress the expression of complementary (idiotypic) antibodies in a dose-dependent fashion, irrespective, as far as the analysis goes, of their isotype. And finally, regulation appears to preferentially affect certain idiotypically defined subsets of antibodies bearing the target idiotope.

4.2. Cellular Basis of Anti-Idiotope-Mediated Regulation

Whereas the cellular basis of idiotope enhancement has not yet been successfully explored in our system, idiotypic suppression, as in other experimental systems (reviewed in Ref. 3), seems to involve regulatory T cells. In our system this was first observed in the case of adult suppression,[36] but was subsequently more fully investigated in neonatally suppressed animals.[3,18a,36a] From such animals, which had been injected at birth with 100 μg anti-idiotope Ac38, T and B cells were isolated and combined, in a criss-cross fashion, in irradiated hosts *in vivo*. The results showed that the B cells from suppressed animals, in combination with normal T cells, were unable to produce virtually any antibody of the *a* subset. At the level of IgG1 antibodies, the cells also did not produce subset *b* antibodies, although they mounted an anti-NP response of normal size. T cells from the suppressed animals, when combined with normal B cells, mediated a normally sized anti-NP response, but subset *a* antibodies of the IgG1 class were absent from the response. We have recently been able to reproduce this result in an *in vitro* culture system (A. Cumano, and H. Tesch, unpublished data). In Table III we depict some of the results obtained in this system which uses the T-cell-independent type II antigen NIP-polymerized flagellin (NIP-Pol) for anti-

TABLE III
Specificity of Anti-Idiotope-Induced Regulatory T Cells[a]

B cells (5 × 10⁶)	T cells	Antigen (100 ng/ml)	λ1-positive antibodies (ng/ml)[b]		
			NIP-binding	Ac38⁺	Ac146⁺
	NS	NIP-Pol	219	52	27
	NS	—	12	<2	<2
	SS	NIP-Pol	126	6	4
NB	NT 2 × 10⁶	NIP-Pol	450	70	63
NB	ST 2 × 10⁶	NIP-Pol	560	50	<2
NB	NT 1 × 10⁶ ST 1 × 10⁶	NIP-Pol	321	40	5
NB	NT 2 × 10⁶ ST 1 × 10⁵	NIP-Pol	400	53	37
NB	—	NIP-Pol	100	6	5

[a] Abbreviations: NB, NT, NS: B, T, spleen cells from 12-week-old control mice; ST, SS: T, spleen cells from 12-week-old mice given 100 μg antibody Ac38 at birth. Purification of cells as in ref. 28(B) and 18a(T).
[b] B and T cells were cultured for 7 days in the presence of NIP-Pol. λ1-bearing antibodies in the supernatant of these cultures were measured by a radioimmunoassay.[17] The experiments were carried out by A Cumano and H. Tesch in this laboratory.

genic stimulation. Clearly, the T cells from suppressed animals do not allow the production of subset *a* antibodies (this time mostly of the IgM class), and they inhibit this capacity in normal T cells, if combined with the latter in equal proportions. Since B cells from the suppressed animals are also most severely impaired in their capacity to produce subset *a* antibodies, we hypothesize that in the suppressed animal the regulatory T cells control and select the functional antibody repertoire at the level of the B-cell precursors.[18a,20] It should be mentioned, however, that in the *in vivo* transfer experiments B cells from suppressed animals prevented idiotope expression by normal B cells, so that B cells may also play a regulatory role.[18a]

4.3. Mechanism of Idiotypic Regulation

The fact that we can suppress subset *a* antibodies by four different anti-idiotope antibodies, each reacting with a separate idiotope of the subset, is evidence for the view[14] that the primary target of the anti-idiotopes is the variable region of the subset *a* antibodies themselves. Similar evidence has recently been obtained in the T15 idiotypic system.[38,39] We think that the anti-idiotope antibody complexes its idiotypic target on the surface of the B cells by which it is produced and that these complexes induce regulatory T and possibly B cells interfering with idiotype expression.[20] Idiotype–anti-idiotope complexes might also be formed in the circulation and presented to T cells via antigen-presenting cells.

A schematic representation of this mechanism is given in Fig. 1, in which it is also suggested that the enhancement of idiotype expression by low doses of anti-idiotype may follow the same general scheme. The latter suggestion is based on our finding that idiotype enhancement and suppression appear to express the same peculiar specificity (affecting, in our system, mainly subset *a* antibodies) which might be imprinted into the system by the T-cell receptor repertoire. The determination of the effector function of anti-idiotypic antibodies by the dose applied to the animals remains unexplained at present. However, the scheme in Fig. 1 depicts two different pathways of activation by which different types of regulatory cells could be induced by different doses of antigen.

The scheme in Fig. 1 suggests that the regulatory I cells are activated by the target idiotype only if it is "labeled" by anti-idiotype. In the case of activation via macrophages or dendritic cells this appears straightforward since these cells are known to selectively pick up complexed immunoglobulin. In the case of activation via B-cell-associated idiotype, "labeling" might reflect activation of the B cell such that it becomes susceptible to interaction with T cells, through the mechanism suggested by Hünig.[40] Alternatively, the regulatory T cells might see "processed" idiotypes[41,42] and thus idiotypic determinants which might differ to some extent from the idiotopes seen by antibodies. In any case, the regulatory cells would only be induced as long as anti-idiotope (or a corresponding antigen) is present in the system. Indeed, as we have observed in the case of neonatal suppression (see above), the system is released from suppression as soon as the anti-idiotope concentration falls below a critical threshold. Inherent in these considerations is the general concept that network-controlled T–B-cell interactions require a prior "activation" of the system by ligand–receptor interactions, in line with data of Cerny and Caulfield[43] and the model proposed by Richter many years ago.[44]

4.4. Idiotype Suppression as a General Model of Self Tolerance

We can look at the scheme in Fig. 1 as a model for self tolerance.[20] A self antigen (the anti-idiotope in the model) appearing at a certain concentration in the system binds to receptors complementary to it and this leads to the induction of anti-idiotypic suppression of those receptors, through regulatory idiotype-specific cells. It should be stressed that anti-idiotypic suppression could similarly be induced against ligand-bound T-cell receptors, so that the scheme in Fig. 1 could be considered a general model for the induction of self tolerance through the idiotypic network, in both the T- and the B-cell compartment. Jerne has himself alluded to the possibility that low-zone tolerance might be network-controlled.[1]

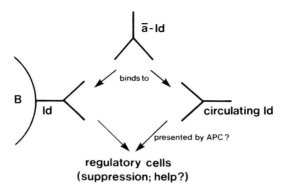

FIGURE 1. Mechanism of idiotype (Id) suppression and enhancement by anti-idiotype (a-Id). APC, antigen-presenting cell. For further explanation see text.

The mechanism depicted in Fig. 1 appears also to make physiological sense in the case of the particular ligand used in our experimental system, the antibody molecule itself.[4,20,45] If an antibody (the anti-idiotope in the experimental system) appears in the organism in microgram concentrations (as antibodies usually do in the course of immune responses), then, according to the model, self tolerance for the variable region of this antibody is established through idiotypic suppression. The immune system is able to stabilize in this way its expressed antibody repertoire. Indeed, experiments have been reported by our group[15] and by others[46-49] indicating that injection of an antibody called "idiotypic" in those experiments) can lead to the enhanced expression of idiotypically related antibodies by the recipient. This phenomenon, which might play an important role in the generation of immunological memory ("idiotypic memory"[15]), may in part be due to the induction of suppression for complementary binding sites and hence represent escape of the "idiotype" from suppression by those sites. The concept that immune responses represent escape from idiotypic suppression is part of the original network hypothesis[1] and is discussed in much detail in Chapter 16 by Fey and colleagues in this volume.

4.5. Idiotype Enhancement as a Mechanism of Network-Driven Diversification of the Antibody Repertoire

The enhancement of idiotype expression by low concentrations of anti-idiotypic antibody (concentrations in the range of "natural" antibodies in the blood[50]) can be seen as a general phenomenon, occurring continuously in the immune system which is constantly exposed to antibodies in the environment. The immune system is known to produce antibodies spontaneously in low concentrations, and initially in ontogeny the spontaneously produced antibodies may largely represent the germline-encoded repertoire. As far as this repertoire represents an idiotypic network, the enhancing mechanism would play its role in the system from the beginning and may contribute to the maturation of B cells into a population of functionally mature cells (possibly those of the long-lived, recirculating B-cell pool[51]), expressing a diverse and interconnected repertoire of antibody binding sites. In fact, the system would thus select in ontogeny the products of those antibody structural genes which are able to encode binding sites complementary to others generated in parallel, and a mechanism for the selection and the maintenance of a diverse set of antibody structural genes in the germ line would be at hand.[52]

It remains to be elucidated, however, whether the germline indeed encodes a functional idiotypic network. If it does not, then the enhancing mechanism would be able to operate only at a second level, namely the interplay of the repertoire generated by the rearrangement of germline genes with somatic mutants of those rearranged genes as they are known to be generated continuously in the system.[53] The enhancing mechanism would keep somatic mutants that happen to be complementary to germline-encoded structures in the system and would thus mediate a continuous "learning" process in the system by which a diverse and selected functional repertoire of antibody binding sites is gradually built up. Maternally transmitted antibodies might then play a role in initiating the expression of (part of?) the germline-encoded antibody repertoire in the offspring. These problems which can be approached experimentally in a straightforward way have been discussed in more detail elsewhere and I refer the reader to the literature.[3,45]

4.6. The Idiotypic Network and T–B Collaboration: Idiotypic Mimicry of T- and B-Cell Receptors

In concluding this chapter, I would like to briefly mention some possible implications of the occurrence of T–B interactions in the frame of the idiotypic network. Such interactions clearly do occur, and a striking example of such a case has been discussed above, in the analysis of the regulatory function of T cells isolated from idiotypically suppressed animals. Depending on the extent to which such interactions occur under physiological conditions (and this would have to be considerable if idiotypic interactions are involved in the generation of self tolerance) and on whether they also occur within the T-cell compartment (for which there is considerable evidence, discussed in many chapters in this volume), one would expect that in ontogeny the T- and B-cell receptor repertoire is selected for a certain degree of idiotypic similarity—a phenomenon amply observed in the past.[3,54,55] The control of B- *and* T-cell idiotypes by genes in the *Igh* locus could then reflect simply a dominant role of B-cell idiotypes in selecting, through idiotypic interactions, part of the T-cell repertoire (discussed in detail in Ref. 3), rather than the participation of V_H genes in *encoding* T-cell receptors, against which there is now considerable experimental evidence.

It is still, however, an enigma, what T cells really see in the world of idiotypes. Together with other experimental work, reviewed in Ref. 3, the data in Section 3 (preferential regulation of a particular subset of anti-NP antibodies by T cells) may point to restrictions of the T-cell repertoire in idiotype recognition which may influence the functional B-cell repertoire more than has so far been anticipated.

ACKNOWLEDGMENTS. The work summarized in this chapter represents the joint effort of a large group of people. I wish to mention specifically R. S. Jack and T. Imanishi-Kari, who defined the NP^b idiotype in this laboratory, M. Reth, who established the experimental system of monoclonal idiotypic and anti-idiotypic antibodies, A. L. M. Bothwell, M. Paskind, and D. Baltimore at MIT, who identified the NP^b V_H gene family through the analysis of the anti-NP antibody-producing hybridomas, T. Takemori, G. Kelsoe, C. E. Müller, S. Nishikawa, H. Tesch, F. Smith, and A. Cumano, who performed regulatory experiments, R. Dildrop. M. Brüggemann, J. Bovens, S. Zaiss, C. Kappen, K. Beyreuther, and A. Radbruch, who did structural work and isolated and characterized idiotope mutants, and G. von Hesberg, S. Irlenbusch, C. Uthoff-Hachenberg, and K. Neifer, who provided expert technical help. I am particularly grateful to T. Takemori, H. Tesch, and A. Cumano for helping me with the present chapter and furnishing unpublished experimental data, and to A. Böhm for typing the manuscript. The work was supported by the Deutsche Forschungsgemeinschaft through SFB 74.

References

1. Jerne, N. K., 1974, Towards a network theory of the immune system, *Ann. Immunol. (Inst. Pasteur).* **125C:**373–389.
2. Köhler, G., and Milstein, C., 1975, Continuous cultures of fused cells secreting antibody of predefined specificity, *Nature* **256:**495–497.

3. Rajewsky, K., and Takemori, T., 1983, Genetics, expression, and function of idiotypes, *Annu. Rev. Immunol.* **1**:569–607.
4. Imanishi, T., and Mäkelä, O., 1973, Strain differences in the fine specificity of mouse anti-hapten antibodies, *Eur. J. Immunol.* **3**:323–330.
5. Imanishi, T., and Mäkelä, O., 1974, Inheritance of antibody specificity. I. Anti-(4-hydroxy-3-nitrophenyl) acetyl of the mouse primary response, *J. Exp. Med.* **140**:1498–1510.
6. Jack, R. S., Imanishi-Kari, T., and Rajewsky, K., 1977, Idiotypic analysis of the response of C57BL/6 mice to the (4-hydroxy-3-nitrophenyl)acetyl group, *Eur. J. Immunol.* **7**:559–565.
7. Mäkelä, O., and Karjalainen, K., 1977, Inherited immunoglobulin idiotypes of the mouse, *Immunol. Rev.* **34**:119–138.
8. Reth, M., Imanishi-Kari, T., Jack, R. S., Cramer, M., Krawinkel, U., Hämmerling, G. J., and Rajewsky, K., 1977, The variable portion of T and B cell receptors for antigen: Binding sites for the hapten (4-hydroxy-3-nitrophenyl) acetyl in C57BL/6 mice, in: *Regulatory Genetics of the Immune System: ICN–UCLA Symposia on Molecular and Cellular Biology*, Volume VI (E. E. Sercarz, L. A. Herzenberg, and C. F. Fox, eds.), Acedemic Press, New York, pp. 139–149.
9. Reth, M., Hämmerling, G. J., and Rajewsky, K., 1978, Analysis of the repertoire of anti-NP antibodies in C57BL/6 mice by cell fusion. I. Characterization of antibody families in the primary and hyperimmune response, *Eur. J. Immunol.* **8**:393–400.
10. Bothwell, A. L. M., Paskind, M., Reth, M., Imanishi-Kari, T., Rajewsky, K., and Baltimore, D., 1981, Heavy chain variable region contribution to the NP^b family of antibodies: Somatic mutation evident in a λ2a variable region, *Cell* **24**:625–637.
11. Bothwell, A. L. M., Paskind, M., Reth, M., Imanishi-Kari, T., Rajewsky, K., and Baltimore, D., 1982, Somatic variants of murine immunoglobulin λ light chains, *Nature* **298**:380–382.
11a. Dildrop, R., Bovens, J., Siekevitz, M., Beyreuther, K., and Rajewsky, K., 1984, A V-region determinant (idiotope) expressed at high frequency in B lymphocytes is encoded by a large set of antibody structural genes, *EMBO J.* **3**:517–523.
12. Reth, M., Imanishi-Kari, T., and Rajewsky, K., 1979, Analysis of the repertoire of anti-(4-hydroxy-3-nitrophenyl) acetyl (NP) antibodies in C57BL/6 mice by cell fusion. II. Characterization of idiotopes by monoclonal anti-idiotope antibodies, *Eur. J. Immunol.* **9**:1004–1013.
13. Rajewsky, K., Takemori, T., and Reth, M., 1981, Analysis and regulation of V gene expression by monoclonal antibodies, in: *Monoclonal Antibody and T Cell Hybridoma: Perspective and Technical Advances* (G. J. Hämmerling, U. Hämmerling, and J. F. Kearney, eds.), Elsevier/North-Holland, Amsterdam, pp. 399–409.
14. Rajewsky, K., Reth, M., Takemori, T., and Kelsoe, G., 1981, A glimpse into the inner life of the immune system, in: *The Immune System* (C. M. Steinberg and I. Lefkovits, eds.), Karger, Basel, pp. 1–11.
15. Kelsoe, G., Reth, M., and Rajewsky, K., 1981, Control of idiotope expression by monoclonal anti-idiotope and idiotope-bearing antibody, *Eur. J. Immunol.* **11**:418–423.
16. Brüggemann, M., Radbruch, A., and Rajewsky, K., 1982, Immunoglobulin V region variants in hybridoma cells. I. Isolation of a variant with altered idiotypic and antigen-binding specificity, *EMBO J.* **1**:629–634.
17. Takemori, T., Tesch, H., Reth, M., and Rajewsky, K., 1982, The immune response against anti-idiotype antibodies. I. Induction of idiotope-bearing antibodies and analysis of the idiotope repertoire, *Eur. J. Immunol.* **12**:1040–1046.
18. Reth, M., Kelsoe, G., and Rajewsky, K., 1981, Idiotypic regulation by isologous monoclonal anti-idiotope antibodies, *Nature* **290**:257–259.
18a. Takemori, T., and Rajewsky, K., 1984, Specificity, duration and mechanism of idiotype suppression induced by neonatal injection of monoclonal anti-idiotope antibodies into mice, *Eur. J. Immunol.* in press.
19. Tesch, H., Takemori, T., and Rajewsky, K., 1983, The immune response against anti-idiotope antibodies. II. The induction of antibodies bearing the target idiotope (Ab3β) depends on the frequency of the corresponding B cells, *Eur. J. Immunol.* **13**:726–732.
19a. Müller, C. E., and Rajewsky, K., 1984, Idiotope regulation by isotype switch variants of two monoclonal anti-idiotope antibodies, *J. Exp. Med.* **159**:758–772.
20. Rajewsky, K., Takemori, T., and Müller, C. E., 1984, Self tolerance through idiotype suppression, in: *Progress in Immunology V* (Y. Yamamura and T. Tada, eds.), Academic Press Japan, Tokyo, p. 533.

21. Le Guern, C., Ben Aïssa, F., Juy, D., Mariamé, B., Buttin, G., and Cazenave, P. -A., 1979, Expression and induction of MOPC-460 idiotopes in different strains of mice, *Ann. Immunol. (Inst. Pasteur)* **130C:**293–302.
22. Urbain, J., Wikler, M., Franssen, J. D., and Colignon, C., 1977, Idiotypic regulation of the immune system by the induction of antibodies against anti-idiotypic antibodies, *Proc. Natl. Acad. Sci. USA* **74:**5126–5130.
23. Jerne, N. K., Roland, J., and Cazenave, P. -A., 1982, Recurrent idiotopes and internal images, *EMBO J.* **1:**243–247.
24. Padlan, E. A., Davies, D. R., Pecht, I., Givol, D., and Wright, C., 1976, Model-building studies of antigen-binding sites: The hapten-binding site of MOPC-315, *Cold Spring Harbor Symp. Quant. Biol.* **42:**627–637.
25. Dwek, R. A., Wain-Hobson, S., Dower, S., Gettins, P., Sutton, B., Perkins, S. J., and Givol, D., 1977, Structure of an antibody combining site by magnetic resonance, *Nature (London)* **266:**31–37.
26. Reth, M., Bothwell, A. L. M., and Rajewsky, K., 1981, Structural properties of the hapten binding site and Idiotopes in the NP^b antibody family, in: *Immunoglobulin idiotypes: ICN–UCLA Symposia on Molecular and Cellular Biology,* Volume XX (C. A. Janeway, Jr., E. E. Sercarz, and H. Wigzell, eds.), Academic Press, New York, pp. 169–178.
27. Weigert, M., and Riblet, R., 1976, Genetic control of antibody variable regions in the mouse, *Cold Spring Harbor Symp. Quant. Biol.* **41:**837–846.
28. Tesch, H., Smith, F. I., Müller-Hermes, W. J. P., and Rajewsky, K., 1984, Heterogeneous and monoclonal helper T cells induce similar anti-NP antibody populations in the primary adoptive response. I. Isotype distribution, *Eur. J. Immunol.* **14:**188–194.
29. Smith, F. I., Tesch, H., and Rajewsky, K., 1984, Heterogeneous and monoclonal helper T cells induce similar anti-(4-hydroxy-3-nitrophenyl)acetyl (NP) antibody populations in the primary adoptive response, *Eur. J. Immunol.* **14:**195–200.
30. Loh, D. Y., Bothwell, A. L. M., White-Scharf, M. E., Imanishi-Kari, T., and Baltimore, D., 1983, Molecular basis of mouse strain-specific anti-hapten response, *Cell* **33:**85–93.
31. Rocca-Serra, J., Tonnelle, C., and Fougereau, M., 1983, Two monoclonal antibodies against antigens using the same V_H germ-line gene, *Nature* **304:**353–355.
32. Nishikawa, S., Takemori, T., and Rajewsky, K., 1983, The expression of a set of antibody variable regions in LPS reactive B cells at various stages of ontogeny and its control by anti-idiotypic antibody, *Eur. J. Immunol.* **13:**318–325.
33. Eichmann, K., 1974, Idiotype suppression. I. Influence of the dose and of the effector functions of anti-idiotypic antibody on the production of an idiotype, *Eur. J. Immunol.* **4:**296–302.
34. Eichmann, K., and Rajewsky, K., 1975, Induction of T and B cell immunity by anti-idiotypic antibody, *Eur. J. Immunol.* **5:**661–666.
35. Kelsoe, G., Reth, M., and Rajewsky, K., 1980, Control of idiotope expression by monoclonal anti-idiotope antibodies, *Immunol. Rev.* **52:**75–88.
36. Kelsoe, G., Takemori, T., Reth, M., and Rajewsky, K., 1981, Generation of specific regulatory T cells with monoclonal anti-idiotope antibody: Induction of suppressor T cells, in: *B Lymphocytes in the Immune Response: Functional, Developmental and Interactive Properties* (N. R. Klinman, D. E. Mosier, I. Sher, and E. S. Vitetta, eds.), Elsevier/North-Holland, Amsterdam, pp. 423–430.
36a. Takemori, T., and Rajewsky, K., 1984, Mechanism of neonatally induced idiotype suppression and its relevance for the acquisition of self tolerance, *Immunol. Rev.* **79:**103–117.
37. Eichmann, K., 1975, Idiotype suppression. II. Amplification of a suppressor T cell with anti-idiotypic activity, *Eur. J. Immunol.* **5:**511–515.
38. Cerney, J., Cronkhite, R., and Heusser, C., 1983, Antibody response of mice following neonatal treatment with a monoclonal anti-receptor antibody: Evidence for B cell tolerance and T suppressor cells specific for different idiotopic determinants, *Eur. J. Immunol.* **13:**244–248.
39. Berek, C., 1983, Antibodies specific for different T15 idiotopes induce neonatal suppression of the T15 idiotype, *Eur. J. Immunol.* **13:**766–772.
40. Hünig, T., 1983, The role of accessory cells in polyclonal T cell activation. II. Induction of interleukin 2 responsiveness requires cell–cell contact, *Eur. J. Immunol.* **13:**596–601.
41. Unanue, E. R., 1981, The regulatory role of macrophages in antigenic stimulation. Part two: Symbiotic relationship between lymphocytes and macrophages, *Adv. Immunol.* **31:**1–136.

42. Chestnut, R. W., and Grey, H. M., 1981, Studies on the capacity of B cells to serve as antigen-presenting cells, *J. Immunol.* **126**:1075–1079.
43. Cerny, J., and Caulfield, M. J., 1981, Stimulation of specific antibody-forming cells in antigen-primed nude mice by the adoptive transfer of syngeneic anti-idiotypic T cells, *J. Immunol.* **126**:2262–2266.
44. Richter, R. H., 1975, A network theory of the immune system, *Eur. J. Immunol.* **5**:350–354.
45. Rajewsky, K., 1983, Symmetry and asymmetry in idiotypic interactions, *Ann. Immunol. (Inst. Pasteur)* **134D**:133–141.
46. Wikler, M., Demeur, C., Dewasme, G., and Urbain, J., 1980, Immunoregulatory role of maternal idiotypes: Ontogeny of immune networks, *J. Exp. Med.* **152**:1024–1035.
47. Rubinstein, L. J., Yeh, M., and Bona, C. A., 1982, Idiotype–anti-idiotype network. II. Activation of silent clones by treatment at birth with idiotypes is associated with the expansion of idiotype-specific helper T cells, *J. Exp. Med.* **156**:506–521.
48. Ivars, F., Holmberg, D., Forni, L., Cazenave, P. -A., and Coutinho, A., 1982, Antigen-independent IgM-induced antibody responses: Requirement for "recurrent" idiotypes, *Eur. J. Immunol.* **12**:146–151.
49. Ortiz-Ortiz, L., Weigle, W. O., and Parks, D. L., 1982, Deregulation of idiotype expression: Induction of tolerance in an anti-idiotypic response, *J. Exp. Med.* **156**:898–911.
50. Jormalainen, S., and Mäkelä, O., 1971, Anti-hapten antibodies in normal sera, *Eur. J. Immunol.* **1**:471–478.
51. Sprent, J., 1973, Circulating T and B lymphocytes of the mouse. II. Life span, *Cell Immunol.* **7**:40–59.
52. Eichmann, K., Falk, I., and Rajewsky, K., 1978, Recognition of idiotypes in lymphocyte interactions. II. Antigen-independent cooperation between T and B lymphocytes that possess similar and complementary idiotypes, *Eur. J. Immunol.* **8**:853–857.
53. Gearhart, P.-J., 1982, Generation of immunoglobulin variable gene diversity, *Immunol. Today* **3**:107–112.
54. Rajewsky, K., and Eichmann, K., 1977, Antigen receptors of T helper cells, *Contemp. Top. Immunobiol.* **7**:69–112.
55. Binz, H., and Wigzell, H., 1977, Antigen-binding idiotypic T-lymphocyte receptors, *Contemp. Top. Immunobiol.* **7**:113–177.

31

The Role of Idiotype in T-Cell Regulatory Events

ADAM LOWY, JOHN MONROE, HANS-DIETER ROYER, AND
MARK I. GREENE

1. Introduction

In his original proposal of an immunoregulatory network of lymphocytes, Jerne proposed that the naive immune system is in a negatively regulated state.[1] Before the introduction of antigen, a lymphocyte specific for a certain antigenic determinant (epitope) is held in check by another lymphocyte's anti-idiotypic receptor. In this network all antibodies represent anti-idiotypes. The appearance of antigen perturbs this homeostatic down-regulation and an immune response is generated. As a consequence of the immune response to the individual epitopes, the amount of antigen is reduced below a threshold level whereupon the systems returns to homeostasis. In recent years, the mechanism by which the immune response is regulated has been investigated. Antigen-specific[2] and nonspecific[3] T-suppressor (Ts) cells play a critical role in this regulation. Further, idiotype–anti-idiotype interactions may be important in both Ts–target cell and Ts–Ts interactions. However, rather than existing in a down-regulated state before the appearance of an antigen, the immune system can be thought of as a complex set of dynamically activated and regulated cellular elements. Antigen stimulates an immune response (postive) and then initiates immunoregulatory (negative) events, instead of simply perturbing homeostatic regulation. Differential antigen presentation to T-helper (Th) and Ts cells by specific antigen-presenting cells (APCs) may shift this delicate balance from immunity to immune regulation. It appears that presentation of antigen by an I-A$^+$ I-J$^-$ APC activates Th[4] cells, while

ADAM LOWY, JOHN MONROE, AND MARK I. GREENE • Department of Pathology, Harvard Medical School, Boston, Massachusetts 02115.   HANS-DIETER ROYER • Department of Biological Chemistry, Harvard Medical School, Boston, Massachusetts 02115.

an I-J$^+$ I-A$^-$ APC activates Ts cells.[5] Moreover, differential expression of *I-A-* or *I-J-* encoded molecules on APCs might mediate these processes. On the other hand, T-cell idiotypes may serve as cell interaction molecules in immunoregulatory events subsequent to Ts activation.[6]

2. The Azobenzenearsonate System

The azobenzenearsonate (ABA) system has proven useful for studying the generation and regulation of immunity. This hapten stimulates antibodies, a large proportion of which express a serologically detected cross-reactive idiotype (CRI).[7] The idiotype expression is linked to genes associated with the *Igh-1* gene complex[8] and *Igk* genes.[9] In addition, appropriate administration of hapten can preferentially activate Ts cells which bear determinants which serologically cross-react with the B-cell idiotype.[10] This review will primarily cover the regulation of ABA-specific T-cell-mediated responses. Although idiotype does not seem to be significant in the generation of ABA-specific T-cell immunity, as evidenced by our inability to detect CRI-like structures on Th or T$_{DTH}$ cells, the Ts cells regulating these events do bear receptor structures which cross-react with the idiotype and anti-idiotype on ABA-specific antibodies. Possible explanations for this phenomenon will be discussed.

Administration of ABA coupled to various protein carriers results in a humoral response which, in *Igh-1^d* and *Igh-1^e* strains of mice, is marked by a CRI on 30–70% of all anti-ABA antibodies.[11] Naive A strain mice may contain antibodies which may be CRI positive, although these may be difficult to demonstrate consistently.[12] Detection of idiotype-bearing proteins in naive mice may be due to some endogenous antigen which induces a humoral response. Certain CRI-positive T cells may also be activated by such endogenous antigens[13]; however, their significance in ABA-specific regulatory events remains unclear.

Ts cells can specifically regulate the idiotype-positive fraction of the ABA-specific humoral response.[14] Because the effector Ts cells involved in these regulatory events were originally thought to be anti-idiotypic, it was proposed that CRI–anti-CRI interactions are responsible for idiotype-specific regulation.[16] A similar phenomenon occurring in the nitrophenyl system is discussed elsewhere in this volume (Sherr *et al.*, Chapter 28).

3. Regulation of Cellular Immunity by Idiotypic Elements

Studies of the generation and regulation of T-cell-mediated anti-ABA responses have revealed a more puzzling picture than the idiotype-specific regulatory events of the humoral response. Subcutaneous administration of ABA coupled to syngeneic spleen cells induces significant DTH[16] and cytolytic T-lymphocyte[17] responses. It appears that recognition of ABA in the context of *I-A* subregion-encoded molecules is critical for the generation of these responses.[15] The I-A$^+$ APC responsible for Th activation has been characterized; it is sensitive to low doses of ultraviolet radiation[18] but is resistant to low doses of cyclophosphamide.[5] Conversely, intravenous administration of identically prepared ABA-coupled cells does not activate T$_{DTH}$ or T$_{CTL}$ cells but rather activates ABA-specific Ts cells.[16] For activation of Ts cells, recognition of ABA in the context of *I-J*-encoded molecules is critical.[19] In contradistinction from the I-A$^+$ APC required for Th activation, the I-J$^+$ APC is relatively resistant to ultraviolet radiation (R. Granstein, A. Lowy, and M. I. Greene, unpublished data) yet sensitive to low doses of cyclophosphamide.[5] Collectively, I-A- and I-J-bearing APCs appear to be critical in the generation of either immune or immunoregulatory events. Indeed, it might also be considered that one set of APCs are capable of expressing either *I-A-* or *I-J*-encoded determinants upon appropriate stimulus by T-cell mediators and may be able to stimulate either Th or Ts depending on whether Ia or I-J structures are expressed on the surface.

4. Suppressor Molecules in Regulating Cellular Immunity

Subsequent to the intravenous administration of ABA-coupled cells, afferent-acting Ts$_1$ cells can be recovered from the spleens of recipient mice.[15] These Ts$_1$ cells are Lyt-1$^+$2$^-$ and secrete a soluble mediator TsF$_1$.[10] This factor binds ABA, is positive for *I-J*-encoded determinants, and, when induced in mice capable of producing CRI$^+$ antibodies, is CRI$^+$.[10] However, whereas the antibody molecule requires certain V$_H$ and V$_\kappa$ structures to induce a CRI configuration, the TsF molecule uses only a V$_H$ epitope similar to that used in the framework and is not antigen binding site related.[20] Hence, T-cell idiotype is conformationally related to a region of V$_H$ linked to *Igh-1* genes, but is not identical to B-cell idiotype.

Administration of TsF$_1$ molecules or B-cell idiotype coupled to cell surface proteins[15] to naive mice activates efferently acting Ts$_2$ cells. These cells are Lyt-1$^+$2$^+$ and I-J$^+$. Interestingly, although Ts$_2$ and TsF$_2$ are anti-CRI$^+$, these anti-CRI$^+$ molecules can be induced in any strain of mouse—even in those unable to produce CRI$^+$ structures. Hence, the genetic linkage between expression of CRI on T and B cells to *Igh-1* genes does not hold true for anti-CRI expression. Thus, B-cell idiotype can stimulate T-cell anti-idiotypic elements, indicating that immunoglobulin can influence T-cell specificities as predicted by Jerne.[1]

The inability of anti-CRI$^+$ TsF$_2$ molecules to suppress the anti-ABA response in Cri$^-$ strains of mice led us to predict that complementary (CRI-like) positive Ts$_3$ cells are the target of the TsF$_2$. Mice unable to synthesize a CRI-like structure would not be able to accept the TsF$_2$ and hence could not suppress the anti-ABA response. This was found to be the case.[11] The Lyt-1$^-$2$^+$ Ts$_3$ cell, after receiving the anti-CRI signal of the TsF$_2$ and an antigen signal, is activated and can subsequently suppress the anti-ABA response in an efferent manner.[21] In addition to the anti-idiotypic TsF$_2$, an antigen signal is required. We have found that presentation of antigen to the Ts$_3$ cell is restricted by *I-J*-encoded molecules on the I-J$^+$ APC.[5,19]

In addition to antigen, antibodies bearing CRI determinants as well as anti-CRI antibodies are able to prime Ts cells which suppress the CTL and DTH responses to ABA. Sy *et al.*[22,23] have demonstrated that intact anti-idiotype antibodies (anti-CRI) as well as idiotype-coupled spleen cells, when given intravenously, are able to suppress the DTH response to ABA. In support of the presence of Igh-restricted idiotype-like structures on T cells involved in immunity to ABA, Sy *et al.*[23] have shown that subcutaneous injection of anti-idiotype can prime for ABA-specific DTH upon subsequent challenge with ABA. These studies are further evidence that B-cell products can influence the T-cell response.

5. Anti-Idiotypic Antibodies and Regulation

We have recently begun characterizing, in detail, the suppressor cell induced by anti-idiotype. Results so far indicate that cells activated by anti-idiotype are able to efferently suppress both DTH and CTL responses to ABA. Further, this cell appears to suppress the ABA-specific T-cell-mediated responses in cyclophosphamide-pretreated mice. Taken together, these results suggest that anti-idiotype is able to directly induce a Ts_3-like cell. If so, these results appear distinct from our previous ones, indicating an absolute requirement for both an antigen-induced signal and an anti-idiotype (TsF_2)-like signal for induction of Ts_3 cells. Kim[25] has shown that the *in vitro* generation of suppressor cells by anti-idiotype requires both anti-idiotype and antigen signals. It is possible that in our case, our heterologous anti-CRI antibodies contain a significant population of antibodies bearing ABA internal image which could mimic antigen for suppressor cell induction, and another population capable of mediating the TsF_2 signal.

Lastly, the ability to prime for Ts cells with anti-CRI, in our experience, is limited to murine strains able to produce CRI^+ humoral responses (i.e., *Igh-1^d*, *Igh-1^e* strains). However, Thomas *et al.*[26] have been able to induce efferent-acting, ABA-specific suppressor cells by anti-CRI in mice with no detectable CRI^+ serum antibodies. It is unclear why mice, unable to express CRI^+ antibodies, are still affected by treatment with anti-CRI. It is possible that certain monoclonal anti-CRI antibodies selected for inhibition of ligand to idiotype may provide an especially strong internal image-induced signal, hence activating the Ts_3 cell without the usual Igh-restricted signal. This result would then be analogous to those of Arnold *et al.*[27] These investigators found that T_{DTH} could be activated with some monoclonal anti-idiotypic antibodies without the usual genetic restrictions required for T_{DTH} cell activation.

6. Igh-Linked T-Cell Structures as Cell Interaction Molecules

Recently, we have focused on the role of CRI-like structures and Igh-linked restrictive elements in Ts_1 function. As mentioned above, although CRI does not appear to be critical in the generation of ABA-specific T-cell immunity, the Ts cells are CRI^+ and anti-CRI^+. While studies from other laboratories[28] may be interpreted to suggest the existence of CRI^+ or anti-CRI^+ Th cells, in our hands, anti-CRI antibodies cannot block ABA-induced T_{DTH} function. Hence, it may be that CRI-like structures are critical only in the suppressor cell-mediated regulation of T-cell-mediated responses. If this is the case, it follows that Ts cells may not exert their regulatory effects via CRI–anti-CRI interactions between Ts–Th cells, but rather these structures act as cell interaction molecules for Ts–Ts-cell communication. This idea would be consistent with work from our laboratory (unpublished observations) and from Gershon's laboratory.[29]

7. Idiotypic Self Restriction Molecules

To support this hypothesis, we have analyzed the possible roles of idiotype in Ts interactions. ABA- and SRBC-specific suppressor molecules are composed of two subunits, one binding antigen and one I-J$^+$.[29] Further, in the SRBC system, it has been demonstrated that the I-J$^+$ molecule bears structures[30] which are expressed in an Igh-linked manner. As both sets of TsF$_1$ molecules act in an Igh-linked restricted manner, we were interested to investigate which subunit was critical in mediating this apparent Igh restriction. Hybrid synthetic suppressor molecules built using the ABA binding fragment and the I-J$^+$ fragment of the SRBC-specific factor suppressed the anti-ABA but not the anti-SRBC response. Further, the genetic restriction of such molecules was guided by the I-J$^+$ *non-antigen-binding* fragment. Although the role of CRI in this event remains unclear, it is clear that the Igh-linked restrictive element for ABA Ts function does not bind antigen. This argues that such *Igh*-linked T-cell-derived molecules do not act as antigen-binding structures but rather act as restriction elements, and indicates that the aforementioned antigen-binding site fragment-shared conformation between Igh-1-linked V$_H$ B-cell structures and TsF elements is even more special than thought. Consistent with this idea we have observed that the suppression function derived from anti-CRI-induced suppressor cells is antigen nonspecific but Igh restricted in its activity (Monroe, Lowy, Drebin, and Greene, in preparation). These findings suggest that structures responsible for Igh restriction are not involved in antigen binding. If this interpretation is correct, these results imply that Igh-linked structures on T regulatory cells may serve as cell interaction molecules in regulatory circuits.

The evidence described above suggests that the CRI-like structure on Ts cells and their factors may play a unique role in T-cell interactions. Its role might not be to bind antigen but rather to restrict Ts–Ts interactions. This is somewhat surprising when one considers the tight genetic linkage between CRI on B and T cells. The CRI on ABA-specific antibodies does appear to be related to the antigen-binding structures. However, molecular studies by our laboratory (Royer, Maxam, Greene *et al.*, in preparation) and others[31–33] indicate that T-cell hybridomas which secrete idiotype-like-bearing structure do not have B-cell V$_H$ genes in a rearranged configuration. Hence, idiotype-like structures on T cells may only serologically cross-react with B-cell idiotypic structures.

If Igh-1-linked CRI-like structures do not mediate antigen binding, and subserve self restriction elements operative in Ts cells, then one can make certain predictions about this interaction mechanism. Since interaction elements are V$_H$-like, B-cell products may influence T-cell idiotype expression in the same way that Jerne predicted. Secondly, one would predict that unlike self restriction for *H-2*-determined structures mediated through adaptive differentiation in the thymus, cells which express idiotype-like molecules need not necessarily be influenced by the thymus in the same manner. If these studies of V$_H$-like structures on T cells are clarified chemically, then we may develop insight into related gene families that have evolved to govern cellular communication in higher vertebrates.

References

1. Jerne, N. K., 1974, Towards a network theory of the immune system, *Ann. Immunol. (Inst. Pasteur)* **125C**:373.
2. Germain, R. N., and Benacerraf, B., 1981, A single major pathway of T lymphocyte interactions in antigen specific immune suppression, *Scand. J. Immunol.* **13**:1.
3. Asherson, G. L., and Zembala, M., 1982, The role of the T acceptor cell in suppressor systems: Antigen

specific T suppressor factor acts via a T acceptor cell; this releases a nonspecific inhibitor of the transfer of contact sensitivity when exposed to antigen in the context of I-J, *Ann. N. Y. Acad. Sci.* **392**:71.

4. Sprent, J., Korngold, R., and Molnar-Kimber, K., 1980, T cell recognition of antigen *in vivo:* Role of the H-2 complex, *Springer Semin. Immunopathol.* **3**:215.

5. Lowy, A., Tominaga, A., Drebin, J., Benacerraf, B., and Greene, M. I., 1983, Identification of an I-J positive antigen presenting cell required for third order T suppressor cell activation, *J. Exp. Med.* **157**:353.

6. Green, D. R., Flood, P. M., and Gershon, R. K., 1983, Immunoregulatory T cell pathway, *Annu. Rev. Immunol.* **1**:439.

7. Kuettner, M. G., Wang, A., and Nisonoff, A., 1972, Quantitative investigations of idiotype antibodies. VI. idiotype specificity as a potential genetic marker for the variable regions of mouse immunoglobulin polypeptide chains, *J. Exp. Med.* **135**:579.

8. Pawlak, L. L., Hart, D. A., and Nisonoff, A., 1973, Requirements for prolonged suppression of an idiotypic specificity in adult mice, *J. Exp. Med.* **137**:1442.

9. Brown, A. R., and Nisonoff, A., 1981, An intrastrain cross reactive idiotype associated with anti p-azophenylarsonate antibodies of A/J and BALB/c mice, *J. Immunol.* **126**:1263.

10. Dietz, M. H., Sy, M.-S., Greene, M. I., Nisonoff, A., Beneacerraf, B., and Germain, R. N., 1980, Antigen-and-receptor-driven regulatory mechanisms. VI. Demonstration of cross-reactive idiotypic determinants of azobenzenearsonate specific antigen-binding suppressor cells producing soluble suppressor factor(s), *J. Imunol.* **125**:2374.

11. Greene, M. I., Nelles, M. J., Sy, M.-S., and Nisonoff, A., 1982, Regulation of immunity to the azobenzenearsonate hapten, *Adv. Immunol.* **32**:253.

12. Hornbeck, P. V., and Lewis, G. K., 1983, Idiotype connection in the immune system. I. Expression of a cross-reactive idiotype on induced anti-p-azophenylarsonate antibodies and on endogenous antibodies not specific for arsonate, *J. Exp. Med.* **157**:1116.

13. Clark, F., and Capra, J. D., 1982, Ubiquitous nonimmunoglobulin p-azobenzenearsonate-binding molecules from lymphoid cells, *J. Exp. Med.* **155**:611.

14. Hirai, Y., and Nisonoff, A., 1980, Selective suppression of the major idiotypic component of an anti-hapten response by soluble T cell derived factors with idiotypic or anti-idiotypic receptors, *J. Exp. Med.* **151**:1213.

15. Sy, M.-S., Dietz, M. H., Germain, R. N., Benacerraf, B., and Greene, M. I., 1980, Antigen-and receptor-driven regulatory mechanisms. IV. Idiotype bearing I-J suppressor T cell factors induce second order suppressor T cells which express anti-idiotypic receptors, *J. Exp. Med.* **150**:1183.

16. Bach, B. A., Sherman, L., Benacerraf, B., and Greene, M. I., 1978, Mechanisms of regulation of cell mediated immunity. II. Induction and suppression of delayed type hypersensitivity to azobenzenearsonate-coupled syngeneic cells, *J. Immunol.* **121**:1460.

17. Sherman, L.,Burakoff, S. J., and Benacerraf, B., 1978, The induction of cytolytic T lymphocytes with specificity of *p*-azophenylarsonate-coupled syngeneic cells, *J. Immunol.* **121**:1432.

18. Greene, M. I., Sy, M.-S., Kripke, M., and Benacerraf, B., 1979, Impairment of antigen presenting cell function by ultraviolet radiation, *Proc. Natl. Acad. Sci. USA* **76**:6591.

19. Takaoki, M., Sy, M.-S.,Tominaga, A., Lowy, A., Tsurifuji, M., Finberg, R., Benacerraf, B., and Greene, M. I., 1982, I-J restricted interactions in the generation of azobenzenearsonate specific T suppressor cells, *J. Exp. Med.* **156**:1325.

20. Sy, M.-S., Brown, A., Bach, B. A., Benacerraf, B., Gottlieb, P. D., Nisonoff, A., and Greene, M. I., 1981, Genetic and serological analysis of the expression of cross reactive idiotypic determinants on anti-p-azobenzenearsonate antibodies and p-azobenzenearsonate specific suppressor T cell factors, *Proc. Natl. Acad. Sci. USA* **78**:1143.

21. Sy, M.-S., Nisonoff, A., Germain, R. N., Benacerraf, B., and Greene, M. I., 1981, Antigen-and-receptor-driven regulatory mechanisms. VIII. Suppression of idiotype negative ABA specific T cells results from the interaction of an anti-idiotypic Ts-2 with a CRI$^+$ primed T cell target, *J. Exp. Med.* **153**:1415.

22. Sy, M.-S., Bach, B. A., Dohi, Y., Nisonoff, A., Benacerraf, B., and Greene, M. I., 1979, Antigen-and-receptor-driven regulatory mechanisms. I. Induction of suppressor T cells with anti-idiotypic antibodies, *J. Exp. Med.* **150**:1216.

23. Sy, M.-S., Bach, B. A., Brown, A., Nisonoff, A., Benacerraf, B., and Greene, M. I., 1979, Antigen-and-receptor-driven regulatory mechanisms. II. Induction of suppressor T cells with idiotype-coupled syngeneic spleen cells, *J. Exp. Med.* **150**:1229.

24. Sy, M. -S., Brown, A. R., Benacerraf, B., and Greene, M. I., 1980, Antigen-and receptor-driven regulatory

mechanisms. III. Induction of delayed-type hypersensitivity to azobenzenearsonate with anti-cross-reactive idiotypic antibodies, *J. Exp. Med.* **151**:896.

25. Kim, G. S., 1979, Mechanisms of idiotype suppression. I. In vitro generation of idiotype-specific suppressor T cells by anti-idiotype antibodies and specific antigen, *J. Exp. Med.* **149**:1371.
26. Thomas, W. R., Morahan, G., and Miller, J. F. A. P., 1983, Induction of suppressor T cells by monoclonal anti-idiotype antibody in strains of mice not expressing the idiotype in hyperimmune serum, *J. Immunol.* **130**:2079.
27. Arnold, B., Wallich, R., and Hammerling, G. J., 1982, Elicitation of delayed type hypersensitivity to phosphorylcholine by monoclonal anti-idiotypic antibodies in an allogeneic environment, *J. Exp. Med.* **156**:670.
28. Miyagawa, N., Miyagawa, S., and Leskowitz, S., 1983, ABA specific helper T cells in A/J mice bear the major cross reactive idiotype, *Cell. Immunol.* **77**:120.
29. Flood, P., Lowy, A., Tominaga, A., Chue, B., Greene, M. I., and Gershon, R. K., 1983, The nature of Igh-V region restricted T cell interactions: Genetic restrictions of an antigen specific suppressor inducer factor is imparted by an I-J$^+$ antigen nonspecific molecule, *J. Exp. Med.* **158**:1938.
30. Yamauchi, K., Murphy, D. B., Cantor, H., and Gershon, R. K., 1981, Analysis of antigen specific Ig restricted cell free material made by I-J$^+$ Lyt -1 cells (Ly -1 TsiF) that induces Ly 2$^+$ cells to express suppressive activity, *Eur. J. Immunol.* **11**:905.
31. Kemp, D. J., Adams, J. M., Mottram, P. L., Thomas, W. R., Walker, I. D., and Miller, J. F. A. P., 1982, A search for messenger RNA molecules bearing immunoglobulin V$_H$ nucleotide sequences in T cells, *J. Exp. Med.* **156**:1848.
32. Kraig, E., Kronenberg, M., Kapp, J. A., Pierce, C. W., Abruzzini, A. F., Sorensen, C. M., Samelson, L. E., Schwartz, R. H., and Hood, L. E., 1983, T and B cells that recognize the same antigen do not transcribe similar heavy chain variable region gene segments, *J. Exp. Med.* **158**:192.
33. Kronenberg, M., Kraig, E., Siv, G., Kapp, J. A., Kappler, J., Marrach, P., Pierce, C. W., and Hood, L., 1983, Three T cell hybridomas do not contain detectable heavy chain variable gene transcripts, *J. Exp. Med.* **158**:210.

Index